Molecular Pathology and Diagnostics of Cancer

Cancer Growth and Progression

Volume 16

Founding Editor

Hans E. Kaiser†, D. Sc.

Series Editors

Aejaz Nasir, M.D., M.Phil., FCAP
Senior Medical Advisor,
Molecular Oncologic Pathologist & Surgical Pathology Lead,
Diagnostic & Experimental Pathology & Tailored Therapeutics,
Eli Lilly & Company, Indianapolis, IN, USA

Timothy J. Yeatman, M.D.
President, Gibbs Research Institute Director,
Gibbs Cancer Center, Gibbs Research Institute and Cancer Center,
Spartanburg, SC, USA

For further volumes:
http://www.springer.com/series/5721

Domenico Coppola
Editor

Molecular Pathology and Diagnostics of Cancer

Springer

Editor
Domenico Coppola
Anatomic Pathology
Moffitt Cancer Center
University of South Florida
Tampa, FL, USA

ISBN 978-94-007-7191-8 ISBN 978-94-007-7192-5 (eBook)
DOI 10.1007/978-94-007-7192-5
Springer Dordrecht Heidelberg New York London

Library of Congress Control Number: 2013951807

Printed on acid-free paper

Springer is part of Springer Science+Business Media (www.springer.com)

Preface

This volume is a comprehensive update on the most common molecular tests currently available to facilitate the diagnosis of challenging pathologic lesions. This book includes recent advances in the field of diagnostic techniques including, among others, fluorescence in situ hybridization (FISH), microarray, proteomics, mutational analysis, and others. The book is structured by organ sites (brain, thyroid and parathyroid, breast, pulmonary, esophago-gastric, hepatocellular, pancreatic, gastroentero-pancreatic/neuroendocrine, prostate, kidney and bladder, male genital, gynecologic and ovarian, soft tissue, pediatric, cutaneous, and lymphoid and myeloid neoplasms). This state-of-the-science reference will provide the practicing pathologists, oncologists, cancer researchers, postgraduates and students of cancer science with the latest information to help with the diagnosis of difficult lesions. In this era where personalized medicine is becoming a reality, we also provided, for each chapter, information about prognostic molecular tests able to predict patient prognosis and/or therapy response. The broad range of topics will make this text a source of easily accessible information on a variety of tumor types for practicing pathologists whether in academic or clinical practice.

Contents

Chapter 1
Molecular Pathology and Diagnostics of Gliomas

Jesse Kresak and Yuan (Frank) Shan

Contents

J. Kresak
University of South Florida, Tampa, FL, USA

Y. (Frank) Shan, M.D. (✉)
Department of Anatomic Pathology, Moffitt Cancer Center & Research Institute, 12902 Magnolia Drive, Tampa, FL 33612, USA
e-mail: Yuan.Shan@moffitt.org

D. Coppola (ed.), *Molecular Pathology and Diagnostics of Cancer*, Cancer Growth and Progression 16, DOI 10.1007/978-94-007-7192-5_1,

Abstract Gliomas are the most common primary malignancy in the central nervous system. With recent advancements in molecular pathology, pathologists now have additional tools for histologic analysis of these brain tumors. Genomic and proteomic studies may aid in the diagnosis of gliomas, as well as have utility in prognostication and response to treatment options. Presented are the most current molecular studies utilized in neuropathology of gliomas, as well as a glimpse to future potential biomarkers.

Keywords Gliomas • Genomics • Proteomics • IDH1 • p53 • 1p/19q • EGFR

Abbreviations

2HG	(R)-2-hydroxyglutarate
COBRA	Combined bisulfite restriction analysis
EGFR	Epidermal growth factor receptor
FISH	Fluorescent in situ hybridization
IDH	Isocitrate dehydrogenase
LOH	Loss of heterozygosity
MALDI-TOF	Matrix assisted laser desorption ionization—time of flight
MAPK	Mitogen-activated protein kinase
MGMT	O^6-methylguanine-DNA methyltransferase
miRNA	microRNA
MMP	Matrix metalloproteinase
MS	Mass spectroscopy
MS-MLPA	Methylation-specific multiplex ligation-dependent probe amplification
PTEN	Phosphatase and tensin homolog
RT-PCR	Reverse transcription-polymerase chain reaction
SELDI-TOF	Surface enhanced laser desorption ionization—time of flight
WHO	World Health Organization

1.1 Introduction

Tumors of the central nervous system account for approximately 1 % of tumors in the body. Glial tumors are the most frequent primary tumor of the central nervous system and are classified as astrocytic, oligodendroglial, mixed oligoastrocytic, or ependymal according to the criteria of the World Health Organization (WHO) [1]. Astrocytomas are the most frequent primary brain neoplasm and range in grade from I to IV based on morphology. Oligodendrogliomas and mixed oligoastrocytomas are graded as either II or III and ependymomas have varieties ranging from grades I to III (Table 1.1).

Table 1.1 Glial tumor grades

		I	II	III	IV
Astrocytomas	Pilocytic	X			
	Diffuse		X		
	Anaplastic			X	
	Glioblastoma				X
	Gliosarcoma				X
Oligodendroglial tumors	Oligodendroglioma		X		
	Anaplastic oligodendroglioma			X	
Mixed tumors	Oligoastrocytoma		X		
	Anaplastic oligoastrocytoma			X	
Ependymomas	Ependymoma		X		
	Anaplastic ependymoma			X	

Based on WHO Classification, 2007 [1]

Although pathologists can classify and stratify central nervous system tumors histologically, one cannot predict the clinical outcome of a particular tumor on morphology alone. Tumors within the same histopathologic entity may behave substantially different. For example, a glioblastoma, the most common and aggressive glial tumor, can be subclassified as primary or secondary, although they are histologically indistinguishable. Primary glioblastomas arise de novo, whereas secondary arise from a pre-existing lesser grade glioma. These two subtypes should be considered as two distinct entities having unique pathogenetic pathways with different behaviors and treatment targets.

Focus has shifted to the molecular level in order to further subclassify glial tumors. Molecular alterations leading to gliogenesis can be genetic or epigenetic, resulting in altered expression of genes and their protein products. Knowledge of the molecular changes in the various types and malignancy grades of gliomas has increased dramatically over the past decade. The goal of such research is to identify biomarkers with clinical utility in establishing diagnosis, predicting prognosis, guiding treatment choices, as well as providing new cellular therapeutic targets.

1.2 Genetic Profiling

1.2.1 IDH1/IDH2

Isocitrate dehydrogenases, IDH1 and IDH2, are homologous, NADP+−dependent cytoplasmic and mitochondrial enzymes, respectively. The role of these enzymes is the conversion of isocitrate to α-ketoglutarate with the simultaneous reduction of NADP+to NADPH. IDH1 has recently been discovered to be mutated in a vast majority of astrocytic, oligodendroglial, and oligoastrocytic gliomas (WHO grades II–III), as well as in secondary glioblastomas (WHO grade IV). IDH1 mutation is very rare in primary glioblastoma and is not involved in pilocytic astrocytomas.

The most common mutation is a heterozygous point mutation with substitution of arginine by histidine at codon 132 (R132H), located in the substrate binding site. This IDH1-R132 mutation has a reported frequency of 50–93 % [2, 3]. IDH2 gene mutations affecting the amino acid R172 are much less common than the IDH1 isoform, 3–5 %, yet have been identified in a small subset of gliomas that lack the typical IDH1 mutation with a predominance in oligodendrogliomas [3]. IDH1 and IDH2 genes appear to behave dominantly and are mutually exclusive.

The carcinogenic effect caused by the mutations of IDH1 and IDH2 is not fully understood but appears to be multifactorial. The product and byproduct of the reaction, α-ketoglutarate and NADPH, both defend against cellular oxidative stress. Thus, with decreased quantities of these compounds, the cell may be more susceptible to oxidative damage. In addition to the tumorogenetic property conferred by the inability to perform the conversion, it appears that the IDH mutation confers an enzymatic gain of function. With the IDH mutations, the cancer cell has the gained ability to convert α-ketoglutarate into (R)-2-hydroxyglutarate (2HG) [4]. This reaction will not only further decrease α-ketoglutarate stores, but will also reduce NADPH to NADP+, further increasing the cell's susceptibility to oxidative stress. The increased amount of 2HG in the brain has been associated with an increased risk of brain tumors in patients with an inborn error of 2HG metabolism [5]. Furthermore, there is an association between the IDH mutation and increased hypoxia-inducible factor-1α [6]. Hypoxia-inducible factor-1α is a transcription factor associated with carcinogenic processes, such as the upregulation of vascular endothelial growth factor, and thus promotes angiogenesis.

Mutations in IDH1 and IDH2 have also been observed in up to 22 % of acute myelogenous leukemias, which concurrently display a dramatic increase in 2HG, supporting the neoenzymatic activity [7].

IDH1 mutation has been shown to be a strong, independent prognostic biomarker not only in glioblastomas, but in diffuse gliomas of lesser grades as well [8]. There is no difference yet to be seen in terms of the point mutation, R132H versus others, regarding patient outcome [9]. While the IDH1 mutation conveys a better patient outcome, it does not predict a better response of the glioma to chemotherapy [8, 10]. In addition to its prognostic value, identification of IDH mutations could be used diagnostically. Analysis of IDH1/2 mutations could be utilized in the separation of primary and secondary glioblastomas or in the challenge of differentiating pilocytic astrocytoma from glioblastoma.

Recently, immunohistochemical staining using a specific antibody against mutant IDH1-R132H was developed, which can be applied to routine paraffin-embedded specimens. This has proved to be a tumor-specific marker differentiating reactive from neoplastic cells in grade II and III gliomas [11, 12]. In addition, this marker also identifies tumor cells in post-therapy specimens with extensive reactive gliosis. While this IHC stain is easy to use and convenient, it will neither detect the IDH mutations of other types, nor the IDH2 mutations of equal importance [11, 13]. Detection of IDH1/2 mutations can also be achieved through various polymerase chain reaction (PCR) techniques and direct sequencing.

1.2.2 MGMT Status

The MGMT (O^6-methylguanine-DNA methyltransferase) gene at 10q26 encodes for a DNA repair protein. In gliomas of different grades, the MGMT gene is silenced by promoter hypermethylation, impeding transcription, and thus resulting in a decreased expression of the MGMT protein. This epigenetic modification has been associated with an increased sensitivity to alkylating chemotherapy. In alkylating therapies such as temozolamide, a methyl group is added to the O^6-position of the nucleotide guanine, resulting in DNA damage and apoptosis [14]. A full-functioning MGMT would remove this methyl group; however, with reduced expression of the protein secondary to promoter hypermethylation, the cell has a decreased ability to repair alkylated DNA. Therefore, MGMT expression analysis can be used to predict which tumors may have a more favorable response to alkylating chemotherapeutic agents [15, 16]. Testing of MGMT can be applied to pediatric gliomas as well [17, 18]. MGMT promoter methylation has been found in up to 40 % of primary glioblastomas and 40–60 % of secondary glioblastomas. The aberration is also present in other diffuse gliomas, with preponderance of oligodendrogliomas at 60–93 % [19].

Although studies have shown that MGMT promoter methylation results in a significantly longer survival time for patients with glioblastoma treated with concomitant treatment of temozolomide and radiotherapy, there have been discordant reports regarding MGMT methylation as a predictor for increased survival in patients receiving radiotherapy alone [15, 20, 21]. However, in gliomas of lesser grades, there is a clear prognostic association between MGMT methylation status and sole radiotherapy [10, 22]. The underlying mechanism by which MGMT methylation would offer a favorable prognosis when not in relationship to chemotherapy is a bit more difficult to discern. As mentioned previously, gliomas often contain multiple molecular aberrancies and thus it may be the result of another molecular change, or the summation of several changes, that convey this prognostic significance to radiotherapy.

The most common method utilized to assess the MGMT promoter methylation status is a methylation-specific PCR analysis, which applies primers composed of differing quantities of CpG sites to allow differentiation between methylated and unmethylated DNA [23]. Methylation-specific pyrosequencing has also been employed with strong sensitivity [24]. Other DNA-based methods are available such as combined bisulfite restriction analysis (COBRA) and methylation-specific multiplex ligation-dependent probe amplification (MS-MLPA). Nonmethylation-specific methods have been tested such as immunohistochemical staining, Western blotting, and biochemical enzyme assays; however, they were found to be less reliable due to staining of non-neoplastic cells, which retain MGMT expression and thus give a false result [23].

1.2.3 p53

As far as current genomic data can reveal, p53 is the most frequent genetic alteration in cancer. p53 is a tumor suppressor protein encoded by the TP53 gene located on the short arm of chromosome 17. The innate role of p53 is genomic stability achieved by cell cycle inhibition and induction of apoptosis. In activated states, p53 acts a transcription regulator leading to the upregulation of p21. The protein p21 is the stop protein responsible for binding to the cyclin-dependent kinase and inhibiting the cell from transitioning from the G1 to the S phase of cell division (see Entrez Gene). Thus, a mutated p53 will be unable to prevent cell replication resulting in uncontrolled tumor growth.

p53 is strongly associated with secondary glioblastomas and found significantly less frequently in primary glioblastomas [1].

The majority of mutations involving p53 lead to missense mutations, and there is a resultant accumulation of the protein in the nucleus of the cell. Therefore, immunohistochemical stains for p53 highlight the nuclei of tumor cells and are used as a surrogate marker for identifying cells affected by a mutation in this pathway. This methodology is more economical than PCR analysis; however, interpretation of the stain is not standardized, leading to ambiguity of interpretation [25].

The significance of the detection of p53 overexpression in gliomas is inconsistent. In terms of diagnosis, p53 would be a less favorable marker than others in distinguishing primary from secondary glioblastoma given that p53 overexpression has been reported in up to 25 % of primary glioblastomas [26]. As a prognostic marker, p53 has shown inconsistent results. While some reports indicate a shorter survival time for gliomas overexpressing p53, this finding has not been confirmed by several meta-analyses [25, 27].

1.2.4 1p/19q Deletion

The loss of chromosome arms 1p and 19q is an established genetic hallmark of oligodendroglial tumors [28]. This combined loss is detected in up to 80 % of oligodendrogliomas and up to 60 % in anaplastic oligodendrogliomas, with decreasing frequency in mixed oligoastrocytic tumors [28, 29].

The 1p/19q deletion has proven its use as a prognostic marker conveying a better response to therapy and a longer survival time [22, 29]. This co-deletion carries the same significance regardless of using chemotherapy, radiotherapy, or the combined and therefore cannot be used to guide treatment choice [22, 29]. Although there is a strong correlation between classic oligodendroglioma morphology ("fried eggs" and "chicken wire") and the co-deletion, 1p/19q deletion cannot always be predicted by morphology alone [30].

It should be noted that deletions of the 1p arm other than the 1p/19q co-deletion have different prognostic implications. For example, a partial loss of 1p in an oligodendroglioma has been suggested to be a less favorable clinical outcome [31]. Therefore, the entire chromosomal arm should be evaluated to detect deletions of differing sizes.

Various techniques are available to detect 1p/19q deletions; however, fluorescent in situ hybridization (FISH) is often employed due to its technical ease. FISH can be used directly on formalin-fixed paraffin-embedded tissue and does not require additional specimens from the patient. Another frequently utilized method is loss of heterozygosity (LOH), which is a PCR-based test that compares tumor DNA to the patient's "normal" DNA, usually from peripheral blood.

1.2.5 BRAF Duplication/Fusion

BRAF, which is part of the mitogen-activated protein kinase (MAPK) pathway and located at 7q34, is aberrantly activated in a majority of pilocytic astrocytomas. BRAF is most commonly activated by duplication of the gene with subsequent fusion of the BRAF genes. BRAF aberrancies exist in 60–80 % of pilocytic astrocytomas and are rarely seen in other gliomas [32]. This discrepancy can lend utility in the differentiation of pilocytic astrocytomas and low-grade gliomas [33]. A missense mutation of BRAF, V600E, has also been identified in a minority of extracerebellar pilocytic astrocytomas; however, this mutation is more frequently seen in ganglio-gliomas and pleomorphic xanthoastrocytomas.

Aside from diagnostic utility, BRAF analysis may prove useful in development of therapeutic options in patients with pilocytic astrocytoma. Studies have demonstrated that silencing and inhibition of BRAF or other constituents of the MAPK pathway inhibit growth of the tumor [34].

Detection of BRAF aberrancies is often accomplished through FISH analysis with probes specific to the KIAA1549 and BRAF genes. PCR has also been utilized; however, this method may not allow for detection of variants of this fusion. Immunohistochemistry is available for detection of the BRAF V600E mutation.

1.2.6 MSH6 Mutation

Unfortunately, high-grade gliomas all too often do not respond to alkylating chemotherapeutic treatments. In these treatment-resistant gliomas, MSH6, a mismatch repair gene, has often been found to be mutated. Studies point to the alkylating chemotherapeutic agents as a cause to the somatic mutations in the MSH6 gene [35, 36]. More research into the role of MSH6 and other mismatch repair genes may be helpful in identifying therapy-resistant tumors and provide for a specific target for further treatment.

1.3 Proteomics

Genetic profiling and proteomics fall along on the same spectrum of diagnostic armory; however, they differ in detection methodologies and in clinical utility. In some cases, proteomic data will validate the established genetic alterations, while in others, proteins have been identified with little knowledge of their originating genes.

There is a wide spectrum of proteomic methodologies, ranging from a simple Western blot to 2-dimension gel electrophoresis to advanced mass spectroscopy (MS) techniques. Various MS methods have been employed, including matrix assisted laser desorption ionization—time of flight (MALDI-TOF) MS, surface enhanced laser desorption ionization—time of flight (SELDI-TOF) MS, and nanoliquid chromatography with tandem mass spectroscopy, yielding a different set of tumor proteins than provided by standard immunohistochemistry or Western blotting. The differing results may be a reflection of protein molecular weight and/or protein abundance [37, 38].

As the elucidation of genetic alterations in gliomas advances, proteomic studies will continue to reveal altered proteins. Future research endeavors into the protein-protein interactions and network-analysis may prove useful in solidifying our understanding of proteomic study results.

1.3.1 EGFR

Epidermal growth factor receptor (EGFR) gene, located on chromosome 7p12, codes for EGFR protein, a member of the transmembrane tyrosine kinase receptor family. The EGFR gene is often amplified in primary glioblastomas, up to 40 % [1, 19], resulting in over-expression of the EGFR protein. EGFR plays a role in tumorigenesis by activating MAPK and PI3K-Akt pathways, leading to cell proliferation, decreased apoptosis [39], and angiogenesis and ease of invasion [40].

Aside from overexpression of wild-type EGFR, primary glioblastomas may also harbor mutated EGFR. The most frequent rearrangement leads to a variant of the EGFR gene known as EGFRvIII (delta EGFR) [40]. This mutation is characterized by an 801 base pair (267 amino acid) in-frame deletion of exons 2–7, resulting in a truncated extracellular domain with the inability to bind a ligand. However, the receptor retains ligand-independent constitutive activity and produces tonic activation of the pathway [41]. The EGFRvIII mutation is seen in half of the glioblastoma multiforme cases exhibiting EGFR amplification, yet can also be seen as a standalone mutation as well [40].

The presence of EGFR amplification or EGFRvIII mutation conveys high-grade malignancy and thus may have utility as a diagnostic and prognostic tool. As such, in cases of anaplastic gliomas with equivocal histology, the detection of EGFR/EGFRvIII lends support to a higher-grade malignancy with an associated poorer patient outcome. This prognostication correlates with the finding that EGFR mutations are more frequent in primary versus secondary glioblastomas, of which primary glioblastomas are associated with later onset and aggressive clinical behavior.

Therapeutically, the EGFR pathway has provided a new target for treatment with variable success. Glioblastomas with EGFR or EGFRvIII expression have been more responsive to tyrosine kinase inhibitors most prominently when PTEN is also expressed [41].

Detection of EGFR amplification is most frequently accomplished via FISH analysis. EGFRvIII analysis is usually done via reverse transcription-PCR (RT-PCR).

Table 1.2 Diagnostic molecular panels

	IDH1/2	p53	EGFR	PTEN
Primary glioblastoma vs.	–	–	+	+
Secondary glioblastoma	+	+	–	–
	IDH1/2	**BRAF**		
Pilocytic astrocytoma vs.	–	+		
Higher grade astrocytoma (except 1′ glioblastoma)	+	–		
	IDH1/2	**p53**	**EGFR**	
Astrocytoma vs.	+	+	Strong	
Reactive gliosis	–	+/–	Weak	

1.3.2 PTEN Alterations and 10q LOH

Phosphatase and tensin homolog (PTEN), located at 10q23, is a tumor suppressor gene with an integral role in opposing the PI3K-Akt pathway. In gliomas with a mutant PTEN gene, there is an associated increase in PI3K-Akt pathway signaling, which may contribute to the tumor's ability to invade and infiltrate. There have also been reports to support the theory that mutations in PTEN lead to activation of EGFR via a PI3K-Akt pathway demonstrating that PTEN plays a role in the angiogenesis of glioblastomas as well [42]. Mutations at the PTEN gene are found in 15–40 % of primary glioblastomas, but they are practically absent in secondary glioblastomas and other gliomas [43].

PTEN is often altered by a LOH at 10q. The LOH can occur in various sites aside from 10q23 (PTEN) such as 10q25, or 10q total loss.

PTEN mutations and 10q LOH both carry the same negative prognostication for high-grade gliomas [19]. LOH analysis or FISH can be used for evaluation.

1.3.3 Prohibitin

Prohibitin is a ubiquitous protein located at 17q21, the same location as the BRCA1 gene. Prohibitin has been found to be overexpressed in various tumor tissues, including breast, bladder, prostate, and thyroid. However, it should be noted that in gliomas there are reports of upregulation as well as downregulation of prohibitin [37, 38]. Although the exact mechanism that prohibitin may play in tumorigenesis remains unclear, given its mitochondrial location and chaperon responsibility, it is believed that the protein may have a regulatory role by modulating transcription [44]. Much more research into the mechanisms and prognostic and therapeutic values of this protein marker should be performed before detection of it is commonly employed in practice.

In summary, the knowledge gained thus far in the study of the genomics and proteomics of gliomas has allowed for both diagnostic, as well as prognostic tools when analyzing glial tissue (Tables 1.2 and 1.3). It is important to note that this is an emerging field and thus use of these evaluation methods should be used in clinical context and in reference to the rapid influx in the literature.

Table 1.3 Molecular alterations as prognostic markers

	Positive			Negative	
	IDH1/2	MGMT	1p19q	EGFR	PTEN
Primary glioblastoma		+		+	+
Secondary glioblastoma	+	+		Rare	
Anaplastic astrocytoma	+	+			
Diffuse astrocytoma	+	+			
Pilocytic astrocytoma		+			
Oligodendroglioma		++	++		
Anaplastic oligodendroglioma			+		
Mixed oligoastrocytoma			+/–		

1.3.4 Comprehensive Diagnostics

Gliomas are tumors characterized by multiple genetic alterations (see Fig. 1.1). Evidence is emerging to support an association between compounded molecular and genetic alterations found in gliomas. There is a strong correlation between the presence of IDH1 mutations and genetic mutations such as p53 and 1p/19q deletions. Recent evidence supports the idea that the IDH mutation is an early event occurring in a glial precursor cell and may lead to, or be prerequisite for, the loss of 1p/19q [10, 45, 46]. The presence of IDH1 mutation is also closely associated with p53 mutations and MGMT promoter methylation in gliomas [10]. Interestingly, there is an inverse correlation between IDH1 mutation and the amplification of EGFR. With IDH1 mutations being prevalent in secondary glioblastomas and EGFR amplification being predominant in primary glioblastomas, this inverse association lends support to the theory of primary and secondary glioblastomas being distinct entities [10]. Similarly, pediatric high-grade gliomas rarely exhibit an IDH mutation conveying a fundamental difference from the adult counterpart [47].

1.4 miRNA

The role of microRNAs (miRNAs) in tumorogenesis is a relatively new and exciting field of research. miRNAs are noncoding RNA segments that can bind mRNA to affect translation of genes. In this manner, miRNAs can regulate oncogenes and tumor suppressor genes and thus are associated with tumor growth, including cellular proliferation, angiogenesis, invasion, and apoptosis [48, 49]. However, it was only in 2005 that the first aberrant miRNA expression was report in gliomas [50, 51].

Utilizing Northern blots and microarrays, the miRNAs that were found by these studies to be upregulated in glioblastoma cell lines and tumors included miR-21 [51] and miR-221; those found to be downregulated included miR-128 and miR-181a, miR-181b, and miR-181c [50]. With the use of quantitative RT-PCR, Silber

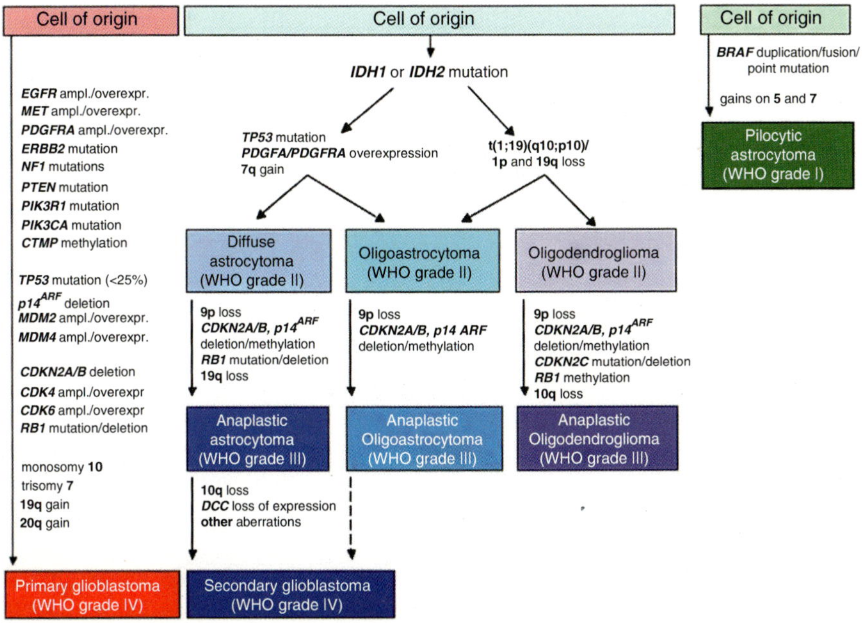

Fig. 1.1 Summary of most frequent molecular alterations in astrocytic, oligodendroglial, and oligoastrocytic gliomas. Primary glioblastomas, the most common gliomas in adults, show complex chromosomal, genetic, and epigenetic alterations targeting genes involved in important cellular pathways, namely the receptor tyrosin kinase/mitogen-activated protein kinase/phosphoinositol 3-kinase pathway (e.g. *EGFR, MET, PDGFRA, ERBB2, NF1, PTEN, PIK3R1, PI3KCA, CTMP*), the p53 pathway (e.g. TP53, *p14^{ARF}, MDM2, MDM4*), and the pRb1 pathway (e.g. *CDKN2A, CDKN2B, CDK4, CDK6, RBI*). In addition, primary glioblastomas frequently show monosomy 10, trisomy 7 and gains of 19q and 20p. Diffuse WHO grade II and III astrocytic, oligodendroglial and oligoastrocytic gliomas and secondary glioblastomas frequently carry mutations in *IDH1* or *IDH2*, suggesting that they share a common, yet to be defined cell of origin. Diffuse astrocytic gliomas often carry additional *TP53* mutations, while oligodendroglial tumors are characterized by 1p/19q deletion. Most oligoastrocytomas have either of these alterations. Molecular changes associated with progression to anaplastic glioma include 9p losses and inactivation of the *CDKN2A*, *P14*^{ARF} and *CDKN2B* genes on 9p21 as well as other changes, while progression to secondary glioblastoma is associated with frequent loss of 10q and *DCC* loss of expression amony others. The majority of pilocytic astrocytomas are characterized by duplication/fusion or point mutation of the *BRAF* gene on 7q34, while other genomic aberrations are rare. From Riemenschneider et al. [16], with kind permission of Springer Science+Business Media

was able to confirm the upregulation of miR21 and to identify the downregulation of miR-124, miR-128a, and miR-137 [52].

The deregulation of miRNAs, much like the ones mentioned above in gliomas, has been implicated in oncogenic pathways of other tumor types. For example, it has been suggested that, in cases of colorectal adenocarcinoma, miR-143 directly binds to KRAS transcripts at the 3′-UTR, thus potentially inhibiting KRAS protein expression [53]. In regard to gliomas, it has been shown that the dual activation of RAS and AKT in progenitor cells can induce the formation of glioblastomas [54].

Given this result and the knowledge that malignant gliomas commonly contain deletions or mutations of the tumor suppressor genes PTEN and p53, which are alterations that may lead to the activation of RAS-MAPK and PI3-AKT pathways, it raises the question to a likely correlation between miRNA deregulation and these oncogenic pathways in the development of central nervous system tumors [55].

Identification of dysregulated miRNAs in tumor tissue may provide a new therapeutic target as it may be possible to modulate miRNA through pre-miRNA molecules or anti-sense oligonucleotides.

1.4.1 miR-21

miR-21 was first noted to be upregulated in glioblastomas and its overexpression has since been documented in numerous solid tumors [48, 51]. Low-grade gliomas have also been found to overly express miR-21. Numerous studies have been conducted to elucidate the significance of increased miR-21 with findings to support the role of miR-21 in multiple oncogenic pathways.

In order to determine the significance of the overexpression, knockdown studies were performed in which glioblastoma cells without miR-21 expression resulted in apoptosis. This would suggest that miR-21 plays an anti-apoptotic role in gliomagenesis [51].

miR-21 indirectly affects the tumor-suppressing p53 pathway by targeting activators, homologs, and cofactors of the system [56]. Chemotherapeutic agents often induce DNA damage in tumor cells leading to apoptosis of the cell. In this way, miR-21 can compromise the p53-mediated apoptosis contributing to drug resistance of glioblastomas. miR-21 also plays a role in the inactivation of TGF-beta and mitochondrial apoptotic pathways [56].

The invasiveness of gliomas may also be attributed to miR-21. RECK and TIMP3, which act as inhibitors to matrix metalloproteinases (MMPs), are direct targets of miR-21. MMPs are peptidases involved in the breakdown of the extracellular matrix, allowing for a tumor to infiltrate with less resistance. MMPs are significantly elevated in gliomas [48, 57].

Expression of miR-21 is not at this time used for diagnosis or prognostication; however, future endeavors into targeted downregulation of miR-21 in gliomas and other tumors may prove to show a great therapeutic promise [48].

1.4.2 miR-221/222

The overexpression of miR-221 has been found in gliomas, exclusive to the high-grade types. miR-221 is often studied and reported in correlation with miR-222 due to their apparent conjunctive function in the cell. miR-221/222 negatively regulates $p27^{Kip1}$, a protein that acts to trigger cell cycle arrest by inhibition of cyclin-dependent kinases [48, 58]. By this means, overexpression of miR-221/222 leads to low levels of $p27^{Kip1}$ and hence continuous glioblastoma cellular proliferation.

1.4.3 *miR-181a and miR-181b*

The downregulation of the miR-181 family has been demonstrated in gliomas [50, 59]. Both miR-181a and miR-181b are under expressed; however, it is only miR-181a that showed a gradient decrease of expression negatively correlating with the tumor grade [59]. Although the exact targets of miR-181 in brain tumors has not been established, studies have shown that normal or overexpression of miR-181a and miR-181b lead to growth inhibition, apoptosis, and decreased invasion. Thus, decreased expression of these miRNAs plays a multifactorial role in tumorogenesis and may very well have more than one target.

1.4.4 *miR-128*

miR-128 is a neuron-specific miRNA that has been found to be downregulated in gliomas, with the most significant decrease of expression in glioblastomas [50]. Two targets of miR-128 have been identified thus far: E2F3a and Bmi-1. E2F3a is a transcription factor responsible for activating genes involved in cellular proliferation. miR-128 negatively regulates this transcription factor; thus decreased expression of miR-128 leads to an unchecked proliferation pathway [48, 60]. Bmi-1 is a factor necessary for the self-renewal of stem cells. Without the inhibition of Bmi-1 by miR-128, glioma cell self-renewal is possible [48, 61]. At the present time, loss of miR-128 could be used as a biomarker for tumorogenesis without significance of therapy or prognosis.

Although it is apparent that miRNAs are differentially expressed in gliomas of varying grades and in comparison to unaffected brain tissue, further investigation into the utilization of miRNA expression signatures as biomarkers for glioma diagnosis, prognosis, and therapeutic targets must still be performed.

1.5 Conclusions

The biology of gliomas is still far from understood and tremendous efforts are still required for further understanding of these complex tumors. The advances in molecular biology of gliomas have resulted in significant progress in the clinical management of patients. For example, a test for co-deletion of chromosomes 1p and 19q in oligodendrogliomas has brought not only a diagnostic tool for pathologists, but treatment options for oncologists, as well as prognostic information for patients. As long as the technique is available, there is potential for genomic tests in the future. From a clinical standpoint, a comprehensive approach using currently available biomarkers may be the best way to decide our patients' diagnosis, therapeutic choice, and prognosis.

References

1. Louis DN, Ohgaki H, Wiestler OD, Cavenee WK, Burger PC, Jouvet A, Scheithauer BW, Kleihues P (2007) The 2007 WHO classification of tumors of the central nervous system. Acta Neuropathol 114:97–109
2. Parsons DW, Jones S, Zhang X, Lin JC, Leary RJ, Angenendt P, Mankoo P, Carter H, Siu IM, Gallia GL, Olivi A, McLendon R, Rasheed BA, Keir S, Nikolskaya T, Nikolsky Y, Busam DA, Tekleab H, Diaz LA Jr, Hartigan J, Smith DR, Strausberg RL, Marie SK, Shinjo SM, Yan H, Riggins GJ, Bigner DD, Karchin R, Papadopoulos N, Parmigiani G, Vogelstein B, Velculescu VE, Kinzler KW (2008) An integrated genomic analysis of human glioblastoma multiforme. Science 321:1807–1812
3. Yan H, Parsons DW, Jin G, McLendon R, Rasheed BA, Yuan W, Kos I, Batinic-Haberle I, Jones S, Riggins GJ, Friedman H, Friedman A, Reardon D, Herndon J, Kinzler KW, Velculescu VE, Vogelstein B, Bigner DD (2009) IDH1 and IDH2 mutations in gliomas. N Engl J Med 360:765–773
4. Dang L, White DW, Gross S, Bennett BD, Bittinger MA, Driggers EM, Fantin VR, Jang HG, Jin S, Keenan MC, Marks KM, Prins RM, Ward PS, Yen KE, Liau LM, Rabinowitz JD, Cantley LC, Thompson CB, Vander Heiden MG, Su SM (2009) Cancer associated IDH1 mutations produce 2-hydroxyglutarate. Nature 462:739–744
5. Aghili M, Zahedi F, Rafiee E (2009) Hydroxyglutaric aciduria and malignant brain tumor: a case report and literature review. J Neurooncol 91:233–236
6. Zhao S, Lin Y, Xu W, Jiang W, Zha Z, Wang P, Yu W, Li Z, Gong L, Peng Y, Ding J, Lei Q, Guan KL, Xiong Y (2009) Glioma-derived mutations in IDH1 dominantly inhibit IDH1 catalytic activity and induce HIF-1alpha. Science 324:261–265
7. Gross S, Cairns RA, Minden MD, Driggers EM, Bittinger MA, Jang HG, Sasaki M, Jin S, Schenkein DP, Su SM, Dang L, Fantin VR, Mak TW (2010) Cancer-associated metabolite 2-hydroxyglutarate accumulates in acute myelogenous leukemia with isocitrate dehydrogenase 1 and 2 mutations. J Exp Med 207:339–344
8. Sanson M, Marie Y, Paris S, Idbaih A, Laffaire J, Ducray F, El Hallani S, Boisselier B, Mokhtari K, Hoang-Xuan K, Delattre JY (2009) Isocitrate dehydrogenase 1 codon 132 mutation is an important prognostic biomarker in gliomas. J Clin Oncol 27:4150–4154
9. Gravendeel LA, Kloosterhof NK, Bralten LB, van Marion R, Dubbink HJ, Dinjens W, Bleeker FE, Hoogenraad CC, Michiels E, Kros JM, van den Bent M, Smitt PA, French PJ (2010) Segregation of non-p.R132H mutations in IDH1 in distinct molecular subtypes of glioma. Hum Mutat 31:E1186–E1199
10. van den Bent MJ, Dubbink HJ, Marie Y, Brandes AA, Taphoorn MJ, Wesseling P, Frenay M, Tijssen CC, Lacombe D, Idbaih A, van Marion R, Kros JM, Dinjens WN, Gorlia T, Sanson M (2010) IDH1 and IDH2 mutations are prognostic but not predictive for outcome in anaplastic oligodendroglial tumors: a report of the European Organization for Research and Treatment of Cancer Brain Tumor Group. Clin Cancer Res 16:1597–1604
11. Kato Y, Jin G, Kuan CT, McLendon RE, Yan H, Bigner DD (2009) A monoclonal antibody IMab-1 specifically recognizes IDH1R132H, the most common glioma derived mutation. Biochem Biophys Res Commun 390:547–551
12. Capper D, Weissert S, Balss J, Habel A, Meyer J, Jäger D, Ackermann U, Tessmer C, Korshunov A, Zentgraf H, Hartmann C, von Deimling A (2009) Characterization of R132H mutation-specific IDH1 antibody binding in brain tumors. Brain Pathol 20:245–254
13. Capper D, Zentgraf H, Balss J, Hartmann C, von Deimling A (2009) Monoclonal antibody specific for IDH1 R132H mutation. Acta Neuropathol 118:599–601
14. Esteller M, Garcia-Foncillas J, Andion E, Goodman SN, Hidalgo OF, Vanaclocha V, Baylin SB, Herman JG (2000) Inactivation of the DNA repair gene MGMT and the clinical response of gliomas to alkylating agents. N Engl J Med 343:1350–1354
15. Hegi ME, Diserens AC, Gorlia T, Hamou MF, de Tribolet N, Weller M, Kros JM, Hainfellner JA, Mason W, Mariani L, Bromberg JE, Hau P, Mirimanoff RO, Cairncross JG,

Janzer RC, Stupp R (2005) MGMT gene silencing and benefit from temozolomide in glioblastoma. N Engl J Med 352:997–1003
16. Reimenschneider M, Jeuken JW, Wesseling P, Reifenberger G (2010) Molecular diagnostics of gliomas: state of the art. Acta Neuropathol 120:567–584
17. Pollack IF, Hamilton RL, Sobol RW, Burnham J, Yates AJ, Holmes EJ, Zhou T, Finlay JL (2006) O6-methylguanine-DNA methyltransferase expression strongly correlates with outcome in childhood malignant gliomas: results from the CCG-945 cohort. J Clin Oncol 24:3431–3437
18. Schlosser S, Wagner S, Muhlisch J, Hasselblatt M, Gerss J, Wolff JE, Frühwald MC (2010) MGMT as a potential stratification marker in relapsed high-grade glioma of children: the HIT-GBM experience. Pediatr Blood Cancer 54:228–237
19. Nikiforova M, Hamilton R (2011) Molecular diagnostics of gliomas. Arch Pathol Lab Med 135:558–568
20. Rivera AL, Pelloski CE, Gilbert MR, Colman H, De La Cruz C, Sulman EP, Bekele BN, Aldape KD (2010) MGMT promoter methylation is predictive of response to radiotherapy and prognostic in the absence of adjuvant alkylating chemotherapy for glioblastoma. Neuro Oncol 12:116–121
21. Stupp R, Mason WP, van den Bent MJ, Weller M, Fisher B, Taphoorn MJ, Belanger K, Brandes AA, Marosi C, Bogdahn U, Curschmann J, Janzer RC, Ludwin SK, Gorlia T, Allgeier A, Lacombe D, Cairncross JG, Eisenhauer E, Mirimanoff RO, European Organisation for Research and Treatment of Cancer Brain Tumor and Radiotherapy Groups, National Cancer Institute of Canada Clinical Trials Group (2005) Radiotherapy plus concomitant and adjuvant temozolomide for glioblastoma. N Engl J Med 352:987–996
22. Wick W, Hartmann C, Engel C, Stoffels M, Felsberg J, Stockhammer F, Sabel MC, Koeppen S, Ketter R, Meyermann R, Rapp M, Meisner C, Kortmann RD, Pietsch T, Wiestler OD, Ernemann U, Bamberg M, Reifenberger G, von Deimling A, Weller M (2009) NOA-04 randomized phase III trial of sequential radiochemotherapy of anaplastic glioma with procarbazine, lomustine, and vincristine or temozolomide. J Clin Oncol 27:5874–5880
23. Weller M, Stupp R, Reifenberger G, Brandes AA, van den Bent MJ, Wick W, Hegi ME (2010) MGMT promotor methylation in malignant gliomas: ready for personalized medicine? Nat Rev Neurol 6:39–51
24. Mikeska T, Bock C, El-Maarri O, Hübner A, Ehrentraut D, Schramm J, Felsberg J, Kahl P, Büttner R, Pietsch T, Waha A (2007) Optimization of quantitative MGMT promoter methylation analysis using pyrosequencing and combined bisulfite restriction analysis. J Mol Diagn 9:368–381
25. Levidou G, El-Habr E, Saetta AA, Bamias C, Katsouyanni K, Patsouris E, Korkolopoulou P (2010) P53 immunoexpression as a prognostic marker for human astrocytomas: a meta-analysis and review of the literature. J Neurooncol 100:363–371
26. Ohgaki H, Kleihues P (2005) Population-based studies on incidence, survival rates, and genetic alterations in astrocytic and oligodendroglial gliomas. J Neuropathol Exp Neurol 64:479–489
27. Nieder C, Petersen S, Petersen C, Thames HD (2000) The challenge of p53 as prognostic and predictive factor in gliomas. Cancer Treat Rev 26:67–73
28. Jeuken JW, von Deimling A, Wesseling P (2004) Molecular pathogenesis of oligodendroglial tumors. J Neurooncol 70:161–181
29. Cairncross G, Jenkins R (2008) Gliomas with 1p/19q codeletion: a.k.a. oligodendroglioma. Cancer J 14:352–357
30. Scheie D, Cvancarova M, Mork S, Skullerud K, Andresen PA, Benestad I, Helseth E, Meling T, Beiske K (2008) Can morphology predict 1p/19q loss in oligodendroglial tumours? Histopathology 53:578–587
31. Idbaih A, Marie Y, Pierron G, Brennetot C, Hoang-Xuan K, Kujas M, Mokhtari K, Sanson M, Lejeune J, Aurias A, Delattre O, Delattre JY (2005) Two types of chromosome 1p losses with opposite significance in gliomas. Ann Neurol 58:483–487
32. Jones DT, Kocialkowski S, Liu L, Pearson DM, Ichimura K, Collins VP (2009) Oncogenic RAF1 rearrangement and a novel BRAF mutation as alternatives to KIAA1549: BRAF fusion in activating the MAPK pathway in pilocytic astrocytoma. Oncogene 28:2119–2123

33. Korshunov A, Meyer J, Capper D, Christians A, Remke M, Witt H, Pfister S, von Deimling A, Hartmann C (2009) Combined molecular analysis of BRAF and IDH1 distinguishes pilocytic astrocytoma from diffuse astrocytoma. Acta Neuropathol 118:401–405
34. Pfister S, Janzarik WG, Remke M, Ernst A, Werft W, Becker N, Toedt G, Wittmann A, Kratz C, Olbrich H, Ahmadi R, Thieme B, Joos S, Radlwimmer B, Kulozik A, Pietsch T, Herold-Mende C, Gnekow A, Reifenberger G, Korshunov A, Scheurlen W, Omran H, Lichter P (2008) BRAF gene duplication constitutes a mechanism of MAPK pathway activation in low-grade astrocytomas. J Clin Invest 118:1739–1749
35. Cahill DP, Levine KK, Betensky RA, Codd PJ, Romany CA, Reavie LB, Batchelor TT, Futreal PA, Stratton MR, Curry WT, Iafrate AJ, Louis DN (2007) Loss of the mismatch repair protein MSH6 in human glioblastomas is associated with tumor progression during temozolomide treatment. Clin Cancer Res 13:2038–2045
36. Yip S, Miao J, Cahill DP, Iafrate AJ, Aldape K, Nutt CL, Louis DN (2009) MSH6 mutations arise in glioblastomas during temozolomide therapy and mediate temozolomide resistance. Clin Cancer Res 15:4622–4629
37. Deighton RF, McGregor R, Kemp J, McColloch J, Whittle I (2010) Glioma pathophysiology: insights emerging from proteomics. Brain Pathol 20:691–703
38. Chumbalkar V, Subhashini C, Dhople VM, Sundaram CS, Jagannadham MV, Kumar KN, Srinivas PN, Mythili R, Rao MK, Kulkarni MJ, Hegde S, Hegde AS, Samual C, Santosh V, Singh L, Sirdeshmukh R (2005) Differential protein expression in human gliomas and molecular insights. Proteomics 5:1167–1177
39. Nagane M, Coufal F, Lin H, Bögler O, Cavenee WK, Huang HJ (1996) A common mutant epidermal growth factor receptor confers enhanced tumorigenicity on human glioblastoma cells by increasing proliferation and reducing apoptosis. Cancer Res 56:5079–5086
40. Gan HK, Kaye AH, Luwor RB (2009) The EGFRvIII variant in glioblastoma multiforme. J Clin Neurosci 16:748–754
41. Mellinghoff IK, Wang MY, Vivanco I, Haas-Kogan DA, Zhu S, Dia EQ, Lu KV, Yoshimoto K, Huang JH, Chute DJ, Riggs BL, Horvath S, Liau LM, Cavenee WK, Rao PN, Beroukhim R, Peck TC, Lee JC, Sellers WR, Stokoe D, Prados M, Cloughesy TF, Sawyers CL, Mischel PS (2005) Molecular determinants of the response of glioblastomas to EGFR kinase inhibitors. N Engl J Med 353:2012–2024
42. Kapoor GS, O'Rourke DM (2003) Receptor tyrosine kinase signaling in gliomagenesis: pathobiology and therapeutic approaches. Cancer Biol Ther 2:330–342
43. Ohgaki H, Kleihues P (2009) Genetic alterations and signaling pathways in the evolution of gliomas. Cancer Sci 100:2235–2241
44. Mishra S, Murphy LC, Murphy LJ (2006) The Prohibitins: emerging roles in diverse functions. J Cell Mol Med 10:353–363
45. Watanabe T, Nobusawa S, Kleihues P, Ohgaki H (2009) DH1 mutations are early events in the development of astrocytomas and oligodendrogliomas. Am J Pathol 174:1149–1153
46. Labussiere M, Idbaih A, Wang XW, Marie Y, Boisselier B, Falet C, Paris S, Laffaire J, Carpentier C, Crinière E, Ducray F, El Hallani S, Mokhtari K, Hoang-Xuan K, Delattre JY, Sanson M (2010) All the 1p19q codeleted gliomas are mutated on IDH1 or IDH2. Neurology 74:1886–1890
47. Paugh BS, Qu C, Jones C, Liu Z, Adamowicz-Brice M, Zhang J, Bax DA, Coyle B, Barrow J, Hargrave D, Lowe J, Gajjar A, Zhao W, Broniscer A, Ellison DW, Grundy RG, Baker SJ (2010) Integrated molecular genetic profiling of pediatric high-grade gliomas reveals key differences with the adult disease. J Clin Oncol 28:3061–3068
48. Novakova J, Slaby O, Vyzula R, Michalek J (2009) MicroRNA involvement in glioblastoma pathogenesis. Biochem Biophys Res Commun 386:1–5
49. Cho WC (2007) OncomiRs: the discovery and progress of microRNAs in cancers. Mol Cancer 6:60
50. Ciafre SA, Galardi S, Mangiola A, Ferracin M, Liu CG, Sabatino G, Negrini M, Maira G, Croce CM, Farace MG (2005) Extensive modulation of a set of microRNAs in primary glioblastoma. Biochem Biophys Res Commun 334:1351–1358

51. Chan JA, Krichevsky AM, Kosik KS (2005) MicroRNA-21 is an antiapoptotic factor in human glioblastoma cells. Cancer Res 65:6029–6033
52. Silber J, James CD, Hodgson JG (2009) MicroRNAs in gliomas: small regulators of a big problem. Neuromolecular Med 11:208–222
53. Chen X, Guo X, Zhang H, Xiang Y, Chen J, Yin Y, Cai X, Wang K, Wang G, Ba Y, Zhu L, Wang J, Yang R, Zhang Y, Ren Z, Zen K, Zhang J, Zhang CY (2009) Role of miR-143 targeting KRAS in colorectal tumorigenesis. Oncogene 28:1385–1392
54. Holland EC, Celestino J, Dai C, Schaefer L, Sawaya RE, Fuller GN (2000) Combined activation of Ras and Akt in neural progenitors induces glioblastoma formation in mice. Nat Genet 25:55–57
55. daFonseca CO, Linden R, Futuro D, Gattass CR, Quiric-Santos T (2008) Ras pathway activation in gliomas: a strategic target for intranasal administration of perillyl alcohol. Arch Immunol Ther Exp 56:267–276
56. Papagiannakopoulos T, Shapiro A, Kosik KS (2008) MicroRNA-21 targets a network of key tumor-suppressive pathways in glioblastoma cells. Cancer Res 68:8164–8172
57. Nakada M, Okada Y, Yamashita J (2003) The role of matrix metalloproteinases in glioma invasion. Front Biosci 8:e261–e269
58. le Sage C, Nagel R, Egan DA, Schrier M, Mesman E, Mangiola A, Anile C, Maira G, Mercatelli N, Ciafrè SA, Farace MG, Agami R (2007) Regulation of the p27(Kip1) tumor suppressor by miR-221 and miR-222 promotes cancer cell proliferation. EMBO J 26:3699–3708
59. Shi L, Cheng Z, Zhang J, Li R, Zhao P, Fu Z, You Y (2008) hsa-mir-181a and hsa-mir-181b function as tumor suppressors in human glioma cells. Brain Res 1236:185–193
60. Zhang Y, Chao T, Li R, Liu W, Chen Y, Yan X, Gong Y, Yin B, Liu W, Qiang B, Zhao J, Yuan J, Peng X (2009) MicroRNA-128 inhibits glioma cells proliferation by targeting transcription factor E2F3a. J Mol Med 87:43–51
61. Godlewski J, Nowicki MO, Bronisz A, Williams S, Otsuki A, Nuovo G, Raychaudhury A, Newton HB, Chiocca EA, Lawler S (2008) Targeting of the Bmi-1 oncogene/stem cell renewal factor by microRNA-128 inhibits glioma proliferation and self-renewal. Cancer Res 68:9125–9130

Chapter 2
Molecular Pathology and Diagnostics of Thyroid and Parathyroid Malignancies

Rodney E. Shackelford and Jason Savell

Contents

R.E. Shackelford
Department of Pathology and Laboratory Medicine, Tulane University School of Medicine, New Orleans, LA 70112-2699, USA

J. Savell, M.D. (✉)
H. Lee Moffitt Cancer Center and Research Institute and University of South Florida, 12902 Magnolia Drive, Tampa, FL 33612, USA
e-mail: Jason.savell@moffitt.org

D. Coppola (ed.), *Molecular Pathology and Diagnostics of Cancer*, Cancer Growth and Progression 16, DOI 10.1007/978-94-007-7192-5_2,

Abstract Malignancies of the thyroid and parathyroid glands are rare oncologic entities that range in clinical behavior from relatively indolent to extremely aggressive malignancies. Presently, establishing a diagnosis and prognosis for thyroid and parathyroid malignancies largely depends on histology supplemented with immunohistochemical analysis. Over the past 20 years, different histologic subtypes of thyroid cancer have been shown to carry specific genetic alterations, which are often preferentially associated with, or unique to, each subtype. In many cases, these genetic alterations have been analyzed via molecular-genetic testing techniques to help establish a diagnosis in cases where histology and immunohistochemistry alone cannot. In addition, such testing has occasionally been used to determine prognosis. Presently, clinical molecular diagnostic testing is not performed on parathyroid tumors. However, differences between parathyroid hyperplasia, adenomas, and carcinomas have been detected via molecular testing. With additional research, these differences may become more fully understood and applied to molecular diagnostics. Thus, although presently not extensively employed, molecular diagnostics of the thyroid and parathyroid are likely to become increasingly important in determining the diagnosis and prognosis of these malignancies, especially for histologically difficult cases. Furthermore, pharmacologic inhibitors of many of the oncogenes mutated in these malignancies are being developed. With time, molecular diagnostic testing for these mutations is likely to be implemented to aid in choosing optimal chemotherapeutic treatment regimens.

Keywords Thyroid • Parathyroid • Malignancies • Tumor papillary • Follicular • Medullary • *BRAF* • *RAS* • *RET* • Molecular diagnostics • *NTRK1* • *PAX8-PPAR* gamma

Abbreviations

ACT	Anaplastic carcinoma of the thyroid
ASA	Allele-specific amplification
ATC	Anaplastic thyroid cancer
FA	Follicular adenomas
FC	Follicular carcinoma
FCT	Follicular carcinoma of the thyroid
FMTC	Familial medullary thyroid cancer
FNA	Fine needle aspirations
HRM	High-resolution melting
HT	Hashimoto's thyroiditis
IR	Ionizing radiation
MEN	Multiple endocrine neoplasia
MTC	Medullary thyroid cancer
PA	Parathyroid adenoma
PC	Parathyroid carcinoma
PCR	Polymerase chair chain reaction
PTC	Papillary thyroid carcinoma
SSCP	Single-strand conformational polymorphism
STAT	Shifted termination assay technology
TC	Thyroid cancers
TSH	Thyroid-stimulating hormone

2.1 Introduction

Cancers of the thyroid and parathyroid are relatively rare oncologic entities for which a straightforward diagnosis, based on histologic grounds and supplemented with immunohistochemistry, is possible in the majority of cases. However, in some cases, distinguishing between benign and malignant neoplasms can be difficult. For example, the follicular variant of papillary thyroid carcinoma (PTC) is easily distinguished from follicular adenomas (FA) or follicular carcinoma (FC) when the typical nuclear features of PTC are distributed diffusely throughout the tumor. However, some PTC cases have only focal and/or poorly developed PTC nuclear features, making the diagnosis of PTC vs. FA and FC quite difficult. Even very experienced thyroid pathologist have had high inter- and intraobserver variability in the diagnosis of difficult cases [1]. Similarly, the use of histology alone to differentiate between parathyroid carcinoma (PC), parathyroid adenoma (PA), and atypical PAs can be difficult or even impossible unless obvious tumor invasion or metastasis is identified [2–4].

Since both thyroid and parathyroid malignancies can cause considerable morbidity and mortality, making the most accurate diagnosis is vital. Recently, molecular diagnostics has begun to play a role in the diagnosis and management of thyroid cancers (TC), especially for cytologically or histologically ambiguous cases. In addition, molecular testing can be valuable in predicting the probable clinical course, allowing risk stratification and possible changes in treatment plans. Lastly, molecular testing as a means of determining the specific chemotherapeutic agents employed in TC treatment is likely to become part of the management of these malignancies. Thus molecular-genetic testing is playing an increasingly important role in the diagnosis and management of thyroid neoplasia and is likely to eventually play a role in the diagnosis and clinical management of PC as well. Here, we will review current molecular-genetic testing for TC and PC with emphasis on the clinical utility of each test.

2.2 Thyroid Cancer: Epidemiology and Risks Factors

TC accounts for ~ 1 % of human malignancies and is the most common of the endocrine neoplasms. Interestingly, an increase in differentiated TC has been found in the United States and other developed countries that cannot be attributed solely to increased medical surveillance and increasingly sensitive diagnostic procedures [5–11]. TC is roughly three times more common in women, is very rare in individuals under age 10 years, and increases with age, having an average age of diagnosis of 40–45 years [12]. Some geographic and ethnic variations are seen with TC, with a low incidence seen in countries like Denmark, Holland, and Slovakia, and higher incidences seen in Iceland and the Hawaiian Islands [12, 13]. Population studies of different ethnic groups moving from low-risk to high-risk areas for TC suggest that both environmental and genetic factors contribute to the development of TC [12, 13]. Risk factors for TC cancer are described below.

2.2.1 Thyroid Cancer Risk Factor: Ionizing Radiation Exposure

Ionizing radiation (IR) exposure has long been known to be a risk factor for TC. Studies of the nuclear bombings of Hiroshima and Nagasaki, the aftermath of the Chernobyl nuclear accident, and effects of external radiotherapy on individuals treated for various head and neck malignancies have all demonstrated that IR to the thyroid significantly increases the TC risk. As expected, the risk for TC increases with higher

IR doses, with exposed children and pediatric patients receiving external IR showing the greatest TC increases. Interestingly, children exposed to the Chernobyl fallout most often presented with the solid and follicular variant of PTC that followed an unusually aggressive clinical course [14–21]. The latency period for TC following IR exposure ranges from a minimum of 4–5 years to a maximum at of 20 years, thereafter declining [21, 22]. Experimental evidence suggests that IR-induced *RET/PTC1* gene rearrangements play an early and important role in IR-induced TC development [14].

2.2.2 Thyroid Cancer Risk Factor: Iodine Deficiency

Areas with chronic dietary iodine deficiency show an increased incidence of benign thyroid nodules and TC, with FC and anaplastic TC (ATC) significantly increased. The underlying molecular mechanism of TC carcinogenesis results, in part, from iodine-deficiency causing increased thyroid-stimulating hormone activity, increased thyroid cell thyroid-stimulating hormone sensitivity with concomitant increased epidermal growth factor-induced cell proliferation, and increased angiogenesis, all of which promote carcinogenesis [23, 24]. Interestingly, some molecular and epidemiologic data have suggested that a high-iodine diet promotes PTC cancer by increasing the incidence of the *BRAF T1799A (V600E)* mutation [25].

2.2.3 Thyroid Cancer Risk Factor: Hormonal Factors

TC shows a strong female predominance that is greater in women in the childbearing years than in post-menopausal women. Additionally, pregnancy causes an increase in thyroid volume and an increased incidence of thyroid nodules and goiters. The reasons for the TC gender differences are poorly understood, although estrogen levels can influence cancer cell growth. In TC, estrogen receptor-alpha agonists promote cell proliferation, whereas estrogen receptor-beta agonists or beta-receptor overexpression suppresses cell proliferation. Several studies have demonstrated that alpha-receptor expression is increased in TC, while the beta-receptor expression is either decreased or absent [26, 27].

2.2.4 Thyroid Cancer Risk Factor: Other Factors

Several other factors influence the incidence of TC. Oddly, current smoking reduces TC risk, whereas alcohol and caffeinated beverages have no effect on TC risk. A diet high in vegetables reduces TC risk, and a high body mass index increases risk [28–30]. Lastly, TC is increased in individuals with benign thyroid nodules and goiters and possibly in individuals with HLA-DR7 [31–33].

2.3 Molecular-Genetic Testing for TC

Molecular testing on TC is not commonly performed, although presently two laboratories offer molecular TC testing within the United States. Testing can usually be performed on fine needle aspirates, paraffin-embedded formalin-fixed tissue, and fresh or frozen tissue. TC has multiple histological variants that range in clinical behavior from the usually indolent and often curable PTC, to anaplastic carcinoma (undifferentiated carcinoma), which almost invariably follows a rapid and lethal course, having a median survival rate of less than 6 months [34–37]. Over the past 20 years, molecular analyses of the different TCs have revealed distinctive gene mutations and expression patterns that correlate with the histological TC type. Additionally, within one histological TC type, specific mutations and gene expression patterns often correlate with a more aggressive clinical course. For example, PTCs with the *BRAF V600E* mutation are more likely to recur and exhibit increased aggressiveness by the recurrent tumor [38]. The molecular alterations seen in TC involve a relatively low number of genes, including *BRAF, RAS, p53, PTEN, NTRK1, RET, CTNNB1,* and the *PAX8/PPAR-gamma* translocation. In the sections, we will review the genetic alterations that occur in the major histological variants of TC and the molecular-genetic tests employed in TC diagnosis and clinical management.

2.4 Papillary Thyroid Carcinoma: Mutations and Molecular Testing

PTC is the most common TC, accounting for ~80 % of TCs in developed countries and up to 90 % of IR-induced TCs. PTC is most commonly composed of cuboidal columnar thyroidal epithelium, usually in papillary projections surrounding fibrovascular cores and often with associated follicles and dense fibrosis. The nuclei are overlapping, vesicular, hypochromatic, and often described as having an "Orphan Annie Eye" appearance, and 50 % of PTC will have psammoma bodies. The usual clinical course is indolent, at least in younger patients, with 98 % of individuals surviving 10 years, a survival rate similar to the general population. Interestingly, cervical lymph node involvement does not alter the prognosis, although etrathyroidal and/or extranodal tumor extension and loss of radioiodine avidity predict a poorer survival. Additionally, local lymph node metastasis is common, whereas hematogenous dissemination is rare. PTC has many variants, including conventional, solid, tall cell, Warthin-like, oncocytic, nodular fasciitis, microcarcinoma, macrofollicular, follicular, columnar cell, encapsulated follicular, diffuse sclerosing encapsulated, diffuse follicular, and cribiform-morular [39–42].

PTC is characterized by a number of different gene mutations, most of which are almost always mutually exclusive of each other and which often correlate with different histological subtypes and clinical courses. At present, there have been no defined mutations found in a subset of PTC (~25 %), indicating the likely presence of unknown genetic alterations or the use of inadequate molecular testing methods [42].

2.4.1 BRAF Mutation Testing

BRAF somatic mutations are found in ~45 % of PTCs [43–45]. *BRAF* is found at 7q34 and consists of 19 exons. It is also known as the V-raf murine sarcoma viral oncogene homolog B1 (B-raf-1) and functions as a serine/threonine kinase. Under normal conditions, BRAF is phosphorylated and activated by KRAS, leading to an increase in cyclins D1-3, mdm2, and c-myc levels, promoting tumorigenesis via promotion of cell cycle entrance, increased growth potential, and apoptosis inhibition. BRAF is commonly constitutively activated in multiple human malignancies, including colorectal carcinomas, low-grade serous ovarian adenocarcinomas, and PTC [45–48]. More than 40 different *BRAF* mutations have been identified in PTC, with ~90 % of mutations involving a T→A transversion at position 1,779 in exon 15, causing a valine→glutamate substitution at residue 600 (V600E). The resulting mutant BRAF kinase is ~500-fold more active than the wild-type kinase and has ablated GTPase activity, allowing the kinase to be constitutively active [49]. Studies on thyroid cell lines and animal models have suggested that the *BRAF V600E* mutation promotes genomic instability, dedifferentiation, metastasis, proliferation, and transformation [50–53].

TCs with *BRAF V600E* often show a worse clinical course than TCs without the mutation and are associated with extrathyroidal extension, advanced disease stages III and IV, recurrence, loss of radioiodine avidity, and distant metastases. Interestingly, *BRAF V600E* mutations are more common in the tall cell, conventional, and Follicular variants of PTC, the three variants that exhibit the most aggressive clinical courses [54]. The *BRAF V600E* mutation is rare in FC [43].

Clinical *BRAF* mutation testing in TC has been performed via many different molecular techniques. Because the V600E mutation makes up the majority of mutations, many testing methods specifically target the 1,779 position T→A transversion. For example, allele-specific amplification polymerase chain reaction (ASA-PCR) and Shifted Termination Assay Technology (STAT) both use the one base-pair difference to detect *BRAF V600E* mutations.

2.4.2 Allele-Specific Amplification-PCR

Also known as amplification refractory mutation system-PCR and allele-specific oligonucleotide-PCR, this method is useful for detecting one to several base-pair changes (transversion or transitions) by taking advantage of the different initiation rates for the *Taq* polymerase from matched vs. mismatched template-primer

3′-termini, with the latter 10^{-3} to 10^{-6} less efficient depending on the mismatch type. ASA-PCR employs multiple primers with 3′ ends, often three base pairs from the 3′-terminus that match either the wild-type or the mutant sequence [55]. Mutation detection is based on the detection of an amplified wild-type or mutant sequence. Amplicon detection methods include the degradation of a probe labeled with a quencher held adjacent to a fluorescent dye. Upon probe degradation by the 5′–3′ exonuclease activity of the *Taq* polymerase, the quencher and fluorescent dye are no longer held in close proximity, allowing fluorescent dye emission detection and hence amplicon detection. Samples can be run multiplexed with different probes carrying different fluorophores or can be run separately with one primer pair, depending on the requirements of the test. Alternatively, other systems can be employed, such as Scorpion technology for amplicon detection. Due to the extremely specific base pairing requirements of the *Taq* polymerase, ASA-PCR can detect as little as one mutant in a background of 10^{-4} wild-type alleles [56]. Due to the low amplification that occurs from mismatched primer-templates with the *Taq* polymerase, ASA-PCR can produce amplicons at very high Cp values. Therefore, to be counted as mutant positive, some testing protocols using ASA-PCR require Cp values (rounds of primer annealing, extension, and denaturation) of 35 or lower [57]. Additionally, ASA-PCR with only one nucleotide difference requires very exact annealing temperatures for both the wild-type and mutant primers to optimize specific primer annealing [58].

Sapio et al. [57] employed ASA-PCR to examine *BRAF* mutations in PTC. One reverse primer was employed, with two forward primers differing at the mutant base pair: 5′-GTGATTTTGGTCTAGCTACAG*T*-3′ (wild type) and 5′-GTGATTTTGGTCTAGCTACAG*A*-3′ (mutant). Analysis of 43 archival PTCs revealed that 44.2 % harbored *BRAF V600E* mutations. No *BRAF* mutations were identified in 35 benign lesions or FCs. Interestingly, when single-strand conformational polymorphism (SSCP) and DNA sequencing testing methods were compared to ASA-PCR, SSCP and DNA sequencing both required more than 40 % mutant DNA to be present for mutation detection, showing a relatively low sensitivity, whereas ASA-PCR demonstrated two to threefold greater sensitivity.

2.4.3 STAT

ASA-PCR has drawbacks, including requiring extremely precise annealing temperatures and giving false-positive results at high Cp values [57, 58]. One technique that partially overcomes these limitations is STAT. With STAT, a detection primer is designed that is complementary to the target DNA, with the 3′-terminal detection primer binding site ending just before the mutant target base. A labeled detection primer then binds to the target sequence. A primer extension reaction is then performed. If the first target base is present in the wild type DNA, the detection primer is not extended. If there is mutational change by any type of mutation, including point mutations, deletions, insertions, or translocations, a primer extension reaction will continue through the target base position, incorporating multiple labeled nucleotides. Colorimetric, fluorometric, or chemiluminescent detection systems can be used to quantify the amount of the mutant transcript. STAT is very sensitive and can detect as little as 1 % mutant DNA [59].

STAT has been employed to analyze PTC *BRAF V600E* mutations with good results. For example, Cohen et al. [60] employed STAT to analyze *BRAF V600E* mutations in 95 excised PTCs and 42 corresponding fine needle aspirations (FNAs). In this study, 100 ng genomic tumor/aspirate DNA was isolated and the region surrounding exon 15 carrying the V600E mutations was amplified via 39 cycles of standard PCR. Both STAT and automated DNA sequencing were performed on 10 μm of the resulting amplicon. *BRAF* mutations were detected in 67 % of the resected PTC and only 12 % of the FC, with only two ATC showing *BRAF* mutations in both the differentiated and undifferentiated areas. Forty-nine preoperative FNAs, which corresponded to the resected PTCs, were analyzed for *BRAF V600E* mutations. A 94 % concordance was found for *BRAF* status. Of three discordant samples, two were sparsely cellular; thus STAT testing is useful for aspirate analysis. Further analysis of a large number of FNAs revealed that clearly benign aspirates had no *BRAF* mutations, 39 % of the clearly malignant aspirates had mutations, as did 16 % of the indeterminate group. Thus STAT *BRAF* testing can be used to identify PTC within the indeterminate group. When STAT testing and DNA sequencing were compared, a 100 % correlation was found between the two methods. Thus STAT testing is comparable to sequencing in accuracy and reliability and has greater sensitivity.

2.4.4 Single Strand Conformation Polymorphism Testing

SSCP testing has been used to detect TC *BRAF* mutations [61]. In SSCP, wild-type and DNA undergoing mutation testing are PCR amplified, along with a known wild-type control. The two DNA samples are heat denatured, rapidly renatured, and subjected to electrophoresis. A ssDNA segment carrying a mutation, even if a single base pair change, will assume different secondary and tertiary structures, which will cause a different migration pattern compared to the wild-type control(s). SSCP has worked well and has the advantage of detecting more than the single *V600E BRAF* mutation, although it does not identify which specific base pair(s) is altered. It is also less sensitive than the ASA-PCR or STAT testing and is often technically challenging to perform. It does have use as an initial mutation-screening tool, which if initially positive, can be followed up by more accurate testing methods. Additionally, SSCP can initially use either genomic DNA or RNA, which is converted into DNA via reverse transcriptase and then PCR amplified. Conformation strand gel electrophoresis thyroid *BRAF* mutation testing, similar to SSCP, has not often been employed in thyroid *BRAF* mutation testing.

Fugazzola et al. [61] employed DNA sequencing and SSCP to analyze *BRAF* mutations in a large multicentric study. *BRAF* RNA was isolated, and cDNA was made via reverse transcriptase with radon hexamer primers. The cDNA immediately around the *V600E BRAF* mutation was PCR amplified with the forward and reverse primers 5′-CATTGCACGAQCAGACTGCAC-3′ and 5′-TCTGACTGAAAGCTGTATGG-3′ and subjected to both SSCP and direct DNA sequencing using ABI PRISM big dye terminators and run on an ABI PRISM 310 genetic analyzer. *BRAF V660E* mutations were found in 38 % of PTCs in an Italian population, with a tendency for the mutation frequency to increase with increasing patient age.

2.4.5 DNA Sequencing

DNA sequencing has often been employed in *BRAF* mutation analyses [58, 61]. Although considered the gold standard in molecular testing, especially Sanger sequencing, direct sequencing has several disadvantages: (1) it can be relatively expensive, especially for longer sequences; (2) other techniques such as ASA-PCR and STAT have higher sensitivity; and (3) it can give false results when applied to formalin-fixed tissue [62, 63]. Direct sequencing has the advantage of interrogating all possible nucleic acid sequences analyzed, thus it identifies rare mutations missed by ASA-PCR and STAT.

2.4.6 High-Resolution Melting Analysis in BRAF Mutation Analysis

High-resolution melting (HRM) analysis is performed on dsDNA. Most often a specific nucleic acid sequence containing the possible mutation of interest is PCR amplified. It is then mixed with a fluorescent dye, such as SYBR green, which emits strongly when bound to dsDNA and poorly in the presence of ssDNA. The amplified dsDNA is then heated, and the transition from dsDNA to ssDNA is followed via the loss of florescence at the DNA melting point. Typically, the data are presented as the negative first derivative of the melting curve, as this makes it easier to identify the exact temperature of dissociation.

Rowe et al. [64] analyzed 42 archival formalin-fixed, paraffin-embedded thyroidal samples, 37 PTC, and 5 benign lesions. The region around the *BRAF V600E* mutation was PCR amplified with 5′-CTC TTCATAATGCTTGCTCTGATAGG-3′ and 5′-TAGTAA CTCAGCAGCATCTCAGG-3′ forward and reverse primer for 45 cycles. The resulting amplicon was cooled and then heated at 0.1 °C/s from 45 °C to 95 °C, with fluorescent peaks determined by plotting the negative derivative of fluorescence with respect to temperature. Of the PTC samples, 62.2 % had the *BRAF V600E* mutation, whereas 0 % of the benign thyroid samples had mutations.

In this study, when HRM was compared to DNA sequencing, a 100 % concordance was revealed. Although useful in detecting *BRAF* mutations, the authors did note that HRN had poor sensitivity and required at least 50 % mutant DNA present to be accurate. Thus, HRM as a testing method is useful, but requires very pure tumor DNA to ensure testing accuracy.

There are several advantages of HRM: (1) it is often cost effective, thus allowing a large number of samples to be interrogated simultaneously; (2) it has a relatively short turn-around time and high accuracy; and (3) once "up and running," the assay is relatively simple to run and analyze. Disadvantages of HRM are that it does not identify the specific base pair(s) mutated and requires pure concentrated samples.

2.4.7 *BRAF2*

BRAF mutation testing is complicated by the closely related *BRAF2* pseudogene located at Xq13.3. The two genes are similar, and careful primer design is required to avoid pseudogene amplification during *BRAF* testing [65, 66]. *BRAF2* is often expressed in *BRAF* mutation-negative PTCs. Additionally, it is expressed in tumorigenic nude mice, it activates MAP kinases, and it can transform NIH3T3 cells [67]. Presently, molecular genetic testing is not performed for *BRAF2,* although this could change, as one study showed nearly 50 % of classic PTC had *BRAF2* expression [67].

2.4.8 *RET/PTC* Mutation Testing

The *RET* oncogene, also known as *ret-proto-oncogene*, is located at 10q11.2, has 21 exons, and has three main isoforms of 1,114, 1,106, and 1,072 amino acids, encoding a protein of ~ 124 kDa. The RET protein has an extracellular domain that binds extracellular ligands, a single transmembrane domain, and an intracellular domain that contains a tyrosine kinase. The physiologic RET ligands all belong to the glial-derived neurotrophic factor family: peresphin, artemin, neurturin, and glial-derived neurotrophic factor. *RET* has multiple functions; for example, it is required for the development of the sympathetic, parasympathetic, and enteric neurons, the kidneys, and male germ cells. Not surprisingly germline loss of *RET* function can cause colonic congenital aganglionosis (Hirschsprung's disease), whereas germline *RET* activation can lead to medullary thyroid cancer (MTC) or multiple endocrine neoplasia type two (MEN2A/B) [68].

For PTC, 20–30 % carry *RET* gene mutations. Unlike the point mutations that activate BRAF and KRAS or the activating *RET* point mutations seen in hereditary MTC or MEN2A/B, *RET* mutations in PTC are typically activating intra- and interchromosomal rearrangements and are unique to PTC. Most rearrangements are in-frame fusions of the RET C-terminal/tyrosine kinase domain with the 5′ end of many heterologous donor genes, of which ~90 % involve the *RET/PTC1* and *RET/PTC3* genes, which result from fusion with the H4 (*D10S170*) gene and the NCOA4 (*ELE1, RFG*, or *ARA70*) genes, respectively [69, 70]. The molecular mechanisms by which these RET rearrangements cause tumorigenesis are incompletely understood, although the fusions lead to constitutive activation of the RET tyrosine kinase. Additionally, the rearrangements induce the nuclear changes typical of PTC, which are found in occult PTCs (making them an early event in PTC tumorigenesis) and induce TC resembling human PTC when expressed in the thyroid tissue of transgenic mice [71–73].

2.4.8.1 Real-Time PCR (RT-PCR) for RET/PTC Rearrangements

RT-PCR is useful for detecting gene rearrangements, as primers can be designed to amplify gene fusion regions (nucleic acid sequences likely unique to the particular tumor type and not found in normal cells). As in the case of the *BCR-abl* gene fusion characterizing chronic myelogenous leukemia, the initial analytic step is purifying RNA, priming with radon heximers, and employing reverse transcriptase to produce a cDNA library. The specific fusion can be PCR amplified and quantified through the use of fusion region flanking primers and a labeled probe.

Zhu et al. [74] used RT-PCR to analyze *RET/PCT1* and *RET/PCT3* rearrangements in 65 snap-frozen PTC samples. Total RNA was isolated with Trizol reagent, and a cDNA library was made via Superscript reverse transcription of 3 μg of RNA primed with radon heximers. The *RET/PTC1* and *RET/PTC3* gene fusions were detected by RT-PCR employing a common reverse primer of 5′-GCAGGTCTCAAGCTCACTC-3′ and RET/PTC1 and RET/PTC3-specific forward primers of 5′-CAAGAGAACAAGGTGCTGAAG-3′ and 5′-CGGTATTGTAGCTGTCCCTTTC-3′, respectively. Appropriately labeled probes were employed for amplicon detection. In PTCs, 22 % showed RET/PTC rearrangements.

Interestingly, the authors compared the ability of standard-sensitivity RT-PCR, high-sensitivity RT-PCR, real-time LightCycler RT-PCR, Southern blotting, and fluorescence *in situ* hybridization FISH to detect *RET/PCT1* and *RET/PCT3* rearrangements [74]. High-sensitivity RT-PCR detected the 14 *RET/PCT* rearrangements detected by standard PCR and 12 additional cases, for a 40 % detection rate. LightCycler RT-PCR detected 12 rearrangements, Southern blot 11, and FISH 14. Overall, 14 % of PTC had rearrangements detected by all five methods. Twelve (18 %) of PTCs had nonclonal rearrangements detected only by high-sensitivity RT-PCR. The authors concluded that the prevalence of different *RET/PTC* rearrangement seen in the literature is in part due to different molecular detection methods and tumor heterogeneities. Other techniques, such as DNA sequencing, have also been used to analyze these rearrangements [75]. However, different RT-PCR protocols are most commonly employed.

2.4.9 RAS Family Proteins and PTC

HRAS, NRAS, and *KRAS* are members of a superfamily of GTPases which has more than 150 members and is divided into five different groups: Ras, Rho, Ran, Rab, and Arf. Members of this group share a conserved G box motif, which transiently binds GTP, resulting in kinase activation and concomitant downstream signaling events that promote cell survival and proliferation. Under normal conditions, RAS proteins rapidly hydrolyze GTP to GDP, rendering the kinase inactive [76, 77]. A number of specific point mutations in codons 12, 13, and 61 ablate the GTPase activity, rendering the kinases constitutively active and oncogenic [76–80]. RAS point mutations are found in 10–20 % of PTC [81–83].

Molecular testing for RAS mutations in PTC has been done by multiple methods. For example, Vasko et al. [82] examined *NRAS* point mutations in 10 FA, 9 atypical follicular tumors, 10 FC, and 10 follicular variants of PTC. The tumors on slides were microdissected, genomic DNA was extracted and purified, and 500 ng was PCR amplified with primers specific for NRAS exon 2. The resulting amplicon was sequenced with an Applied Biosystem 373XL sequencer. No *NRAS* mutations were detected in any FA. Exon 2 *NRAS* mutations were identified in 33 % of the atypical follicular tumors, 20 % of the FC, and 20 % of the follicular variant PTC. Ezzat et al. [83] used SSCP testing and DNA sequencing to examine point mutations in exons 12, 13, and 61 of *HRAS* and *NRAS*. These exons were PCR amplified from 100 ng genomic DNA, and the DNA was heat denatured and analyzed by PAGE. Of 45 histologically characterized TC, adenomas, and hyperplastic nodules, one *HRAS* at codon 13 mutation was identified in one PTC and two PTC and one FA carried the *NRAS* codon 61 mutation. No tumors carried *KRAS* mutations.

2.4.10 NTRK1 Mutation in PTC

NTRK1, also known as *TrkA*, is found at 1q21-22 and has at least 17 exons that encode a 796-amino acid glycosylated protein of ~ 140 kDa. NTRK1 is widely expressed in neuronal and non-neuronal tissues and functions as a nerve growth factor receptor tyrosine kinase. Roughly 5–25 % of PTCs carry *NTRK1* mutations, depending on the population examined [84–87]. Similar to *RET, NTRK1* is constitutively activated by rearrangements involving at least three other genes, with the 3′ terminus of *NTRK1* fusing with the 5′ of genes, such as TPM3, TPR, and TFG. All rearrangements lead to constitutive NTRK1 tyrosine kinase activation [85, 88–92]. Once activated, NTRK1 activates RAS, RAC, PI3K, PLC-gamma, and MAPK, leading to cell proliferation [92].

NTRK1 has been analyzed by multiple methods, with PCR amplification of tumor-derived reverse transcribed RNA, followed by amplicon sequencing being a commonly used technique. Beimfohr et al. [93] used this technique with multiplex PCR and Sanger sequencing to examine 81 pediatric PTCs from children who had been exposed to the Chernobyl fallout. All tumors were previously determined to be devoid of *RET* rearrangements of types PTC1 to PTC5. *TPM3/NTRK1* fusions were identified in five tumors. Reciprocal *NTRK1/TPM3* transcripts were found in four of five of these tumors. Tumors with the *TPM3/NTRK1* fusions were histologically no different than other post-Chernobyl childhood PTCs. The authors concluded that, compared to the high number of *RET* mutations seen in this population [14], NTRK1 rearrangements play a small role in Chernobyl fallout-induced pediatric PTCs. Presently, clinical testing for *NTRK1* mutations/rearrangements in TC is not routinely performed.

2.4.11 c-MET *Mutation in PTC*

c-MET is located at 7q31.2, consists of 21 exons, and encodes a hepatocyte growth factor/scatter factor receptor with tyrosine kinase activity. c-Met is synthesized as a 170 kDa single-chain precursor that is cleaved post-translationally to yield an internal 145 kDa beta-subunit and a 45 kDa extracellular alpha-subunit domain [94]. c-MET is overexpressed in ovarian, colorectal, pancreatic, renal cell, non-small lung, and thyroid malignancies [95–101]. Inappropriate ligation of c-MET by the hepatocyte growth factor increases epithelial cell growth and division and causes epithelial cells to acquire increased motility and invasive capacities [94, 95, 102]. Hence, c-MET expression is likely to play an important role in PTC acquiring invasive/metastatic potential [97].

c-MET is barely detected in normal thyroid or thyroid tissue affected by non-neoplastic disease. c-MET expression is increased roughly 100-fold in thyroid carcinomas, and its overexpression strongly correlates with locally advanced disease and/or distant metastases [103]. Immunohistochemical studies of benign thyroid tissue revealed that c-MET is usually located along the basal membrane, occasionally found with the cytoplasm, and not found at the apical cell membrane. In PTC, these analyses identified increased c-MET immunoreactivity in the cytoplasm and apical membrane, with loss of reactivity seen along the basal membrane. In PTC, c-MET was co-localized with tight junction protein zona occludens-1 in the cytoplasmic/apical membrane locations. These findings indicate that a change in cell polarity occurs in PTC expressing c-MET, which likely relates to the increased invasive/metastatic abilities of PTC overexpressing c-MET [102, 104]. c-MET overexpression did not increase PTC Ki-67 levels or increase tumor cell proliferation, and is reduced or absent in poorly differentiated tumors. c-MET is overexpressed in roughly 77 % of PTCs and 70 % of Hürthle cell tumors [102]. Interestingly, c-Met expression is significantly higher in the most aggressive PTC subtype, Tall Cell PTC, where its increased expression correlates with extracapsular spread, skeletal muscle invasion, and lymphatic invasion [105].

Currently clinical molecular diagnostic testing in not routinely preformed for c-MET overexpression. c-MET expression has been detected in PTC via immunohistochemistry, Western blotting, tissue microarray, cDNA expression arrays, and quantitative real-time PCR, typically as basic research tools [106–108]. Most likely c-MET detection methods will be developed that will be applicable to molecular diagnostics as c-MET inhibitors, including monoclonal antibodies, and small-molecule tyrosine kinase inhibitors have shown encouraging results in *in vitro* studies, animal models, and in human phase I and II clinical trials [109, 110].

2.4.12 **p53** *and* **CTNNB1** *Mutations in PTC*

PTC rarely carries mutations of the *p53* and *CTNNB1* genes [111]. Presently, no clinical molecular testing is performed for mutations or changes in these genes in PTC.

2.4.13 Hashimoto's Thyroiditis Versus PTC

Hashimoto's thyroiditis (HT) can present with different histological patterns, such as the classic features of chronic autoimmune thyroiditis, or HT associated with hyperplastic/adenomatous lesions, or even HT associated with concurrent TC. HT can be nodular, sometimes with one or more large, so-called "dominant nodules," which histologically can have some features of PTC, including nuclear membrane irregularities, nuclear clearing, and increased size. In some cases, differentiating between reactive and malignant morphologic changes can be difficult. Sadow et al. [112] examined 28 cases of HT with a dominant nodule and looked for *BRAF, RET, KRAS, NRAS,* and *HRAS* mutations and *RET/PTC1* and *RET/PTC3* rearrangements within the dominant nodule. No *BRAF* or *RAS* mutations or *RET/PTC* rearrangements were detected in the dominant HT nodules, even in those with atypical, worrisome histological features. BRAF V600E mutations were only identified in HT with concomitant PTC. Thus dominant nodules in HT are neither malignant, nor precursor lesions, and molecular testing can separate even very atypical HT from PTC.

2.4.14 Conclusions on Molecular Testing for PTC

Molecular testing for PTC can be performed on resected thyroidal lesions and FNAs. Although not presently widely used in the clinical setting, molecular testing of the thyroid can be useful for histologically ambiguous cases and FNAs deemed indeterminate or suspicious for malignancy. Testing such as *BRAF* mutational analysis also has pronostic value. In particular, simultaneous testing for *BRAF V600E* and *RET/PTC* mutations, which together cover ~70–80 % of PTCs, is a useful aid in the diagnosis of PTC, especially for cytologically/histologically difficult cases, as these two mutations are almost exclusively found in PTC [1, 14].

2.5 Anaplastic Carcinoma of the Thyroid

Anaplastic carcinoma of the thyroid (ACT) accounts for roughly <2 % of TCs. ACT is one of the most aggressive human malignancies and carries a dismal prognosis, with a median survival of 6 months and a 5-year survival rate ranging from 1 % to 7.1 %. These tumors are so aggressive that the original diagnosis is often questioned in long-term survivors; in addition, despite its low incidence, it accounts for 50 % of deaths due to TC. ACT usually presents with symptoms related to a rapidly growing thyroid mass that shows extensive local invasion and early metastases to the bones, liver, lungs, and brain. Although it is rarely seen in younger individuals, it is usually a malignancy of those in their sixth and seventh decades. Histologically ACT shows extreme cellular pleomorphism and a high mitotic index, often with spindle cells resembling a sarcoma, undifferentiated squamoid cells, and pleomorphic giant cells resembling osteoclasts. The cell types may predominate in any given tumor or may occur in any combination within a tumor [113–118].

ACT carries multiple mutations that occur with different frequencies, including *RAS* (22 %), *BRAF* (26 %), *p53* (55 %), *beta-catanin* (38 %), *Axin* (82 %), *PTEN* (12 %), and *PIK3CA* (17 %). Although several of these mutations occur in well-differentiated TCs, like PTC, mutations of *p53, beta-catanin,* and *PIK3CA* are usually found only in ATC and likely represent late mutational events that contribute to the aggressive course of ATC [119]. The common finding of more differentiated areas with ACTs resembling PTC or follicular carcinoma of the thyroid (FCT), combined with many ACTs carrying the same mutations as PTC and FCT, indicates that many ACTs probably arise from well-differentiated TCs. Clinical molecular diagnostic testing is not commonly performed on ACT; however, because of its lethal clinical course, intensive research into the molecular pathology of ACT is being done in the hope of finding more effective treatments, especially as related to targeted molecular therapies [119].

2.6 Follicular Carcinoma of the Thyroid: Mutations and Molecular Testing

FCT accounts for 5–15 % of TCs, making it the second most common TC. FCT and PTC together make up 90 % of TCs, making up the "differentiated TC" category [111]. The incidence of FCT peaks in the fifth decade, usually presenting as slowly enlarging non-tender nodules and typically following a more aggressive clinical course than PTC. Patients with FCT often show hematogenous metastases to the brain, lung, and bone. Individuals with tumors that do not show capsule invasion have an 86 % 10-year survival rate, whereas those with invasion have a 44 % 10-year survival rate. Histologically, FTCs show follicular epithelial cells with vesicular nuclei and follicles that are often devoid of collagen. Diagnosis of FCT vs. FA rests on the identification of capsular or vascular invasion or the identification of metastases [120, 121].

FCT often have *RAS* mutations (40–50 %), *PAX8-PPAR-gamma* gene rearrangements (~35 %), and less common *PTEN* and *PI3KCA* mutations (7 %). *BRAF* mutations are rare, and *RET* gene alterations have not been identified in FTC (115). Currently, clinical molecular testing is uncommon for FTC; when it is done, testing focuses on *PAX8-PPAR-gamma* gene rearrangements and *RAS* mutations.

2.6.1 RAS Mutations

Molecular testing for *NRAS, KRAS,* and *HRAS* were addressed above (Sect. 2.4 on PTC). However, many testing methods combine two or more standard protocols. For example, Nikiforova et al. [122] analyzed *NRAS, KRAS,* and *HRAS* in a series of 88 TCs consisting of 33 conventional FCTs of the thyroid, 23 conventional FAs, 19 Hürthle cell carcinomas, and 13 Hürthle cell adenomas. *RAS* mutation testing was performed using a combination of RT-PCR and HRM to analyze *NRAS, KRAS,* and *HRAS* activating point mutations at codons 12, 13, and 61. RNA was isolated from paraffin-embedded or frozen tissue, and 3 μg of RNA were converted in a cDNA library by reverse transcriptase with random heximer primers. The resulting cDNA was PCR amplified with two primers specific for each point of mutation being interrogated. Within each PCR reaction were two fluorescently labeled oligonucleotide hybridization probes. The two probes would hybridize internal to the primers such that the two fluorophores would be adjacent at the annealing step. One fluorophore functions as a donor and the other as an acceptor and emitter of a specific light wavelength. After 40 rounds of conventional PCR, the amplicons were cooled to 45 °C and heated at 0.2 °C/s to 95 °C. For detection purposes, one probe spans the mutation site. The wild-type and mutant amplicons are distinguished by different denaturation temperatures, reflecting the thermodynamic stability of complementary vs. point-mismatched probe-target duplexes. Using this technique, the group found 49 % of FCT had *RAS* mutations, whereas 48 %, 11 %, and 8 % of FAs, Hürthle cell carcinomas, and Hürthle cell adenomas had mutations, respectively. Comparison with DNA sequencing demonstrated that the method was both sensitive and accurate.

2.6.2 PAX8-PPAR-Gamma

PAX8-PPAR-gamma rearrangements are found in ~35 % of FTCs and ~55 % of FAs, but not in PTC or ATC [111, 122]. *PAX8-PPAR-gamma* rearrangements result from a t(2;3)(q13;p25) translocation, which encodes a protein that promotes the development of differentiated FTC, but is not sufficient for carcinogenesis [122–124]. PAX8 is a 48-kDa nuclear thyroid-specific paired domain transcription factor found at 2q13 that regulates thyroid follicular cell development and the expression of thyroid-specific genes [125]. *PPAR-gamma* or the peroxisome proliferator-activated receptor-gamma is found at 3p25.2. *PPAR-gamma* is a ligand-activated transcription factor that dimerizes with the retinoic X receptor and is expressed primarily in adipose and lymphoid tissues, colon, liver, and heart. PPAR-gamma activity plays a role in many diseases, including diabetes, atherosclerosis, cancer, and metabolic syndrome. Additionally, PPAR-gamma binds antihyperglycemic/antidiabetic agents such as the thiazolidinediones [121].

PAX8-PPAR-gamma rearrangements have been detected with many different methods, including interphase FISH, immunohistochemistry, Northern blotting, sequencing, and reverse-transcriptase-PCR [123, 124]. Most commonly reverse-transcriptase PCR is employed, as this technique is highly specific and sensitive for the *PAX8-PPAR-gamma* rearrangement. Cheung et al. [123] analyzed *PAX8-PPAR-gamma* rearrangements by isolating total tumor RNA and producing a mixture of cDNAs with Superscript II reverse transcriptase. The *PAX8-PPAR-gamma* rearrangement was then PCR amplified with primers specific for *PAX8* exon 6, 5′-CGCGGATCCGCATTGACTCACAGAGCA-3′, and exon 1 of *PPAR-gamma,* 5′-CCGGAATTCGAAGTCAACAGTAGTGAA-3′. The integrity of the RNA was tested by simultaneous amplification of the beta$_2$-microglobulin RNA. Additionally, other primers were employed to amplify other *PAX8* exons sometimes involved in variants of the *PAX8-PPAR-gamma* translocation. Amplicons were measured and resolved by 5 % acrylamide gel electrophoresis. The identities of the amplicons were then checked via sequencing. *PAX8-PPAR-gamma* rearrangements and *RAS* mutations are found together in FTC at a low rate of ~3 % [126]. Interestingly, some data exist indicating that *PAX8-PPAR-gamma* rearrangements may be specific to some ethnic groups and not to others [127].

2.6.3 p53 *Mutations in FTC*

p53 mutations are a late event in thyroid carcinogenesis and are associated with the progression of differentiated TC to ACT [111, 128, 129]. *p53* mutations are only rarely found in FTC, and analysis of its mutation has little value in the molecular diagnostics of FTC.

2.6.4 *PTEN and CTNNB1 Mutations in FTC*

PTEN, also known as phosphatase and tensin homolog, is located at 10q23.3 and functions as a tumor suppressor via dephosphorylation of protein tyrosine, serine, and threonine phosphates, as well as by catalyzing the removal of the D3 phosphate of phosphatidylinositol 3,4,5-trisphosphate. These activities antagonize the PI3K-AKT/PBK signaling pathway, thereby attenuating signaling that promotes cell cycle progression and cell survival [130]. *PTEN* is mutated in about 7 % of FTC, but not FAs [131, 132]. *CTNNB1* mutations are rare in FTC [111]. Interestingly, down-regulation of unmutated CTNNB1 membrane expression in FTC is associated with progressive loss of tumor differentiation, while *CTNNB1* mutation is associated with poorly or undifferentiated carcinomas [111, 133]. Molecular diagnostic testing is not routinely performed for *PTEN* or *CTNNB1* mutations in FTC.

2.7 Hürthle Cell Tumors

Hürthle or oxyphillic cell carcinoma accounts for ~5 % of differentiated TC. Hürthle cell tumors arise from follicular cell cells and are defined as encapsulated thyroid lesions consisting of at least 75 % Hürthle cells, which typically have very few or no lymphocytes, scant or no colloid, and large polygonal cell cells with indistinct cell borders, pleomorphic hyperchromatic nuclei with a prominent nucleus, and pink finely granular cytoplasm on hematoxylin-eosin staining due to abundant cytoplasmic mitochondria [120, 134]. Roughly 30 % of these tumors are malignant and hence show an invasive growth pattern and/or distant metastases. Interestingly, features such as pleomorphism, anaplasia, and atypia are seen in benign as well as malignant Hürthle cell tumors and are of no value in determining malignancy. The aggressiveness of these tumors is poorly defined with some studies showing them to be more aggressive than FTC and other equally of less aggressive [134]. Hürthle cell tumors show somatic mitochondrial, GRIM-19, RET/PTC gene mutations, and chromosomal gains at 5p and losses at 2q and 9q [120, 134, 135]. Presently, molecular resting is not performed on Hürthle cell tumors.

2.8 Medullary Thyroid Cancer: Mutations and Molecular Testing

Medullary thyroid cancer (MTC) accounts for ~4 % of TCs and arises from neural crest-derived parafollicular C-cells of the thyroid, giving them the clinical and histological features of neuroendocrine tumors such as carcinoid and islet-cell tumors; 25–30 % of MTCs occur in inherited autosomal dominant disorders that are usually preceded by bilateral, multicentric C-cell hyperplasia/calitonin-producing lesions. Hereditary MTCs occur in younger individuals and are often associated with other endocrine tumors, usually in well-defined genetic syndromes such as MEN2 and MENB (see below). The remaining MTCs are sporadic, occurring at an older age than hereditary MTCs and having a poorer prognosis. Histologically, MTCs consist of small polygonal to spindled cells in a solid or trabecular patterns, often with associated amyloids. MTC nearly always occurs in the lateral thyroidal lobes, with other thyroidal locations being far less common [136, 137]. Interestingly, residual C-cell hyperplasia near an MTC often indicates that a particular MTC is hereditary, although C-cell hyerplasia can rarely occur next to sporadic MTC or other benign and malignant thyroid lesions [138]. MTC has a worse prognosis than other TCs such as PTC, due to early metastases, with about half of affected individuals having local lymph node involvement at diagnosis. Distant metastases are common, often to the adrenal glands, lungs, liver, and bones. The 5-year survival rate is 60–70 %, and the 10-year survival rate is 40–50 %. Presently, establishing a diagnosis and prognosis of MTC depends largely on histologic analysis combined with immunostaining for calcitonin, and in some cases analysis of serum calcitonin and carcinoembryonic antigen levels, both of which are secreted by MTC [136–139]. Molecular diagnostic testing has an import role in patient care for these tumors.

Both sporadic and hereditary MTC are characterized by activating or "gain of function" *RET* mutations and less by *RET* gene rearrangements, as are found in PTC [69, 70]. Molecular diagnostic testing is mainly performed for possible hereditary MTC, as testing results are an important part of establishing a diagnosis (in conjunction with clinical data) and determining whether kindred testing is required. About 98 % of individuals with hereditary MTC syndromes carry germline *RET* mutations, whereas 40–50 % of sporadic cases carry *RET* mutations [140–146]. Last, about 4–11 % of individuals with apparently sporadic MTC actually carry germline *RET* gene mutations. Thus screening sporadic MTC cases for germline *RET* mutations can identify kindreds who can benefit from early medical intervention, such as prophylactic thyroidectomy [145–148].

Since the *RET* mutations in MTC are activating, they typically involve single or a few nucleotide changes that cause constitutive tyrosine kinase activation via loss of normal kinase inhibitory mechanisms, as are also found in other proto-oncogenes such as *KRAS* and *BRAF*. For example, 23–85 % of sporadic MTCs have an exon 16, codon 918 (ATGACG; MetThr) activating mutation, and this mutation along with exon 15, codon 833 (GCTTTT; ArgCys) accounts for more than 98 % of MEN2B cases [140–148]. *RET* mutations have been detected by many different molecular methods, including SSCP, microarrays, sequencing, temperature gradient capillary electrophoresis, denaturing gradient gel electrophoresis, and HRM of PCR products [149–154].

2.8.1 *RET DNA Sequencing*

Since one or a few *RET* mutations often characterize a specific MEN syndrome, mutation-specific *RET* testing is often performed. However, mutation-specific testing will not locate unknown or novel mutations. To find such mutations, DNA sequencing works well. Ahmed et al. [153] employed PCR and sequencing to identify nine infrequent novel *RET* gene variants; 6,700 cases of suspected MEN2A or familial MTC (FMTC) or a family history of MEN2A of or FMTC were analyzed. Genomic DNA was extracted from peripheral blood leukocytes and amplified via PCR employing a sense primer; 5′-CAACATTTGCCCTCAGGACTG-3′, and an antisense primer; 5′-CTTGAAGGCATCCACGGAGA-3′. The resulting 1,785-base pair amplicon was analyzed for variants by forward and reverse sequencing using a radiolabeled terminator cycle sequencing kit (Thermo Sequenase no. US79770; Amersham Life Science, Piscataway, NJ). Although sequencing identifies all possible mutations/variants within an amplified DNA sequence, it is also relatively expensive compared to other methods and has lower sensitivity than techniques such as ASA-PCR.

2.8.2 HRN Analysis of *RET* Mutations with Asymmetric PCR

RET gene analysis lends itself to mutation-specific testing, allowing more sensitive, lower cost tests to be employed than sequencing. For example, Margraf et al. [154] used modified HRN and PCR to identify RET codon 883 and 918 mutations in individuals with suspected MEN2B. Normal and codon 883 and 918 heterozygous mutants DNA samples were obtained, the DNA purified, and PCR amplified with primer sets that cover the codons mutated in MEN2B. Unlabeled oligonucleotide probes were added to the mix that had incorporated 3′ amino modifiers that prevent DNA polymerase extension during PCR. The unlabeled oligonucleotide probes carried the wild type of mutant probe sequences, corresponding to the known MEN2B *RET* mutations. LCGreen dye was added to the reaction. The PCR reaction was carried out with an excess of the primer for the strand targeted for amplification over 55 PCR cycles. Asymmetric PCR results in the accumulation of ssDNA, facilitating later HRN analysis. At the end of the PCR reaction, the reaction tube was heated to 95 °C for 30 s and cooled to 50 °C to generate probe-ssDNA duplexes. HRN data were collected by heating the reaction chambers to 95 °C at 30 acquisitions/s while analyzing LCGreen emission with a 450 nm excitation and 500-nm emission filter combination. All samples were later sequenced for assay validification. This technique allowed rapid and accurate identification of MEN2B mutations in a closed-tube system that is less time-consuming and expensive than sequencing.

2.8.3 Reverse Transcriptase-PCR in the Diagnosis of MTC

Thyroid tumors are often diagnosed by cytologic examination of FNAs. In some cases a diagnosis is not possible due to inadequate FNA sampling, poor fixation, or a lack of epithelial cells. To facilitate diagnosis in such cases Takano et al. [155] developed a new molecular technique termed aspiration biopsy-reverse transcriptase-PCR. In this technique, cells left over in the FNA needle are used for reverse transcriptase-PCR of genes specifically expressed in one TC type. *RET* proto-oncogene, calcitonin, and carcinoembryonic antigen expression is restricted to MTC [156–158]. Takano et al. [155] examined 35 thyroid tissue samples consisting of 6 normal thyroids, 3 adenomatous goiters, 6 FAs, 7 PTCs, 2 FTCs, and 11 MTCs. Total RNA was extracted and reverse transcribed with

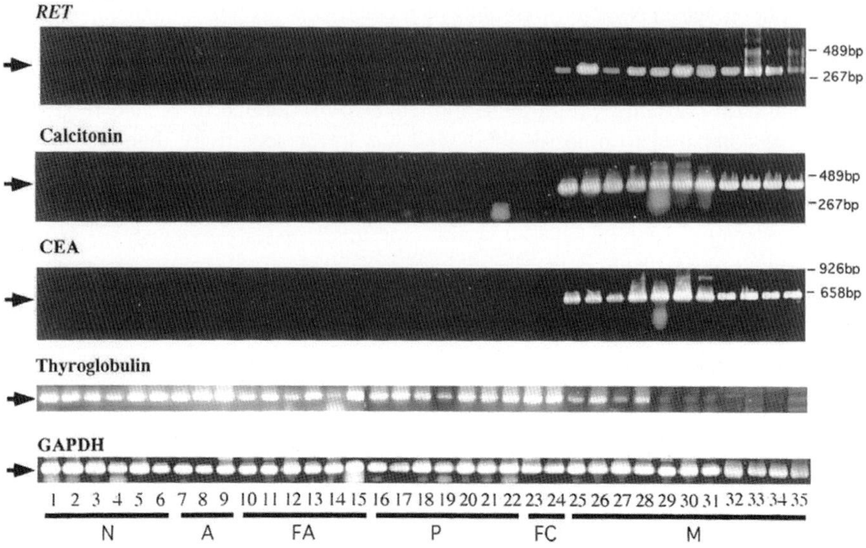

Fig. 2.1 Aspiration biopsy-reverse transcriptase-PCR analysis by Takano et al. [155] of the expression of RET, calcitonin, and CEA mRNAs. Six normal thyroid tissues samples (*N*), three adenomatous goiters (*A*), six follicular adenomas (*FA*), seven papillary carcinomas (*P*), two follicular carcinomas (*FC*), and 11 MTCs (*M*). *Arrows* indicate the expected positions of the PCR products

M-MLV reverse transcriptase. One microliter of the resulting cDNAs were PCR amplified with the following primers over 30 cycles and analyzed by gel electrophoresis:

- *RET:* 5′ (5′-GCAGCATTGTTGGGGGACA) (codon 588–594)
- *RET:* 3′ (5′-CACCGGAAGAGGAGTAGCTG) (codon 685–692)
- Calcitonin: 5′ (59-CCTTCCTGGCTCTCAGCATC) (base 57–76)
- Calcitonin: 3′ (5′-GAGTTTAGTTGGCATTCTGG) (base 445–464)
- Carcinoembryonic antigen: 5′ (5′-ACAAGGATGCTGTGGCCTTC) (base 1,658–1,677)
- Carcinoembryonic antigen: 3′ (5′-AGGGCTGCTATATCAGAGCA) (base 2,211–2,)
- Thyroglobulin: 5′ (5′-GTTGGCAACCTCATCGT) (base 7,011–7,027)
- Thyroglobulin: 3′ (5′-AATTCTGCAGTGCCTGGT) (base 7,657–7,674)
- GAPDH: 5′ (5′-CCATGGAGAAGGCTGGGG) (base 371–388)
- GAPDH: 3′ (5′-CAAAGTTGTCATGGATGACC) (base 546–565)

GAPDH was detected in all samples. Thyroglobulin was detected in all normal thyroid tissue, the adenomatous goiters, FAs, and PTCs and weakly in 4 of the 11 MTCs. RET, calcitonin, and carcinoembryonic antigen expression was detected in all 11 MTCs and in none of the non-MTC samples (Fig. 2.1). This technique was confirmed to work well for left over cells in FNA needles. Thus aspiration biopsy-reverse transcriptase-PCR can be a useful molecular diagnostic test where standard cytologic sampling is inadequate.

2.9 Hereditary Thyroid Cancer Syndromes

Several hereditary TC-prone syndromes have been identified, including MEN2A, MEN2B, FMTC, and hereditary PTC. Molecular diagnostic testing plays a role in the first three syndromes, where once identified in a proband, kindred analysis and subsequent early medical intervention can significantly reduce mortality and morbidity in affected individuals. Here, we will briefly discuss each syndrome.

Multiple endocrine neoplasia type 2A and 2B and familial MTC (MEN2A, MEN2B, and FMTC, respectively) syndromes are all characterized by an autosomal dominant inheritance pattern, activating *RET* gene mutations, and MTC. Virtually all individuals with these syndromes will develop C-cell hyperplasia followed by MTC. In fact, MTC is typically the first clinical manifestation of these syndromes, and, without medical intervention, the most common cause of death in individuals with these syndromes. Once germline *RET* gene mutations are identified in individuals with one of these syndromes, prophylactic thyroidectomy is recommended to prevent MTC development [159].

2.9.1 MEN2A

MEN2A or Sipple's syndrome is an autosomal dominant disorder characterized by MTC and pheochromocytomas and hyperparathyroidism in about 50 % and 30 % of affected individuals, respectively. Other less common manifestations of MEN2A include cutaneous lichen amyloidosis and Hirschsprung's disease [159]; 97 % of MEN2A is caused by activating missense germline *RET* mutations in exon 10, codons 609, 611, 618, and 620, and in exon 11, codons 630 and 634, all of which enhance receptor dimerization, with increased receptor autophosphorylation and hence increased kinase activity [139–148, 160]. Molecular diagnostic testing for MEN2A is usually directed at these specific mutations with methods described above.

2.9.2 MEN2B

MEN2B or Wermer's syndrome is characterized by MTC, pheochromocytoma, mucosal neuromas (of the tongue, lips, conjuctivae), ganglioneuromas of the intestines, characterized by special facial appearance, and marfanoid habitus.

Interestingly, the MTC of MEN2B is more aggressive than those seen in MEN2A or FMTC; 98 % of MEN2B carry *RET* mutations in either exon 16, codon 918, or exon 15, codon 833 [140–148, 160]. Directed testing for these mutations is the most sensitive, rapid, and accurate method for identifying individuals with MEN2B [154].

2.9.3 FMTC

MTC is the only manifestation of FMTC and typically follows a very indolent course. A kindred should have 10 or more *RET* mutation carriers with MTC and sufficient history to rule out pheochromocytoma or hyperparathyroidism [159]. FMTC is characterized by the same mutations as are found in MEN2A, with a few individuals having germline mutations in codons 768, 790, 791, 804, and 891 in *RET* exons 13, 14, and 15 [139–148, 160]. Molecular diagnostic testing is usually directed at the more frequently occurring of these mutations.

2.9.4 TC and MicroRNA Expression Profiling

Although not presently employed in TC molecular diagnostic testing, differences have been detected in the levels of specific microRNAs in PTC, ATC, MTC, oncocytic tumors, and FTC, with each histopathological TC type showing a unique microRNA expression pattern [161–164]. Additionally, the microRNA expression pattern changed with concomitant *BRAF, RET/PTC,* and *PAX8-PPAR-gamma*, but not with *RAS* mutations, showing possible microRNA expression pattern alterations with mutational status [164]. Although not presently employed in the molecular diagnostics of TC, different microRNA patterns are well established in TC and are likely to be incorporated into TC molecular testing in the future. Interestingly, microRNA studies have proven valuable in increasing our understanding of some thyroid lesions. For example, the hyalinizing trabecular adenoma is a distinctive thyroid neoplasm that shows some morphological features of PTC, including similar nuclear characteristics, psammoma bodies, and *RET/PTC* rearrangements [165–167]. Sheu et al. [168] analyzed microRNA expression and *BRAF V600E* mutation and *RET/PTC-1* and *-3* rearrangements in 18 hyalinizing trabecular adenomas. They found that microRNAs -146b, -181b, -21, -221, and -222, which are all significantly up-regulated in PTC, were suppressed in hyalinizing trabecular adenomas. Additionally, no *BRAF V600E* mutation and *RET/PTC-1* and *-3* rearrangements were detected. Based on this, the authors concluded that the hyalinizing trabecular adenoma and PTC are separate entities. The reasons for the discrepant findings of this study vs. previous studies concerning *RET/PTC-1* and *-3* rearrangements were not explained [167, 168].

2.10 Parathyroid Cancer: Mutations and Molecular Testing

Parathyroid cancer (PC) is a rare malignancy with an incidence of 0.4–4 % in all patients surgically treated for primary hyperparathyroidism [169, 170]. The majority of patients present with hypercalcemia, often found during a routine health screening, leading to a diagnosis of primary hyperparathyroidism. Typically, the clinical features will include high serum calcium levels (>14 mg/mL), parathyroid hormone levels at least five times above normal, a palpable lesion, bone symptoms, and operative findings suggestive of invasive growth. Histologic features of PC include broad intersecting fibrous bands within the tumor, increased mitotic index, stromal invasion, and angiolymphatic/perineural invasion. A definitive histological diagnosis of PC requires obvious tissue invasion or metastasis [169–171]. Interestingly, up to 86 % of PCs are not recognized as such intraoperatively and do not receive adequate surgical resection. In addition, in one series, half of all metastatic and recurrent PCs were initially diagnosed as benign [172, 173]. Currently there are no molecular diagnostic tests that can differentiate parathyroid adenoma (PA) from PC. Since clinically diagnosing a tumor as malignant based on metastasis is unacceptable, there is a strong need for such tests. Several areas of research appear promising.

2.10.1 Parafibromin Immunoreactivity

HRPT2 is a recently identified PC tumor suppressor found at 1q25 and has 17 exons that encode a 61 kDa nuclear protein parafibromin [174]. Germline mutations of the gene have been identified in kindreds with hyperparathyroidism-jaw tumor syndrome, which is characterized by childhood parathyroid hyperplasia, fibro-osseous jaw tumors, renal lesions, with a ~ 15 % lifetime chance of developing PC [175, 176]. Howell et al. [177] analyzed 60 parathyroid tumors , including five from individuals with hyperparathyroidism-jaw tumor syndrome, three with familial isolated hyperparathyroidism, three with MEN1, one with MEN2A, 25 sporadic PAs, 17 hyperplastic parathyroid glands, two lithium-associated tumors, and four sporadic PCs. All 17 exons and intron-exon boundaries were PCR amplified and analyzed by denaturing high-performance liquid chromotography. *HRPT2* mutations were found in all four sporadic PCs, all five tumors from individuals with hyperparathyroidism-jaw tumor syndrome, and in one of the two tumors from individuals with familial isolated hyperparathyroidism. The authors hypothesized that *HRPT2* mutation is an early event in PC carcinogenesis and may be a potential marker for both familial and sporadic PCs. Interestingly, parafibromin immunostaining is reduced in PCs compared to PA, with positive parafibromin nuclear staining largely excluding carcinoma and reduced staining likely indicating carcinoma or rare PAs with low staining [178, 179].

2.10.2 Cyclin D1

Cyclin D1 or *PRAD1* is located at 11q13 and encodes a cyclin-dependent kinase that plays a central role in regulating and promoting G_1S phase cell cycle progression [180]. Chromosomal rearrangements of the *cyclin D1* regulatory region have been detected in 8 % of PAs and 20–40 % of PCS, and 31 % of hyperplastic parathyroid glands overexpress cyclin D1 [181, 182]. The overexpression appears to result from the effects of growth factor stimulation and calcium-sensing receptor activation [183].

2.10.3 Cellular Proliferation Markers

Ki-67 and PCNA immunohistochemical staining may have some value in separating PC from benign hyperplasia and adenomas, although the literature is contradictory and due to the rarity of PC most studies include relatively few cases [184, 185]. Last, the proapototic gene product FHIT appears to be preferentially mutated in PC compared to hyperplastic or adenomatous parathyroid lesions [185].

2.10.4 Chromosomal Changes

PC and PAs show gains and losses in specific chromosomal locations, often where tumor suppressor genes (at 1p, 3q, 4q, 13q, and 21q) and oncogenes are located (at 1q, 5q, 9q, 16p, 19p, and Xq). Interestingly, these areas tend to be different between PCs and PAs, likely indicating a different molecular pathogenesis of these neoplasms [186]. Presently, none of the above molecular alterations identified in PC, PA, or hyperplasia are used in molecular diagnostics, and many of these alterations appear to be quite similar between PC and PAs. Further research is required before molecular diagnostic tests for parathyroid neoplastic lesions can be implemented.

2.11 Conclusion

Over the past 20 years, different histopathologically defined thyroid malignancies have been shown to have mutation and gene expression patterns that allow them to be clearly distinguished via molecular analysis. In many cases, such analyses allow a clear diagnosis where the histology is ambiguous [1, 14]. Additionally, in many cases, as with PTC *BRAF* and *c-MET*, these mutations give useful prognostic information. Last, inhibitors for many of the constitutively active mutated kinases found in the TCs are being developed, which will eventually necessitate molecular diagnostic testing, as is currently done for *KRAS* mutations in colorectal carcinoma (see Chap. 5, Molecular Pathology and Diagnostics of Colorectal Cancer). Thus molecular diagnostics applied to these TCs are likely to increase. Currently, there are few molecular diagnostic procedures applied to parathyroid malignancies. However, there is a strong need for diagnostic tests that can differentiate PAs from PCs. Testing should become available as our knowledge of the molecular pathology underlying this malignancy increases.

Acknowledgement We would like to thank Miss Jennifer Burton for her help in manuscript preparation and proofreading.

References

1. Elsheikh TM, Asa SL, Chan JK, DeLellis RA, Heffess CS, LiVolsi VA, Wenig BM (2008) Interobserver and intraobserver variation among experts in the diagnosis of thyroid follicular lesions with borderline nuclear features of papillary carcinoma. Am J Clin Pathol 130:736–744
2. Fernandez-Ranvier GG, Khanafshar E, Jensen K, Zarnegar R, Lee J, Kebebew E, Duh QY, Clark OH (2007) Parathyroid carcinoma, atypical parathyroid adenoma, or parathyromatosis? Cancer 110:255–264
3. DeLellis RA (1993) Tumors of the parathyroid gland. In: Rosai J, Sobin LH (eds) Atlas of tumor pathology. 3rd series, fascicle 6. Armed Forces Institute of Pathology, Washington, DC, pp 3–63
4. Clayman GL, Gonzalez HE, El-Naggar A, Vassilopoulou-Sellin R (2004) Parathyroid carcinoma: evaluation and interdisciplinary management. Cancer 100:900–905
5. Enewold L, Zhu K, Ron E, Marrogi AJ, Stojadinovic A, Peoples GE, Devesa SS (2009) Rising thyroid cancer incidence in the United States by demographic and tumor characteristics, 1980-2005. Cancer Epidemiol Biomarkers Prev 18:784–791
6. Burgess JR, Tucker P (2006) Incidence trends for papillary thyroid carcinoma and their correlation with thyroid surgery and thyroid fine-needle aspirate cytology. Thyroid 16:47–53
7. Colonna M, Guizard AV, Schvartz C et al (2007) A time trend analysis of papillary and follicular cancers as a function of tumour size: a study of data from six cancer registries in France (1983–2000). Eur J Cancer 43:891–900
8. Leenhardt L, Grosclaude P, Cherie-Challine L (2004) Increased incidence of thyroid carcinoma in France: a true epidemic or thyroid nodule management effects? Report from the French Thyroid Cancer Committee. Thyroid 14:1056–1060
9. Liu S, Semenciw R, Ugnat AM, Mao Y (2001) Increasing thyroid cancer incidence in Canada, 1970–1996: time trends and age-period-cohort effects. Br J Cancer 85:1335–1339
10. Smailyte G, Miseikyte-Kaubriene E, Kurtinaitis J (2006) Increasing thyroid cancer incidence in Lithuania in 1978–2003. BMC Cancer 6:284
11. Franceschi S, Boyle P, Maisonneuve P et al (1993) The epidemiology of thyroid carcinoma. Crit Rev Oncog 4:25–52
12. Nagataki S, Nyström E (2002) Epidemiology and primary prevention of thyroid cancer. Thyroid 12:889–896
13. Mizuno T, Iwamoto KS, Kyoizumi S, Nagamura H, Shinohara T, Koyama K, Seyama T, Hamatani K (2000) Preferential induction of RET/PTC1 rearrangement by X-ray irradiation. Oncogene 19:438–443
14. Ron E, Lubin JH, Shore RE, Mabuchi K, Modan B, Pottern LM, Schneider AB, Tucker MA, Boice JD Jr (1995) Thyroid cancer after exposure to external radiation: a pooled analysis of seven studies. Radiat Res 141:259–277

15. Williams D (1994) Epidemiology. Chernobyl, eight years on. Nature 371:556
16. Hancock SL, McDougall IR, Constine LS (1995) Thyroid abnormalities after therapeutic external radiation. Int J Radiat Oncol Biol Phys 31:1165–1170
17. Mabuchi K, Soda M, Ron E, Tokunaga M, Ochikubo S, Sugimoto S, Ikeda T, Terasaki M, Preston DL, Thompson DE (1994) Cancer incidence in atomic bomb survivors. Part I: use of the tumor registries in Hiroshima and Nagasaki for incidence studies. Radiat Res 137:S1–S16
18. Thompson DE, Mabuchi K, Ron E, Soda M, Tokunaga M, Ochikubo S, Sugimoto S, Ikeda T, Terasaki M, Izumi S et al (1994) Cancer incidence in atomic bomb survivors. Part II: solid tumors, 1958-1987. Radiat Res 137:S17–S67
19. Nikiforov Y, Gnepp DR (1994) Pediatric thyroid cancer after the Chernobyl disaster. Pathomorphologic study of 84 cases (1991-1992) from the Republic of Belarus. Cancer 74:748–766
20. Pui CH, Cheng C, Leung W, Rai SN, Rivera GK, Sandlund JT, Ribeiro RC, Relling MV, Kun LE, Evans WE, Hudson MM (2003) Extended follow-up of long-term survivors of childhood acute lymphoblastic leukemia. N Engl J Med 349:640–649
21. Hancock SL, Cox RS, McDougall IR (1991) Thyroid diseases after treatment of Hodgkin's disease. N Engl J Med 325:599–605
22. Knobel M, Medeiros-Neto G (2007) Relevance of iodine intake as a reputed predisposing factor for thyroid cancer. Arq Bras Endocrinol Metabol 51:701–712
23. Belfiore A, La Rosa GL, La Porta GA, Giuffrida D, Milazzo G, Lupo L, Regalbuto C, Vigneri R (1992) Cancer risk in patients with cold thyroid nodules: relevance of iodine intake, sex, age, and multinodularity. Am J Med 93:363–369
24. Guan H, Ji M, Bao R, Yu H, Wang Y, Hou P, Zhang Y, Shan Z, Teng W, Xing M (2009) Association of high iodine intake with the T1799A BRAF mutation in papillary thyroid cancer. J Clin Endocrinol Metab 94:1612–1617
25. Negri E, Dal Maso L, Ron E, La Vecchia C, Mark SD, Preston-Martin S, McTiernan A, Kolonel L, Yoshimoto Y, Jin F, Wingren G, Rosaria Galanti M, Hardell L, Glattre E, Lund E, Levi F, Linos D, Braga C, Franceschi S (1999) A pooled analysis of case-control studies of thyroid cancer. II. Menstrual and reproductive factors. Cancer Causes Control 10:143–155
26. Chen GG, Vlantis AC, Zeng Q, van Hasselt CA (2008) Regulation of cell growth by estrogen signaling and potential targets in thyroid cancer. Curr Cancer Drug Targets 8:367–377
27. Mack WJ, Preston-Martin S, Dal Maso L, Galanti R, Xiang M, Franceschi S, Hallquist A, Jin F, Kolonel L, La Vecchia C, Levi F, Linos A, Lund E, McTiernan A, Mabuchi K, Negri E, Wingren G, Ron E (2003) A pooled analysis of case-control studies of thyroid cancer: cigarette smoking and consumption of alcohol, coffee, and tea. Cancer Causes Control 14:773–785
28. Bosetti C, Negri E, Kolonel L, Ron E, Franceschi S, Preston-Martin S, McTiernan A, Dal Maso L, Mark SD, Mabuchi K, Land C, Jin F, Wingren G, Galanti MR, Hallquist A, Glattre E, Lund E, Levi F, Linos D, La Vecchia C (2002) A pooled analysis of case-control studies of thyroid cancer. VII. Cruciferous and other vegetables (International). Cancer Causes Control 13:765–775
29. Dal Maso L, La Vecchia C, Franceschi S, Preston-Martin S, Ron E, Levi F, Mack W, Mark SD, McTiernan A, Kolonel L, Mabuchi K, Jin F, Wingren G, Galanti MR, Hallquist A, Glattre E, Lund E, Linos D, Negri E (2000) A pooled analysis of thyroid cancer studies. V. Anthropometric factors. Cancer Causes Control 11:137–144
30. Pacini F, Elisei R, Di Coscio GC, Anelli S, Macchia E, Concetti R, Miccoli P, Arganini M, Pinchera A (1988) Thyroid carcinoma in thyrotoxic patients treated by surgery. J Endocrinol Invest 11:107–112
31. Farbota LM, Calandra DB, Lawrence AM, Paloyan E (1985) Thyroid carcinoma in Graves' disease. Surgery 98:1148–1153
32. Sridama V, Hara Y, Fauchet R, DeGroot LJ (1985) Association of differentiated thyroid carcinoma with HLA-DR7. Cancer 56:1086–1088
33. Hundahl SA, Fleming ID, Fremgen AM, Menck HR (1998) A national cancer data base report on 53 856 cases of thyroid carcinoma treated in the US. Cancer 83:2638–2648

34. Gilliland FD, Hunt WC, Morris DM, Key CR (1997) Prognostic factors for thyroid carcinoma. A population-based study of 15 698 cases from the surveillance, epidemiology and end results (SEER) Program 1973–1991. Cancer 79:564–573
35. Kitamura Y, Shimizu K, Nagahama M, Sugino K, Ozaki O, Mimura T, Ito K, Ito K, Tanaka S (1999) Immediate causes of death in thyroid carcinoma: clinicopathological analysis of 161 fatal cases. J Clin Endocrinol Metabol 84:4043–4049
36. Are C, Shaha AR (2006) Anaplastic thyroid carcinoma: biology, pathogenesis, prognostic factors and treatment approaches. Ann Surg Oncol 13:453–464
37. Xing M, Westra WH, Tufano RP, Cohen Y, Rosenbaum E, Rhoden KJ, Carson KA, Vasko V, Larin A, Tallini G, Tolaney S, Holt EH, Hui P, Umbricht CB, Basaria S, Ewertz M, Tufaro AP, Califano JA, Ringel MD, Zeiger MA, Sidransky D, Ladenson PW (2005) BRAF mutation predicts a poorer clinical prognosis for papillary thyroid cancer. J Clin Endocrinol Metab 90:6373–6379
38. Ito Y, Hirokawa M, Jikuzono T, Higashiyama T, Takamura Y, Miya A, Kobayashi K, Matsuzuka F, Kuma K, Miyauchi A (2007) Extranodal tumor extension to adjacent organs predicts a worse cause-specific survival in patients with papillary thyroid carcinoma. World J Surg 31:1194–1201
39. Ain KB (1995) Papillary thyroid carcinoma. Etiology, assessment, and therapy. Endocrinol Metab Clin North Am 24:711–760
40. Pelizzo MR, Merante Boschin I, Toniato A, Pagetta C, Casal Ide E, Mian C, Rubello D (2008) Diagnosis, treatment, prognostic factors and long-term outcome in papillary thyroid carcinoma. Minerva Endocrinol 33:359–379
41. Isarangkul W (1993) Dense fibrosis. Another diagnostic criterion for papillary thyroid carcinoma. Arch Pathol Lab Med 117:645–646
42. Adeniran AJ, Zhu Z, Gandhi M, Steward DL, Fidler JP, Giordano TJ, Biddinger PW, Nikiforov YE (2006) Correlation between genetic alterations and microscopic features, clinical manifestations, and prognostic characteristics of thyroid papillary carcinomas. Am J Surg Pathol 30:216–222
43. Kimura ET, Nikiforova MN, Zhu Z et al (2003) High prevalence of BRAF mutations in thyroid cancer: genetic evidence for constitutive activation of the RET/PTC-RAS-BRAF signaling pathway in papillary thyroid carcinoma. Cancer Res 63:1454–1457
44. Cohen Y, Xing M, Mambo E et al (2003) BRAF mutation in papillary thyroid carcinoma. J Natl Cancer Inst 95:625–627
45. Barault L, Veyrie N, Jooste V, Lecorre D, Chapusot C, Ferraz JM, Lièvre A, Cortet M, Bouvier AM, Rat P, Roignot P, Faivre J, Laurent-Puig P, Piard F (2008) Mutations in the RAS-MAPK, PI(3)K (phosphatidylinositol-3-OH kinase) signaling network correlate with poor survival in a population-based series of colon cancers. Int J Cancer 122:2255–2259
46. Loupakis F, Ruzzo A, Cremolini C, Vincenzi B, Salvatore L, Santini D, Masi G, Stasi I, Canestrari E, Rulli E, Floriani I, Bencardino K, Galluccio N, Catalano V, Tonini G, Magnani M, Fontanini G, Basolo F, Falcone A, Graziano F (2009) KRAS codon 61, 146 and BRAF mutations predict resistance to cetuximab plus irinotecan in KRAS codon 12 and 13 wild-type metastatic colorectal cancer. Br J Cancer 101:715–721
47. Benvenuti S, Sartore-Bianchi A, Di Nicolantonio F, Zanon C, Moroni M, Veronese S, Siena S, Bardelli A (2007) Oncogenic activation of the RAS/RAF signaling pathway impairs the response of metastatic colorectal cancers to anti-epidermal growth factor receptor antibody therapies. Cancer Res 67:2643–2648
48. Wan PT, Garnett MJ, Roe SM, Lee S, Niculescu-Duvaz D, Good VM, Jones CM, Marshall CJ, Springer CJ, Barford D, Marais R (2004) Mechanism of activation of the RAF-ERK signaling pathway by oncogenic mutations of B-RAFBRAF. Cell 116:855–867
49. Mitsutake N, Knauf JA, Mitsutake S, Mesa C Jr, Zhang L, Fagin JA (2005) Conditional BRAFV600E expression induces DNA synthesis, apoptosis, dedifferentiation, and chromosomal instability in thyroid PCCL3 cells. Cancer Res 65:2465–2473
50. Knauf JA, Ma X, Smith EP, Zhang L, Mitsutake N, Liao XH, Refetoff S, Nikiforov YE, Fagin JA (2005) Targeted expression of BRAFV600E in thyroid cells of transgenic mice results in papillary thyroid cancers that undergo dedifferentiation. Cancer Res 65:4238–4245

51. Liu D, Liu Z, Condouris S, Xing M (2007) BRAF V600E maintains proliferation, transformation, and tumorigenicity of BRAF-mutant papillary thyroid cancer cells. J Clin Endocrinol Metab 92:2264–2271
52. Ouyang B, Knauf JA, Smith EP, Zhang L, Ramsey T, Yusuff N, Batt D, Fagin JA (2006) Inhibitors of Raf kinase activity block growth of thyroid cancer cells with RET/PTC or BRAF mutations in vitro and in vivo. Clin Cancer Res 12:1785–1793
53. Xing M (2007) BRAF mutation in papillary thyroid cancer: pathogenic role, molecular bases, and clinical implications. Endocr Rev 28:742–762
54. Huang MM, Arnheim N, Goodman MF (1992) Extension of base mispairs by Taq DNA polymerase: implications for single nucleotide discrimination in PCR. Nucleic Acids Res 20:4567–4573
55. Kimura H, Kasahara K, Kawaishi M, Kunitoh H, Tamura T, Holloway B, Nishio K (2006) Detection of epidermal growth factor receptor mutations in serum as a predictor of the response to gefitinib in patients with non-small-cell lung cancer. Clin Cancer Res 12:3915–3921
56. Franklin WA, Haney J, Sugita M, Bemis L, Jimeno A, Messersmith WA (2010) KRAS mutation: comparison of testing methods and tissue sampling techniques in colon cancer. J Mol Diagn 12:43–50
57. Sapio MR, Posca D, Troncone G, Pettinato G, Palombini L, Rossi G, Fenzi G, Vitale M (2006) Detection of BRAF mutation in thyroid papillary carcinomas by mutant allele-specific PCR amplification (MASA). Eur J Endocrinol 154:341–348
58. Shackelford W, Deng S, Murayama K, Wang J (2004) A new technology for mutation detection. Ann N Y Acad Sci 1022:257–262
59. Cohen Y, Rosenbaum E, Clark DP, Zeiger MA, Umbricht CB, Tufano RP, Sidransky D, Westra WH (2004) Mutational analysis of BRAF in fine needle aspiration biopsies of the thyroid: a potential application for the preoperative assessment of thyroid nodules. Clin Cancer Res 10:2761–2765
60. Fugazzola L, Puxeddu E, Avenia N, Romei C, Cirello V, Cavaliere A, Faviana P, Mannavola D, Moretti S, Rossi S, Sculli M, Bottici V, Beck-Peccoz P, Pacini F, Pinchera A, Santeusanio F, Elisei R (2006) Correlation between B-RAFV600E mutation and clinico-pathologic parameters in papillary thyroid carcinoma: data from a multicentric Italian study and review of the literature. Endocr Relat Cancer 13:455–464
61. Gilbert MT, Haselkorn T, Bunce M, Sanchez JJ, Lucas SB, Jewell LD, Van Marck E, Worobey M (2007) The isolation of nucleic acids from fixed, paraffin-embedded tissues-which methods are useful when? PLoS One 2:e537
62. Williams C, Pontén F, Moberg C, Söderkvist P, Uhlén M, Pontén J, Sitbon G, Lundeberg J (1999) A high frequency of sequence alterations is due to formalin fixation of archival specimens. Am J Pathol 155:1467–1471
63. Rowe LR, Bentz BG, Bentz JS (2007) Detection of BRAF V600E activating mutation in papillary thyroid carcinoma using PCR with allele-specific fluorescent probe melting curve analysis. J Clin Pathol 60:1211–1215
64. McGivern A, Wynter CV, Whitehall VL, Kambara T, Spring KJ, Walsh MD, Barker MA, Arnold S, Simms LA, Leggett BA, Young J, Jass JR (2004) Promoter hypermethylation frequency and BRAF mutations distinguish hereditary non-polyposis colon cancer from sporadic MSI-H colon cancer. Fam Cancer 3:101–107
65. Eychene A, Barnier JV, Apiou F, Dutrillaux B, Calothy G (1992) Chromosomal assignment of two human B-raf (Rmil) proto-oncogene loci: B-raf-1 encoding the p94Braf/Rmil and B-raf-2, a processed pseudogene. Oncogene 7:1657–1660
66. Zou M, Baitei EY, Alzahrani AS, Al-Mohanna F, Farid NR, Meyer B, Shi Y (2009) Oncogenic activation of MAP kinase by BRAF pseudogene in thyroid tumors. Neoplasia 11:57–65
67. Wells SA Jr, Santoro M (2009) Targeting the RET pathway in thyroid cancer. Clin Cancer Res 15:7119–7123
68. Santoro M, Dathan NA, Berlingieri MT, Bongarzone I, Paulin C, Grieco M, Pierotti MA, Vecchio G, Fusco A (1994) Molecular characterization of RET/PTC3; a novel rearranged version of the RET proto-oncogene in a human thyroid papillary carcinoma. Oncogene 9:509–516

69. Bongarzone I, Butti MG, Coronelli S, Borrello MG, Santoro M, Mondellini P, Pilotti S, Fusco A, Della Porta G, Pierotti MA (1994) Frequent activation of ret protooncogene by fusion with a new activating gene in papillary thyroid carcinomas. Cancer Res 54:2979–2998
70. Jhiang SM, Sagartz JE, Tong Q, Parker-Thornburg J, Capen CC, Cho JY, Xing S, Ledent C (1996) Targeted expression of the ret/PTC1 oncogene induces papillary thyroid carcinomas. Endocrinology 137:375–378
71. Fischer AH, Bond JA, Taysavang P, Battles OE, Wynford-Thomas D (1998) Papillary thyroid carcinoma oncogene (RET/PTC) alters the nuclear envelope and chromatin structure. Am J Pathol 153:1443–1450
72. Viglietto G, Chiappetta G, Martinez-Tello FJ, Fukunaga FH, Tallini G, Rigopoulou D, Visconti R, Mastro A, Santoro M, Fusco A (1995) RET/PTC oncogene activation is an early event in thyroid carcinogenesis. Oncogene 11:1207–1210
73. Zhu Z, Ciampi R, Nikiforova MN, Gandhi M, Nikiforov YE (2006) Prevalence of RET/PTC rearrangements in thyroid papillary carcinomas: effects of the detection methods and genetic heterogeneity. J Clin Endocrinol Metab 91:3603–3610
74. Hamatani K, Eguchi H, Ito R, Mukai M, Takahashi K, Taga M, Imai K, Cologne J, Soda M, Arihiro K, Fujihara M, Abe K, Hayashi T, Nakashima M, Sekine I, Yasui W, Hayashi Y, Nakachi K (2008) RET/PTC rearrangements preferentially occurred in papillary thyroid cancer among atomic bomb survivors exposed to high radiation dose. Cancer Res 68:7176–7182
75. Wennerberg K, Rossman KL, Der CJ (2005) The Ras superfamily at a glance. J Cell Sci 118:843–846
76. Schubbert S, Shannon K, Bollag G (2006) Hyperactive Ras in disorders and cancer. Nat Rev Cancer 7:295–308
77. Kislitsin D, Lerner A, Rennert G, Lev Z (2002) K-ras mutations in sporadic colorectal tumors in Israel: unusual high frequency of codon 13 mutations and evidence for nonhomogeneous representation of mutation subtypes. Dig Dis Sci 47:1073–1079
78. Breivik J, Meling GI, Spurkland A, Rognum TO, Gaudernack G (1994) K-ras mutation in colorectal cancer: relations to patient age, sex and tumour location. Br J Cancer 69:367–371
79. Vogelstein B, Fearon ER, Hamilton SR, Kern SE, Preisinger AC, Leppert M, Nakamura Y, White R, Smits AM, Bos JL (1988) Genetic alterations during colorectal-tumor development. N Engl J Med 319:525–532
80. Namba H, Rubin SA, Fagin JA (1990) Point mutations of ras oncogenes are an early event in thyroid tumorigenesis. Mol Endocrinol 4:1474–1479
81. Vasko W, Gaudart J, Savchenko V et al (2004) Thyroid follicular adenomas may display features of carcinoma and follicular variant of papillary carcinoma. Eur J Endocrinol 151:779–786
82. Ezzat S, Zheng L, Kolenda A et al (1996) Prevalence of activating ras mutations in morphologically characterized thyroid nodules. Thyroid 6:409–416
83. Wajjwalku W, Nakamura S, Hasegawa Y, Miyazaki K, Satoh Y, Funahashi H, Matsuyama M, Takahashi M (1992) Low frequency of rearrangements of the ret and trk proto-oncogenes in Japanese thyroid papillary carcinomas. Jpn J Cancer Res 83:671–675
84. Bongarzone I, Fugazzola L, Vigneri P, Mariani L, Mondellini P, Pacini F, Basolo F, Pinchera A, Pilotti S, Pierotti MA (1996) Age-related activation of the tyrosine kinase receptor protooncogenes RET and NTRK1 in papillary thyroid carcinoma. J Clin Endocrinol Metab 81:2006–2009
85. Greco A, Pierotti MA, Bongarzone I, Pagliardini I, Lanzi C, Della-Porta G (1992) Trk-T1 is a novel oncogene formed by the fusion of tpr and trk genes in human papillary thyroid carcinomas. Oncogene 7:237–242
86. Delvincourt C, Patey M, Flament JB, Suarez HG, Larbre H, Jardillier JC, Delisle MJ (1996) Ret and trk proto-oncogene activation in thyroid papillary carcinomas in French patients from the Champagene-Ardenne region. Clin Biochem 29:267–271
87. Lomen-Hoerth C, Shooter EM (1995) Widespread neurotrophin receptor expression in the immune system and other nonneuronal rat tissues. J Neurochem 64:1780–1789

88. Koizumi H, Morita M, Mikami S, Shibayama E, Uchikoshi T (1998) Immunohistochemical analysis of TrkA neurotrophin receptor expression in human non-neuronal carcinomas. Pathol Int 48:93–101
89. Sozzi G, Bongarzone I, Miozzo M et al (1992) Cytogenetic and molecular genetic characterization of papillary thyroid carcinomas. Genes Chromosomes Cancer 5:212–218
90. Greco A, Mariani C, Miranda C et al (1995) The DNA rearrangement that generates the TRK-T3 oncogene involves a novel gene on chromosome 3 whose product has a potential coiled-coil domain. Mol Cell Biol 15:6118–6127
91. Greco A, Miranda C, Pierotti MA (2010) Rearrangements of NTRK1 gene in papillary thyroid carcinoma. Mol Cell Endocrinol 321:44–49
92. Beimfohr C, Klugbauer S, Demidchik EP, Lengfelder E, Rabes HM (1999) NTRK1 rearrangement in papillary thyroid carcinomas of children after the Chernobyl reactor accident. Int J Cancer 80:842–847
93. Lin JC, Naujokas M, Zhu H, Nolet S, Park M (1998) Intron-exon structure of the MET gene and cloning of an alternatively-spliced Met isoform reveals frequent exon-skipping of a single large internal exon. Oncogene 16:833–842
94. Scarpino S, Stoppacciaro A, Colarossi C et al (1999) Hepatocyte growth factor (HGF) stimulates tumour invasiveness in papillary carcinoma of the thyroid. J Pathol 189:570–575
95. Di Renzo MF, Olivero M, Giacomini A et al (1995) Overexpression and amplification of the met/HGF receptor gene during the progression of colorectal cancer. Clin Cancer Res 1:147–154
96. Di Renzo MF, Olivero M, Katsaros D et al (1994) Overexpression of the Met/HGF receptor in ovarian cancer. Int J Cancer 58:658–662
97. Di Renzo MF, Olivero M, Fero S et al (1992) Overexpression of the c-MET/HGF receptor gene in human thyroid carcinomas. Oncogene 7:2549–2553
98. Ichimura E, Maeshima A, Nakajima T, Nakamura T (1996) Expression of c-met/HGF receptor in human non-small cell lung carcinomas in vitro and in vivo and its prognostic significance. Jpn J Cancer Res 87:1063–1069
99. Natali PG, Prat M, Nicotra MR et al (1996) Overexpression of the met/HGF receptor in renal cell carcinomas. Int J Cancer 69:212–217
100. Di Renzo MF, Poulsom M, Olivero M, Comoglio PM, Lemoine NR (1995) Expression of the Met/hepatocyte growth factor receptor in human pancreatic cancer. Cancer Res 55:1129–1138
101. Weidner KM, Behrens J, Vandekerckhove J, Birchmeier W (1990) Scatter factor: molecular characteristics and effect on the invasiveness of epithelial cells. J Cell Biol 111:2097–2108
102. Nardone HC, Ziober AF, LiVolsi VA, Mandel SJ, Baloch ZW, Weber RS, Mick R, Ziober BL (2003) c-Met expression in tall cell variant papillary carcinoma of the thyroid. Cancer 98:1386–1393
103. Fluge Ø, Haugen DR, Lillehaug JR, Varhaug JE (2001) Difference in patterns of Met expression in papillary thyroid carcinomas and nonneoplastic thyroid tissue. World J Surg 25:623–631
104. Ruco LP, Ranalli T, Marzullo A, Bianco P, Prat M, Comoglio PM, Baroni CD (1996) Expression of Met protein in thyroid tumours. J Pathol 180:266–270
105. Chen BK, Furihata M, Takeuchi T, Iwata J, Liang SB, Sonobe H (1999) Overexpression of c-Met protein in human thyroid tumors correlated with lymph node metastasis and clinicopathologic stage. Pathol Res Pract 195:427–433
106. Siraj AK, Bavi P, Abubaker J, Jehan Z, Sultana M, Al-Dayel F, Al-Nuaim A, Alzahrani A, Ahmed M, Al-Sanea O, Uddin S, Al-Kuraya KS (2007) Genome-wide expression analysis of Middle Eastern papillary thyroid cancer reveals c-MET as a novel target for cancer therapy. J Pathol 213(2):190–199
107. Sculte KM, Antoch G, Ellrichmann M, Finken-Eigen M, Köhrer K, Simon D, Goretzki PE, Röher HD (1998) Regulation of the HGF-receptor c-met in the thyroid gland. Exp Clin Endocrinol Diabetes 106:310–318

108. Chattopadhyay C, El-Naggar AK, Williams MD, Clayman GL (2008) Small molecule c-MET inhibitor PHA665752: effect on cell growth and motility in papillary thyroid carcinoma. Head Neck 30:991–1000
109. Eder JP, Vande Woude GF, Boerner SA, LoRusso PM (2009) Novel therapeutic inhibitors of the c-Met signaling pathway in cancer. Clin Cancer Res 15:2207–2214
110. Giusti F, Falchetti A, Franceschelli F, Marini F, Tanini A, Brandi ML (2010) Thyroid cancer: current molecular perspectives. J Oncol 351:679
111. Sadow PM, Heinrich MC, Corless CL et al (2010) Absence of BRAF, NRAS, KRAS, HRAS, mutations, and RET/PTC gene rearrangements distinguishes dominant nodules in Hashimoto thyroiditis from papillary thyroid carcinomas. Endocr Pathol 21:73–79
112. Lam KY, Lo CY, Chan KW, Wan KY (2000) Insular and anaplastic carcinoma of the thyroid: a 45-year comparative study at a single institution and a review of the significance of p53 and p21. Ann Surg 231:329–338
113. Venkatesh YS, Ordonez NG, Schultz PN, Hickey RC, Goepfert H, Samaan NA (1990) Anaplastic carcinoma of the thyroid. A clinicopathologic study of 121 cases. Cancer 66:321–330
114. Nel CJ, van Heerden JA, Goellner JR, Gharib H, McConahey WM, Taylor WF, Grant CS (1985) Anaplastic carcinoma of the thyroid: a clinicopathologic study of 82 cases. Mayo Clin Proc 60:51–58
115. Schaefer CJ (1988) Long-term survival in anaplastic thyroid cancer. Md Med J 37:873–874
116. Rosai J, Saxen EA, Woolner L (1985) Undifferentiated and poorly differentiated carcinoma. Semin Diagn Pathol 2:123–136
117. Nusynowitz ML (1991) Differentiating anaplastic thyroidcarcinomas. J Nucl Med 32:1363–1364
118. Smallridge RC, Copland JA (2010) Anaplastic thyroid carcinoma: pathogenesis and emerging therapies. Clin Oncol 22(6):486–497
119. Lo CY, Chan WF, Lam KY, Wan KY (2005) Follicular thyroid carcinoma: the role of histology and staging systems in predicting survival. Ann Surg 242:708–715
120. Parameswaran R, Brooks S, Sadler GP (2010) Molecular pathogenesis of follicular cell derived thyroid cancers. Int J Surg 8:186–193
121. Nikiforova MN, Lynch RA, Biddinger PW, Alexander EK, Dorn GW 2nd, Tallini G, Kroll TG, Nikiforov YE (2003) RAS point mutations and PAX8-PPAR gamma rearrangement in thyroid tumors: evidence for distinct molecular pathways in thyroid follicular carcinoma. J Clin Endocrinol Metab 88:2318–2326
122. Cheung L, Messina M, Gill A, Clarkson A, Learoyd D, Delbridge L, Wentworth J, Philips J, Clifton-Bligh R, Robinson BG (2003) Detection of the PAX8-PPAR gamma fusion oncogene in both follicular thyroid carcinomas and adenomas. J Clin Endocrinol Metab 88:354–357
123. Krol TG, Sarraf P, Pecciarini L, Chen CJ, Mueller E, Spiegelman BM, Fletcher JA (2000) PAX8-PPARgamma1 fusion oncogene in human thyroid carcinoma. Science 289:1357–1360
124. Mansouri A, Chowdhury K, Gruss P (1998) Follicular cells of the thyroid gland require Pax8 gene function. Nat Genet 19:87–90
125. Willson TM, Cobb JE, Cowan DJ, Wiethe RW, Correa ID, Prakash SR, Beck KD, Moore LB, Kliewer SA, Lehmann JM (1996) The structure-activity relationship between peroxisome proliferator-activated receptor-gamma agonism and the antihyperglycemic activity of thiazolidinediones. J Med Chem 39:665–668
126. Hibi Y, Nagaya T, Kambe F, Imai T, Funahashi H, Nakao A, Seo H (2004) Is thyroid follicular cancer in Japanese caused by a specific t(2; 3)(q13; p25) translocation generating Pax8-PPAR gamma fusion mRNA? Endocr J 51:361–366
127. Pollina L, Pacini F, Fontanini G, Vignati S, Bevilacqua G, Basolo F (1996) bcl-2, p53 and proliferating cell nuclear antigen expression is related to the degree of differentiation in thyroid carcinomas. Br J Cancer 73:139–143

128. Donghi R, Longoni A, Pilotti S, Michieli P, Della Porta G, Pierotti MA (1993) Gene p53 mutations are restricted to poorly differentiated and undifferentiated carcinomas of the thyroid gland. J Clin Invest 91:1753–1760
129. Xing M (2010) Genetic alterations in the phosphatidylinositol-3 kinase/Akt pathway in thyroid cancer. Thyroid 20:697–706
130. Hou P, Liu D, Shan Y, Hu S, Studeman K, Condouris S, Wang Y, Trink A, El-Naggar AK, Tallini G, Vasko V, Xing M (2007) Genetic alterations and their relationship in the in the phospatidylinositol 3-kinase pathway in thyroid cancer. Clin Cancer Res 13:1161–1170
131. Wang Y, Hou P, Yu H, Wang W, Ji M, Zhao S, Yan S, Sun X, Liu D, Shi B, Zhu G, Condouris S, Xing M (2007) High prevalence and mutual exclusivity of genetic alterations in the phosphatidylinositol-3-kinase pathway in thyroid tumors. J Clin Endocrinol Metab 92:2387–2390
132. Garcia-Rostan G, Camp RL, Herrero A, Carcangiu ML, Rimm DL, Tallini G (2001) Beta-catenin dysregulation in thyroid neoplasms: down-regulation, aberrant nuclear expression, and CTNNB1 exon 3 mutations are markers for aggressive tumor phenotypes and poor prognosis. Am J Pathol 158:987–996
133. Barnabei A, Ferretti E, Baldelli R, Procaccini A, Spriano G, Appetecchia M (2009) Hurthle cell tumours of the thyroid. Personal experience and review of the literature. Acta Otorhinolaryngol Ital 29:305–311
134. MaÅLximo V, Sobrinho-Simoes M (2000) Hurthle cell tumours of the thyroid. A review with emphasis on mitochondrial abnormalities with clinical relevance. Virchows Arch 437:107–115
135. Ljungberg O (1972) On medullary carcinoma of the thyroid. APMIS Suppl A 80:1–57
136. Papotti M, Sambataro D, Pecchioni C, Bussolati G (1996) The pathology of medullary carcinoma of the thyroid: review of the literature and personal experience on 62 cases. Endocr Pathol 7:1–20
137. Komminoth P, Roth J, Saremaslani P et al (1994) Polysialic acid of the neural cell adhesion molecule in the human thyroid: a marker for medullary thyroid carcinoma and primary C-cell hyperplasia. Am J Surg Pathol 18:399–411
138. Correia-Deur JE, Toledo RA, Imazawa AT, Lourenco DM Jr, Ezabella MC, Tavares MR, Toledo SP (2009) Sporadic medullary thyroid carcinoma: clinical data from a university hospital. Clinics (Soa Paulo) 64:379–386
139. Jijiwa M, Fukuda T, Kawai K, Nakamura A, Kurokawa K, Murakumo Y, Ichihara M, Takahashi M (2004) A targeting mutation of tyrosine 1062 in Ret causes a marked decrease of enteric neurons and renal hypoplasia. Mol Cell Biol 24:8026–8036
140. Segouffin-Cariou C, Billaud M (2000) Transforming ability of MEN2A-RET requires activation of the phosphatidylinositol 3-kinase signaling pathway. J Biol Chem 275:3568–3576
141. Scott RP, Eketjäll S, Aineskog H, Ibáñez CF (2005) Distinct turnover of alternatively spliced isoforms of the RET kinase receptor mediated by differential recruitment of the Cbl ubiquitin ligase. J Biol Chem 280:13442–13449
142. Acton DS, Velthuyzen D, Lips CJ, Höppener JW (2000) Multiple endocrine neoplasia type 2B mutation in human RET oncogene induces medullary thyroid carcinoma in transgenic mice. Oncogene 19:3121–3125
143. Donis-Keller H, Dou S, Chi D, Carlson KM, Toshima K, Lairmore TC, Howe JR, Moley JF, Goodfellow P, Wells SA Jr (1993) Mutations in the RET proto-oncogene are associated with MEN 2A and FMTC. Hum Mol Genet 2:851–856
144. Erdogan MF, Gürsoy A, Ozgen G, Cakir M, Bayram F, Ersoy R, Algün E, Cetinars B, Cömlekçi A, Kadioglu P, Balci MK, Yetkin I, Kabalak T, Erdogan G (2005) Ret proto-oncogene mutations in apparently sporadic Turkish medullary thyroid carcinoma patients: Turkmen study. J Endocrinol Invest 28:806–809
145. Elisei R, Romei C, Cosci B, Agate L, Bottcic V, Molinaro E, Sculli M, Miccoli P, Basolo F, Grasso L, Pacini F, Pinchera A (2007) RET genetic screening in patients with medullary thyroid cancer and their relatives: experience with 807 individuals at one center. J Clin Endocrinol Metab 92:4725–4729

146. Hedayati M, Nabipour I, Rezaei-Ghaleh N, Azizi F (2006) Germline RET mutations in exons 10 and 11: an Iranian survey of 57 medullary thyroid carcinoma cases. Med J Malaysia 61:564–569
147. Bugalho MJ, Domingues R, Santos JR, Catarino AL, Sobrinho L (2007) Mutation analysis of the RET proto-oncogene and early thyroidectomy: results of a Portuguese cancer centre. Surgery 141:90–95
148. Ceccherini I, Hofstra RM, Luo Y, Stulp RP, Barone V, Stelwagen T, Bocciardi R, Nijveen H, Bolino A, Seri M et al (1994) DNA polymorphisms and conditions for SSCP analysis of the 20 exons of the ret protooncogene. Oncogene 9:3025–3029
149. Kruckeberg KE, Thibodeau SN (2004) Pyrosequencing technology as a method for the diagnosis of multiple endocrine neoplasia type 2. Clin Chem 50:522–529
150. Kim IJ, Kang HC, Park JH, Ku JL, Lee JS, Kwon HJ, Yoon KA, Heo SC, Yang HY, Cho BY, Kim SY, Oh SK, Youn YK, Park DJ, Lee MS, Lee KW, Park JG (2002) RET oligonucleotide microarray for the detection of RET mutations in multiple endocrine neoplasia type 2 syndromes. Clin Cancer Res 8:457–463
151. Blank RD, Sklar CA, Martin ML (1996) Denaturing gradient gel electrophoresis to diagnose multiple endocrine neoplasia type 2. Clin Chem 42:598–603
152. Ahmed SA, Snow-Bailey K, Highsmith WE, Sun W, Fenwick RG, Mao R (2005) Nine novel gremlin gene variants in the RET proto-oncogene identified in twelve unrelated cases. J Mol Diagn 7:283–288
153. Margraf RL, Mao R, Witter CT (2008) Rapid diagnosis of MEN2B using unlabeled probe melting analysis and the LightCycler 480 instrument. J Mol Diagn 10:123–128
154. Takano T, Miyauchi A, Matsuzuka F, Liu G, Higashiyama T, Yokozawa T, Kuma K, Amino N (1999) Preoperative diagnosis of medullary thyroid carcinoma by RT-PCR using RNA extracted from leftover cells within a needle used for fine needle aspiration biopsy. J Clin Endocrinol Metab 84:951–955
155. Santoro M, Rosati R, Grieco M et al (1990) The RET proto-oncogene is consistently expressed in human pheochromocytomas and thyroid medullary carcinomas. Oncogene 5:1595–1598
156. Lloyd RV, Sisson JC, Marangos PJ (1983) Calcitonin, carcinoembryonic antigen, and neuron-specific enolase in medullary thyroid carcinoma. Cancer 51:2234–2239
157. Zajac JD, Penschow J, Mason T, Tregear G, Coghlan J, Martin TJ (1986) Identification of calcitonin and calcitonin gene-related peptide messenger ribonucleic acid in medullary thyroid carcinomas by hybridization histochemistry. J Clin Endocrinol Metab 62:1037–1043
158. Lakhani VT, You YN, Wells SA (2007) The multiple endocrine neoplasia syndromes. Annu Rev Med 58:253–265
159. Eng C, Clayton D, Schuffenecker I et al (1996) The relationship between specific RET proto-oncogene mutations and disease phenotype in multiple endocrine neoplasia type 2: International RET mutation consortium analysis. JAMA 276:1575–1579
160. He H, Jazdzewski K, Li W, Liyanachchi S, Nagy R, Volinia S, Calin GA, Liu CG, Franssila K, Suster S, Kloos RT, Crcoe CM, de la Chapelle A (2005) The role of microRNA genes in papillary thyroid carcinoma. Proc Natl Acad Sci USA 102:19075–19080
161. Weber F, Teresi RE, Broelsch CE, Frilling A, Eng C (2006) A limited set of human microRNA is deregulated in follicular thyroid carcinoma. J Clin Endocrinol Metab 91:3584–3591
162. Visone R, Pallante P, Vecchione A, Cirombella R, Ferracin M, Ferraro A, Volinia S, Coluzzi S, Leone V, Borbone E, Liu CG, Petrocca F, Troncone G, Calin GA, Scarpa A, Colato C, Tallini G, Santoro M, Croce CM, Fusco A (2007) Specific microRNAs are downregulated in human thyroid anaplastic carcinomas. Oncogene 26:7590–7595
163. Nikiforova MN, Tseng MN, Steward D, Diorio D, Nikiforov YE (2008) MicroRNA expression profiling of thyroid tumors: biological significance and diagnostic utility. J Clin Endocrinol Metab 93:1600–1608
164. Carney JA, Volante M, Papotti M, Asa S (2004) Hyalinizing trabecular tumour. In: DeLellis RA, Lloyd RV, Heitz P, Eng C (eds) World Health Organization classification of tumours. Pathology & genetics. Tumours of endocrine organs. IARC Press, Lyon, pp 104–105

165. Katoh R, Jasani B, Williams ED (1989) Hyalinizing trabecular adenoma of the thyroid. A report of three cases with immunohistochemical and ultrastructural studies. Histopathology 15:211–224
166. Cheung CC, Boerner SL, MacMillan CM, Ramyar L, Asa SL (2000) Hyalinizing trabecular tumor of the thyroid: a variant of papillary carcinoma proved by molecular genetics. Am J Surg Pathol 24:1622–1626
167. Sheu SY, Vogel E, Worm K, Grabellus F, Schwertheim S, Schmid KW (2010) Hyalinizing trabecular tumour of the thyroid-differential expression of distinct miRNAs compared with papillary thyroid carcinoma. Histopathology 56:632–640
168. Levin KE, Galante M, Clark OH (1987) Parathyroid carcinoma versus parathyroid adenoma in patients with profound hypercalcaemia. Surgery 101:649–660
169. Shortell CK, Andrus CH, Phillips CE Jr, Schwartz SI (1991) Carcinoma of the parathyroid gland: a 30-year experience. Surgery 110:704–708
170. Hunt JL (2008) Molecular diagnosis in head and neck: what a surgical pathologist must know. Head Neck Pathol 2:99–102
171. Hundahl SA, Fleming ID, Fremgen AM, Menck HR (1999) Two hundred eighty-six cases of parathyroid carcinoma treated in the U.S. between 1985–1995: a National Cancer Data Base Report. The American College of Surgeons Commission on Cancer and the American Cancer Society. Cancer (Phila) 86:538–544
172. Sandelin K, Tullgren O, Farnebo LO (1994) Clinical course of metastatic parathyroid cancer. World J Surg 18:594–598
173. Carpten JD, Robbins CM, Villablanca A et al (2002) HRPT2, encoding parafibromin, is mutated in hyperparathyroidism-jaw tumor syndrome. Nat Genet 32:676–680
174. Howell VM, Haven CJ, Kahnoski K, Khoo SK, Petillo D, Chen J, Fluren GJ, Robinson BG, Delbridge LW, Philips J, Nelson AE, Krause U, Hammje K, Dralle H, Hoang-Vu C, Gimm O, March DJ, Morreau H, The BT (2003) HRPT2 mutations are associated with malignancy in sporadic parathyroid tumours. J Med Genet 40:657–663
175. Szabo J, Heath B, Hill VM, Jackson CE, Zarbo RJ, Mallette LE, Chew SL, Besser GM, Thakker RV, Huff V et al (1995) Hereditary hyperparathyroidism-jaw tumour syndrome: the endocrine tumour gene HRPT2 maps to chromosome 1q21-q31. Am J Hum Genet 56:944–950
176. Teh BT, Farnebo F, Kristoffersson U, Sundelin B, Cardinal J, Axelson R, Yap A, Epstein M, Heath H, Cameron D 3rd, Larsson C (1996) Autosomal dominant primary hyperparathyroidism and jaw tumour syndrome associated with renal hamartomas and cystic kidney disease: linkage to 1q21-q32 and loss of the wild type allele in renal hamartomas. J Clin Endocrinol Metab 81:4204–4211
177. Juhlin CC, Villablanca A, Sandelin K, Haglund F, Norderström J, Forsberg L, Bränström R, Obara T, Arnold A, Larsson C, Höög A (2007) Parafibromin immunoreactivity: its use as an additional diagnostic marker for parathyroid tumor classification. Endocr Relat Cancer 14:501–512
178. Tan MH, Morrison C, Wang P, Yang X, Haven CJ, Zhang C, Zhao P, Tertiaova MS, Korpi-Hyovalti E, Burgess JR, Soo KC, Cheah WK, Cao B, Resau J, Morreau H, Teh BT (2004) Loss of parafibromin immunoreactivity is a distinguishing feature of parathyroid carcinoma. Clin Cancer Res 10:6629–6637
179. Shackelford RE, Kaufman WK, Paules RS (1999) Cell cycle control, checkpoint mechanisms, and genotoxic stress. Environ Health Perspect 107(Suppl 1):5–24
180. Westin G, Björklund P, Akersröm G (2009) Molecular genetics of parathyroid disease. World J Surg 33:2224–2233
181. Shane E, Bilezkina JP (1982) Parathyroid carcinoma: a review of 62 patients. Endocr Rev 3:218–226
182. Corbette S, Eller-Vainicher C, Vicentini L, Lania A, Mantovani G, Beck-Peccoz P, Spada A (2007) Modulation of cyclin D1 expression in human tumoral parathyroid cells: effects of growth factors and calcium sensing receptor activation. Cancer Lett 255:34–41

183. Kameyama K, Takami H, Umemura S, Osamura YR, Wada N, Sugino K, Mimura T, Ito K (2000) PCNA and Ki-67 as prognostic markers in human parathyroid carcinomas. Ann Surg Oncol 7:301–304
184. Thomopoulou GE, Tseleni-Balafouta S, Lazaris AC, Koutselini H, Kavantzas N, Davaris PS (2003) Immunohistochemical detection of cell cycle regulators, Fhit protein and apoptotic cells in parathyroid lesions. Eur J Endocrinol 148:81–87
185. Kulkarni PS, Parkh PM (2004) The carcinoma of parathyroid gland. Indian J Cancer 41:51–59
186. Palanisamy N, Imanishi Y, Rao PH, Tahara H, Chaganti RSK, Arnold A (1998) Novel chromosomal abnormalities identified by comparative genomic hybridization in parathyroid adenomas. J Clin Endocrinol Metabol 83:1766–1770. doi:10.1210/jc.83.5.1766

Chapter 3
Molecular Pathology and Diagnostics of Breast Cancer

William Kong, Ted Richards, Jin Q. Cheng, and Domenico Coppola

Contents

Abstract Proper treatment of breast cancer often depends on timely and accurate diagnosis. Due to the heterogeneic nature of breast cancer, it is important to continually develop diagnostic methods and tools that strive to provide consistent and reliable results for optimal patient specific care. Early microscopic observations of tumor sections have revealed that specific morphological structures of the mammary gland, such as luminal or basal layers, are often mimicked by cancer cells. This has resulted in a hypothesis that hyperplastic cells originate from their respective anatomical sites. Newer findings now suggest breast cancer arises from mammary stem

W. Kong
Stanford University School of Medicine, Stanford, CA 94305-5101, USA

T. Richards • J.Q. Cheng • D. Coppola, M.D. (✉)
Department of Anatomic Pathology and Oncological Sciences,
H. Lee Moffitt Cancer Center & Research Institute and University
of South Florida, 12902 Magnolia Drive, Tampa, FL 33612, USA
e-mail: Domenico.coppola@moffitt.org

D. Coppola (ed.), *Molecular Pathology and Diagnostics of Cancer*,
Cancer Growth and Progression 16, DOI 10.1007/978-94-007-7192-5_3,

or progenitor cells, which then differentiate into various lineages by molecular mechanisms not yet fully understood. Subtypes of breast cancers are reliably labeled aggressive, including triple negative and hereditary breast cancers. Molecular diagnosis is currently available through various platforms, including: MammaPrint®, Veridex®, Theros®, and Oncotype DX®, which have improved the resolution of diagnosis. Significant advancements in a variety of scientific disciplines in basic research, integration of next-generation sequencing technologies, and innovative computational and mathematical methods in integration of diverse data types on a large scale will likely translate into clinical applications such as breast cancer diagnosis.

Keywords Molecular diagnosis • Breast cancer • Mammary development • miR-155 • BRCA

Abbreviations

ER	Estrogen receptor
HER2/NEU	Human epidermal growth factor receptor 2
miRNA	microRNA
NMuMG	Normal mouse mammary gland epithelial cells
PR	Progesterone receptor
RS	Recurrence score

3.1 Introduction

Breast cancer is a heterogeneous disease first appreciated by histopathologists when they noted a large diversity of phenotypes while observing specimens under the microscope [1–3]. It was also apparent that different phenotypes often associated with different biological and clinical behaviors; leading to early diagnostic schemes based on appearance. Under the microscope, specimens had features that resembled microanatomical structures of the normal mammary gland, misleading histopathologists to hypothesize that breast cancer likely arises from these structures; hence, the terms ductal and lobular carcinomas were coined [4]. The first part of this chapter will provide background information on mammary gland development from the embryonic stages to post-pregnancy involution. It is important to grasp this concept to fully appreciate the original classification schemes of breast cancer. Then, we will briefly discuss the importance of histological grading and estrogen receptor (ER), progesterone receptor (PR), and human epidermal growth factor receptor 2 (HER2/neu) status. This is the foundation for understanding use of microarray technology to diagnose breast cancer, since it was proposed that phenotype is reflected by its gene expression signature. Numerous platforms, such as MammaPrint®,

Oncotype DX®, Theros®, have been developed in recent years to serve this purpose. Rapid development in breast cancer research utilizing various approaches ranging from biology to genetics and covering specific areas of interest including normal and cancer stem cell identification, protein-protein interaction(s), non-coding regulatory RNAs, genetics and epigenetics may provide improvements to current diagnostic approaches in the future.

3.2 Mammary Gland Development

The murine model has been utilized dependably to study basic mechanisms of mammary development. Development can be classified into stages: embryonic, pre/post-puberty, pregnancy, and involution. Each pregnancy begins a cycle of alveolar differentiation, milk production, and then involution. During embryonic development, the first significant event is marked by formation of the bilateral milk lines on embryonic day 10. These lines fragment and coalesce into five pairs of mammary placodes, forming elevated buds by embryonic day 11. The mammary buds then invaginate below the epithelial surface into a bulb and induce transformation of their underlying stroma into the mammary mesenchyme. Next, sprouts appear from each bud and penetrate into the mammary mesenchyme, forming a primitive tree-like structure by embryonic day 18 [5]. The sprouts extend, forming hollow ducts comprising an inner layer luminal epithelial cells surrounded by outer layer of basal myoepithelial cells. These layers play important functional roles during pregnancy where luminal epithelial cells and basal epithelial cells provide a niche for progenitors of alveolar sacs, while myoepithelial cells give rise to contractile cells for milk secretion [6, 7]. Different types of breast cancer were originally believed to arise from these distinct microanatomical structures of the normal breast, hence giving origin to the terminology of ductal and lobular carcinomas [8–10].

Mammary development seizes until puberty, where production of ovarian steroids initiates a second phase of growth that drives expansion and further branching of the ductal system. Terminal end buds, a structure resembling Edison's incandescent glass bulb, are located at the ends of each duct. Stem cells are believed to be located within this structure and are housed in a niche environment that enables them to self-renew and remain undifferentiated and quiescent [5–7]. Some stem cells located within the terminal end buds are programmed to undergo progenitor commitment and further differentiation as the ducts elongate, branch, and invade into the outer borders of the mammary fat pad. Additionally, both stem and progenitor cells are seeded along the ducts as sources of alveolar differentiation for each pregnancy event. After weaning is completed, these alveolar sacs undergo involution, returning the mammary gland back into a mostly ductile organ while adipogenesis fills in the voids to replenish the mammary fat pad [4, 6, 11, 12] (Fig. 3.1). It is believed that most in situ precursors lesions and invasive breast cancers arise from stem/progenitor cells and are able to give rise to all histological types [4, 13, 14]; therefore, the luminal and basal resemblance that have long since been appreciated by histopathologists.

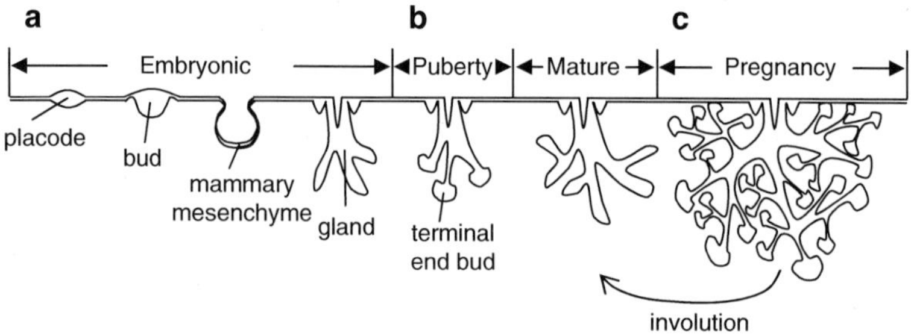

Fig. 3.1 Murine mammary gland development. (**a**) During embryonic development, bilateral milk lines are established by embryonic day 10 (E10). The milk line breaks up and coalesces into individual mammary placodes which transform into elevated buds by E11. Each bud continually develops and invaginates below the epithelial surface to form a bulb structure that condenses the underlying stroma and pushes into the mammary mesenchyme towards the fat pad. Sprouts branch from the bulb and penetrate into the mammary mesenchyme in formation of a primitive tree like structure by E18. (**b**) Formation of the mature mammary gland begins in the presence of circulating steroid and peptide hormones systemically produced at the onset of puberty. (**c**) Each pregnancy cycle involves the formation of milk producing alveolar sacs. The mammary gland undergoes post-lactational involution after weaning

3.3 ER, PR, HER2/neu, BRCA1/2, Grade, Stage, and Lymph Node Status

Current diagnosis emphasize standard clinical features such as the tumor size, extent of lymph node involvement, and distant metastasis and have all been integrated into the American Joint Committee on Cancer TNM classification standard and still play a central role in determining prognosis and treatment course by the physician [15–20]. Similarly, ER and PR status have been defined as important markers of breast cancer pathology decades ago, but now are gold standards in prescribing adjuvant therapy [21–28]. Another important marker for therapy response of breast cancer is the amplification of HER2/neu. Testing for this marker has become routine before prescribing Herceptin therapy. HER2/neu is a cell membrane surface-bound receptor tyrosine kinase belonging to the epidermal growth factor receptor family (ErbB) involved in signal transduction pathways promoting cell growth and differentiation [29–35]. Although its presence indicates aggressive tumor, trastuzumab, a specific antibody that targets the cell surface receptor, is supplemented, so that the receptor can be blocked from receiving growth signals [36–39].

A subtype of aggressive breast cancer, called "triple negative," lacks ER/PR/HER2 expression and grows without the need for external growth hormones [40–46]. It is more prevalent in younger women and characterized by early recurrence and visceral metastasis to the brain [40, 47, 48]. Fortunately, it is still sensitive to conventional chemotherapy and often prescribed concurrently with surgery [40, 41, 49–51]. Although the molecular biology of this breast cancer subtype is not yet fully understood, it has been recently associated with mutations in the two major breast cancer susceptibility genes, BRCA1 and BRCA2 [52–56].

BRCA1 and BRCA2 function as tumor suppressors involved in DNA damage response and DNA repair. Mutation in one copy of either BRCA1 or BRCA2 can increase the risk of hereditary breast and ovarian cancer with a lifetime risk of 50–80 % and 30–50 % for breast and ovarian cancer, respectively. Additionally, cancer development occurs earlier than non-hereditary breast cancer and is often aggressive [57].

Other points in early classification schemes are stage, grade, and lymph node status. Tumor size is used to assign stage, whereas the Nottingham histological grading system defines proliferative activity (mitotic index) and degree of differentiation (tubule formation and nuclear pleomorphism) of the tumor [58, 59]. Assessment of lymph node status is also part of tumor staging, and it can provide prognostic value. However, the combination of all three is often used to predict tumor prognosis. It has been reported that late stage and high grade can override the positive effects of negative node involvement [15, 17, 60–64].

Although determining ER, PR, and HER2 status may seem trivial and often conflicts with classification schemes, it is significant since it allows for targeted therapy. Targeting the ER and widespread use of the selective ER modulator tamoxifen in breast cancer are well-established targeted therapeutic modalities. These are responsible for the major improvements in cure rates, quality of life, and disease prevention for breast cancer observed over the past two decades. Targeting both HER2/neu with trastuzumab and the vascular endothelial growth factor with bevacizumab in combination with chemotherapy has become a further milestone in molecularly targeted therapy of this disease [65–69].

3.4 Gene Expression Arrays

The Stanford group pioneered class discovery through the use of high-throughput technologies and re-emphasized that breast cancer is not a single entity and that it can be classified into at least five groups by their molecular signature: luminal subdivided into luminal A and luminal B; basal-like; HER2; and a least characterized normal breast-like. Luminal tumors, like normal luminal epithelial cells of the breast, express cytokeratins 8/18, and are ER positive. This group is further subdivided into luminal A (lower grade and excellent prognosis) and luminal B (higher grade and poorer prognosis exemplified by higher proliferation rates). The basal-like breast cancers express genes resembling normal basal/myoepithelial mammary cells. For instance, they express cytokeratins 5, 6, 14, and 17, P-cadherin, caveolins 1 and 2, and EGFR. They are often ER, PR, and HER2/neu negative and are of higher histological grade characterized by a high mitotic index. They exhibit necrotic regions with lymphocytic infiltrate and often metastasize. HER2 tumors are ER negative with high HER2/neu expression. This type of breast cancer is aggressive but, unlike the basal like tumors, responds to adjuvant therapy. The last group is the normal breast-like and is not well characterized, but their gene expression profile resembles fibroadenomas and normal breast samples [4, 70–78].

Although classification based on gene expression arrays may seem more objective and straightforward, there are always exceptions. For instance, not all breast tumors that are *HER2* amplified can be categorized into the HER2 group. Some *HER2*-amplified tumors express ER, and their gene expression signature resembles the luminal type. Furthermore, the basal type is not always triple negative (ER, PR, and HER2), and a small subset of triple negative breast cancers is not basal like. Therefore, the use of microarrays to classify breast cancer might not always align with previous histopathological classifications. Nevertheless, MammaPrint®, Oncotype DX®, and Theros® have been developed in recent years for molecular diagnosis of breast cancer gene expression array technologies, and we provide a brief overview below of each [4, 70–82].

3.4.1 MammaPrint®

The first breast cancer classification through utility of gene expression profiles was demonstrated by van't Veer et al. [83]. The original data sets were samples from patients younger than 55 years old, tumor size smaller than 5 cm, and lymph node negative. They analyzed the gene expression signature of samples taken from breast cancer patients who developed metastasis within 5 years after diagnosis and compared these against the gene expression signatures of samples taken from breast cancer patients who were metastasis free during the same time. The analysis identified a 70-gene expression signature that could provide a predictive value for 5 years metastasis. This resulted in administration of proper treatment to patients with aggressive breast cancer.

The results from this study were validated in a subsequent study by Vijver et al. that encompassed more patients. They determined this gene set was an independent predictor of outcome in a multivariate survival analysis. Beyond its ability to demonstrate likelihood of metastasis, this gene expression signature could stratify node-positive patients based on disease outcome prediction. This assay is currently undergoing phase III clinical trial organized by the European Organization for Research and Treatment of Cancer. The trial is setup to profile the 70-gene expression signature and to simultaneously determine the clinicopathological characteristics for 6,000 patients. If the 70-gene expression signature and clinicopathological data agree, patients will be treated accordingly. However, if the two diagnostic tools differ, patients will be randomized and treated according to the results of the 70-gene expression signature or clinicopathological parameters [84–89].

Finally, this 70-gene expression signature has been shown to outperform traditional clinical and histological parameters for providing a prognostic value [90–93]. A downside to this gene expression signature is that it fails to stratify ER-negative or HER2-positive breast cancer since it predicts 96–100 % and 78–95 %, of them, respectively, which will have poor prognosis. For the remaining 5–22 % HER2-positive breast cancers not predicted to be in the high-risk group, the controversial question is whether to provide trastuzumab treatment or not [93–95]. Regardless, this assay received FDA approval for use in patients younger than 61 years old, at stages I/II, node negative, and tumor size smaller than 5 cm [84–89].

3.4.2 *Veridex®*

In the original study, Wang et al. [96] separated 115 lymph node-negative breast cancer samples, from systemic therapy naïve patients, into 35 ER-negative and 80 ER-positive for analyses. From the analyses, samples from patients who were ER-positive with distant metastasis expressed 16 genes differentially, whereas samples from patients who were ER-negative with distant metastasis expressed 60 genes differentially. This resulted in a 76-gene signature that can predict likelihood of metastasis. A subsequent study expanded to examine 171 lymph node-negative tumors from systemic therapy-naïve patients. This gene expression signature was shown to be an independent prognostic factor in multivariate analysis. It should be noted that this gene expression signature failed to provide a predictive value when applied to ER-negative patients [96–99].

3.4.3 *Theros®*

Ma et al. analyzed the gene expression signatures of 60 patients uniformly treated with adjuvant tamoxifen alone. They analyzed the whole tissue sections and laser-capture microdissected samples from patients who responded to tamoxifen treatment and identified three strongly predictive genes: homeobox gene HOXB13, interleukin 17B receptor (IL17BR) and EST AI240933. The study showed expression ratios between HOXB13 and IL17BR were strongly correlated with recurrence and outperformed other clinical pathological predictors. A validation study was carried out from RNA samples extracted from paraffin-embedded tissues from a cohort of 20 patients. Then the HOXB13:IL17BR expression ratio was re-evaluated in a cohort of 206 postmenopausal patients with ER-positive breast cancer who underwent tamoxifen-only treatment from the North Central Cancer Treatment Group (NCCTG) 89-30-52 trial. It was further expanded into a study with a cohort of 852 patients. In these studies, the HOXB13-to-IL17BR ratios were shown to identify ER-positive breast cancer patients that underwent tamoxifen treatment but at high risk of recurrence. It was also shown that the HOXB13-to-IL17BR ratios were a predictor of outcome for ER-positive patients who were either adjuvant naïve or who underwent tamoxifen treatment. Although the HOXB13:IL17BR ratios are practical in these aspects, it appears to have limited ability to predict outcome in lymph node-positive patients. These studies have led to the development of Theros®, a RT-qPCR-based test performed in a central laboratory and commercialized by Biotheranostics. This test is recommended for lymph node negative ER-positive breast cancers patients treated with surgery alone, to define risk of recurrence and benefit from endocrine therapy. At the time of this review, the HOXB13:IL17BR index has not yet been shown to predict adjuvant hormone therapy or chemotherapy benefit and has not been included in the American Society of Clinical Oncology or National Comprehensive Cancer Network guidelines for breast cancer treatment [100–104].

3.4.4 *Oncotype DX®*

The OncotypeDX® platform (Genomic Health Inc., Redwood City, CA, USA) utilizes RT-qPCR to analyze the expression of 16 cancer-related genes: Ki67, STK15, survivin, CCNB1, MYBL2, GRB7, HER2, ER, PGR, BCL2, SCUBE2, MMP11, CTSL2, GSTM1, CD68, and BAG1, in addition to five reference genes (*ACTB*, *GAPDH*, *RPLPO*, *GUS*, and *TFRC*). The test utilizes RNA extracted from formalin-fixed paraffin-embedded ER-positive breast cancer samples. Selection of genes was originally derived from published literature, genomic databases, and microarray data.

OncotypeDX® predicts risk of recurrence in ER-positive, lymph node-negative breast cancer patients and provides treatment guidelines via a quantitative system of continuous Recurrence Score (RS) that ranges between 0 and 100 to predict the risk of recurrence within 10 years. This score has also been shown to be an independent predictor of outcome in multivariate survival analyses where samples are categorized, based on the RS into three risk group: low ($RS < 18$), intermediate ($RS = 18–31$), and high ($RS \geq 31$).

Studies have validated OncotypeDX® and demonstrated that breast cancer patients who are ER-positive with a low RS tend to have a low risk of recurrence and will not benefit much from chemotherapy. On the other hand, breast cancer patients who are ER-positive with a high RS tend to have a high risk of recurrence and can benefit from chemotherapy. This justifies the use of endocrine therapy in addition to chemotherapy for ER-positive patients with a high RS score. This assay has been implemented into the American Society of Clinical Oncology guidelines for the use of tumor markers in breast cancer and into the National Comprehensive Cancer Network guidelines for breast cancer treatment [105–110].

3.5 MicroRNAs

The miRNA paradigm shifted from worm development to cancer when G.A. Calin et al. identified miR-15 and miR-16 as tumor suppressors at 13q14 in chronic lymphocytic leukemia in 2002 [111]. It has been shown that hemizygous or homozygous loss of 13q14 occurs in more than 50 % of B-cell chronic lymphocytic leukemia, mantle cell lymphoma, and prostate cancers and only slightly lower in multiple myeloma; however, detailed genetic analysis of traditional genes located in this region yielded inconclusive evidence. The discovery of miRNA prompted Calin et al. to revisit information coded within this region. They discovered that the genetic code for two miRNAs, miR-15 and miR-16, are indeed located in this area and hypothesized that deletion of 13q14 results in loss of miR-15 and miR-16 expression. This was confirmed when analyses showed 68 % of RNA samples from B-cell chronic lymphocytic leukemia patients do not express these two miRNAs [111]. Shortly after, Michael et al. showed a similarly reduced expression of mature miR-143 and miR-145 in colorectal cancer [112]; Metzler et al. showed an accumulation of miR-155 in Burkitt lymphoma [113], and a similar trend was reported for other types of B-cell lymphomas, including diffuse large B-cell lymphoma [114, 115]. In 2004, Takamizawa et al. showed that let-7 was often lost in lung cancer and had a direct correlation to postoperative survival. They also found that overexpression of exogenous let-7 in lung cancer cell lines leads to growth inhibition [116]. Later, to complement Takamizawa's findings, Johnson et al. published data demonstrating that let-7 is indeed a probable tumor suppressor by targeting oncogenic RAS [117]. These landmark studies established the importance of miRNAs in cancer, leading to an exponential growth in miRNA cancer research. Numerous studies reporting miRNA profiling of cancer specimens were published with the intent to determine the functional significance of individual miRNAs in addition to the speculation that miRNA profiles could have clinical practicality for tumor classification.

3.5.1 Breast Cancer Subtype miRNA Profiles

Early and recent miRNA profiles showed a subset of miRNAs differentially expressed in normal tissues compared to solid tumors including breast cancers. Furthermore, some of these miRNAs were associated with biopathologic features of breast cancer such as ER+/–, PR+/–, cancer stage, nodal status, vascular invasion, proliferation index, and p53 status [118–122]. miRNA profiles were also performed on the different molecular subtypes of breast cancer as defined by gene expression signatures. Furthermore, the use of miRNA profiling was applied to determining a miRNA signature of different mammary cell types [123–128].

Blenkiron et al. showed that 133 miRNAs are differentially expressed in the human breast and in the different molecular subtypes of breast cancer. They first classified 93 cases of primary human breast tumors by gene expression profiling into luminal A, luminal B, basal-like, HER2+, normal-like, and ER+/–. Using a bead-based flow cytometric miRNA expression profiling method, they identified differentially expressed miRNAs in the various molecular subtypes. These miRNAs include pathologically important miRNAs: members within the let-7, miR-200, and miR-10 family; the miR-17–92 and miR-214 clusters; and individual miRNAs such as miR-155, miR-21. Furthermore, they showed miR-100, miR-99a, miR-130a, miR-126*, miR-136, miR-146b, miR-15b, miR-107, and miR-103 can differentiate between the luminal A and luminal B subtypes, in addition to providing a profile for differentiating ER+/– and tumor grade [128].

Sempere et al. used locked nucleic acid array to profile breast cancer cell lines in addition to normal and tumor breast tissue specimens. Then, they implemented an in situ hybridization method to determine the localization of miRNAs within specific cell types of formalin-fixed, paraffin-embedded tissue specimens. The rational was that the miRNAs of interest should be aberrantly expressed within malignant cells rather than the involved stroma, infiltrating lymphocytes, and/or vasculature. They found miR-145 and miR-205 expression in myoepithelial cells of normal mammary epithelial structures, whereas their expression was significantly reduced or eliminated in matching tumor specimens. Let-7a, miR-21, miR-141, and miR-214 were detectable within luminal epithelial cells in normal tissue where let-7a was often decreased while miR-21 was increased in malignant cells. Interestingly, although the authors did not extrapolate on this finding, their heat map indicated elevated expression levels of miR-221, miR-222, miR-214, and miR-21 in ER- tumors [124].

3.5.2 MicroRNA-155

One miRNA rising to prominence in breast cancer is microRNA-155 (miR-155). It was originally identified to be differentially expressed in miRNA profiles [118, 119, 128]. Kong et al. discovered miR-155 may have implications in aggressive, invasive breast cancer using TGFβ induced epithelial to mesenchymal transition in normal mouse mammary gland epithelial cells (NMuMG), an *in vitro* cell line model often used to study mechanisms of breast cancer metastasis. NMuMG expressing miR-155 exhibits greater invasion and migration, whereas NMuMG without miR-155 had the opposite effect. miR-155 expression also induced cellular plasticity that could be rescued with RhoA reconstitution [129]. In another study, Kong et al. showed miR-155 induced breast cancer cell proliferation and chemoresistance by targeting FOXO3a [130]. Furthermore, Blenkiron et al. showed that miR-155 expression is highly elevated in basal-like and high-grade breast cancer [128].

Chang et al. recently published data showing that the tumor suppressor BRCA1 epigenetically controls miR-155 expression. They demonstrated that the R1699Q moderate risk variant, which exhibits a point mutation in the BRCT domain, loses its ability to repress miR-155, explaining how BRCA1-deficient cells express high levels of miR-155. Orthotopic transplantation of BRCA1+ MDA-MB-468 cells ectopically expressing miR-155 into athymic nude mice exhibited accelerated tumor growth relative to control. Analyses of BRCA1-mutant human breast tumors show inverse correlation between BRCA1 and miR-155 expression [131]. The complementation of *in vitro* experiments by Kong et al., with the clinical breast cancer profile work by Blenkiron et al., suggested that miR-155 has important clinical implications in aggressive breast cancer. The data of Chang et al. solidified the physiological importance of miR-155 in the critical BRCA1 mutant breast cancers. This suggests miR-155 could be a potential biomarker in addition to a therapeutic target for specific types of aggressive breast cancers [128–131].

3.6 Conclusions

Diagnosis of breast cancer has evolved from observing the physical appearance of the tumor under the microscope to quantifying expression of genes at the molecular level. Although the latter method may seem less subjective and more quantitative, it is still subject to variations including but not limited to sample handling and reagent lot variations among other factors. Implementation should probably not replace the former method supported by the expertise of a trained pathologist. Molecular diagnosis should probably be used in a combinatorial manner, although the cost of doing so might not justify its implementation. Furthermore, basic research in science now covers a variety of subjects such as epigenetics, regulation by non-coding RNAs, identification of cancer stem cells and understanding their functions from genetics to biology, and a vast variety of other disciplines in between. Furthermore, next-generation sequencing technologies and the technological means to integrate and analyze diverse data types on a large scale, which allows investigation of biological networks in diseased state, will likely drive further changes in molecular diagnosis of not only breast cancers but other diseases.

References

1. Azzopardi JG, Ahmed A, Millis RR (1979) Problems in breast pathology. Major Probl Pathol 11:1–466, i-xvi
2. Tavassoli FA (1992) Classification of metaplastic carcinomas of the breast. Pathol Annu 27(Pt 2):89–119
3. Mourad WA (1998) Book review: Rosen's breast pathology. Ann Saudi Med 18:278
4. Weigelt B, Reis-Filho JS (2009) Histological and molecular types of breast cancer: is there a unifying taxonomy? Nat Rev Clin Oncol 6:718–730
5. Veltmaat JM, Mailleux AA, Thiery JP, Bellusci S (2003) Mouse embryonic mammogenesis as a model for the molecular regulation of pattern formation. Differentiation 71:1–17
6. Tiede B, Kang Y (2011) From milk to malignancy: the role of mammary stem cells in development, pregnancy and breast cancer. Cell Res 21:245–257
7. Woodward WA, Chen MS, Behbod F, Rosen JM (2005) On mammary stem cells. J Cell Sci 118:3585–3594
8. Reis-Filho JS, Lakhani SR (2008) Breast cancer special types: why bother? J Pathol 216:394–398
9. Simpson PT, Reis-Filho JS, Gale T, Lakhani SR (2005) Molecular evolution of breast cancer. J Pathol 205:248–254
10. Vargo-Gogola T, Rosen JM (2007) Modelling breast cancer: one size does not fit all. Nat Rev Cancer 7:659–672
11. Visvader JE (2009) Keeping abreast of the mammary epithelial hierarchy and breast tumorigenesis. Genes Dev 23:2563–2577
12. Petersen OW, Polyak K (2010) Stem cells in the human breast. Cold Spring Harb Perspect Biol 2(5):a003160
13. Wellings SR, Jensen HM (1973) On the origin and progression of ductal carcinoma in the human breast. J Natl Cancer Inst 50:1111–1118
14. Wellings SR, Jensen HM, Marcum RG (1975) An atlas of subgross pathology of the human breast with special reference to possible precancerous lesions. J Natl Cancer Inst 55:231–273

15. Basaran G, Devrim C, Caglar HB, Gulluoglu B, Kaya H, Seber S, Korkmaz T, Telli F, Kocak M, Dane F, Yumuk FP, Turhal SN (2011) Clinical outcome of breast cancer patients with N3a (>/=10 positive lymph nodes) disease: has it changed over years? Med Oncol 28:726–732
16. Colzani E, Liljegren A, Johansson AL, Adolfsson J, Hellborg H, Hall PF, Czene K (2011) Prognosis of patients with breast cancer: causes of death and effects of time since diagnosis, age, and tumor characteristics. J Clin Oncol 29:4014–4021
17. Kuru B (2006) Prognostic significance of total number of nodes removed, negative nodes removed, and ratio of positive nodes to removed nodes in node positive breast carcinoma. Eur J Surg Oncol 32:1082–1088
18. Leitner SP, Swern AS, Weinberger D, Duncan LJ, Hutter RV (1995) Predictors of recurrence for patients with small (one centimeter or less) localized breast cancer (T1a, b N0 M0). Cancer 76:2266–2274
19. Singletary SE, Allred C, Ashley P et al (2002) Revision of the American Joint Committee on Cancer staging system for breast cancer. J Clin Oncol 20:3628–3636
20. Singletary SE, Allred C, Ashley P et al (2003) Staging system for breast cancer: revisions for the 6th edition of the AJCC cancer staging manual. Surg Clin North Am 83:803–819
21. Bodmer A, Castiglione-Gertsch M (2011) Role of hormonal manipulations in patients with hormone-sensitive metastatic breast cancer. Eur J Cancer 47(Suppl 3):S28–S37
22. Higgins MJ, Baselga J (2011) Targeted therapies for breast cancer. J Clin Invest 121:3797–3803
23. Lonning PE, Haynes BP, Straume AH, Dunbier A, Helle H, Knappskog S, Dowsett M (2011) Exploring breast cancer estrogen disposition: the basis for endocrine manipulation. Clin Cancer Res 17:4948–4958
24. Bardou VJ, Arpino G, Elledge RM, Osborne CK, Clark GM (2003) Progesterone receptor status significantly improves outcome prediction over estrogen receptor status alone for adjuvant endocrine therapy in two large breast cancer databases. J Clin Oncol 21:1973–1979
25. Leong AS, Zhuang Z (2011) The changing role of pathology in breast cancer diagnosis and treatment. Pathobiology 78:99–114
26. Thakkar JP, Mehta DG (2011) A review of an unfavorable subset of breast cancer: estrogen receptor positive progesterone receptor negative. Oncologist 16:276–285
27. Delozier T (2010) Hormonal treatment in breast cancer. J Gynecol Obstet Biol Reprod (Paris) 39(8 Suppl):F71–F78
28. Tamaki Y, Miyoshi Y, Noguchi S (2002) Adjuvant hormonal therapy. Breast Cancer 9:185–189
29. Clark GM, McGuire WL (1991) Follow-up study of HER-2/neu amplification in primary breast cancer. Cancer Res 51:944–948
30. Howe LR, Brown PH (2011) Targeting the HER/EGFR/ErbB family to prevent breast cancer. Cancer Prev Res (Phila) 4:1149–1157
31. Gutierrez C, Schiff R (2011) HER2: biology, detection, and clinical implications. Arch Pathol Lab Med 135:55–62
32. Guarneri V, Barbieri E, Dieci MV, Piacentini F, Conte P (2010) Anti-HER2 neoadjuvant and adjuvant therapies in HER2 positive breast cancer. Cancer Treat Rev 36(Suppl 3):S62–S66
33. Mukai H (2010) Treatment strategy for HER2-positive breast cancer. Int J Clin Oncol 15:335–340
34. Leyland-Jones B (2009) Human epidermal growth factor receptor 2-positive breast cancer and central nervous system metastases. J Clin Oncol 27:5278–5286
35. Ross JS, Slodkowska EA, Symmans WF, Pusztai L, Ravdin PM, Hortobagyi GN (2009) The HER-2 receptor and breast cancer: ten years of targeted anti-HER-2 therapy and personalized medicine. Oncologist 14:320–368
36. LoRusso PM, Weiss D, Guardino E, Girish S, Sliwkowski MX (2011) Trastuzumab emtansine: a unique antibody-drug conjugate in development for human epidermal growth factor receptor 2-positive cancer. Clin Cancer Res 17:6437–6447
37. Wong WM (1999) Drug update: trastuzumab: anti-HER2 antibody for treatment of metastatic breast cancer. Cancer Pract 7:48–50

38. Goldenberg MM (1999) Trastuzumab, a recombinant DNA-derived humanized monoclonal antibody, a novel agent for the treatment of metastatic breast cancer. Clin Ther 21:309–318
39. Colomer R, Shamon LA, Tsai MS, Lupu R (2001) Herceptin: from the bench to the clinic. Cancer Invest 19:49–56
40. Anders CK, Carey LA (2009) Biology, metastatic patterns, and treatment of patients with triple-negative breast cancer. Clin Breast Cancer 9(Suppl 2):S73–S81
41. Bosch A, Eroles P, Zaragoza R, Vina JR, Lluch A (2010) Triple-negative breast cancer: molecular features, pathogenesis, treatment and current lines of research. Cancer Treat Rev 36:206–215
42. Kang SP, Martel M, Harris LN (2008) Triple negative breast cancer: current understanding of biology and treatment options. Curr Opin Obstet Gynecol 20:40–46
43. Kobayashi S (2008) Basal-like subtype of breast cancer: a review of its unique characteristics and their clinical significance. Breast Cancer 15:153–158
44. Rakha EA, Ellis IO (2009) Triple-negative/basal-like breast cancer: review. Pathology 41:40–47
45. Reis-Filho JS, Tutt AN (2008) Triple negative tumours: a critical review. Histopathology 52:108–118
46. Anders C, Carey LA (2008) Understanding and treating triple-negative breast cancer. Oncology (Williston Park) 22:1233–1239, discussion 1239–1240, 1243
47. Haffty BG, Yang Q, Reiss M et al (2006) Locoregional relapse and distant metastasis in conservatively managed triple negative early-stage breast cancer. J Clin Oncol 24:5652–5657
48. Hines SL, Vallow LA, Tan WW, McNeil RB, Perez EA, Jain A (2008) Clinical outcomes after a diagnosis of brain metastases in patients with estrogen- and/or human epidermal growth factor receptor 2-positive versus triple-negative breast cancer. Ann Oncol 19:1561–1565
49. Carey LA, Dees EC, Sawyer L et al (2007) The triple negative paradox: primary tumor chemosensitivity of breast cancer subtypes. Clin Cancer Res 13:2329–2334
50. Rodler E, Korde L, Gralow J (2010) Current treatment options in triple negative breast cancer. Breast Dis 32:99–122
51. Yagata H, Kajiura Y, Yamauchi H (2011) Current strategy for triple-negative breast cancer: appropriate combination of surgery, radiation, and chemotherapy. Breast Cancer 18:165–173
52. Lee LJ, Alexander B, Schnitt SJ, Comander A, Gallagher B, Garber JE, Tung N (2011) Clinical outcome of triple negative breast cancer in BRCA1 mutation carriers and noncarriers. Cancer 117:3093–3100
53. Gonzalez-Angulo AM, Timms KM, Liu S, Chen H, Litton JK, Potter J, Lanchbury JS, Stemke-Hale K, Hennessy BT, Arun BK, Hortobagyi GN, Do KA, Mills GB, Meric-Bernstam F (2011) Incidence and outcome of BRCA mutations in unselected patients with triple receptor-negative breast cancer. Clin Cancer Res 17:1082–1089
54. Antoniou AC, Wang X, Fredericksen ZS et al (2010) A locus on 19p13 modifies risk of breast cancer in BRCA1 mutation carriers and is associated with hormone receptor-negative breast cancer in the general population. Nat Genet 42:885–892
55. Atchley DP, Albarracin CT, Lopez A, Valero V, Amos CI, Gonzalez-Angulo AM, Hortobagyi GN, Arun BK (2008) Clinical and pathologic characteristics of patients with BRCA-positive and BRCA-negative breast cancer. J Clin Oncol 26:4282–4288
56. Young SR, Pilarski RT, Donenberg T, Shapiro C, Hammond LS, Miller J, Brooks KA, Cohen S, Tenenholz B, Desai D, Zandvakili I, Royer R, Li S, Narod SA (2009) The prevalence of BRCA1 mutations among young women with triple-negative breast cancer. BMC Cancer 9:86
57. Roy R, Chun J, Powell SN (2011) BRCA1 and BRCA2: different roles in a common pathway of genome protection. Nat Rev Cancer 12:68–78
58. Rakha EA, El-Sayed ME, Lee AH et al (2008) Prognostic significance of Nottingham histologic grade in invasive breast carcinoma. J Clin Oncol 26:3153–3158
59. Elston CW, Ellis IO (1991) Pathological prognostic factors in breast cancer. I. The value of histological grade in breast cancer: experience from a large study with long-term follow-up. Histopathology 19:403–410

60. Galea MH, Blamey RW (1993) Comment on 'Predicting recurrence in axillary node negative breast cancer patients', by Rosner and Lane. Breast Cancer Res Treat 28:299–300
61. Rosner D, Lane WW (1993) Predicting recurrence in axillary-node negative breast cancer patients. Breast Cancer Res Treat 25:127–139
62. Hutter RV (1984) Pathological parameters useful in predicting prognosis for patients with breast cancer. Monogr Pathol 25:175–185
63. Leong AS, Raymond WA (1989) Prognostic parameters in breast cancer. Pathology 21:169–175
64. Reiss M (1989) Prognostic factors in primary breast cancer. Conn Med 53:565–571
65. Le XF, Mao W, Lu C, Thornton A, Heymach JV, Sood AK, Bast RC Jr (2008) Specific blockade of VEGF and HER2 pathways results in greater growth inhibition of breast cancer xenografts that overexpress HER2. Cell Cycle 7:3747–3758
66. Pegram MD, Reese DM (2002) Combined biological therapy of breast cancer using monoclonal antibodies directed against HER2/neu protein and vascular endothelial growth factor. Semin Oncol 29(3 Suppl 11):29–37
67. Perez EA, Spano JP (2012) Current and emerging targeted therapies for metastatic breast cancer. Cancer 118:3014–3025
68. Tortora G, Ciardiello F, Gasparini G (2008) Combined targeting of EGFR-dependent and VEGF-dependent pathways: rationale, preclinical studies and clinical applications. Nat Clin Pract Oncol 5:521–530
69. Wong TW, Lee FY, Emanuel S, Fairchild C, Fargnoli J, Fink B, Gavai A, Hammell A, Henley B, Hilt C, Hunt JT, Krishnan B, Kukral D, Lewin A, Malone H, Norris D, Oppenheimer S, Vite G, Yu C (2011) Antitumor and antiangiogenic activities of BMS-690514, an inhibitor of human EGF and VEGF receptor kinase families. Clin Cancer Res 17:4031–4041
70. Ignatiadis M, Sotiriou C (2008) Understanding the molecular basis of histologic grade. Pathobiology 75:104–111
71. Tibshirani R, Hastie T, Narasimhan B, Chu G (2002) Diagnosis of multiple cancer types by shrunken centroids of gene expression. Proc Natl Acad Sci USA 99:6567–6572
72. Prat A, Ellis MJ, Perou CM (2011) Practical implications of gene-expression-based assays for breast oncologists. Nat Rev Clin Oncol 9:48–57
73. Weigelt B, Pusztai L, Ashworth A, Reis-Filho JS (2011) Challenges translating breast cancer gene signatures into the clinic. Nat Rev Clin Oncol 9:58–64
74. Sotiriou C, Pusztai L (2009) Gene-expression signatures in breast cancer. N Engl J Med 360:790–800
75. Badve S, Nakshatri H (2009) Oestrogen-receptor-positive breast cancer: towards bridging histopathological and molecular classifications. J Clin Pathol 62:6–12
76. Hu Z, Fan C, Oh DS, Marron JS, He X, Qaqish BF, Livasy C, Carey LA, Reynolds E, Dressler L, Nobel A, Parker J, Ewend MG, Sawyer LR, Wu J, Liu Y, Nanda R, Tretiakova M, Ruiz Orrico A, Dreher D (2006) The molecular portraits of breast tumors are conserved across microarray platforms. BMC Genomics 7:96
77. Weigelt B, Baehner FL, Reis-Filho JS (2010) The contribution of gene expression profiling to breast cancer classification, prognostication and prediction: a retrospective of the last decade. J Pathol 220:263–280
78. Dabney AR (2005) Classification of microarrays to nearest centroids. Bioinformatics 21:4148–4154
79. Perou CM, Sorlie T, Eisen MB et al (2000) Molecular portraits of human breast tumours. Nature 406:747–752
80. Reis-Filho JS, Weigelt B, Fumagalli D, Sotiriou C (2010) Molecular profiling: moving away from tumor philately. Sci Transl Med 2:47ps43
81. Sorlie T, Perou CM, Tibshirani R et al (2001) Gene expression patterns of breast carcinomas distinguish tumor subclasses with clinical implications. Proc Natl Acad Sci USA 98:10869–10874
82. Sorlie T, Tibshirani R, Parker J et al (2003) Repeated observation of breast tumor subtypes in independent gene expression data sets. Proc Natl Acad Sci USA 100:8418–8423

83. van't Veer LJ, Dai H, van de Vijver MJ et al (2002) Gene expression profiling predicts clinical outcome of breast cancer. Nature 415:530–536
84. Bogaerts J, Cardoso F, Buyse M et al (2006) Gene signature evaluation as a prognostic tool: challenges in the design of the MINDACT trial. Nat Clin Pract Oncol 3:540–551
85. Cardoso F, Piccart-Gebhart M, Van't Veer L, Rutgers E (2007) The MINDACT trial: the first prospective clinical validation of a genomic tool. Mol Oncol 1:246–251
86. Cardoso F, Van't Veer L, Rutgers E, Loi S, Mook S, Piccart-Gebhart MJ (2008) Clinical application of the 70-gene profile: the MINDACT trial. J Clin Oncol 26:729–735
87. Mook S, Van't Veer LJ, Rutgers EJ, Piccart-Gebhart MJ, Cardoso F (2007) Individualization of therapy using Mammaprint: from development to the MINDACT Trial. Cancer Genomics Proteomics 4:147–155
88. Mook S, Bonnefoi H, Pruneri G et al (2009) Daily clinical practice of fresh tumour tissue freezing and gene expression profiling; logistics pilot study preceding the MINDACT trial. Eur J Cancer 45:1201–1208
89. Rutgers E, Piccart-Gebhart MJ, Bogaerts J, Delaloge S, Veer LV, Rubio IT, Viale G, Thompson AM, Passalacqua R, Nitz U, Vindevoghel A, Pierga JY, Ravdin PM, Werutsky G, Cardoso F (2011) The EORTC 10041/BIG 03–04 MINDACT trial is feasible: results of the pilot phase. Eur J Cancer 47:2742–2749
90. Buyse M, Loi S, van't Veer L, Viale G, Delorenzi M, Glas AM, d'Assignies MS, Bergh J, Lidereau R, Ellis P, Harris A, Bogaerts J, Therasse P, Floore A, Amakrane M, Piette F, Rutgers E, Sotiriou C, Cardoso F, Piccart MJ, TRANSBIG Consortium (2006) Validation and clinical utility of a 70-gene prognostic signature for women with node-negative breast cancer. J Natl Cancer Inst 98:1183–1192
91. Mook S, Schmidt MK, Viale G et al (2009) The 70-gene prognosis-signature predicts disease outcome in breast cancer patients with 1–3 positive lymph nodes in an independent validation study. Breast Cancer Res Treat 116:295–302
92. Bueno-de-Mesquita JM, van Harten WH, Retel VP, van't Veer LJ, van Dam FS, Karsenberg K, Douma KF, van Tinteren H, Peterse JL, Wesseling J, Wu TS, Atsma D, Rutgers EJ, Brink G, Floore AN, Glas AM, Roumen RM, Bellot FE, van Krimpen C, Rodenhuis S, van de Vijver MJ, Linn SC (2007) Use of 70-gene signature to predict prognosis of patients with node-negative breast cancer: a prospective community-based feasibility study (RASTER). Lancet Oncol 8:1079–1087
93. Bueno-de-Mesquita JM, Linn SC, Keijzer R, Wesseling J, Nuyten DS, van Krimpen C, Meijers C, de Graaf PW, Bos MM, Hart AA, Rutgers EJ, Peterse JL, Halfwerk H, de Groot R, Pronk A, Floore AN, Glas AM, Van't Veer LJ, van de Vijver MJ (2009) Validation of 70-gene prognosis signature in node-negative breast cancer. Breast Cancer Res Treat 117:483–495
94. Bueno-de-Mesquita JM, Sonke GS, van de Vijver MJ, Linn SC (2011) Additional value and potential use of the 70-gene prognosis signature in node-negative breast cancer in daily clinical practice. Ann Oncol 22:2021–2030
95. Straver ME, Glas AM, Hannemann J, Wesseling J, van de Vijver MJ, Rutgers EJ, Vrancken Peeters MJ, van Tinteren H, Van't Veer LJ, Rodenhuis S (2010) The 70-gene signature as a response predictor for neoadjuvant chemotherapy in breast cancer. Breast Cancer Res Treat 119:551–558
96. Wang Y, Klijn JG, Zhang Y et al (2005) Gene-expression profiles to predict distant metastasis of lymph-node-negative primary breast cancer. Lancet 365:671–679
97. Desmedt C, Piette F, Loi S, Wang Y, Lallemand F, Haibe-Kains B, Viale G, Delorenzi M, Zhang Y, d'Assignies MS, Bergh J, Lidereau R, Ellis P, Harris AL, Klijn JG, Foekens JA, Cardoso F, Piccart MJ, Buyse M, Sotiriou C, TRANSBIG Consortium (2007) Strong time dependence of the 76-gene prognostic signature for node-negative breast cancer patients in the TRANSBIG multicenter independent validation series. Clin Cancer Res 13:3207–3214
98. Foekens JA, Atkins D, Zhang Y, Sweep FC, Harbeck N, Paradiso A, Cufer T, Sieuwerts AM, Talantov D, Span PN, Tjan-Heijnen VC, Zito AF, Specht K, Hoefler H, Golouh R, Schittulli F, Schmitt M, Beex LV, Klijn JG, Wang Y (2006) Multicenter validation of a gene expression-based

prognostic signature in lymph node-negative primary breast cancer. J Clin Oncol 24:1665–1671
99. Kreike B, van Kouwenhove M, Horlings H, Weigelt B, Peterse H, Bartelink H, van de Vijver MJ (2007) Gene expression profiling and histopathological characterization of triple-negative/basal-like breast carcinomas. Breast Cancer Res 9:R65
100. Goetz MP, Suman VJ, Ingle JN, Nibbe AM, Visscher DW, Reynolds CA, Lingle WL, Erlander M, Ma XJ, Sgroi DC, Perez EA, Couch FJ (2006) A two-gene expression ratio of homeobox 13 and interleukin-17B receptor for prediction of recurrence and survival in women receiving adjuvant tamoxifen. Clin Cancer Res 12:2080–2087
101. Jerevall PL, Ma XJ, Li H, Salunga R, Kesty NC, Erlander MG, Sgroi DC, Holmlund B, Skoog L, Fornander T, Nordenskjöld B, Stål O (2011) Prognostic utility of HOXB13:IL17BR and molecular grade index in early-stage breast cancer patients from the Stockholm trial. Br J Cancer 104:1762–1769
102. Ma XJ, Hilsenbeck SG, Wang W et al (2006) The HOXB13:IL17BR expression index is a prognostic factor in early-stage breast cancer. J Clin Oncol 24:4611–4619
103. Ma XJ, Wang Z, Ryan PD et al (2004) A two-gene expression ratio predicts clinical outcome in breast cancer patients treated with tamoxifen. Cancer Cell 5:607–616
104. Reid JF, Lusa L, De Cecco L et al (2005) Limits of predictive models using microarray data for breast cancer clinical treatment outcome. J Natl Cancer Inst 7:927–930
105. Goldstein LJ, Gray R, Badve S et al (2008) Prognostic utility of the 21-gene assay in hormone receptor-positive operable breast cancer compared with classical clinicopathologic features. J Clin Oncol 26:4063–4071
106. Habel LA, Shak S, Jacobs MK et al (2006) A population-based study of tumor gene expression and risk of breast cancer death among lymph node-negative patients. Breast Cancer Res 8:R25
107. Mina L, Soule SE, Badve S et al (2007) Predicting response to primary chemotherapy: gene expression profiling of paraffin-embedded core biopsy tissue. Breast Cancer Res Treat 103:197–208
108. Paik S (2007) Development and clinical utility of a 21-gene recurrence score prognostic assay in patients with early breast cancer treated with tamoxifen. Oncologist 12:631–635
109. Paik S, Shak S, Tang G et al (2004) A multigene assay to predict recurrence of tamoxifen-treated, node-negative breast cancer. N Engl J Med 351:2817–2826
110. Paik S, Tang G, Shak S et al (2006) Gene expression and benefit of chemotherapy in women with node-negative, estrogen receptor-positive breast cancer. J Clin Oncol 24:3726–3734
111. Calin GA, Dumitru CD, Shimizu M et al (2002) Frequent deletions and down-regulation of micro- RNA genes miR15 and miR16 at 13q14 in chronic lymphocytic leukemia. Proc Natl Acad Sci USA 99:15524–15529
112. Michael MZ, O'Connor SM, van Holst Pellekaan NG, Young GP, James RJ (2003) Reduced accumulation of specific microRNAs in colorectal neoplasia. Mol Cancer Res 1:882–891
113. Metzler M, Wilda M, Busch K, Viehmann S, Borkhardt A (2004) High expression of precursor microRNA-155/BIC RNA in children with Burkitt lymphoma. Genes Chromosomes Cancer 39:167–169
114. Eis PS, Tam W, Sun L, Chadburn A, Li Z, Gomez MF, Lund E, Dahlberg JE (2005) Accumulation of miR-155 and BIC RNA in human B cell lymphomas. Proc Natl Acad Sci USA 102:3627–3632
115. Kluiver J, Poppema S, de Jong D, Blokzijl T, Harms G, Jacobs S, Kroesen BJ, van den Berg A (2005) BIC and miR-155 are highly expressed in Hodgkin, primary mediastinal and diffuse large B cell lymphomas. J Pathol 207:243–249
116. Takamizawa J, Konishi H, Yanagisawa K, Tomida S, Osada H, Endoh H, Harano T, Yatabe Y, Nagino M, Nimura Y, Mitsudomi T, Takahashi T (2004) Reduced expression of the let-7 microRNAs in human lung cancers in association with shortened postoperative survival. Cancer Res 64:3753–3756
117. Johnson SM, Grosshans H, Shingara J, Byrom M, Jarvis R, Cheng A, Labourier E, Reinert KL, Brown D, Slack FJ (2005) RAS is regulated by the let-7 microRNA family. Cell 120:635–647

118. Volinia S, Calin GA, Liu CG, Ambs S, Cimmino A, Petrocca F, Visone R, Iorio M, Roldo C, Ferracin M, Prueitt RL, Yanaihara N, Lanza G, Scarpa A, Vecchione A, Negrini M, Harris CC, Croce CM (2006) A microRNA expression signature of human solid tumors defines cancer gene targets. Proc Natl Acad Sci USA 103:2257–2261
119. Iorio MV, Ferracin M, Liu CG, Veronese A, Spizzo R, Sabbioni S, Magri E, Pedriali M, Fabbri M, Campiglio M, Ménard S, Palazzo JP, Rosenberg A, Musiani P, Volinia S, Nenci I, Calin GA, Querzoli P, Negrini M, Croce CM (2005) MicroRNA gene expression deregulation in human breast cancer. Cancer Res 65:7065–7070
120. Iorio MV, Casalini P, Tagliabue E, Menard S, Croce CM (2008) MicroRNA profiling as a tool to understand prognosis, therapy response and resistance in breast cancer. Eur J Cancer 44:2753–2759
121. Di Leva G, Gasparini P, Piovan C, Ngankeu A, Garofalo M, Taccioli C, Iorio MV, Li M, Volinia S, Alder H, Nakamura T, Nuovo G, Liu Y, Nephew KP, Croce CM (2010) MicroRNA cluster 221–222 and estrogen receptor alpha interactions in breast cancer. J Natl Cancer Inst 102:706–721
122. Volinia S, Galasso M, Sana ME, Wise TF, Palatini J, Huebner K, Croce CM (2012) Breast cancer signatures for invasiveness and prognosis defined by deep sequencing of microRNA. Proc Natl Acad Sci USA 109:3024–3029
123. Valastyan S, Reinhardt F, Benaich N, Calogrias D, Szász AM, Wang ZC, Brock JE, Richardson AL, Weinberg RA (2009) A pleiotropically acting microRNA, miR-31, inhibits breast cancer metastasis. Cell 137:1032–1046
124. Sempere LF, Christensen M, Silahtaroglu A, Bak M, Heath CV, Schwartz G, Wells W, Kauppinen S, Cole CN (2007) Altered MicroRNA expression confined to specific epithelial cell subpopulations in breast cancer. Cancer Res 67:11612–11620
125. Yan LX, Huang XF, Shao Q, Huang MY, Deng L, Wu QL, Zeng YX, Shao JY (2008) MicroRNA miR-21 overexpression in human breast cancer is associated with advanced clinical stage, lymph node metastasis and patient poor prognosis. RNA 14:2348–2360
126. Radojicic J, Zaravinos A, Vrekoussis T, Kafousi M, Spandidos DA, Stathopoulos EN (2011) MicroRNA expression analysis in triple-negative (ER, PR and Her2/neu) breast cancer. Cell Cycle 10:507–517
127. Sieuwerts AM, Mostert B, Bolt-de Vries J, Peeters D, de Jongh FE, Stouthard JM, Dirix LY, van Dam PA, Van Galen A, de Weerd V, Kraan J, van der Spoel P, Ramírez-Moreno R, van Deurzen CH, Smid M, Yu JX, Jiang J, Wang Y, Gratama JW, Sleijfer S, Foekens JA, Martens JW (2011) mRNA and microRNA expression profiles in circulating tumor cells and primary tumors of metastatic breast cancer patients. Clin Cancer Res 17:3600–3618
128. Blenkiron C, Goldstein LD, Thorne NP et al (2007) MicroRNA expression profiling of human breast cancer identifies new markers of tumor subtype. Genome Biol 8:R214
129. Kong W, Yang H, He L, Zhao JJ, Coppola D, Dalton WS, Cheng JQ (2008) MicroRNA-155 is regulated by the transforming growth factor beta/Smad pathway and contributes to epithelial cell plasticity by targeting RhoA. Mol Cell Biol 28:6773–6784
130. Kong W, He L, Coppola M, Guo J, Esposito NN, Coppola D, Cheng JQ (2010) MicroRNA-155 regulates cell survival, growth, and chemosensitivity by targeting FOXO3a in breast cancer. J Biol Chem 285:17869–17879
131. Chang S, Wang RH, Akagi K, Kim KA, Martin BK, Cavallone L, Kathleen Cuningham Foundation Consortium for Research into Familial Breast Cancer (kConFab), Haines DC, Basik M, Mai P, Poggi E, Isaacs C, Looi LM, Mun KS, Greene MH, Byers SW, Teo SH, Deng CX, Sharan SK (2011) Tumor suppressor BRCA1 epigenetically controls oncogenic microRNA-155. Nat Med 17:1275–1282

Chapter 4
Molecular Pathology and Diagnostics of Non-small Cell Lung Carcinoma

Brian Quigley, Steve Ducker, and Farah Khalil

Contents

B. Quigley, M.D. • S. Ducker, M.D. • F. Khalil, M.D. (✉)
Department of Pathology and Cell Biology, University of South Florida, Tampa, FL, USA

Moffitt Cancer Center and Research Institute, 12902 Magnolia Drive,
Tampa, FL 33612, USA
e-mail: farah.khalil@moffitt.org

D. Coppola (ed.), *Molecular Pathology and Diagnostics of Cancer*,
Cancer Growth and Progression 16, DOI 10.1007/978-94-007-7192-5_4,

Abstract Of all the molecular alterations that may have predictive value in non-small cell lung cancer (NSCLC), testing for *EGFR* mutations is usually the first step in determining course of adjuvant therapy. Activation of *EGFR* mutations, and perhaps amplification, predicts the response of NSCLC to tyrosine kinase inhibitors (TKIs). The presence of activating *KRAS* mutations predicts resistance to TKI therapy, but the value of this test is questionable in NSCLC given that the coexistence of both *EGFR* and *KRAS* mutations in the same patient is extremely rare and the presence of a *KRAS* mutation may not have much different significance than the absence of an *EGFR* mutation. In patients who are considered for gemcitabine therapy, measurement of ribonucleotide reductase subunit 1 (RRM1) expression levels may help predict which patients are less likely to respond, as higher levels of RRM1 have been shown to overcome the anti-metabolite of this drug. Similarly, in patients being considered for platinum-based therapy, determination of excision-repair cross complementing-1 protein (ERCC1) expression level may help predict which patients are less likely to respond, given that ERCC1 repairs platinum-induced DNA damage. The use of these predictive factors ideally will help target therapy to individual tumors to achieve the best chance for long-term survival and to avoid side effects from medications that are unlikely to have any effect. Further studies will continue to refine testing and treatment algorithms.

Keywords Cancer • Lung • Carcinoma • Non-small cell • Molecular • Smoker • Squamous cell carcinoma • Adenocarcinoma • EGFR • KRAS • ALK • FISH • ERCC1 • RRM1

Abbreviations

ALK	Anaplastic lymphoma kinase
ARMS	Amplification refractory mutation system analysis
dNTP	Deoxyribonucleoside triphosphate
EGFR	Epidermal growth factor receptor
ELM4	Echinoderm microtubule-associated protein-like 4
ERCC1	Excision-repair cross complementing-1 protein
ERK	Extracellular signal-regulated kinase
FISH	Fluorescence in-situ hybridization
IHC	Immunohistochemistry
LOH 3p	Loss of heterozygosity of 3p
MASI	Mutant allele-specific imbalance
MEK	MAPK/ERK kinase
MRP	Multidrug resistance protein
NSCLC	Non-small cell lung cancer
PI3K	Phosphoinositide 3-kinase
PTEN	Phosphatase and tensin homolog
RRM1	Ribonucleotide reductase subunit 1
SNP	Single-nucleotide polymorphisms
TKI	Tyrosine kinase inhibitors

4.1 Introduction

In the United States, lung cancer is the number one cause of cancer deaths in both men and women [1–3]. Not surprisingly, given this fact, survival from lung cancer is poor. Although most cases of lung carcinoma can be attributed to cigarette smoking, a number of cases occur in people who have never smoked. As could be expected from the different exposure to carcinogens between smoking and non-smoking patients, lung carcinomas in these populations tend to have different molecular abnormalities, supporting the argument for differing mechanisms of carcinogenesis. A consequence of unique molecular alterations is differing responses to targeted therapeutic agents. Predicting responsiveness of a tumor to particular drugs often involves determination of some specific molecular characteristic. Description of such predictive molecular markers with background on their role in tumorigenesis and evidence for their value as predictive markers will be discussed in this chapter.

4.2 Lung Carcinoma Basics

4.2.1 Survival and Response Rates

Across all treatments and tumor stages, the overall survival rate for non-small cell lung cancer (NSCLC) is only 16 % at 5 years [1]. Patients with chemotherapy-treated advanced NSCLC have an 8–10-month median survival compared with only 4 or 5 months when untreated [2]. Response rates for treated metastatic NSCLC are only 17–37 %, with a median survival of only 6.7–11.3 months, 1-year survival rate of only 31–46 %, and 2-year survival rate of 9–21 % [1–4]. Time to progression averages 4–6 months, and response to second-line therapy is far worse at 8 % [5].

4.2.2 Gender, Smoking Status, and Histology

Although 85–90 % of lung cancers in men are attributable to smoking, 25 % of cases in men and women combined are not caused by smoking [6, 7]. Furthermore, lung cancers in smokers and never-smokers have different molecular characteristics, some attributable to carcinogenic agents in cigarette smoke [6–9]. Not only are there often molecular differences between lung cancers in smokers versus never-smokers [6, 8, 10], but frequencies of histologic types vary as well. Depending on the patient population, adenocarcinomas (Image 4.1) account for 62 % of lung cancers in never-smokers but only 19 % of lung cancers in smokers. Squamous cell carcinoma, on the other hand, accounts for 28–52 % of lung cancers in smokers but only 5.9–18 % in never-smokers [8, 11, 12].

Gender differences are present as well. Squamous cell carcinoma accounts for 44 % of lung cancers in men compared to 25 % in women, while adenocarcinomas comprise 28 % of lung cancers in men compared to 42 % in women. Frequencies of small- and large-cell carcinomas are roughly equal between men and women [7]. Part of the gender differences can be explained by the fact that a higher percentage of never-smokers are women [11, 12].

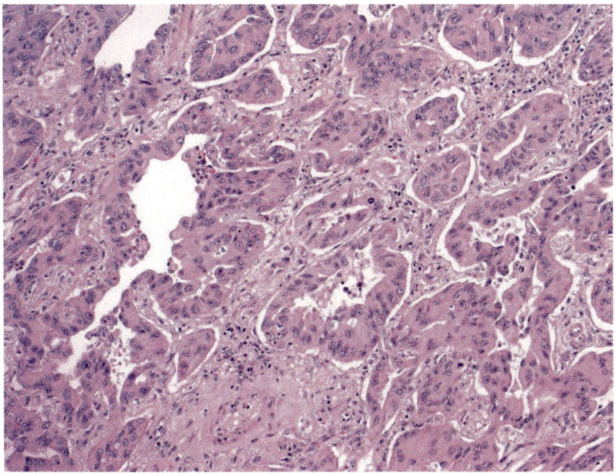

Image 4.1 Adenocarcinoma, 10× magnification

4.2.3 Treatment

The standard treatment for early NSCLC is surgery followed by adjuvant chemotherapy intended to prevent recurrences caused by micrometastases [2]. Advanced-stage or metastatic NSCLC is treated with a doublet chemotherapy regimen, for example, a doublet regimen, including cisplatin or carboplatin plus either docetaxel, paclitaxel, vinorelbine, gemcitabine, or irinotecan; other platinum combinations; or non-platinum combinations [1–4, 13–15]. Older patients or those with poor performance status may be treated with a single agent [14]. It has been shown that adjuvant chemotherapy in resectable NSCLC provides a 5–15 % absolute increase in overall survival [2, 16, 17].

4.2.4 Common Genetic Alterations in Lung Cancer

Various genetic alterations are often present in lung cancers, some of which may have specific prognostic or predictive value. The three most common genetic alterations found across all subtypes of lung cancer are loss of heterozygosity of 3p (LOH 3p), *TP53* mutations, and *PRb* mutations [7, 18–20]. Up to 80 % of cases demonstrate LOH 3p, which is the location of tumor suppressor genes such as *FHIT* [7, 9]. The *TP53* gene, which encodes the p53 tumor suppressor, is mutated in 50 % of NSCLC and 70 % of small cell carcinomas [7, 19]. Some alterations occur in specific histologic types. For example, squamous cell carcinomas frequently overexpress cytokeratins 5, 6, 13, 14, 16, 17, and 19 and infrequently harbor *KRAS* mutations [7]. In contrast, adenocarcinomas contain *KRAS* mutations in up to 30 %

(especially in smokers) [10], contain *TP53* mutations [10], and show overexpression of p27 [9, 21] and Cox-2 [7, 21].

Of the molecular alterations identified in lung carcinomas, some have been shown to have prognostic implications. Never-smoking status, high epidermal growth factor receptor (EGFR) protein expression, and increased *EGFR* gene copy number were all independent prognostic factors in the study by Hirsch et al. [22]. In squamous cell carcinomas, loss of PRb expression portends poor prognosis [7]. TP53 mutation has not been shown to have prognostic significance in squamous cell carcinomas but indicates poor prognosis for those with stage I and II adenocarcinomas [7, 19]. Poor prognosis may also accompany *KRAS* activating mutations and HER-2/neu overexpression [7]. Overexpression of p27 is correlated with well-differentiated tumors and indicates a good prognosis [7] (Fig. 4.1).

4.3 Theory Behind the Use of Molecular Predictive Markers

Despite the fact that, in the population as a whole, chemotherapy provides a survival benefit for NSCLC, not every patient will respond; worse yet, many may only suffer from the adverse effects. This includes death in 1–2 % of patients receiving platinum-based regimens [17]. To avoid treating patients who are unlikely to respond, it would be ideal to have predictive markers to determine whether a patient would be likely to respond to a given regimen [1]. Such predictive markers may be positive, such as the presence of an activating EGFR gene mutation predicting response to tyrosine kinase [22], or negative, such as a *KRAS* mutation predicting resistance to tyrosine kinase inhibitors (TKIs). Predictive markers are not to be confused with prognostic markers or factors that estimate a patient's likely outcome regardless of therapy [1].

Molecular alterations that serve as predictive markers are naturally going to fall into the category of a gene encoding drug metabolism, transmembrane transport, or target proteins [23]. Among the most studied predictive markers in lung cancer are EGFR, excision-repair cross complementing-1 protein (ERCC1), KRAS, and ribonucleotide reductase subunit 1 (RRM1). The following sections will discuss each of these markers, from the mechanisms by which they are thought to influence response to therapy and the clinical evidence supporting their value as molecular predictive markers.

4.4 Epidermal Growth Factor Receptor

4.4.1 Background

The most promising and widely reported molecular predictive factor in NSCLC is EGFR. The epidermal growth factor itself was first identified by Cohen in 1962 [24–26]. After epidermal growth factor binds to the EGFR, the receptor dimerizes, autophosphorylates, and activates several pathways, including MAP kinase, Jak2/STAT3, STAT5, and phosphoinositide 3-kinase (PI3K/Akt), which stimulate proliferation, metastasis, and migration and prevent apoptosis [5, 27–31]. Levels of phosphorylated STAT3 are most significantly correlated with phosphorylated EGFR levels, indicating that most of the signals from activated EGFR are transmitted through the STAT3 pathway [5]. It has also been shown that EGFR that is constitutively active as a result of either an exon 19 deletion or L858R substitution preferentially stimulates STAT and AKT pathways, preventing apoptosis but not promoting proliferation [28, 32]. This is consistent with the observation that there is no association between *EGFR* mutation and stage or metastasis, indicating absence of a link to tumor progression [32].

Because the epidermal growth factor normally favors growth and proliferation, mutations of its receptor that render it constitutively active independent of ligand-binding lead to a malignant phenotype [33, 34]. Increased EGFR gene copy number or overexpression has also been investigated for each of their roles in oncogenesis. It has been suggested that, based on their mechanisms of action, EGFR monoclonal antibodies (such as cetuximab, matuzumab, and panitumab, which bind the extracellular domain of EGFR and prevent ligand binding) should be beneficial to patients with tumors overexpressing surface EGFR, whereas TKIs should benefit patients having tumor proliferation and metastases driven by EGFR autophosphorylation [24, 35, 36]. In the latter case, blocking the catalytic site of the receptor (responsible for activating downstream molecules) could conceivably prevent growth and proliferation and even favor apoptosis in cancer cells. Two promising drugs that target the catalytic domain of the EGFR by competing with ATP are the reversible TKIs erlotinib and gefitinib [5, 36, 37]. Tumors likely to respond to TKIs are the ones that are dependent on aberrant signaling through the EGFR pathway for survival [36, 38].

The TKI erlotinib has been shown in a randomized, placebo-controlled, phase III trial to provide significant survival benefit compared to placebo in unselected, previously treated advanced-stage NSCLC patients [25]. In this trial and in others published before the discovery that lung tumors harboring mutations in the *EGFR* gene are sensitive to TKIs, it was observed that patients with certain demographic characteristics responded better to these agents. Studies had demonstrated that higher response rates to gefitinib were observed in women, Japanese patients, and in those with adenocarcinomas [11, 29, 39, 40]. The higher response rate in Japanese patients and the better outcome in women were not attributable to differences in pharmacokinetics in these populations [40]. It was also known that never-smokers had higher response rates, longer times to progression, and longer median overall survivals when treated with TKIs than smokers [11, 41]. These clinical characteristics (female sex, Asian origin, never-smoking status, and adenocarcinoma histology) have been independently associated with response to erlotinib [25, 42] and gefitinib (never-smoking status and female sex in Japanese patients) [43], and it has been suggested that these clinical characteristics may be of value as surrogate predictors of response to TKIs when molecular profiles are not available [44, 45]. Three articles published in 2004 revealed that *EGFR* mutations are the common factor linking the aforementioned patient demographics with consistent response to TKIs [7, 46].

Although erlotinib was shown to provide survival benefit as compared to placebo in a phase III trial [25], it was disappointing that gefitinib was shown only to be non-inferior to docetaxel in a randomized, placebo-controlled phase III trial, with no benefit over docetaxel even in subgroups of women, patients with adenocarcinomas, never-smokers, or Asian patients [47]. Compared to placebo, however, gefitinib did provide significant survival benefit for never-smokers and Asian patients in the randomized, placebo-controlled ISEL trial [48]. Without this subgroup analysis, survival was not significantly longer with gefitinib even compared to placebo, although response rate was significantly higher with gefitinib in the whole group and most pronounced in subgroups of patients with adenocarcinoma, never-smokers, women, and Asian patients [48].

EGFR activity may be increased in NSCLC by several different mechanisms, which may be assessed separately in the lab. The gene, *EGFR* (located on chromosome 7p12), may be mutated and/or amplified and the EGFR protein may be overexpressed in the presence or absence of either of these abnormalities. Background information and clinical studies regarding the predictive value of each of these aberrations are reviewed in the following sections.

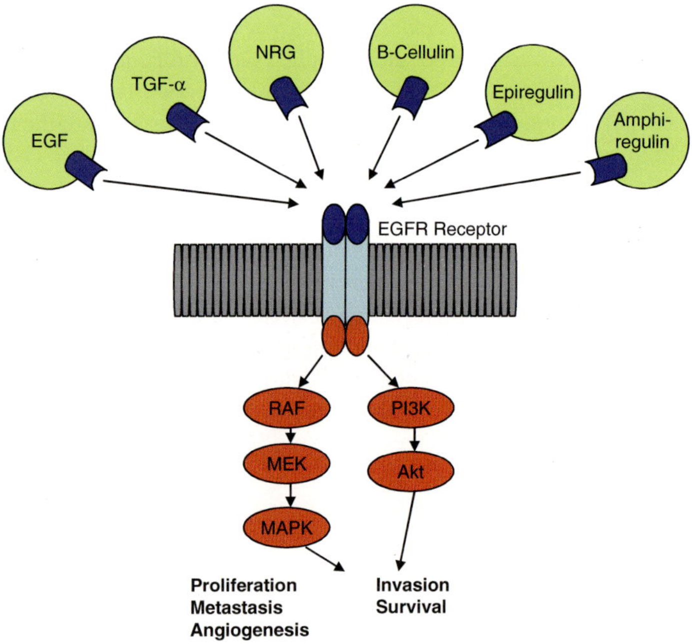

Fig. 4.1 EGFR Receptor involved in tumorigenesis of non-small cell lung cancer. *EGFR* epidermal growth factor receptor, *EGF* epidermal growth factor, *TGF* transforming growth factor, *NRG* neuregulin, *RAF* v-raf 1 murine leukemia viral oncogene homolog 1, *Akt* protein kinase B, *PI3K*, phosphatidylinositol-3-kinase, *MEK*, *MAPK* mitogen-activated protein kinase

4.4.2 EGFR *Mutations*

4.4.2.1 Types of Mutations

Many different types of mutations have been identified in the *EGFR* gene, approximately 90 % of which are either small deletions from exon 19 (codons 746–750) or substitution of arginine for leucine at position 858 in exon 21 (L858R). Another 3 % are substitutions of a variety of amino acids in place of glycine at codon 719 (G719X) and 3 % are in-frame insertions in exon 20 [7, 29, 37, 46, 49–51]. The overall incidence of *EGFR* mutations in NSCLC ranges from 12.1 % to 49 %, depending on the patient population [37, 46, 49–51]. Tyrosine kinase domain mutations of *EGFR* are rare in non-lung tumors [28].

The exon 19 deletions and L858R substitution are activating mutations that result in increased phosphorylation of EGFR independent of ligand stimulation [11, 28, 29, 52]. These mutant EGFRs have greater affinity for TKIs and are susceptible to inhibition by TKIs in vitro [34, 52]. Politi et al. and Ji et al. each showed that expression of either the exon 19 deletion or L858R substitution mutation in *EGFR* causes adenocarcinoma to develop in mice and that the tumors regressed when either expression of the mutant gene was blocked or erlotinib was administered [33–35, 53]. Greulich et al. obtained similar results in cell cultures and confirmed that these mutations result in constitutive ligand-independent receptor activation, which is further enhanced by the addition of ligand stimulation [54]. In summary, *EGFR* genes specifically with activating mutations produce EGFR that demonstrates ligand-independent stimulation of downstream growth and survival pathways that produce the malignant phenotype [5, 11, 33–35, 53, 55].

4.4.2.2 Clinical Characteristics of Patients with *EGFR* Mutations

Since the discovery that NSCLCs with *EGFR* mutations may be more responsive to TKIs, the characteristics of patients and tumors harboring these mutations have been validated again and again. A compilation of data from 2,880 patients generated in the review by Mitsudomi et al. in 2007 shows that *EGFR* mutations are found in 32 % of Asians compared to 7 % of non-Asians, 38 % of females compared to 10 % of males, 47 % of never-smokers compared to 7 % of smokers, and 30 % of adenocarcinomas compared to 2 % of non-adenocarcinomas [29]. Many other studies have also found *EGFR* mutations to be significantly associated with females, Asian origin, never-smoking status, and adenocarcinoma histology [22, 36–38, 41, 42, 45, 46, 51, 56–58], which overlap with characteristics of patients who respond to TKIs [25]. From a different angle, smoking has been shown not to be a risk factor for *EGFR*-mutant NSCLC, whereas female sex is a significant risk factor [59]. A significant association between presence of *EGFR* mutation and younger age was even demonstrated by Eberhard et al. in the phase III TRIBUTE study [49]. Compared to white patients, African Americans are significantly less likely to have activating mutations of *EGFR* [60]. Among Korean patients with adenocarcinomas, the presence of *EGFR* mutations has not been shown to be associated with gender, smoking history, histological grade, age, bronchioloalveolar component, or stage [61]. Despite the statistical associations, it is important to remember that there will be exceptions to the rules. Park et al. in 2009 found that 3 of 20 male patients with squamous cell carcinoma of the lung had *EGFR* mutations, all of which responded to gefitinib, and, in addition, one of the *EGFR*-wild-type patients responded as well [38].

4.4.3 Histology of **EGFR**-*Mutant Tumors*

With respect to histology, it has been shown that, among adenocarcinomas that contain *EGFR* mutations, the majority are of terminal respiratory unit type [28, 62]. This subset of lung adenocarcinomas is characterized by cytologic resemblance to type II pneumocytes, Clara cells, or nonciliated bronchiolar cells [62]. Positive immunohistochemical staining for both thyroid transcription factor-1 and surfactant precursor protein B is a highly sensitive and specific method of identifying TRU-type lung adenocarcinomas [62]. *EGFR* mutations have also been identified in areas of atypical adenomatous hyperplasia, a preneoplastic lesion [62].

4.4.4 Relationship of Smoking Status to **EGFR** *Mutations*

The first molecular alteration that is actually found more often in non-smokers with NSCLC than in smokers is mutation of *EGFR* [28, 35]. Although some studies have shown a significant relationship between *EGFR* mutation presence and non-smoking status [6, 45, 56, 63, 64], and others have shown a trend toward lower *EGFR* mutation incidence with higher cumulative smoke exposure [29], not all studies have found a significant relationship between presence of *EGFR* mutation and smoking status [49, 61]. Even though a given never-smoker may be more likely to have an EGFR mutation than a smoker, *EGFR* mutations are still occasionally identified in smokers. Mitsudomi et al. in 2007 found *EGFR* mutations in 20 % of NSCLC from smokers, explaining that the reason *EGFR* mutations are found in a smaller percentage of tumors from smokers is that they are diluted by tumors arising from different smoking-induced mechanisms not usually present in never-smokers [30, 31, 35, 59]. To further investigate the relationship between smoke exposure and *EGFR* mutation status, Lee et al. examined the incidence of *EGFR* mutations in never-smokers with and without environmental tobacco smoke exposure, finding a significantly lower incidence of *EGFR* mutations in those with environmental tobacco smoke exposure than in those without. They also found a trend toward lower response to TKIs in patients with environmental tobacco smoke exposure compared to those without [64].

4.4.5 EGFR *Mutation as a Molecular Predictor of Response to TKIs*

The heart of determining the usefulness of *EGFR* mutation status as a predictive factor for response to TKIs lies in the clinical trials and retrospective studies investigating this relationship. In 2004, Lynch et al. was one of the first groups to demonstrate that *EGFR* mutations are associated with clinical response to gefitinib and to show in vitro that *EGFR* mutants were more sensitive to gefitinib. No mutations were present in patients who did not respond to gefitinib. In vitro, both the exon 19 deletion mutants and L858R mutants were more sensitive to gefitinib than tumors with wild-type *EGFR*. All eight mutants they identified were heterozygotes, indicating that these mutations act in a dominant manner (as do other oncogenes) [46]. Paez et al. promptly confirmed these results [41] and Pao et al. soon added that *EGFR* mutations were also identified in tumors sensitive to erlotinib [45]. Since then, many studies have confirmed association between *EGFR* mutation status and response to TKIs, and a review of the literature by Mitsudomi et al. in 2007 compiling data from 1,335 patients showed that EGFR TKI response was observed in 70 % of *EGFR* mutant tumors compared to only 10 % of patients with *EGFR* wild-type tumors [15, 29, 43, 58, 63, 65, 66]. In the phase II IDEAL trial, *EGFR* mutant tumors responded better to gefitinib than those with wild-type *EGFR* [58]. Kalikaki et al. demonstrated that patients with classic activating *EGFR* mutations treated with gefitinib had significantly longer median overall survival than those with wild-type EGFR. This relationship was not present in patients with other types of *EGFR* mutations [55]. Significantly higher objective tumor response to TKIs in *EGFR* mutants compared to wild-type has been demonstrated by several studies [37, 50, 65, 67], although others have found no relationship [42].

Differential response to treatment between the different types of *EGFR* mutations have been observed by some authors. Mitsudomi et al. reported that deletional mutations had higher response rates to gefitinib than other mutations, especially L858R [29]. Along those lines, Hirsch et al. found that patients who only had exon 19 deletions had significantly higher objective response than patients with exon 21 mutations [22]. On the contrary, Pao et al. found in vitro that wild-type *EGFR* and exon 19 deletion mutants responded similarly to gefitinib and erlotinib, whereas L858R mutants were about 10 times as sensitive [45]. As of yet, there has been no report of response to TKIs in a patient with an exon 20 insertion [29].

Not all patients with activating mutations of *EGFR* respond to TKIs [68]. Conversely, some patients without *EGFR* mutations still respond to TKIs [7, 67, 68]. In 2009, Yoshioka et al. published a phase II prospective study with *EGFR* mutation status determination followed by erlotinib treatment and determined that *EGFR* wild-type tumors have "modest" response to erlotinib without irreversible toxicity [69]. Some of the mechanisms by which patients harboring *EGFR* mutations become resistant to TKI therapy are discussed later in this chapter.

4.4.6 EGFR *Mutation as Molecular Predictor of Response to Chemotherapy*

TKIs are not FDA approved for use as first-line therapy for NSCLC in the United States [36]. Because first-line therapy is limited to conventional chemotherapy (a doublet regimen: for example, cisplatin or carboplatin plus either docetaxel, paclitaxel, vinorelbine, gemcitabine, or irinotecan; other platinum combinations; or non-platinum combinations) [2–4, 13, 14] (as mentioned previously), naturally the impact of *EGFR* mutation status on response to initial chemotherapy has been investigated. Results of such studies have been conflicting, with many studies reporting no association, while Hotta et al. showed that *EGFR* mutations were associated with longer overall and progression-free survival but not better response to front-line chemotherapy (consisting of various regimens, including both platinum- and non-platinum based) and other studies showed that only patients who carried deletions in exon 19 of *EGFR* had response to initial chemotherapy [15, 55]. Kalikaki et al. found a higher objective response rate to initial chemotherapy (particularly platinum-based regimens) in patients with classic activating EGFR mutations compared to wild-type *EGFR* [55]. First-line cytotoxic chemotherapy response was not correlated with *EGFR* mutation status in the study by Yoshida et al. (the exact chemotherapy regimens were not specified in this study) [69].

4.4.7 *TKIs Versus Chemotherapy in* EGFR *Mutant Tumors*

Although many studies have shown a benefit of erlotinib over placebo in *EGFR-mutation* positive patients, differential responses between TKIs and conventional chemotherapy have been more difficult to demonstrate. In the phase III TRIBUTE study, erlotinib did not provide any survival, objective response rate, time to progression, or duration of response advantage over carboplatin plus paclitaxel alone in *unselected* patients [44, 49]. Similarly, gefitinib did not provide any survival advantage compared to docetaxel in unselected patients or subgroups with clinical characteristics associated with *EGFR* mutations or *EGFR* mutations themselves in the phase III INTEREST trial [47]. However, patients with *EGFR*-mutant tumors had significantly improved objective response rate compared to wild-type tumors when treated with erlotinib plus carboplatin plus paclitaxel in the TRIBUTE study [49]. There was even a non-significant trend toward better response to erlotinib plus carboplatin plus paclitaxel compared to carboplatin plus paclitaxel alone in *EGFR-mutant* patients [49]. Regardless of treatment arm in this study, patients with *EGFR*-mutant tumors had significantly better response rate and longer median time to progression than those with wild-type tumors [49]. The randomized, placebo-controlled INTACT trials did not show added benefit from gefitinib in addition to chemotherapy alone in unselected patients [58]. In at least one study, higher objective response rate was observed in *EGFR* mutation-positive patients treated with gefitinib compared to docetaxel, although mutation status did not predict better survival [70].

4.4.8 *Impact of* EGFR *Mutation on Survival*

Impact of *EGFR* mutation status on treatment response is of great importance, but may have little meaning to patients unless there is a concomitant impact on survival. Longer median survival (but not progression-free survival) after first-line chemotherapy was observed in patients with *EGFR* mutations [71]. Overall and progression-free survival following first-line chemotherapy were also significantly longer in patients with *EGFR*-mutant tumors than in those with wild-type *EGFR* in the study by Hotta et al. [15]. With respect to TKI (gefitinib) treatment, use of this agent as first- or second-line therapy resulted in significantly longer progression-free survival in *EGFR*-mutant patients than in those treated with chemotherapy [71]. In a series of 397 patients by Kosaka et al. in 2009, patients with *EGFR* mutations survived significantly longer than those with wild-type mutations, with no survival difference between exon 19 deletion and L858R substitution [51].

4.4.9 *Molecular Prognostic Value of* EGFR *Mutations*

Because subset analyses of the TRIBUTE and INTACT trials have shown that better response was observed in patients with *EGFR* mutations patients even on chemotherapy alone (not just with chemotherapy plus TKI), it has been argued that *EGFR* mutations are prognostic factors instead of predictive [35, 49, 58]. Other studies have confirmed that patients with *EGFR* mutations (or clinical characteristics classically associated with *EGFR* mutations) have longer survival on chemotherapy even without TKIs [47, 49, 55, 58, 71]. Marks et al. found a trend toward longer overall survival in patients with *EGFR* mutations and stage I disease compared to patients with *EGFR* wild-type or *KRAS*-mutant tumors [72]. On the other hand, both Kosaka et al. and Shigematsu et al. showed that *EGFR* mutation was not a significant prognostic factor in patients treated with surgery alone [35, 51, 57]. In 2009, Kosaka et al. again showed in their series of 397 patients that neither the exon 19 deletion nor the L858R substitution mutation was an independent prognostic factor [51]. It has been suggested that, because of the characteristics of patients who tend to have *EGFR* mutations, they have better prognosis regardless of treatment given [7, 47].

4.4.10 *Sensitivity of* EGFR *Mutation Detection Methods*

As important as detection of *EGFR* mutations may be for patients with NSCLC, currently implemented detection methods may be missing a large portion of positive cases. Hirsch et al. compared two methods to detect *EGFR* mutations: direct sequencing and amplification refractory mutation system analysis (ARMS). ARMS uses allele-specific PCR to detect the exon 21 L858R point mutation and the most common exon 19 deletion (del G2235-A2249). They concluded that ARMS is more sensitive than sequencing (for detecting the most common mutations) because 10 of the 17 mutations detected by ARMS were missed by sequencing. However, since sequencing is not restricted to detecting specific known mutations, it identified overall 10 different mutations that were missed by ARMS; therefore, it is useful in detecting novel or uncommon mutations [37].

4.5 *EGFR* Gene Copy Number

4.5.1 *Background and Clinical Associations with* EGFR *Amplification*

EGFR gene copy number has also been investigated for its possible predictive and prognostic values in NSCLC. In general, a gene's copy number may be increased as a result of true amplification or it may accompany polysomy of its entire chromosome. Gene copy number in either case is determined using fluorescence in-situ hybridization (FISH) [73, 74]. The frequency of FISH positivity for *EGFR* ranges from 30 % to 50 % in NSCLCs and is more frequent in older patients and women in some studies [22, 37, 50, 58, 60, 63, 70]. In the IDEAL and INTACT trials, the demographic characteristics that are similar between patients with *EGFR* mutations and those that respond to TKIs (female, never-smokers, adenocarcinoma, Asian origin) were not associated with *EGFR* amplification [58]. In one study, *EGFR* FISH positivity was observed significantly more often in African Americans than whites, which was entirely attributable to the cases with high polysomy [60]. Never-smokers have been shown to more often have high *EGFR* gene copy numbers than smokers [22, 63, 70].

4.5.2 *Relationship Between* EGFR *Mutation and Amplification*

Scholl et al. reported on a significant relationship between *EGFR* gene amplification and exon 19 deletions [75]. In a study of 99 pulmonary adenocarcinomas from chemotherapy-naïve, never-smoking east Asian women, significantly more exon 19 deletions were present in tumors with *EGFR* amplification than in those with *EGFR* disomy or low or high polysomy [75]. Further, only the mutated, not the wild-type allele, was amplified [75]. They concluded that *EGFR* amplification only occurs in tumors with exon 19 deletions of *EGFR* and not other types of mutations or wild-type *EGFR* [75]. Other studies have found other mutations associated with *EGFR* amplification; however, in patients treated with prior chemotherapy [75], gene amplification is more often associated with *EGFR* mutations than is polysomy [73].

They further reported that, in tumors with exon 19 deletions, constitutive activation of EGFR occurs only in the presence of amplification [75]. In cells with the L858R substitution, constitutive activation was observed regardless of gene amplification [75]. Other studies have confirmed association between *EGFR* mutation of unspecified type and *EGFR* FISH positivity [63, 66, 67]. Increased EGFR expression by immunohistochemistry (IHC) was also significantly associated with FISH positivity but not mutation status [63, 76].

4.5.3 EGFR *FISH: Criteria and Special Considerations*

Varella-Garcia et al. have proposed the following criteria to define FISH positivity for *EGFR*: at least 40 % of the cells must have at least 4 copies of the *EGFR* signal, or the *EGFR* to centromere enumeration probe for chromosome 7 (CEP7) ratio must be at least two (averaged over all nuclei), or there must be gene clusters (at least 4 spots) in at least 10 % of tumors cells, or there must be at least 15 copies of the *EGFR* gene in at least 10 % of the tumor cells [74]. The result is equivocal if none of the above criteria is met but at least 25 % of the cells have at least four signals; in this case, if a second reviewer calls it positive, it is reported as positive; otherwise the test is reported as negative [74].

Several reports state that TKIs may benefit patients with either *EGFR* amplification or 7p polysomy. However, gene amplification is more often associated with *EGFR* mutations than is polysomy [73]. Since the two mechanisms of increased *EGFR* gene copy number may have different predictive values, a method has been proposed to more reliably distinguish true gene amplification from chromosome 7 polysomy. The *EGFR* gene itself lies on chromosome 7p12, which is close enough to the centromere of chromosome 7 that gene amplification of this region may also amplify parts of the centromere, giving the false impression that the whole chromosome has been duplicated (polysomy 7). The 7q31 region is sufficiently far from both the centromere and the *EGFR* locus that identification of this region may help distinguish signals from *EGFR* amplification and signals from the centromere [73].

4.5.4 Molecular Predictive Value of EGFR *Gene Copy Number Versus Mutation*

Most of the studies assessing the predictive value of *EGFR* amplification compare this to the predictive value of *EGFR* mutation. Capuzzo et al. were the first to report that survival following gefitinib was best predicted by increased *EGFR* gene copy number compared to *EGFR* mutation status or EGFR expression by IHC [29, 44, 63]. At least three other groups found *EGFR* gene copy number to be a better predictor of response to TKIs than *EGFR* mutation status [29, 35, 37, 42, 44, 71, 77]. In one study, *EGFR* FISH positivity was even associated with significant survival benefit from erlotinib, which was not observed for tumors with wild-type *EGFR*, mutant *EGFR*, or those that were *EGFR* FISH-negative [50]. A significantly better response to gefitinib compared to docetaxel was seen in patients with high *EGFR* gene copy number in another study, although gene copy number was not associated with better survival in this study [70].

In the Hirsch study, patients whose tumors were *EGFR* negative by both FISH and IHC had poor response to gefinitib regardless of *EGFR* mutation status. Inversely, patients positive for *EGFR* by both FISH and IHC had excellent outcome independent of *EGFR* or *KRAS* mutations. These findings suggest that *EGFR* gene copy number is a better predictor of response to gefitinib than *EGFR* mutation status [22, 35, 37, 71]. Hirsch et al. determined that the combination of *EGFR* gene copy number and protein expression by IHC is the most predictive of response to gefitinib and concluded that "*EGFR* gene copy number is a predictor of survival benefit with gefitinib compared with placebo" [22, 37]. Takano et al. found after multivariate analysis that response to gefitinib in Japanese patients could be predicted by either high *EGFR* gene copy number or *EGFR* mutation alone but pointed out that the significance of increased copy number is clouded by the observation that mutation presence predicts response whether increased copy number is present or not [67].

On the other hand, at least three groups found *EGFR* mutation status to be a better predictor of response to TKIs than *EGFR* gene copy number [43, 66, 68, 71]. Variations in the demographics of the study populations may be partly responsible for the conflicting results. In fact, Gerber has pointed out that *EGFR* gene copy number seems to have more predictive value in Caucasian populations (who have low *EGFR* mutation frequency) [42, 63], whereas *EGFR* mutation status holds more predictive value in East Asian populations (who have higher *EGFR* mutation frequency) [36, 42, 58, 63, 67].

Not all studies have found evidence to support the predictive role of *EGFR* FISH positivity. Both the INTEREST and INVITE phase III studies failed to show association of *EGFR* FISH positivity with prediction of benefit from gefitinib compared to chemotherapy [47, 60, 78]. Although *EGFR* FISH positivity was associated with TKI response in univariate analysis in the studies by Han et al. in 2006 and Ichihara et al. in 2007, in multivariate analysis, the only factor that independently predicted both response and survival from gefitinib was gefitinib-sensitive *EGFR* mutation [35, 43, 66, 71]. Further, while *EGFR* FISH positivity may predict response to TKIs, it has no predictive value for response to chemotherapy [76].

4.5.5 Molecular Prognostic Value of EGFR *FISH Positivity*

In contrast to its association with favorable response to TKIs, *EGFR* FISH positivity may be a negative prognostic factor [7, 63, 76]. Zhu et al. in 2008 found that *EGFR* FISH positivity was a poor prognostic marker by multivariate analysis [50]. Sholl et al. also found significantly worse outcome (shorter disease-free survival and higher stage at presentation) in patients with *EGFR* amplification [75]. In the Hirsch study, there was a nonsignificant trend toward worse outcome in patients with high *EGFR* gene copy number compared to low gene copy number in the placebo group [22]. To reiterate, this is in contrast to the better outcome predicted by EGFR FISH positivity in patients treated with gefitinib [37]. Tsao et al. and Dziadziuszko et al. did not find *EGFR* gene copy number to have prognostic value [42, 76]. However, at least one study has suggested a contradictory prognostic implication of *EGFR* FISH positivity [77].

4.6 EGFR Protein Expression Levels

4.6.1 Background

The last mechanism of increased EGFR activity to be discussed is protein overexpression, determined using IHC. Up to 90 % of NSCLCs strongly express EGFR protein by IHC [37, 70, 79], more frequently in squamous cell carcinomas than in adenocarcinomas [39, 40, 76], which is notably the opposite histologic association found with *EGFR* mutations. Although the overexpression of wild-type EGFR does not result in the malignant phenotype [31, 53], and many studies have not demonstrated a relationship between EGFR protein expression and response to TKIs [27, 39, 47, 79, 80], other studies have shown better response to TKIs in tumors expressing EGFR by IHC [7, 22, 37, 42, 44, 50, 63].

Ethnicity-associated EGFR genotypes may underlie some of the predictive value of EGFR overexpression. *EGFR* gene transcriptional activity and EGFR expression are related to the number of CA repeats contained in intron 1, with a higher number of repeats correlating with lower *EGFR* transcription, lower levels of EGFR mRNA, and lower EGFR protein expression [7, 81, 82]. The 20-repeat allele has only approximately 20 % the EGFR transcription activity of the 16-repeat allele [7, 81, 83]. Assuming for a moment that EGFR protein expression may affect response to TKIs, differences in the number of CA repeats may account for some of the racial differences in response to TKIs in EGFR-positive tumors; for example, higher response rates in Japanese patients treated with TKIs may be because in Asia the 20-repeat allele is the most common, whereas Caucasians and African Americans more commonly have the 16-repeat allele [7, 61, 83].

4.6.2 Molecular Predictive and Prognostic Value of EGFR Overexpression

Based on evidence that activating mutations or amplification of *EGFR* predicts response to TKIs, one may suspect that EGFR overexpression may have similar predictive value. Indeed, Tsao et al. found expression of EGFR by IHC to be associated with response to erlotinib but not with survival [42]. Parra et al. also found that, within a subset of patients with adenocarcinoma, response to gefitinib was significantly associated with high EGFR expression by IHC [39]. Whereas some authors have suggested that EGFR overexpression by IHC may predict response to TKIs, the evidence that overexpression may be related to response to conventional chemotherapy is limited [76, 84]. Comparing response to a TKI and conventional chemotherapy, there was no differential survival between gefitinib treatment and docetaxel treatment with respect to EGFR expression status in the phase III INTEREST trial [47]. Evidence for any predictive value of EGFR overexpression is sparse; in fact, it has been reported that EGFR overexpression actually correlates more with the occurrence of skin toxicity resulting from TKIs than to response of the tumor [7]. Although at least one study demonstrated significant poor prognostic value of high EGFR expression by IHC [39], neither the predictive nor the prognostic value of EGFR protein expression has been established [39, 42, 63, 76, 79, 80, 85].

Results of studies comparing EGFR expression to therapy response are dependent on the method of protein detection (i.e., the specific antibody used), and such differences between studies may account for some of the conflicting results [39, 79]. Comparing results from four different antibody kits, Mathieu et al. found three kits to yield 80 % positivity in a series of cases, while the fourth kit yielded only 68 % positivity [79]. Additionally, biopsies were more often positive than surgical or cytology specimens using one particular kit, while metastases were more often negative than primary tumors using another kit [79].

4.7 *EGFR* Summary

Over time, differing opinions have existed on whether there is enough data to confirm the predictive value of *EGFR* mutations. In 2005, the authors of the TRIBUTE study believed that the use of *EGFR* mutation status as a marker predicting benefit to erlotinib plus chemotherapy was not clear because, although *EGFR* mutants had significantly better objective response rates than wild-type *EGFR* when treated with erlotinib plus carboplatin and paclitaxel, adding erlotinib to carboplatin plus paclitaxel did not improve response in *EGFR* mutants compared to carboplatin and paclitaxel alone [49]. Later publications have stated a more definitive predictive value, which likely arose from more and more data confirming the superiority of *EGFR* mutational analysis over IHC and FISH. In 2006, Han et al. found that, in multivariate analysis, the only factor that independently predicted both response and survival from gefitinib was gefinitib-sensitive *EGFR* mutations [35, 66]. Kalikaki et al. in 2009 went as far as to show that classical activating mutations of *EGFR* are an independent factor predicting response to first-line chemotherapy [55]. Thus, although amplification and overexpression of EGFR may have some predictive value, their analysis has not been employed clinically as often as mutation analysis.

Even though the presence of an activating mutation of *EGFR* may indicate that a patient is more likely to respond to TKIs, some patients without mutations do respond. With this in mind, a patient with a good performance status who does not respond to first-line chemotherapy may wish to pursue TKI therapy regardless of *EGFR* mutation status. EGFR testing can also help with estimating prognosis in some patients.

Testing is not warranted in all patients, especially when the test result (e.g. *EGFR* mutation status) is not going to change clinical management (e.g., administration of a TKI). Other patients who may not require testing for *EGFR* mutations include patients who come for second opinions and are already taking TKIs and showing response, patients with such poor performance status and for whom systemic therapy would not even be considered, and patients in whom initial biopsy material is insufficient for testing and risk of re-biopsy outweighs benefit. In addition, difficulties arise for patients who lack insurance or have insurance issues and thus may have difficulties paying for testing and/or treatment (Dr. Jhanelle Gray, telephone interview). For these types of issues, individuals should seek help from assistance programs.

In summary, patients with activating *EGFR* mutations are more likely to respond to TKI therapy and probably have improved prognosis independent of therapy.

4.8 Tyrosine Kinase Inhibitors

4.8.1 Adverse Effects of Tyrosine Kinase Inhibitors as Predictors of Response

As might be expected from its name, epidermal growth factor is critical for mediating differentiation and proliferation of keratinocytes, explaining why a rash often develops with its inhibition [31, 86, 87]. In some studies, the development of acneiform rash has been quite convincingly correlated with better tumor responses and improved overall and progression-free survival with TKI treatment, likely because skin toxicity is related to systemic drug concentration and activity [5, 80, 86, 88, 89]. There has also been a significant correlation between grade of rash and degree of tumor response to erlotinib [89]. Accordingly, some authors consider skin toxicity to be a predictive marker of response to TKIs [88].

4.8.2 Molecular Alterations Conferring Resistance to TKIs

Although many tumors with *EGFR* mutations initially respond to TKIs, disease progression invariably occurs (usually within 6–12 months), commonly by selective survival of tumor cells with acquired mutations conferring resistance to these agents

[29, 35, 90, 91]. Even small clones of tumor cells containing a mutation that confers resistance to TKIs may have a significant clinical impact [91, 92]. The following section discusses the mechanisms behind several molecular alterations that unfortunately predict resistance to TKI therapy.

4.8.2.1 T790M

The most common secondary *EGFR* mutation leading to TKI resistance is substitution of methionine in place of threonine at codon 790 (T790M), independently identified by Pao et al. and Kobayashi et al. in 2005 [35, 90, 93–95]. After identifying the presence of the T790M point mutation in a patient who was initially sensitive to gefitinib but later became resistant, Kobayashi et al. demonstrated in vitro that introducing the T790M mutation into previously gefitinib-sensitive NSCLC cells harboring either wild-type, exon 19 deletion, or L858R substitution *EGFR* genotypes induced resistance to gefitinib [94]. Pao et al. also demonstrated in vitro that NSCLC cells harboring the T790M mutation with otherwise wild-type or mutated *EGFR* (either exon 19 deletion or L858R substitution) did not respond to either erlotinib or gefitinib [93].

Structural analysis performed by Kobayashi et al. showed that the T790M point mutation of *EGFR* changes the tyrosine in the catalytic domain to methionine, which is bulkier and prevents erlotinib (and presumably gefitinib) from binding [7, 35, 94, 96]. Not only does the T790M mutation alter TKI binding, but it also enhances kinase activity of EGFR (when coupled with the L858R mutation), offering cells with this mutation a survival advantage [11, 29, 52, 97]. Another missense mutation, D761Y, has been reported to confer a milder degree of TKI resistance, which may still be clinically relevant [98]. Greater resistance to gefitinib is produced when the T790M mutation occurs on the same DNA strand as the *EGFR* activating mutation (L858R or exon 19 deletion) [99], which is the most common scenario [100]. This can be explained by understanding that only the mutant allele will code for the mutant, constitutively active EGFR; likewise, binding of TKIs to these mutant, constitutively active EGFRs will only be altered if the resistance mutation has occurred on the mutant allele.

The T790M point mutation has been identified in approximately 50 % of patients who had activating *EGFR* mutations and later acquired resistance to EGFR TKIs [35, 44, 91, 95, 96, 98]. Engelman et al. demonstrated in vitro that malignant cells with activating mutations of *EGFR* that are initially sensitive to gefitinib become resistant after prolonged exposure to gefitinib and may acquire the T790M mutation in *EGFR* [44, 99]. Even so, the question arises as to whether TKI treatment itself induces the resistance mutation or if it merely results in selection of resistant clones [96]. Considering that the T790M mutation is found in 0.5–3.6 % (depending on the sensitivity of the assay; highest with mutant-enriched PCR) of patients who have never been treated with TKIs [29, 91], it is likely that TKIs merely result in selection of resistant clones rather than induce the T790M mutation themselves [29, 91].

4.8.2.2 Exon 20 Insertion Mutation

The exon 20 insertion mutation of *EGFR* (D770insNPG) has been demonstrated by Greulich et al. to confer erlotinib and gefitinib resistance in vitro. Response was obtained, however, from the irreversible EGFR inhibitor CL-387,785 [54]. Two patients harboring this mutation (who incidentally were both never-smoking women with adenocarcinomas) both progressed despite gefitinib treatment [66]. Intermediate sensitivity to erlotinib or gefitinib was observed in G719S of exon 18. The authors suggested that sensitivity may be related to the specific mutation present [35, 44, 54].

4.8.2.3 Low PTEN Expression

Low phosphatase and tensin homolog (PTEN) expression is a major reason why tumors become resistant to TKIs [101, 102]. PTEN normally functions to down-regulate the PI3K pathway (downstream of EGFR; mediates growth, proliferation, and survival). Loss of PTEN leads to persistent activation of the PI3K pathway independent of EGFR signaling, making this proliferation signal unresponsive to EGFR blockade [101, 102]. Bianco et al. demonstrated that, in gefitinib-resistant cells lacking PTEN, reconstitution of PTEN reversed EGFR-independent PI3K pathway activity and restored gefitinib sensitivity [102]. Zhuang et al. demonstrated that irradiating TKI-resistant tumors with low PTEN expression may help reverse the resistance by increasing PTEN expression levels [101]. Although low PTEN expression may induce resistance to TKIs, there may not be a relationship between PTEN expression and survival [27].

4.8.2.4 MET Amplification

Some authors have reported acquired resistance to EGFR TKIs in tumors with MET amplification [29, 99, 103]. It has also been suggested that MET activation (which may be induced by hepatocyte growth factor binding, overexpression, or structural alterations) may be used in place of MET amplification to determine sensitivity to TKIs [103]. The results of an in vitro study by Rho et al. suggested that sensitivity to TKIs was not associated with MET activation in the absence of MET amplification [103].

4.8.3 Methods to Overcome Resistance Mutations

Methods to overcome T790M-induced EGFR TKI resistance are of clinical interest. Murine and in vitro studies reveal some agents that may be beneficial. Although T790M makes cells resistant to gefitinib and erlotinib (which are reversible TKIs), the effect of irreversible TKIs (which covalently bind the EGFR kinase domain) is not changed by T790M. Irreversible TKIs include EKB-569, HKI-272, CI-1033, CL-387,785, and BIBW2992 [29, 94, 96, 98, 99]. The irreversible EGFR inhibitor CL-387,785 inhibits EGFR and downstream molecules more potently than gefitinib or erlotinib in cells harboring the T790M mutation, although not nearly to the degree that would be observed in cells without the T790M mutation [94, 99, 103]. Regales et al. demonstrated in mice that tumors harboring the T790M TKI resistance mutation had the most shrinkage (and complete response in most tumors) when treated with a combination of two drugs: BIBW-2992 (which is an irreversible EGFR TKI) and cetuximab (which is an EGFR-specific antibody). This combination resulted in lower total and phosphorylated EGFR. Neither agent alone induced complete response in any of the tumors in the study [90]. Another study has shown that, in mouse xenograft models of NSCLC with *EGFR* T790M mutations, CUDC-305 (a heat-shock protein 90 inhibitor) inhibits tumor growth [104].

Blocking signaling molecules downstream of EGFR has the potential to overcome resistance induced by a variety of mutations that alter binding of drugs to EGFR [53, 105]. Src is one such downstream signaling molecule that is vital to maintaining the malignant phenotype of *EGFR* mutant cells [53]. In vitro, Src inhibitors have been shown to prevent oncogenesis caused by *EGFR* mutations, suggesting that these may be of clinical benefit in TKI-resistant *EGFR*-mutated NSCLCs [53]. Faber et al. demonstrated in vitro that blocking two major pathways downstream from EGFR resulted in tumor shrinkage even in cell lines with various TKI resistance mutations including T790M [105].

4.9 Excision-Repair Cross-Complementation Group 1 (ERCC1)

4.9.1 Background

Whereas most of the discussion on molecular predictive factors in NSCLC has focused on response to TKIs, the ERCC1 enzyme may predict resistance to platinum-based therapy [7, 106–109]. Overexpression of ERCC1 occurs in 31–68 % of NSCLCs and is significantly associated with older age, squamous cell rather than adenocarcinoma histology, and pleural invasion [2, 13, 106, 110–112]. ERCC1 repairs platinum-DNA adducts (which cause inter- and intra-strand cross links) caused by platinum-based agents in cancer cells [7, 13, 106, 112–114]. This enzyme first recognizes the DNA damage and then removes the damaged nucleotides [115]. If the defects caused by the cytotoxic agent are not repaired, the cell will undergo apoptosis, which is, of course, the goal of administration of anti-cancer therapy. Through its DNA-repair action, ERCC1 reverses damage caused by certain chemotherapeutics on cancer cells, thus providing resistance to their anti-cancer effects [13, 113, 114, 116]. It is the expression level of ERCC1 that has been studied for its predictive value, since it has been established that ERCC1 mRNA levels correlate with DNA repair capacity [117].

4.9.2 Evidence for Molecular Predictive Value of ERCC1

Based on its normal biological function, ERCC1 has been studied for its relationship to chemotherapy resistance. In a phase III trial, patients were prospectively randomized to either a control arm, where all patients were treated with docetaxel plus cisplatin regardless of ERCC1 mRNA level, or a genotypic arm, where patients with low ERCC1 mRNA received docetaxel plus cisplatin. Those with high ERCC1 mRNA received docetaxel plus gemcitabine. The objective response rate was significantly higher in patients assigned to the genotypic arm than in those in the control arm group [65, 118]. It is interesting to note that patients in the genotypic arm responded better, even though gemcitabine was used for patients with high ERCC1 expression, which is correlated with high RRM1 expression. High RRM1 expression has been shown to predict resistance to gemcitabine treatment (to be discussed further in the following section) [118]. The results of this study clearly demonstrate the clinical utility of ERCC1 mRNA levels for determination of appropriate chemotherapy regimen for patients with advanced NSCLC [118].

Many other studies have confirmed better response or survival following chemotherapy for NSCLC in patients with low ERCC1 expression. The IALT study demonstrated that patients with ERCC1-negative tumors had prolonged survival with adjuvant cisplatin, whereas those with ERCC1-positive tumors did not, suggesting that adjuvant cisplatin-based chemotherapy may be beneficial in completely resected ERCC1-negative NSCLCs [1, 2, 106]. Ikeda et al. drew similar conclusions from their study [2]. Ceppi et al. also found higher median survival time in chemotherapy-treated patients with low ERCC1 mRNA than in those with high [85]. Azuma et al. found longer median progression-free and overall survival in carboplatin/paclitaxel-treated patients with ERCC1-negative tumors compared to those with ERCC1-positive tumors [110]. Further, significantly longer progression-free survival was seen in patients with tumors negative for both ERCC1 and class III beta tubulin compared with tumors positive for either or both of these markers [110]. A randomized, phase III trial found a significant association between expression levels of ERCC1 and response to gemcitabine, although no relation to survival was appreciated [119]. Wang et al. negatively correlated ERCC1 expression with tumor response to platinum-based chemotherapy, concluding that it may be a useful marker to predict response to platinum-based chemotherapy in Chinese patients with advanced NSCLC [120]. Lee et al. found ERCC1 expression to be significantly associated with shorter overall survival in patients with advanced NSCLC treated with platinum-based chemotherapy [111]. At least two groups found low ERCC1 mRNA levels to correlate significantly with longer median overall survival but not with tumor response to platinum-based chemotherapy in patients treated with these chemotherapeutics [30, 65, 121]. Other studies have failed to find a relationship between expression of ERCC1 and response to platinum-containing agents altogether [108, 121–123]. The collective evidence suggests ERCC1 expression may be a useful predictive factor indicating resistance of NSCLCs to platinum-based chemotherapy [1]. On the contrary, many other studies [1, 106, 124] have shown that high rather than low ERCC1 mRNA correlated with longer survival in untreated patients [30].

4.9.3 Molecular Predictive Value of ERCC1 Polymorphisms

Some polymorphisms in the *ERCC1* gene are associated with differential response to platinum-based agents [7, 106–108, 117]. Such differences may be attributable to variation in ERCC1 mRNA levels, mRNA stability, or protein function, depending on the genotype [107, 108]. It has been demonstrated that patients with polymorphic *ERCC1* genes (harboring either CT or TT genotype at codon 118) had significantly shorter survival and time to progression following docetaxel-cisplatin treatment compared to those with the wild-type (CC) genotype [108, 117]. Response to docetaxel-cisplatin, on the other hand, was not associated with *ERCC1* genotype [108]. On the other hand, Zhou et al. did not find any relationship between polymorphisms in codon 118 and survival following treatment with platinum-based chemotherapy [107]. In their study, a different polymorphism, C8092A, was associated with lower survival in patients with stage III disease treated with platinum-based chemotherapy, with significantly lower survival seen for each 8092A allele present [107]. The total number of variant alleles between *ERCC1* and *XRCC1* (possible 0–4) also correlated with overall survival among non-smoking Han Chinese women with stage III or IV adenocarcinoma (the greater the number of variant alleles, the shorter the median survival time) [117]. Tibaldi et al. found that patients with the *ERCC1* C118T genotype and treated with cisplatin-gemcitabine had significantly better clinical benefit, but there was no association with treatment response, time to progression, or survival [125].

Evidence supporting the role of *ERCC* genes in NSCLC carcinogenesis comes from the observation that some *ERCC* genotypes impart a higher risk for development of adenocarcinomas. Yin et al. found that non-smoking women who are heterozygous or homozygous for the 751C variant allele of *ERCC2* have a significantly higher risk of developing lung adenocarcinoma compared to homozygous wild-type. Heterozygous variant alleles of *ERCC1* 118 did not correlate with increased risk of development of adenocarcinoma but combining the heterozygous/homozygous group did reach significance. Some other studies have either not confirmed these results or have suggested the opposite relationship [115].

4.9.4 Molecular Prognostic Value of ERCC1 Expression

In contrast to the negative impact that high ERCC1 expression has on platinum-based-chemotherapy-treated patients, higher ERCC1 expression is actually significantly associated with *longer* median survival in patients not treated with chemotherapy [1, 106, 124]. These data suggest that high ERCC1 expression may be a favorable prognostic marker [1]. Other groups have also found positive prognostic value from ERCC1 expression [13, 85, 126]. A possible explanation for the favorable prognostic association is that patients with higher DNA-repair capacity may be less likely to relapse following surgical treatment, as fewer oncogenic mutations may be allowed to occur [13, 124]. In some studies, ERCC1 expression did not have any molecular prognostic value [1, 106, 127].

4.9.5 ERCC1 Summary

High expression of ERCC1, which functions to repair platinum-DNA adducts, predicts resistance of NSCLCs to platinum-based chemotherapeutics (which are first-line agents). Determination of ERCC1 levels would seem to hold the most value in patients with poor performance status who would be likely to suffer the most risk from taking systemic therapy that is unlikely to help. Polymorphisms in the *ERCC1* gene, which alter the expression levels or function, correlate with resistance of NSCLCs through their relationship to the level of repair activity by ERCC1. Although high expression of ERCC1 counteracts the effects of platinum-based chemotherapeutics, a high degree of DNA repair activity should naturally be beneficial and could conceivably reduce the risk of development of additional tumors in the future. This may account for the favorable prognosis observed in NSCLC patients with high ERCC1 expression who are not treated with chemotherapy.

4.10 Ribonucleotide Reductase (RRM1)

4.10.1 Background

Ribonucleotide reductase, constitutively expressed in all dividing cells, is responsible for converting ribonucleotides into deoxyribonucleotides via a reduction reaction [128], which is the rate-limiting step in *de novo* deoxyribonucleoside triphosphate (dNTP) biosynthesis [129, 130]. Ribonucleotide reductase is composed of two subunits, designated R1 and R2, each with a specific function in nucleotide synthesis. The R1 subunit is encoded by the *RRM1* gene, and the two closely-related R2 subunits are encoded by the *RRM2* and *RRM2b (p53R2)* genes, respectively [129, 131, 132]. The larger R1 subunit is considered the catalytic and regulatory site, whereas the smaller R2 subunit contains two iron moieties used in the generation of free radicals, important in the reduction of the hydroxyl group of the ribose sugar [67, 128, 129, 132]. The *p53R2* gene is induced by p53 expression, which occurs in the presence of DNA damage; thus, p53R2 is an important mediator of p53-regulated DNA repair [67, 129, 132]. As the rate-limiting step in dNTP synthesis, activity of ribonucleotide reductase ultimately determines the relative intracellular concentrations of the four dNTPs, which is controlled through a specificity site on the R1 subunit [129, 133–136]. As such, ribonucleotide reductase is critical to maintaining replication fidelity, considering that higher rates of base misinsertion and lower proofreading activity during DNA replication occur when nucleotide concentrations are abnormal [129, 135, 136]. This suggests that overexpression of ribonucleotide reductase may cause abnormal nucleotide concentrations resulting in mutations, which may occur in growth regulatory genes [129, 135].

4.10.2 Role in Carcinogenesis

Overexpression of *RRM1* (which acts as a tumor suppressor gene) [129, 137–139] has been shown to reduce chemical carcinogenesis in the lung [129, 140] and prevent lung cancer metastases [137, 139, 141]. In contrast, overexpression of either *RRM2* or *p53R2* results in higher mutation rates in cultured cells and in the development of lung neoplasms in mice [129]. RRM2 overexpression in particular is associated with the largest tumor size, greatest tumor multiplicity, and the most pathologically advanced neoplasms [129]. The higher incidence of lung neoplasms in transgenic mice with *RRM2* or *p53R2* overexpression in the study by Xu et al. was accompanied by a particular activating *KRAS* mutation (codon 12 G to T transversion) in some of the neoplasms that was not found in neoplasms of control mice or transgenic mice overexpressing *RRM1* [129]. This suggests a different mechanism of mutagenesis and carcinogenesis in tumors that arise in the setting of *RRM2* or *p53R2* overexpression compared to *RRM1* overexpression or spontaneous development in wild-type mice [129]. Free radicals, a normal product of RRM2 activity, may have contributed to the development of the G to T transversions seen in the neoplasms of mice overexpressing these proteins in the Xu study [129]. p53R2, on the other hand, has antioxidant activity [141, 142] and might be expected to be protective against malignancy. In fact, it has been shown that p53R2 binds MAPK/ERK kinase 2 (MEK2) (and much less MEK1), preventing phosphorylation of MEK1/2 and likewise its downstream effector extracellular signal-regulated kinase-1/2 (ERK1/2), thereby inhibiting tumor cell transformation and invasion (considering that ERK1/2 activates cell motility and disrupts adhesions) [141].

4.10.3 Molecular Predictive Value of RRM1 Expression

RRM1 is expressed in approximately 40 % of NSCLC [143], and there has been no correlation between RRM1 mRNA levels and age, gender, performance status, or stage [144], although expression levels of RRM1 are significantly associated with expression of ERCC1 [85, 145]. Gemcitabine is an antimetabolite chemotherapeutic agent that competitively inhibits DNA polymerase as well as ribonucleotide reductase, thereby preventing DNA synthesis and cell division [47, 85, 144–148]. High levels of RRM1 expression overcome the antimetabolite effect of gemcitabine and therefore may be used as a predictive marker of gemcitabine resistance [1, 139, 146, 149, 150].

Conversely, lower expression has been associated with better survival after cisplatin plus gemcitabine combination [7, 109, 145, 151]. Indeed, higher expression of RRM1 by IHC has been associated with shorter overall and progression-free survival as well as lower disease control following gemcitabine treatment in cases of locally advanced or metastatic NSCLC [85, 144, 146]. This is in contrast to the survival-enhancing effect that high RRM1 expression has on early stage NSCLC following curative surgery, presumably for its ability to repair DNA damage and prevent recurrence [139, 146, 152]. Bepler et al. in 2006 also showed that there is a positive relationship between the expression of RRM1 and resistance of NSCLC to gemcitabine plus platinum combination therapy [150]. Since expression of RRM1 and ERCC1 are correlated, it is worthy of mention that the relationship between ERCC1 and resistance to this chemotherapeutic regimen was similar, although to a lesser degree [150]. Bepler et al. confirmed the results of previous studies that tumor shrinkage in response to gemcitabine was significantly inversely correlated with RRM1 expression [17]. In a study by Rosell et al., high RRM1 expression correlated with worse survival in patients treated with the gemcitabine/cisplatin combination, but had no significant impact on survival when vinorelbine was added to this combination [145]. Therefore, a gemcitabine/cisplatin combination could be used in patients with low RRM1 expression levels while vinorelbine could be added when RRM1 expression levels are high [145].

Many other studies have detected significant relationships between RRM1 expression and response or survival but did not find this to be an independent molecular predictive or prognostic factor. Wang et al. found RRM1 expression to correlate with poor tumor response, but this was not an independent predictive factor [143]. In cisplatin/gemcitabine-treated patients, longer median survival time was observed with low RRM1 expression compared to high RRM1 expression, although RRM1 expression was not an independent prognostic factor in this study [85]. Other studies have not demonstrated a relationship between RRM1 expression levels and response to cisplatin, carboplatin, or gemcitabine [122]. Souglakos et al. found RRM2 expression to be an independent predictor of response to docetaxel/gemcitabine in lung adenocarcinomas, but RRM1 had neither predictive nor prognostic value in this study [144]. Overall, the evidence is in support of the molecular predictive value of RRM1 expression-level determination.

4.10.4 Molecular Prognostic Value of RRM1 Expression

Bepler and colleagues have extensively researched the use of the RRM1 component of ribonucleotide reductase (located on chromosome 11p15.5) as a molecular predictive and prognostic marker for NSCLC [42, 149, 153]. Given the tumor suppressor activity of RRM1, it becomes clear how loss of heterozygosity of 11p15.5 (which is reportedly common in NSCLC) contributes to carcinogenesis and survivability of this cancer [42]. Sure enough, patients with NSCLC who only have one copy of the *RRM1* gene (instead of two) have shorter survival [1].

In addition to the above synthetic functions of RRM1, it has been proposed to also suppress cell migration, invasion, and metastasis through induction of PTEN expression [36, 81, 137, 139, 151–154]. In a 2004 study, Bepler et al. found that high RRM1 expression was strongly correlated with a better overall and disease-free survival in resectable NSCLC [153]. They concluded that the mechanism behind improved survival was that RRM1 acted as an inducer for, and in concert with, PTEN, a known tumor suppressor gene [153]. Therefore, high levels of both RRM1 and PTEN may impart a more favorable outcome in patients with resectable NSCLC [153].

In a related study in 2007, Zheng et al. examined tumor specimens from 187 patients with resectable, stage 1 NSCLC [139]. They quantitatively determined the levels of RRM1, PTEN, and ERCC1 and found that both the median disease-free and overall survival were significantly higher in patients with high expression of either RRM1 or ERCC1 [139]. Expression of RRM1 and ERCC1 are correlated, and patients with high expression of both proteins had significantly longer median overall and disease-free survivals than patients with high expression of only one or neither of the proteins [139, 151]. Of note, there was a lack of association between RRM1 and PTEN expressions in this study, which is in contrast to a prior study by Bepler et al. as described above [139, 151, 153].

4.10.5 RRM1 Single-Nucleotide Polymorphisms

As was discussed for ERCC1, single-nucleotide polymorphisms (SNPs) that have an impact on expression levels of a protein that has predictive or prognostic implications may be used as a surrogate to expression level determination. In one study, although there was no relationship between RRM1 mRNA levels or RRM1 SNPs and response to gemcitabine, one SNP located within the promoter region (C(−)37A) was associated with significantly longer progression-free survival following gemcitabine treatment [155]. Curiously, higher RRM1 expression levels have previously been associated with this particular SNP [155, 156]. The highest response to gemcitabine treatment has been associated with the RR37AC-RR524CT allelotype (found in 29.9 % of cases), which has been shown to be associated with low RRM1 expression in vitro [47, 157, 158]. With respect to platinum-based chemotherapy, the (−)524CT allelotype is associated with the highest response rate; again, this finding may be related to the expression level of RRM1, which was not assessed in this study [157]. In patients with resectable NSCLC, the allelotype associated with the highest promoter activity and thus RRM1 expression levels (RR37CC- RR524TT) was associated with the longest disease-free and overall survival [47, 158]. Although these results suggest that RRM1 genotype may have predictive or prognostic value, the above-mentioned SNPs do not seem to correlate with RRM1 expression levels in vivo, and therefore may harbor their predictive or prognostic value independent from correlation with expression levels [158].

4.10.6 RRM1 Summary

RRM1 catalyzes the rate-limiting step in nucleotide synthesis (which will be highly active in NSCLCs) and is competitively inhibited by the antimetabolite gemcitabine. Competitive inhibition is overcome by increased levels of RRM1 (found in 40 % of NSCLCs), which may be related to polymorphisms in thc *RRM1* gene. Studies have shown that NSCLCs with high RRM1 levels respond poorly to gemcitabine. RRM1 is thought to induce expression of the tumor suppressor PTEN, and this may account for the observation that high levels of RRM1 correlate with better survival in resectable NSCLC. Expression of RRM1 and ERCC1 are correlated, so it comes as no surprise that NSCLCs with high levels of RRM1 (and thus ERCC1) respond poorly to the combination of gemcitabine (which inhibits RRM1) and cisplatin (which causes DNA damage that ERCC1 can repair). It is promising that, in at least one study, adding vinorelbine to the gemcitabine/cisplatin combination eliminated the association of high RRM1 levels with poor tumor response [145].

4.11 KRAS

Ras proteins are plasma membrane-associated 21-kDa GTPases encoded by the *RAS* gene on chromosome 12p12.1 [159]. The family of *RAS* genes includes three subtypes: *HRAS*, *KRAS*, and *NRAS* [159]. Initially discovered as genes from human cancer cell lines that transformed mouse cells in vitro [159, 160], *HRAS* and *KRAS* were later found to be homologous to retroviral oncogenes (of the Harvey-rat sarcoma virus and Kirsten-rat sarcoma virus, respectively) [159, 161]. *NRAS* was later identified in human neuroblastoma cells [159, 162]. *KRAS* mutations, found in approximately 16 % of NSCLCs, account for the majority of *RAS* mutations in human lung cancers [11, 22, 37, 49, 50, 66, 70, 159, 163, 164]. In contrast to *RAS* genes present in normal tissue, those present in cancer usually possess a missense mutation in codon 12 or 13 (accounting for 97 % of *KRAS* mutations) or less commonly codon 61 [10, 159, 165]. These mutations impair the GTPase activity of the RAS protein, resulting in constitutive activation and perpetual transmission of downstream signals [10, 159, 166].

RAS proteins, initially activated following activation and autophosphorylation of EGFR, transmit signals through a variety of pathways with a wide array of seemingly antagonistic endpoints [159]. For example, the RAS-RAF-MEK-ERK pathway culminates in cell proliferation [159] and the PI3K/Akt, STAT3, and STAT5 pathways have anti-apoptotic effects [159], whereas RAS-related activation of p38, p53, and p16/INK4a leads to senescence [159, 167, 168]. It seems that p16 is not activated when Ras is only moderately activated (i.e., expressed at levels comparable to wild-type *KRAS*) [159, 169], allowing pathways favoring survival and proliferation to dominate, explaining the oncogenic effects of mutant *KRAS* [159, 167].

4.11.1 KRAS *Copy Number Gain*

As is the case with *EGFR*, *KRAS* is frequently amplified in NSCLC [159, 170, 171], with mutant allele-specific imbalance (MASI) occurring in 58 % of tumors with *KRAS* mutations [100, 159]. However, whereas the mechanism of MASI with *EGFR* is typically copy number gain, MASI with *KRAS* usually results from uniparental disomy of the mutant allele without copy number gain [100, 159]. Similar to *EGFR*, copy number gains of *KRAS* are found more frequently in tumors with mutant *KRAS* [100]. Found in only 10 % of 288 lung adenocarcinomas, *KRAS* copy number gains in the absence of *KRAS* mutations showed only a non-significant trend toward association with worse prognosis in the study by Soh et al. [100]. Although few studies have examined the impact of KRAS amplification, copy number gain, or MASI on treatment response or survival, it is known that higher levels of active, GTP-bound KRAS are found in tumors with either *KRAS* mutations or MASI; GTPase activity is highest when both alterations are present [100, 159].

4.11.2 KRAS *Mutation Background*

In 1984, the association between somatic *KRAS* mutations and lung carcinoma was discovered [159], and as early as 1990 it was reported that activating mutations of the *KRAS* oncogene indicated poor prognosis in NSCLC [29]. Mice with induced *KRAS* mutations prematurely develop tumors in many organs, especially the lung, where the tumors resembled well-differentiated human papillary adenocarcinomas of alveolar type II pneumocyte origin [172]. In contrast to *EGFR* mutations, which are identified in never-smoking women of Asian origin, *KRAS* mutations and copy number gains [100] tend to occur in Caucasians with smoking histories, although mutations in either oncogene are most commonly found in adenocarcinomas [7, 11, 29, 37, 49, 50, 159, 163]. With respect to histology, mucinous or goblet-cell patterns of bronchioloalveolar carcinoma more frequently harbor *KRAS* mutations than the non-mucinous type [159, 164, 173–175]. Tumors that are KRAS-dependent tend to be well-differentiated and have *KRAS* copy number gain and KRAS overexpression [159, 176]. Even though they did not find a significant association between *KRAS* mutation status and smoking history or cumulative smoke exposure, Riely et al. found that *KRAS* mutations in smokers were significantly more often G to T or G to C transversions rather than the G to A transitions found in never smokers, providing further evidence of distinct molecular alterations in lung cancers of smokers [10].

4.11.3 *Molecular Predictive Value of* KRAS *Mutations*

Strategies to block mutant *KRAS* signaling in NSCLC have not been met with success [100, 176], because unlike the case of *EGFR* mutations, tumors with mutant *KRAS* are not always dependent upon KRAS for signaling so that targeted blockade of KRAS results in little to no tumor shrinkage [159, 177]. Consequently, the molecular predictive value of *KRAS* mutations lies in their association with resistance to TKIs [55]. The first report of EGFR-TKI resistance in NSCLC patients with *KRAS* mutations was by Pao et al. in 2005 [35, 97]. Recalling the position of KRAS as a second-messenger of EGFR signaling, it becomes clear why constitutive activation of KRAS (such as by mutation) leads to proliferation independent of blockade of EGFR signaling at the level of EGFR itself. However since mutations of both *KRAS* and *EGFR* are found in the same patient [7, 11, 37, 50, 61, 66], it is debatable whether it is the presence of the *KRAS* mutation or the absence of an *EGFR* mutation that is responsible for the lack of response to TKIs in *KRAS*- mutant tumors [159]. In fact, among patients without *EGFR* mutation treated with first-line EGFR-TKIs, the *KRAS* status has no impact on overall survival [159, 177].

Supporting the role of *KRAS* mutation status in determining responsiveness clinically, in vitro evidence provided by Park et al. demonstrated that NSCLC cells with *KRAS* mutations are resistant to gefitinib. Furthermore, down-regulation of *KRAS* through lovastatin administration led to significantly more cytotoxicity compared to gefitinib alone in these resistant cells [38]. Most clinical studies have found lower response to TKIs and even conventional chemotherapy in *KRAS*-mutant tumors as well as decreased overall and progression-free survival in these patients [7, 10, 66, 92, 96]. Miller et al. demonstrated a significantly higher response rate to EGFR TKIs for wild-type *KRAS* patients compared to *KRAS* mutants [44, 68]. Patients with wild-type but not mutant *KRAS* derived significant survival benefit from erlotinib in the BR.21 study [50]. Adjuvant chemotherapy significantly prolonged survival in patients with tumors harboring wild-type *KRAS*, but it did not prolong survival in patients with mutant *KRAS* [2]. Many other studies showed nonsignificant trends toward decreased survival or decreased response to chemotherapy or TKIs in patients harboring *KRAS* mutations [37, 49, 77]. Other studies revealed no association between *KRAS* mutation status and response to TKIs or conventional chemotherapy whatsoever [22, 50, 51, 55, 70, 178].

Although there are conflicting opinions, *KRAS* mutation is generally accepted as a predictor of resistance to TKI therapy [10, 163]. Further, there is evidence that detection of *KRAS* mutations by methods more sensitive than direct sequencing has an even higher predictive value [92]. In the study by Marchetti et al., *KRAS* mutation detected by mutant-enriched sequencing was an independent predictive factor of response to TKIs [92]. The power of the results from the Marchetti study suggests that failure of some other groups to detect the predictive ability of *KRAS* mutations may lie in their failure to detect a large portion of the actual mutations themselves. In their own study, Marchetti et al. found that *KRAS* mutation status as detected by direct sequencing alone (the standard, less sensitive method) was not an independent predictive factor for resistance to TKIs; independent predictive value was only held by *KRAS* mutation status as detected by the more sensitive mutant-enriched sequencing (which in this study detected *KRAS* mutations in approximately twice as many tumors compared to direct sequencing). Highlighting the importance of mutations in minor clones, patients with tumors harboring *KRAS* mutations had the same survival outcome whether the mutation was detected by direct sequencing or by mutant-enriched sequencing alone, indicating that mutations detected by mutant-enriched sequencing alone are equally as clinically significant as those detected by both methods. The clinical impact of selection of minor clones harboring resistance mutations was discussed earlier [92].

4.11.4 **KRAS** *Summary*

In summary, *KRAS* mutations are useful in predicting resistance of NSCLCs to TKIs; further studies are required to determine the impact on response to conventional chemotherapy. Although tumors with *KRAS* copy number gain have higher levels of activated KRAS, suggesting that copy number gain may have molecular predictive value similar to that of *KRAS* mutation, the predictive value needs to be validated clinically. Finally, *KRAS* mutations are thought to hold negative prognostic value [11, 42, 49, 68, 96].

4.12 *ALK* Gene Rearrangements

4.12.1 Background

First linked to lung cancer when it was identified as a transforming agent from a pulmonary adenocarcinoma in 2007, the *ELM4-ALK* fusion gene (found in approximately 3.8 % of NSCLCs) has become of interest as a possible therapeutic target in NSCLC [179, 180]. It is interesting to note that the ELM4-ALK rearrangement in NSCLC was discovered in the same manner as Ras proteins originally (as transforming agents) [179]. The anaplastic lymphoma kinase (ALK; originally discovered in anaplastic lymphomas in 1994) [179, 181, 182] is a receptor tyrosine kinase that is a member of the insulin receptor family [179, 181, 183]. Similar to other receptor tyrosine kinases including EGFR, ligand binding triggers dimerization of ALK receptors followed by autophosphorylation and precipitation of downstream signals through the RAS-ERK, JAK3-STAT3, and PI3K/Akt pathways, which, as mentioned previously, affects cell proliferation, survival, and migration [179, 184]. A common rearrangement partner with ALK, echinoderm microtubule-associated protein-like 4 (ELM4) is a cytosolic protein critical to microtubule formation [179, 185, 186].

ALK (on chromosome 2p21) and *ELM4* (on chromosome 2p23) are located only 12.7 megabases apart [179]. Inversion of this part of the short arm of chromosome 2 [Inv(2)(p21p23)] creates a fusion between these two genes, with resultant disregulation of transcription and constitutive activation of ALK [179, 180]. At least 11 other variants of the ELM4-ALK rearrangement have been described [187], and *ALK* can also fuse with *TFG* and *KIF5B* in NSCLC [187–189]. Rearrangements of the ALK gene can be detected by FISH, IHC, or real-time polymerase chain reaction [179].

4.12.2 Demographic and Histologic Associations

Similar to the case with EGFR mutations, ALK rearrangements are usually found in adenocarcinomas of non- or light-smokers [179, 180, 187, 190–192], although the patients tend to be younger and with more advanced tumors [187, 190, 193]. Despite these similar clinicopathologic characteristics between EGFR mutations and ALK rearrangements, these molecular alterations are almost always mutually exclusive, which is also the case between ALK rearrangements and KRAS mutations [179, 187, 190–194]. Certain histologic patterns have been reported to be associated with ALK rearrangements in NSCLCs. In Asian populations, ALK-rearranged lung adenocarcinomas usually have an acinar pattern [187, 188, 193]. Approximately 60 % of ALK-rearranged lung adenocarcinomas in Western populations harbor solid growth patterns containing at least 10 % signet-ring cells, a pattern uncommonly found in ELM4-ALK wild type tumors [187, 191, 195].

4.12.3 Role in Carcinogenesis and Molecular Predictive Value

As is the case with constitutively active EGFR and KRAS, constitutively activated ALK resulting from the ELM4-ALK fusion leads to the development of adenocarcinomas in mice, which regressed upon administration of ALK inhibitors [179, 180, 194]. Recognition of ALK rearrangements in NSCLC led to the trial of the ALK inhibitor PF02341066 (crizotinib), which in one study led to partial response in 17 of 29 patients [179, 187, 196]. In contrast to EGFR, where the targeted therapy (TKIs) was first discovered followed by identification of EGFR mutations as the predictive factor, the discovery of ELM4-ALK rearrangement in NSCLC was followed by trials of targeted therapies. In vitro studies have shown crizotinib to stop growth in cancers harboring ALK translocations [187, 197, 198]. ALK rearrangements do not seem to predict response to platinum-based chemotherapy. In 12 patients with NSCLC containing ALK rearrangements, both response and survival following platinum-based chemotherapy were similar to results experienced by patients with *EGFR* mutations only or double-wild-type tumors [187, 191]. Response to erlotinib in patients with tumors containing ALK rearrangements was similar to that in patients lacking *EGFR* mutations [187, 191].

4.12.4 ALK Rearrangement Summary

Certain ALK rearrangements lead to constitutive activation of ALK, triggering downstream pathways that disregulate cellular growth and survival. Just like activating *EGFR* mutations, activating ALK rearrangements have been shown to cause pulmonary adenocarcinomas in mice. After the discovery of ALK rearrangements in some NSCLCs, trials with the ALK inhibitor crizotinib were initiated, the results of which are promising that ALK rearrangements may predict response to crizotinib.

4.13 Multidrug Resistance Proteins

Multidrug resistance proteins (MRPs) have been investigated for their possible predictive value in lung carcinoma. It is not yet clear whether MRPs have predictive or prognostic implications. Although Li et al. found that response to cisplatin correlated with expression of MRP1 and that higher MRP1 expression levels correlated with shorter progression-free and overall survival, MRP1 expression was not an independent prognostic factor [126]. In contrast, MRP1 did not predict response to cisplatin nor did it correlate with overall survival in the study by Filipits et al. [199]. Other reports have found worse outcome associated with MRP1 overexpression and at least one found longer overall survival [199]. RRM2 expression levels were an independent prognostic factor for completely resected NSCLC in one study, but it still did not predict response to cisplatin [199].

4.14 BRCA1

BRCA1 has been shown to correlate with risk of breast and ovarian cancer development in women [1, 7]. Much like ERCC1, BRCA1 is involved in nucleotide excision repair, one of the mechanisms for repairing platinum and alkylating agent-induced DNA adducts. In accordance with their related functions, expression of BRCA1 is significantly associated with expression of both ERCC1 and RRM1 (all of which are expressed at higher levels in squamous cell carcinoma) [1, 7, 127]. Dysfunctional BRCA1 may fail to repair damage induced by these chemotherapeutics, leading to drug sensitivity. This suggests that decreased BRCA1 function may serve as a predictive marker [7, 111, 139, 200, 201]. Some studies have demonstrated that patients with low BRCA1 expression have better response to neoadjuvant cisplatin-gemcitabine [1, 7, 120, 200, 201]. Other studies have not found any association between BRCA1 expression and tumor response to cisplatin-gemcitabine or epirubicin-gemcitabine [123]. The association of BRCA1 overexpression with poor prognosis was confirmed by Rosell et al. [127]. The true predictive and prognostic values of BRCA1 in NSCLC are not yet established.

4.15 p53

TP53 is the gene encoding the p53 tumor suppressor gene. Studies report varying associations of p53 expression and *TP53* mutations with treatment response and prognosis in NSCLC. In the JBR.10 study, p53 overexpression (demonstrated in 132/253 cases) was associated with significantly shorter overall survival. However, p53-positive tumors did benefit significantly from adjuvant chemotherapy, whereas p53-negative tumors did not [2]. In the study by Kosaka et al., *TP53* mutations were not associated with prognosis in Japanese patients with lung adenocarcinomas treated surgically [51].

4.16 Gene Expression Profiling

Given the wide array of molecular alterations that may impact on treatment response, gene expression profiling may hold the most promise for a comprehensive estimate of a given patient's response to treatment and prognosis. Gene expression profiling uses databases of expression profiles that are associated with sensitivity or resistance to various agents [7]. Potti et al. have developed a gene expression profile that estimates prognosis even more accurately than clinical or pathologic stage, which helps identify specifically high-risk patients from within stage 1A who may benefit from adjuvant chemotherapy [1, 202]. Chen et al. also found a five-gene panel (consisting of *DUSP6*, *MMD*, *STAT1*, *ERBB3*, and *LCK*) independently associated with both progression-free and overall survival in NSCLC [1, 203].

Acknowledgements We thank Dr. Jhanelle Gray, Assistant Member, Department of Thoracic Oncology and Experimental Therapeutics Program at Moffitt Cancer Center, for her help with the EGFR Summary.

References

1. Bepler G, Begum M, Simon GR (2008) Molecular analysis-based treatment strategies for non-small cell lung cancer. Cancer Control 15(2):130–139
2. Ikeda N, Nagase S, Ohira T (2009) Individualized adjuvant chemotherapy for surgically resected lung cancer and the roles of biomarkers. Ann Thorac Cardiovasc Surg 15(3):144–149
3. Kelly K et al (2001) Randomized phase III trial of paclitaxel plus carboplatin versus vinorelbine plus cisplatin in the treatment of patients with advanced non–small-cell lung cancer: a Southwest Oncology Group trial. J Clin Oncol 19(13):3210–3218
4. Schiller JH et al (2002) Comparison of four chemotherapy regimens for advanced non-small-cell lung cancer. N Engl J Med 346(2):92–98
5. Emery IF et al (2009) Response to gefitinib and erlotinib in non-small cell lung cancer: a retrospective study. BMC Cancer 9:333
6. Seike M et al (2009) MiR-21 is an EGFR-regulated anti-apoptotic factor in lung cancer in never-smokers. Proc Natl Acad Sci U S A 106(29):12085–12090
7. Mountzios G et al (2010) Histopathologic and genetic alterations as predictors of response to treatment and survival in lung cancer: a review of published data. Crit Rev Oncol Hematol 75(2):94–109
8. Helland A, Brustugun OT (2009) Lung cancer in smokers and never-smokers. Tidsskr Nor Laegeforen 129(18):1859–1862
9. Subramanian J, Govindan R (2008) Molecular genetics of lung cancer in people who have never smoked. Lancet Oncol 9(7):676–682
10. Riely GJ, Marks J, Pao W (2009) KRAS mutations in non-small cell lung cancer. Proc Am Thorac Soc 6(2):201–205

11. Rudin CM et al (2009) Lung cancer in never smokers: molecular profiles and therapeutic implications. Clin Cancer Res 15(18):5646–5661
12. Toh CK et al (2006) Never-smokers with lung cancer: epidemiologic evidence of a distinct disease entity. J Clin Oncol 24(15):2245–2251
13. Holm B et al (2009) Different impact of excision repair cross-complementation group 1 on survival in male and female patients with inoperable non-small-cell lung cancer treated with carboplatin and gemcitabine. J Clin Oncol 27(26):4254–4259
14. Sheth S (2010) Current and emerging therapies for patients with advanced non-small-cell lung cancer. Am J Health Syst Pharm 67(1 Suppl 1):S9–S14
15. Hotta K et al (2007) Clinical significance of epidermal growth factor receptor gene mutations on treatment outcome after first-line cytotoxic chemotherapy in Japanese patients with non-small cell lung cancer. J Thorac Oncol 2(7):632–637
16. Pignon JP et al (2008) Lung adjuvant cisplatin evaluation: a pooled analysis by the LACE Collaborative Group. J Clin Oncol 26(21):3552–3559
17. Bepler G et al (2008) Clinical efficacy and predictive molecular markers of neoadjuvant gemcitabine and pemetrexed in resectable non-small cell lung cancer. J Thorac Oncol 3(10):1112–1118
18. Toloza EM, Roth JA, Swisher SG (2000) Molecular events in bronchogenic carcinoma and their implications for therapy. Semin Surg Oncol 18(2):91–99
19. Hommura F et al (1999) Predictive value of expression of p16INK4A, retinoblastoma and p53 proteins for the prognosis of non-small-cell lung cancers. Br J Cancer 81(4):696–701
20. Mohamed S et al (2007) Prognostic implications of cell cycle-related proteins in primary resectable pathologic N2 nonsmall cell lung cancer. Cancer 109(12):2506–2514
21. Kim SJ et al (2010) Phosphorylated epidermal growth factor receptor and cyclooxygenase-2 expression in localized non-small cell lung cancer. Med Oncol 27(1):91–97
22. Hirsch FR et al (2007) Combination of EGFR gene copy number and protein expression predicts outcome for advanced non-small-cell lung cancer patients treated with gefitinib. Ann Oncol 18(4):752–760
23. Toffalorio F et al (2010) Expression of gemcitabine- and cisplatin-related genes in non-small-cell lung cancer. Pharmacogenomics J 10(3):180–190
24. Modjtahedi H, Essapen S (2009) Epidermal growth factor receptor inhibitors in cancer treatment: advances, challenges and opportunities. Anticancer Drugs 20(10):851–855
25. Shepherd FA et al (2005) Erlotinib in previously treated non-small-cell lung cancer. N Engl J Med 353(2):123–132
26. Cohen S (1962) Isolation of a mouse submaxillary gland protein accelerating incisor eruption and eyelid opening in the new-born animals. J Biol Chem 237:1555–1562
27. Cetin Z et al (2010) Evaluation of PTEN and Mcl-1 expressions in NSCLC expressing wild-type or mutated EGFR. Med Oncol 27(3):853–860
28. Mitsudomi T, Yatabe Y (2010) Epidermal growth factor receptor in relation to tumor development: EGFR gene and cancer. FEBS J 277(2):301–308
29. Mitsudomi T, Yatabe Y (2007) Mutations of the epidermal growth factor receptor gene and related genes as determinants of epidermal growth factor receptor tyrosine kinase inhibitors sensitivity in lung cancer. Cancer Sci 98(12):1817–1824
30. Lord RV et al (2002) Low ERCC1 expression correlates with prolonged survival after cisplatin plus gemcitabine chemotherapy in non-small cell lung cancer. Clin Cancer Res 8(7):2286–2291
31. Yarden Y, Sliwkowski MX (2001) Untangling the ErbB signalling network. Nat Rev Mol Cell Biol 2(2):127–137
32. Sordella R et al (2004) Gefitinib-sensitizing EGFR mutations in lung cancer activate anti-apoptotic pathways. Science 305(5687):1163–1167
33. Ji H et al (2006) The impact of human EGFR kinase domain mutations on lung tumorigenesis and in vivo sensitivity to EGFR-targeted therapies. Cancer Cell 9(6):485–495
34. Politi K et al (2006) Lung adenocarcinomas induced in mice by mutant EGF receptors found in human lung cancers respond to a tyrosine kinase inhibitor or to down-regulation of the receptors. Genes Dev 20(11):1496–1510

35. Uramoto H, Mitsudomi T (2007) Which biomarker predicts benefit from EGFR-TKI treatment for patients with lung cancer? Br J Cancer 96(6):857–863
36. Gerber DE (2008) EGFR inhibition in the treatment of non-small cell lung cancer. Drug Dev Res 69(6):359–372
37. Hirsch FR et al (2006) Molecular predictors of outcome with gefitinib in a phase III placebo-controlled study in advanced non-small-cell lung cancer. J Clin Oncol 24(31):5034–5042
38. Park IH et al (2009) Lovastatin overcomes gefitinib resistance in human non-small cell lung cancer cells with K-Ras mutations. Invest New Drugs 28(6):791–799
39. Parra HS et al (2004) Analysis of epidermal growth factor receptor expression as a predictive factor for response to gefitinib ('Iressa', ZD1839) in non-small-cell lung cancer. Br J Cancer 91(2):208–212
40. Fukuoka M et al (2003) Multi-institutional randomized phase II trial of gefitinib for previously treated patients with advanced non-small-cell lung cancer (The IDEAL 1 Trial) [corrected]. J Clin Oncol 21(12):2237–2246
41. Paez JG et al (2004) EGFR mutations in lung cancer: correlation with clinical response to gefitinib therapy. Science 304(5676):1497–1500
42. Tsao MS et al (2005) Erlotinib in lung cancer – molecular and clinical predictors of outcome. N Engl J Med 353(2):133–144
43. Ichihara S et al (2007) The impact of epidermal growth factor receptor gene status on gefitinib-treated Japanese patients with non-small-cell lung cancer. Int J Cancer 120(6):1239–1247
44. Bonomi PD, Buckingham L, Coon J (2007) Selecting patients for treatment with epidermal growth factor tyrosine kinase inhibitors. Clin Cancer Res 13(15 Pt 2):s4606–s4612
45. Pao W et al (2004) EGF receptor gene mutations are common in lung cancers from "never smokers" and are associated with sensitivity of tumors to gefitinib and erlotinib. Proc Natl Acad Sci U S A 101(36):13306–13311
46. Lynch TJ et al (2004) Activating mutations in the epidermal growth factor receptor underlying responsiveness of non-small-cell lung cancer to gefitinib. N Engl J Med 350(21):2129–2139
47. Kim SO et al (2008) Efficacy of gemcitabine in patients with non-small cell lung cancer according to promoter polymorphisms of the ribonucleotide reductase M1 gene. Clin Cancer Res 14(10):3083–3088
48. Thatcher N et al (2005) Gefitinib plus best supportive care in previously treated patients with refractory advanced non-small-cell lung cancer: results from a randomised, placebo-controlled, multicentre study (Iressa Survival Evaluation in Lung Cancer). Lancet 366(9496):1527–1537
49. Eberhard DA et al (2005) Mutations in the epidermal growth factor receptor and in KRAS are predictive and prognostic indicators in patients with non-small-cell lung cancer treated with chemotherapy alone and in combination with erlotinib. J Clin Oncol 23(25):5900–5909
50. Zhu CQ et al (2008) Role of KRAS and EGFR as biomarkers of response to erlotinib in National Cancer Institute of Canada Clinical Trials Group Study BR.21. J Clin Oncol 26(26):4268–4275
51. Kosaka T et al (2009) Prognostic implication of EGFR, KRAS, and TP53 gene mutations in a large cohort of Japanese patients with surgically treated lung adenocarcinoma. J Thorac Oncol 4(1):22–29
52. Mulloy R et al (2007) Epidermal growth factor receptor mutants from human lung cancers exhibit enhanced catalytic activity and increased sensitivity to gefitinib. Cancer Res 67(5):2325–2330
53. Chung BM et al (2009) The role of cooperativity with Src in oncogenic transformation mediated by non-small cell lung cancer-associated EGF receptor mutants. Oncogene 28(16):1821–1832
54. Greulich H et al (2005) Oncogenic transformation by inhibitor-sensitive and -resistant EGFR mutants. PLoS Med 2(11):e313
55. Kalikaki A et al (2010) Clinical outcome of patients with non-small cell lung cancer receiving front-line chemotherapy according to EGFR and K-RAS mutation status. Lung Cancer 69(1):110–115

56. Toyooka S et al (2007) The impact of sex and smoking status on the mutational spectrum of epidermal growth factor receptor gene in non small cell lung cancer. Clin Cancer Res 13(19):5763–5768
57. Shigematsu H et al (2005) Clinical and biological features associated with epidermal growth factor receptor gene mutations in lung cancers. J Natl Cancer Inst 97(5):339–346
58. Bell DW et al (2005) Epidermal growth factor receptor mutations and gene amplification in non-small-cell lung cancer: molecular analysis of the IDEAL/INTACT gefitinib trials. J Clin Oncol 23(31):8081–8092
59. Matsuo K et al (2007) Risk factors differ for non-small-cell lung cancers with and without EGFR mutation: assessment of smoking and sex by a case–control study in Japanese. Cancer Sci 98(1):96–101
60. Leidner RS et al (2009) Genetic abnormalities of the EGFR pathway in African American Patients with non-small-cell lung cancer. J Clin Oncol 27(33):5620–5626
61. Jang TW et al (2009) EGFR and KRAS mutations in patients with adenocarcinoma of the lung. Korean J Intern Med 24(1):48–54
62. Yatabe Y et al (2005) EGFR mutation is specific for terminal respiratory unit type adenocarcinoma. Am J Surg Pathol 29(5):633–639
63. Capuzzo F et al (2005) Epidermal growth factor receptor gene and protein and gefitinib sensitivity in non-small-cell lung cancer. J Natl Cancer Inst 97(9):643–655
64. Lee YJ et al (2010) Impact of environmental tobacco smoke on the incidence of mutations in epidermal growth factor receptor gene in never-smoker patients with non-small-cell lung cancer. J Clin Oncol 28(3):487–492
65. Adams VR, Harvey RD (2010) Histological and genetic markers for non-small-cell lung cancer: customizing treatment based on individual tumor biology. Am J Health Syst Pharm 67(1 Suppl 1):S3–S9, quiz S15–S16
66. Han SW et al (2006) Optimization of patient selection for gefitinib in non-small cell lung cancer by combined analysis of epidermal growth factor receptor mutation, K-ras mutation, and Akt phosphorylation. Clin Cancer Res 12(8):2538–2544
67. Takano T et al (2005) Epidermal growth factor receptor gene mutations and increased copy numbers predict gefitinib sensitivity in patients with recurrent non-small-cell lung cancer. J Clin Oncol 23(28):6829–6837
68. Miller VA et al (2008) Molecular characteristics of bronchioloalveolar carcinoma and adenocarcinoma, bronchioloalveolar carcinoma subtype, predict response to erlotinib. J Clin Oncol 26(9):1472–1478
69. Yoshioka H et al (2010) A phase II trial of erlotinib monotherapy in pretreated patients with advanced non-small cell lung cancer who do not possess active EGFR mutations: Okayama Lung Cancer Study Group trial 0705. J Thorac Oncol 5(1):99–104
70. Douillard JY et al (2010) Molecular predictors of outcome with gefitinib and docetaxel in previously treated non-small-cell lung cancer: data from the randomized phase III INTEREST trial. J Clin Oncol 28(5):744–752
71. Yoshida K et al (2010) Clinical outcomes of advanced non-small cell lung cancer patients screened for epidermal growth factor receptor gene mutations. J Cancer Res Clin Oncol 136(4):527–535
72. Marks JL et al (2008) Prognostic and therapeutic implications of EGFR and KRAS mutations in resected lung adenocarcinoma. J Thorac Oncol 3(2):111–116
73. Casorzo L et al (2009) Evaluation of 7q31 region improves the accuracy of EGFR FISH assay in non small cell lung cancer. Diagn Pathol 4:36
74. Varella-Garcia M et al (2009) EGFR fluorescence in situ hybridisation assay: guidelines for application to non-small-cell lung cancer. J Clin Pathol 62(11):970–977
75. Sholl LM et al (2009) Lung adenocarcinoma with EGFR amplification has distinct clinicopathologic and molecular features in never-smokers. Cancer Res 69(21):8341–8348
76. Dziadziuszko R et al (2007) Epidermal growth factor receptor gene copy number and protein level are not associated with outcome of non-small-cell lung cancer patients treated with chemotherapy. Ann Oncol 18(3):447–452

77. Schneider CP et al (2008) Epidermal growth factor receptor-related tumor markers and clinical outcomes with erlotinib in non-small cell lung cancer: an analysis of patients from German centers in the TRUST study. J Thorac Oncol 3(12):1446–1453
78. Crino L et al (2008) Gefitinib versus vinorelbine in chemotherapy-naive elderly patients with advanced non-small-cell lung cancer (INVITE): a randomized, phase II study. J Clin Oncol 26(26):4253–4260
79. Mathieu A et al (2010) Comparison of four antibodies for immunohistochemical evaluation of epidermal growth factor receptor expression in non-small cell lung cancer. Lung Cancer 69(1):46–50
80. Perez-Soler R et al (2004) Determinants of tumor response and survival with erlotinib in patients with non–small-cell lung cancer. J Clin Oncol 22(16):3238–3247
81. Gebhardt F, Zanker KS, Brandt B (1999) Modulation of epidermal growth factor receptor gene transcription by a polymorphic dinucleotide repeat in intron 1. J Biol Chem 274(19):13176–13180
82. Etienne-Grimaldi MC et al (2005) Analysis of the dinucleotide repeat polymorphism in the epidermal growth factor receptor (EGFR) gene in head and neck cancer patients. Ann Oncol 16(6):934–941
83. Liu W et al (2003) Interethnic difference in the allelic distribution of human epidermal growth factor receptor intron 1 polymorphism. Clin Cancer Res 9(3):1009–1012
84. Schittenhelm MM et al (2009) Molecular determinants of response to matuzumab in combination with paclitaxel for patients with advanced non-small cell lung cancer. Mol Cancer Ther 8(3):481–489
85. Ceppi P et al (2006) ERCC1 and RRM1 gene expressions but not EGFR are predictive of shorter survival in advanced non-small-cell lung cancer treated with cisplatin and gemcitabine. Ann Oncol 17(12):1818–1825
86. Alexandrescu DT, Kauffman CL, Dasanu CA (2009) Persistent hair growth during treatment with the EGFR inhibitor erlotinib. Dermatol Online J 15(3):4
87. Peus D, Hamacher L, Pittelkow MR (1997) EGF-receptor tyrosine kinase inhibition induces keratinocyte growth arrest and terminal differentiation. J Invest Dermatol 109(6):751–756
88. Giovannini M et al (2009) Clinical significance of skin toxicity due to EGFR-targeted therapies. J Oncol 2009:849051
89. Wacker B et al (2007) Correlation between development of rash and efficacy in patients treated with the epidermal growth factor receptor tyrosine kinase inhibitor erlotinib in two large phase III studies. Clin Cancer Res 13(13):3913–3921
90. Regales L et al (2009) Dual targeting of EGFR can overcome a major drug resistance mutation in mouse models of EGFR mutant lung cancer. J Clin Invest 119(10):3000–3010
91. Inukai M et al (2006) Presence of epidermal growth factor receptor gene T790M mutation as a minor clone in non-small cell lung cancer. Cancer Res 66(16):7854–7858
92. Marchetti A et al (2009) Clinical implications of KRAS mutations in lung cancer patients treated with tyrosine kinase inhibitors: an important role for mutations in minor clones. Neoplasia 11(10):1084–1092
93. Pao W et al (2005) Acquired resistance of lung adenocarcinomas to gefitinib or erlotinib is associated with a second mutation in the EGFR kinase domain. PLoS Med 2(3):e73
94. Kobayashi S et al (2005) EGFR mutation and resistance of non-small-cell lung cancer to gefitinib. N Engl J Med 352(8):786–792
95. Kosaka T et al (2006) Analysis of epidermal growth factor receptor gene mutation in patients with non-small cell lung cancer and acquired resistance to gefitinib. Clin Cancer Res 12(19):5764–5769
96. Pao W et al (2005) KRAS mutations and primary resistance of lung adenocarcinomas to gefitinib or erlotinib. PLoS Med 2(1):e17
97. Vikis H et al (2007) EGFR-T790M is a rare lung cancer susceptibility allele with enhanced kinase activity. Cancer Res 67(10):4665–4670

98. Balak MN et al (2006) Novel D761Y and common secondary T790M mutations in epidermal growth factor receptor-mutant lung adenocarcinomas with acquired resistance to kinase inhibitors. Clin Cancer Res 12(21):6494–6501
99. Engelman JA et al (2006) Allelic dilution obscures detection of a biologically significant resistance mutation in EGFR-amplified lung cancer. J Clin Invest 116(10):2695–2706
100. Soh J et al (2009) Oncogene mutations, copy number gains and mutant allele specific imbalance (MASI) frequently occur together in tumor cells. PLoS One 4(10):e7464
101. Zhuang HQ et al (2009) The drug-resistance to gefitinib in PTEN low expression cancer cells is reversed by irradiation in vitro. J Exp Clin Cancer Res 28:123
102. Bianco R et al (2003) Loss of PTEN/MMAC1/TEP in EGF receptor-expressing tumor cells counteracts the antitumor action of EGFR tyrosine kinase inhibitors. Oncogene 22(18):2812–2822
103. Rho JK et al (2009) The role of MET activation in determining the sensitivity to epidermal growth factor receptor tyrosine kinase inhibitors. Mol Cancer Res 7(10):1736–1743
104. Bao R et al (2009) Targeting heat shock protein 90 with CUDC-305 overcomes erlotinib resistance in non-small cell lung cancer. Mol Cancer Ther 8(12):3296–3306
105. Faber AC et al (2009) Differential induction of apoptosis in HER2 and EGFR addicted cancers following PI3K inhibition. Proc Natl Acad Sci U S A 106(46):19503–19508
106. Olaussen KA et al (2006) DNA repair by ERCC1 in non-small-cell lung cancer and cisplatin-based adjuvant chemotherapy. N Engl J Med 355(10):983–991
107. Zhou W et al (2004) Excision repair cross-complementation group 1 polymorphism predicts overall survival in advanced non-small cell lung cancer patients treated with platinum-based chemotherapy. Clin Cancer Res 10(15):4939–4943
108. Isla D et al (2004) Single nucleotide polymorphisms and outcome in docetaxel-cisplatin-treated advanced non-small-cell lung cancer. Ann Oncol 15(8):1194–1203
109. West H et al (2009) Molecular analysis-based treatment strategies for the management of non-small cell lung cancer. J Thorac Oncol 4(9 Suppl 2):S1029–S1039, quiz S1041–S1042
110. Azuma K et al (2009) Expression of ERCC1 and class III beta-tubulin in non-small cell lung cancer patients treated with carboplatin and paclitaxel. Lung Cancer 64(3):326–333
111. Lee HW et al (2009) Expression of excision repair cross-complementation group 1 protein predicts poor outcome in advanced non-small cell lung cancer patients treated with platinum-based doublet chemotherapy. Lung Cancer 65(3):377–382
112. Jeong SH et al (2010) Expression of Bcl-2 predicts outcome in locally advanced non-small cell lung cancer patients treated with cisplatin-based concurrent chemoradiotherapy. Lung Cancer 68(2):288–294
113. Rabik CA, Dolan ME (2007) Molecular mechanisms of resistance and toxicity associated with platinating agents. Cancer Treat Rev 33(1):9–23
114. de Laat WL, Jaspers NG, Hoeijmakers JH (1999) Molecular mechanism of nucleotide excision repair. Genes Dev 13(7):768–785
115. Yin Z et al (2009) ERCC2, ERCC1 polymorphisms and haplotypes, cooking oil fume and lung adenocarcinoma risk in Chinese non-smoking females. J Exp Clin Cancer Res 28:153
116. Martin LP, Hamilton TC, Schilder RJ (2008) Platinum resistance: the role of DNA repair pathways. Clin Cancer Res 14(5):1291–1295
117. Yin Z et al (2009) Association between polymorphisms in DNA repair genes and survival of non-smoking female patients with lung adenocarcinoma. BMC Cancer 9:439
118. Cobo M et al (2007) Customizing cisplatin based on quantitative excision repair cross-complementing 1 mRNA expression: a phase III trial in non-small-cell lung cancer. J Clin Oncol 25(19):2747–2754
119. Reynolds C et al (2009) Randomized phase III trial of gemcitabine-based chemotherapy with in situ RRM1 and ERCC1 protein levels for response prediction in non-small-cell lung cancer. J Clin Oncol 27(34):5808–5815
120. Wang X et al (2010) Positive expression of ERCC1 predicts a poorer platinum-based treatment outcome in Chinese patients with advanced non-small-cell lung cancer. Med Oncol 27(2):484–490

121. Ota S et al (2009) Immunohistochemical expression of BCRP and ERCC1 in biopsy specimen predicts survival in advanced non-small-cell lung cancer treated with cisplatin-based chemotherapy. Lung Cancer 64(1):98–104
122. Shimizu J et al (2008) mRNA expression of RRM1, ERCC1 and ERCC2 is not associated with chemosensitivity to cisplatin, carboplatin and gemcitabine in human lung cancer cell lines. Respirology 13(4):510–517
123. Wachters FM et al (2005) ERCC1, hRad51, and BRCA1 protein expression in relation to tumour response and survival of stage III/IV NSCLC patients treated with chemotherapy. Lung Cancer 50(2):211–219
124. Simon GR et al (2005) ERCC1 expression is a predictor of survival in resected patients with non-small cell lung cancer. Chest 127(3):978–983
125. Tibaldi C et al (2008) Correlation of CDA, ERCC1, and XPD polymorphisms with response and survival in gemcitabine/cisplatin-treated advanced non-small cell lung cancer patients. Clin Cancer Res 14(6):1797–1803
126. Li J et al (2009) Expression of MRP1, BCRP, LRP, and ERCC1 in advanced non-small-cell lung cancer: correlation with response to chemotherapy and survival. Clin Lung Cancer 10(6):414–421
127. Rosell R et al (2007) BRCA1: a novel prognostic factor in resected non-small-cell lung cancer. PLoS One 2(11):e1129
128. Berg J (2002) Deoxyribonucleotides synthesized by the reduction of ribonucleotides through a radical mechanism. In: Biochemistry. W.H. Freeman, New York, pp 702–704
129. Xu X et al (2008) Broad overexpression of ribonucleotide reductase genes in mice specifically induces lung neoplasms. Cancer Res 68(8):2652–2660
130. Nordlund P, Reichard P (2006) Ribonucleotide reductases. Annu Rev Biochem 75:681–706
131. Tanaka H et al (2000) A ribonucleotide reductase gene involved in a p53-dependent cell-cycle checkpoint for DNA damage. Nature 404(6773):42–49
132. Nakano K et al (2000) A ribonucleotide reductase gene is a transcriptional target of p53 and p73. Oncogene 19(37):4283–4289
133. Chabes A et al (2003) Survival of DNA damage in yeast directly depends on increased dNTP levels allowed by relaxed feedback inhibition of ribonucleotide reductase. Cell 112(3):391–401
134. Reichard P et al (2000) Cross-talk between the allosteric effector-binding sites in mouse ribonucleotide reductase. J Biol Chem 275(42):33021–33026
135. Caras IW, Martin DW Jr (1988) Molecular cloning of the cDNA for a mutant mouse ribonucleotide reductase M1 that produces a dominant mutator phenotype in mammalian cells. Mol Cell Biol 8(7):2698–2704
136. Mathews CK (2006) DNA precursor metabolism and genomic stability. FASEB J 20(9):1300–1314
137. Gautam A, Li ZR, Bepler G (2003) RRM1-induced metastasis suppression through PTEN-regulated pathways. Oncogene 22(14):2135–2142
138. Fan H et al (1997) The R1 component of mammalian ribonucleotide reductase has malignancy-suppressing activity as demonstrated by gene transfer experiments. Proc Natl Acad Sci U S A 94(24):13181–13186
139. Zheng Z et al (2007) DNA synthesis and repair genes RRM1 and ERCC1 in lung cancer. N Engl J Med 356(8):800–808
140. Gautam A, Bepler G (2006) Suppression of lung tumor formation by the regulatory subunit of ribonucleotide reductase. Cancer Res 66(13):6497–6502
141. Piao C et al (2009) Ribonucleotide reductase small subunit p53R2 suppresses MEK-ERK activity by binding to ERK kinase 2. Oncogene 28(21):2173–2184
142. Xue L et al (2006) Structurally dependent redox property of ribonucleotide reductase subunit p53R2. Cancer Res 66(4):1900–1905
143. Wang W et al (2009) Crosstalk to stromal fibroblasts induces resistance of lung cancer to epidermal growth factor receptor tyrosine kinase inhibitors. Clin Cancer Res 15(21):6630–6638

144. Souglakos J et al (2008) Ribonucleotide reductase subunits M1 and M2 mRNA expression levels and clinical outcome of lung adenocarcinoma patients treated with docetaxel/gemcitabine. Br J Cancer 98(10):1710–1715
145. Rosell R et al (2004) Ribonucleotide reductase messenger RNA expression and survival in gemcitabine/cisplatin-treated advanced non-small cell lung cancer patients. Clin Cancer Res 10(4):1318–1325
146. Lee JJ et al (2010) The immunohistochemical overexpression of ribonucleotide reductase regulatory subunit M1 (RRM1) protein is a predictor of shorter survival to gemcitabine-based chemotherapy in advanced non-small cell lung cancer (NSCLC). Lung Cancer 70(2):205–210
147. Plunkett W et al (1995) Gemcitabine: metabolism, mechanisms of action, and self-potentiation. Semin Oncol 22(4 Suppl 11):3–10
148. Giovannetti E et al (2006) Transcription analysis of human equilibrative nucleoside transporter-1 predicts survival in pancreas cancer patients treated with gemcitabine. Cancer Res 66(7):3928–3935
149. Davidson JD et al (2004) An increase in the expression of ribonucleotide reductase large subunit 1 is associated with gemcitabine resistance in non-small cell lung cancer cell lines. Cancer Res 64(11):3761–3766
150. Bepler G et al (2006) RRM1 modulated in vitro and in vivo efficacy of gemcitabine and platinum in non-small-cell lung cancer. J Clin Oncol 24(29):4731–4737
151. Schettino C et al (2008) The potential role of pharmacogenomic and genomic in the adjuvant treatment of early stage non small cell lung cancer. Curr Genomics 9(4):252–262
152. Bepler G et al (2004) RRM1 and PTEN as prognostic parameters for overall and disease-free survival in patients with non-small-cell lung cancer. J Clin Oncol 22(10):1878–1885
153. Bepler G et al (2002) Prognostic significance of molecular genetic aberrations on chromosome segment 11p15.5 in non-small-cell lung cancer. J Clin Oncol 20(5):1353–1360
154. Pitterle DM et al (1999) Lung cancer and the human gene for ribonucleotide reductase subunit M1 (RRM1). Mamm Genome 10(9):916–922
155. Dong S et al (2010) RRM1 single nucleotide polymorphism −37CA correlates with progression-free survival in NSCLC patients after gemcitabine-based chemotherapy. J Hematol Oncol 3:10
156. Bepler G, Sharma S, Gautam A, Smith P, Zheng Z, Hofmann J, Simonet G (2002) Tumor genotype, RRM1 expression and outcome of patients with lung cancer. Eur J Cancer 38:S82–S83
157. Feng JF et al (2009) Polymorphisms of the ribonucleotide reductase M1 gene and sensitivity to platin-based chemotherapy in non-small cell lung cancer. Lung Cancer 66(3):344–349
158. Bepler G et al (2005) Ribonucleotide reductase M1 gene promoter activity, polymorphisms, population frequencies, and clinical relevance. Lung Cancer 47(2):183–192
159. Suda K, Tomizawa K, Mitsudomi T (2010) Biological and clinical significance of KRAS mutations in lung cancer: an oncogenic driver that contrasts with EGFR mutation. Cancer Metastasis Rev 29(1):49–60
160. Krontiris TG, Cooper GM (1981) Transforming activity of human tumor DNAs. Proc Natl Acad Sci U S A 78(2):1181–1184
161. Der CJ, Krontiris TG, Cooper GM (1982) Transforming genes of human bladder and lung carcinoma cell lines are homologous to the ras genes of Harvey and Kirsten sarcoma viruses. Proc Natl Acad Sci U S A 79(11):3637–3640
162. Shimizu K et al (1983) Three human transforming genes are related to the viral ras oncogenes. Proc Natl Acad Sci U S A 80(8):2112–2116
163. Mao C et al (2010) KRAS mutations and resistance to EGFR-TKIs treatment in patients with non-small cell lung cancer: a meta-analysis of 22 studies. Lung Cancer 69(3):272–278
164. Marchetti A et al (1996) Bronchioloalveolar lung carcinomas: K-ras mutations are constant events in the mucinous subtype. J Pathol 179(3):254–259
165. Forbes S et al (2006) COSMIC 2005. Br J Cancer 94(2):318–322
166. Bos JL (1989) Ras oncogenes in human cancer: a review. Cancer Res 49(17):4682–4689

167. Karnoub AE, Weinberg RA (2008) Ras oncogenes: split personalities. Nat Rev Mol Cell Biol 9(7):517–531
168. Sun P et al (2007) PRAK is essential for ras-induced senescence and tumor suppression. Cell 128(2):295–308
169. Tuveson DA et al (2004) Endogenous oncogenic K-ras(G12D) stimulates proliferation and widespread neoplastic and developmental defects. Cancer Cell 5(4):375–387
170. Weir BA et al (2007) Characterizing the cancer genome in lung adenocarcinoma. Nature 450(7171):893–898
171. Kendall J et al (2007) Oncogenic cooperation and coamplification of developmental transcription factor genes in lung cancer. Proc Natl Acad Sci U S A 104(42):16663–16668
172. Johnson L et al (2001) Somatic activation of the K-ras oncogene causes early onset lung cancer in mice. Nature 410(6832):1111–1116
173. Kobayashi T et al (1990) Association of point mutation in c-Ki-ras oncogene in lung adenocarcinoma with particular reference to cytologic subtypes. Cancer 66(2):289–294
174. Tsuchiya E et al (1995) High K-ras mutation rates in goblet-cell-type adenocarcinomas of the lungs. J Cancer Res Clin Oncol 121(9–10):577–581
175. Yatabe Y et al (2004) CK20 expression, CDX2 expression, K-ras mutation, and goblet cell morphology in a subset of lung adenocarcinomas. J Pathol 203(2):645–652
176. Singh A et al (2009) A gene expression signature associated with "K-Ras addiction" reveals regulators of EMT and tumor cell survival. Cancer Cell 15(6):489–500
177. Jackman DM et al (2009) Impact of epidermal growth factor receptor and KRAS mutations on clinical outcomes in previously untreated non-small cell lung cancer patients: results of an online tumor registry of clinical trials. Clin Cancer Res 15(16):5267–5273
178. Loriot Y et al (2009) Are RAS mutations predictive markers of resistance to standard chemotherapy? Nat Rev Clin Oncol 6(9):528–534
179. Solomon B, Varella-Garcia M, Camidge DR (2009) ALK gene rearrangements: a new therapeutic target in a molecularly defined subset of non-small cell lung cancer. J Thorac Oncol 4(12):1450–1454
180. Soda M et al (2007) Identification of the transforming EML4-ALK fusion gene in non-small-cell lung cancer. Nature 448(7153):561–566
181. Morris SW et al (1995) Fusion of a kinase gene, ALK, to a nucleolar protein gene, NPM, in non-Hodgkin's lymphoma. Science 267(5196):316–317
182. Shiota M et al (1994) Hyperphosphorylation of a novel 80 kDa protein-tyrosine kinase similar to Ltk in a human Ki-1 lymphoma cell line, AMS3. Oncogene 9(6):1567–1574
183. Iwahara T et al (1997) Molecular characterization of ALK, a receptor tyrosine kinase expressed specifically in the nervous system. Oncogene 14(4):439–449
184. Chiarle R et al (2008) The anaplastic lymphoma kinase in the pathogenesis of cancer. Nat Rev Cancer 8(1):11–23
185. Houtman SH et al (2007) Echinoderm microtubule-associated protein like protein 4, a member of the echinoderm microtubule-associated protein family, stabilizes microtubules. Neuroscience 144(4):1373–1382
186. Pollmann M et al (2006) Human EML4, a novel member of the EMAP family, is essential for microtubule formation. Exp Cell Res 312(17):3241–3251
187. Sasaki T et al(2010) The biology and treatment of EML4-ALK non-small cell lung cancer. Eur J Cancer, 46(10): 1773–1780
188. Takeuchi K et al (2009) KIF5B-ALK, a novel fusion oncokinase identified by an immunohistochemistry-based diagnostic system for ALK-positive lung cancer. Clin Cancer Res 15(9):3143–3149
189. Rikova K et al (2007) Global survey of phosphotyrosine signaling identifies oncogenic kinases in lung cancer. Cell 131(6):1190–1203
190. Wong DW et al (2009) The EML4-ALK fusion gene is involved in various histologic types of lung cancers from nonsmokers with wild-type EGFR and KRAS. Cancer 115(8):1723–1733

191. Shaw AT et al (2009) Clinical features and outcome of patients with non-small-cell lung cancer who harbor EML4-ALK. J Clin Oncol 27(26):4247–4253
192. Koivunen JP et al (2008) EML4-ALK fusion gene and efficacy of an ALK kinase inhibitor in lung cancer. Clin Cancer Res 14(13):4275–4283
193. Inamura K et al (2009) EML4-ALK lung cancers are characterized by rare other mutations, a TTF-1 cell lineage, an acinar histology, and young onset. Mod Pathol 22(4):508–515
194. Soda M et al (2008) A mouse model for EML4-ALK-positive lung cancer. Proc Natl Acad Sci U S A 105(50):19893–19897
195. Rodig SJ et al (2009) Unique clinicopathologic features characterize ALK-rearranged lung adenocarcinoma in the western population. Clin Cancer Res 15(16):5216–5223
196. Kwak E (2009) Clinical activity observed in a phase I dose escalation trial of an oral c-met and ALK inhibitor, PF-02341066. J Clin Oncol 27(suppl):152, abstr 3509
197. McDermott U et al (2008) Genomic alterations of anaplastic lymphoma kinase may sensitize tumors to anaplastic lymphoma kinase inhibitors. Cancer Res 68(9):3389–3395
198. Christensen JG et al (2007) Cytoreductive antitumor activity of PF-2341066, a novel inhibitor of anaplastic lymphoma kinase and c-Met, in experimental models of anaplastic large-cell lymphoma. Mol Cancer Ther 6(12 Pt 1):3314–3322
199. Filipits M et al (2007) Multidrug resistance proteins do not predict benefit of adjuvant chemotherapy in patients with completely resected non-small cell lung cancer: International Adjuvant Lung Cancer Trial Biologic Program. Clin Cancer Res 13(13):3892–3898
200. Reguart N et al (2008) BRCA1: a new genomic marker for non-small-cell lung cancer. Clin Lung Cancer 9(6):331–339
201. Taron M et al (2004) BRCA1 mRNA expression levels as an indicator of chemoresistance in lung cancer. Hum Mol Genet 13(20):2443–2449
202. Potti A et al (2006) A genomic strategy to refine prognosis in early-stage non-small-cell lung cancer. N Engl J Med 355(6):570–580
203. Chen HY et al (2007) A five-gene signature and clinical outcome in non-small-cell lung cancer. N Engl J Med 356(1):11–20

Chapter 5
Molecular Pathology and Diagnostics of Colorectal Cancer

Rodney E. Shackelford, Aejaz Nasir, Ardeshir Hakam, David Shibata, Timothy Yeatman, and Domenico Coppola

Contents

R.E. Shackelford
Department of Pathology and Laboratory Medicine, Tulane University School of Medicine, 1430 Tulane Avenue, SL-79, New Orleans, LA 70112, USA

A. Nasir
Diagnostic & Experimental Pathology & Tailored Therapeutics Program, Eli Lilly & Company, Indianapolis, IN, USA

A. Hakam • D. Coppola, M.D. (✉)
Department of Anatomic Pathology and Oncological Sciences, H. Lee Moffitt Cancer Center & Research Institute and University of South Florida, 12902 Magnolia Drive, Tampa, FL 33612, USA
e-mail: Domenico.coppola@moffitt.org

D. Shibata
Department of Surgical Oncology, H. Lee Moffitt Cancer Center & Research Institute and University of South Florida, 12902 Magnolia Drive, Tampa, FL 33612, USA

T. Yeatman
Gibbs Research Institute and Cancer Center, Spartanburg, SC 29303

D. Coppola (ed.), *Molecular Pathology and Diagnostics of Cancer*, Cancer Growth and Progression 16, DOI 10.1007/978-94-007-7192-5_5,

Abstract Colorectal carcinoma (CRC) is the third most common malignancy in the United States and is the second leading cause of cancer deaths. Over the past 20 years, our knowledge of this CRC carcinogenesis has enormously increased; presently, several molecular diagnostic tests are commonly employed to analyze stage IV CRC and familiar CRC syndromes to determine treatment options and CRC inheritance and risk. More recently the number of CRC diagnostic tests has enormously expanded as our knowledge of CRC carcinogenesis has increased. Here, we review the standard tests employed in CRC, such as KRAS and Braf analyses, and also include less commonly employed tests related to familiar CRC and microsatellite instability. Last, we focus on possible future CRC genetic tests and testing modalities, focusing on techniques such as microarray and mass spectrophotometry.

Keywords Colorectal carcinoma • KRAS • BRAF • FAP • UGT1A1 • NHPCC • PJS • APC • Mutation • Hamartomatous polyposis syndromes

Abbreviations

8-oxo-G	7,8-dihydro-8-oxo-deoxyguanosine
AFAP	Attenuated familial adenomatous polyposis
APC	Adenomatous polyposis
ARMS	Amplification resistant mutation system
CRC	Colorectal carcinoma
CSGE	Conformation strand gel electrophoresis
EGFR	Epidermal growth factor receptor
FAP	Familial adenomatous polyposis
GTP	Guanosine-5′-triphosphate
HNPCC	Polyposis hereditary nonpolyposis colon cancer
HRM	High-resolution melting
JPS	Juvenile polyposis syndrome
MAP	MYH-associated polyposis
mCRC	Metastatic CRC
MLH1	MutL homolog 1
MLH3	MutS homolog 3
MLPA	Multiplex ligation-dependent probe amplification
MSH2	MutS homolog 2
MSH6	MutS homolog 6
MSI	Microsatellite instability
NCCN	National Comprehensive Cancer Network
PCR	Polymerase chain reaction

PJS	Peutz-Jeghers syndrome
PMS2	Postmeiotic segregation increased 2
PTT	Protein truncation test
SSCP	Single strand conformation polymorphism
T-ARMS-PCR	Tetra-primer amplification refractory mutation system PCR

5.1 Introduction

Colorectal carcinoma (CRC) is the third most common malignancy in the United States, with nearly 150,000 new cases annually, accounting for roughly 15 % of all US malignancies, and is currently the second leading cause of cancer-related deaths for both sexes [1]. CRC shows a peak incidence between the ages of 70 and 79 years and by 70 years roughly 50 % of the population in high-risk areas for CRC will have some form of colorectal neoplasia, spanning the continuum from adenomatous polyps to CRC [1, 2]. The average life-time risk for CRC in the US for individuals who lack a personal or family history of this malignancy is ~6 %, ~20 % for individuals with an effected first-degree relative, and 80–100 % for individuals with a hereditary CRC syndrome [1–3].

5.2 Environmental Versus Genetic Factors in Colorectal Cancer Risk

CRC shows a 20-fold variation among different geographic locations, with low incidences in India and Africa and a higher incidence in the US and Western Europe. Migration studies from low-risk to high-risk areas indicate that environmental factors play an important role in CRC risk [1, 2, 4]. Several studies have addressed the relative roles of heritable factors vs. shared and nonshared environmental factors in CRC risk and estimate the percentage of CRCs resulting from statistically significant heritable causes to range between 15 and 35 % [5–8]. The largest of these studies analyzed 44,788 mono-and dizygotic twin pairs and found heritable causes accounted for approximately 35 % of the risk for CRC, with the remaining risk due to environmental factors. Interestingly, hereditary factors played a slightly greater role in younger individuals with CRC than in older individuals [5].

Environmental risk factors for CRC include a diet high in red meat and fat, increasing age, a family history of CRC, the Metabolic Syndrome, a personal history of inflammatory bowel disease or a heritable CRC syndrome, smoking, physical inactivity, heavy alcohol consumption, a history of nightshift work, and a diet low in fiber and plants [9–13]. Conversely, physical activity, a diet high in vegetables and fruits, and nonsteroidal anti-inflammatory drug use are associated with a lower CRC risk, with nonsteroidal anti-inflammatory drugs reducing colonic adenomatous polyp numbers [9].

5.3 Molecular-Genetic Testing in CRC

Over the past 15 years, the diagnosis, analysis, and treatment of CRC have dramatically changed. Until relatively recently, the establishment of a CRC diagnosis and prognostic indicator analysis depended on hematoxylin-eosin stained slide examination supplemented with immunohistochemical analysis. Within the past few years, molecular-genetic testing has become increasingly important in the diagnosis and management of hereditary CRC syndromes and in determining the treatment options for de novo metastatic CRC (mCRC), particularly as related to panitumumab and cetuximab use [14–17].

5.4 EGFR, *KRAS*, and De Novo CRC

The epidermal growth factor receptor (EGFR) is a 170-kDa transmembrane glycoprotein and member of the ErbB family of growth factor receptor tyrosine kinase family, which consists of four closely related receptors. The EGFR has six major ligands that are expressed to various degrees in different tissues: heparin binding EGF, transforming growth factor-α, betacellulin, amphiregulin, heregulin, and EGF [18, 19]. EGFR is overexpressed in a variety of tumors, including ~70 % of individuals with mCRC, with its overexpression linked to a poorer prognosis [20–23]. Not surprisingly, EGFR overexpression is often associated with EGFR ligand overexpression by CRC cells, forming a malignancy-promoting autocrine regulatory loop [24–26].

EGFR binding leads to receptor homodimerization, subsequent tyrosine kinase domain activation with receptor cytoplasmic tail autophosphorylation, the recruitment of intracellular signaling proteins such as growth factor receptor-bound protein (GRB2), son of sevenless (SOS), with eventual KRAS activation [27]. *KRAS* is the human homologue of the Kirsten rat sarcoma virus [28, 29]. *KRAS* encodes the KRAS protein, a member of the Ras small guanine nucleotide-binding proteins, which functions in signal transduction cascades initiated by the ligation of several cell surface receptors, including EGFR, hepatocyte growth factor (c-Met), and insulin-like growth factor receptors [30, 31].

Upon activation, KRAS binds guanosine-5′-triphosphate (GTP) and activates a number of down-stream signaling proteins, including Raf, Braf, mTOR, MEK, ERK, and PIK3CA, resulting in the expression of gene products promoting cell growth, differentiation, and proliferation and which exert anti-apoptotic and pro-angiogenic effects [19, 32]. KRAS is a GTPase that hydrolyzes GTP to guanosine-5′-diphosphate resulting in KRAS inactivation. The GTPase activity of KRAS is accelerated by the GTPase-activating proteins, which attenuate KRAS signaling. Thus, the growth-promoting effects of EGFR and KRAS are tightly regulated under normal conditions, while constitutive EGFR and KRAS signaling promotes CRC growth and neoplastic progression [19, 23, 32–34].

Recently, two anti-EGFR monoclonal antibodies, panitumumab (Vectibix) and cetuximab (Erbitux), have demonstrated efficacy in the treatment of mCRC. Cetuximab is a chimeric mouse-human monoclonal IgG1 antibody with proven second-or third-line efficacy for treating CRC and head and neck cancers [35–38]. Cetuximab binds the EGFR with an affinity ~fivefold higher than physiological EGFR ligands, preventing EGFR homodimerization, tyrosine kinase activation, and subsequent signaling [39, 40]. Cetuximab binding also causes the cetuximab-EGFR complex to be internalized and degraded, thus both EGFR signaling and receptor availability are lowered [41, 42]. Last, cetuximab mediates antibody-dependent cellular cytotoxicty against the EGFR in a murine tumor model; this mechanism of action may also contribute to its efficacy [43].

Panitumumab is a fully humanized IgG2 monoclonal antibody that binds the EGFR with high affinity ($Kd = 5 \times 10^{-11}$ M). Upon binding, panitumumab blocks EGFR, EGF, and transforming growth factor-α binding, blocking tyrosine kinase activation, attenuating tumor cell activation and proliferation, and stimulating receptor internalization. In vitro panitumumab administration causes cell cycle arrest at the G_0/G_1 interphase, inhibiting tumor colony formation. Last, like cetuximab, panitumumab also initiates complement-dependent and antibody-dependent cell-mediated cytotoxicities [43, 44].

Immunohistochemical EGFR positivity was initially employed as an entry criterion for studies evaluating the efficacy of these antibodies in CRC treatment. However, many studies demonstrated that EGFR expression is a poor biomarker for anti-EGFR antibody response, with responses seen in individuals with low, high, or even no EGFR expression [35, 45–47]. These results necessitated alternative biomarker testing for the evaluation of clinical cetuximab and panitumumab use. Since EGFR signaling promotes and maintains the CRC malignant phenotype [20–26], mutations causing constitutive activation of a down-stream EGFR signaling proteins are likely to be involved in CRCs refractory to cetuximab and panitumumab treatment. Several studies demonstrated constitutive activating *KRAS, BRAF,* and *PIK3CA* mutations in CRC, with *KRAS* mutations being most frequent at 27–45 % [35, 47–50]. Interestingly, activating *KRAS* mutations appear early in the genesis of CRC, with mutations found in adenomatous polyps [50]. Most activating *KRAS* mutations exhibit GTPase activity loss combined with GTPase-activating protein insensitivity [32]. Roughly 90 % of *KRAS* activating mutations occur in codons 12 and 13 of exon 2, with rare mutations seen in codons 59 and 61 of exon 3 [32, 51–53]. Interestingly, not all *KRAS* mutations are the same; CRCs with microsatellite instability (MSI) combined with the G13D *KRAS* mutation have a significantly improved prognosis [54]. Additionally, a recent study has demonstrated that patients with the G13D KRAS mutation still respond well to cetuximab [55]. Thus, evidence is accumulating that not all activating KRAS mutations are the same and not all render patients refractory to anti-EGFR antibodies.

5.5 KRAS Mutation Testing in De Novo CRC

Activating *KRAS* mutations are strongly linked to loss of anti-EGFR antibody response, and individuals carrying these mutations experience no survival benefit from cetuximab or panitumumab. Additionally, this treatment may be detrimental to individuals with *KRAS* mutations. Last, cetuximab and panitumumab treatment is costly at roughly $10,000 per month [47, 56–59]. Thus molecular testing for *KRAS* mutations is important in patient care and for cost-effective healthcare delivery; it is also currently recommended by the National Comprehensive Cancer Network (NCCN) for all patients with mCRC being considered for anti-EGFR therapy [60]. Currently, there are several different molecular protocols employed in *KRAS* mutation testing. Three common ones are amplification resistant mutation system (ARMS) for identifying specific mutations, various sequencing methods, and high-resolution melting analysis (HRM). Each of these techniques has specific advantages and disadvantages, and they are often combined.

5.5.1 Tissue Preparation

Sample preparation for *KRAS* testing in mCRC is more elaborate than for many other molecular tests. Mutation analysis typically begins with formalin-fixed or formalin-fixed, paraffin-embedded tissue. DNA from these samples require special preparation given that (1) it is usually fragmented and cross-linked to other biomolecules, making amplification (especially of longer DNA sequences) difficult, (2) it contains polymerase chain reaction (PCR) inhibitors, which must be thoroughly removed prior to amplification, (3) formalin fixation can introduce DNA sequence alterations, and (4) tumor tissue containing possible *KRAS* mutations is usually intermixed with areas of benign tissue and/or benign stromal elements, often necessitating histological examination and microdissection of the slide to increase the portion of tumor within the sample [50–63].

DNA purification usually begins with histological identification of CRC on a glass slide, often followed by removal and purification of DNA from the malignant component, from an unstained recut or core taken from a tumor-bearing portion of the paraffin block. Removal with a needle or scalpel is possible where a clear boundary exists between malignant and benign tissue. Alternatively, laser microdissection allows the isolation of small cell clusters or even single cells if extremely pure tumor DNA is required [63]. The resulting tumor-enriched sample is often deparaffinized in xylene, digested with protinase K, and the DNA is isolated via robotic instrumentation or commercial DNA purification columns [63]. Once purified DNA is obtained, *KRAS* mutational status may be analyzed by several different molecular tests. Where an instrument such as a microtome is used to cut and dissect slides, the instrument should be carefully cleaned between runs to prevent cross contamination (30 min with 30 % bleach, followed by washing with dH_2O and ethanol has been used to clean all cutting surfaces).

5.5.2 Direct Sequencing

Direct DNA sequencing is commonly used in *KRAS* mutation analysis for mCRC. Typically purified temple DNA is amplified via PCR employing forward and reverse primers spanning the activating mutations in codons 12 and 13 of exon 2. The amplified product is purified and sequenced usually via a commercial automated sequencer and analyzed with special attention given to any changes in codons 12 or 13. While pyrosequencing is commonly used, Sanger sequencing is considered the gold standard and requires that the tumor-derived DNA template contains at least 20 % mutant *KRAS* DNA for detection [64–67]. Most automated sequencers employ software programs to assist in the analysis of the statistical significance of low level base pair changes [64–66]. A clear advantage of direct DNA sequencing is that all base pairs are examined within the amplified sequence.

5.5.3 ARMS

The *Taq* DNA polymerase initiates the PCR reaction poorly from mismatched template-primer 3′-termini; with a 10^{-3}–10^{-6} lower amplification efficiency depending on the mismatch type [68]. ARMS PCR takes advantage of this *Taq* property by using multiple primers with 3′ ends, which match *KRAS* codons 12 and 13 mutations. Increased *KRAS* mutations are detected via technologies such as labeled probe degradation in real-time PCR or via the use of similar Scorpion primers [69, 70]. An advantage of ARMS is that it can detect very small concentrations of mutant *KRAS* since it employs mutation-specific primers. In some systems, ARMS technology can detect one mutant allele in a background of 10^4 wild-type alleles [71]. Additionally, since most tumors with mutations will have some component of unmutated *KRAS*, amplifying unmutated *KRAS* can serve as a useful PCR positive control. One disadvantage of ARMS PCR is that 3′ mismatched primers will initiate amplification at a low rate from a wild-type *KRAS* template [68], thus "*KRAS* mutations" that appear only at very high Cp values should not be considered valid mutations. Comparison to a wild-type *KRAS* amplification controls can be useful. Positive ARMS PCR results have been used where the Cp value is 35 or lower [70].

5.5.4 HRM

HRM involves PCR amplification of the KRAS genomic DNA with primers spanning codons 12 and 13 of exon 2. The amplified DNA is mixed with a fluorophore that emits more strongly bound to dsDNA than ssDNA. The amplified dsDNA is then heated from a low to a high temperature and fluorescent intensity is measured and compared to a wild-type control. Multiple data acquisitions (~25) are taken per degree temperature increase [70]. As the temperature increases, the dsDNA denatures to ssDNA, lowering fluorescent signal intensity, producing a sigmoid curve. Amplified KRAS sequences with denaturation points different than the wild-type control are mutated [71]. HRM is quick to perform but also relatively expensive and does not identify specific mutations [72].

5.5.5 *Comparing Direct Sequencing, ARMS, and HRM*

In general, KRAS mutation analysis via DNA sequencing, HRM, ARMS, and other PCR-based detection methodologies give similar results and all are clinically useful [70–72]. Franklin et al. [70] compared these techniques and found some interesting differences. HRM gave the highest frequency of KRAS mutations with 54 % of samples showing denaturation point abnormalities, while DNA sequencing and ARMS gave 36 % and 43 % mutation rates, respectively. Sequencing of the HRM samples with denaturation point abnormalities revealed that only 61 % actually had KRAS mutations. ARMS identified mutations where 100 % detected by HRM, indicating 100 % sensitivity. Additionally, ARMS was 100 % accurate with single round testing. DNA sequencing detected 17 % fewer mutations than ARMS due to lower sensitivity and required a 20–50 % greater concentration of mutant DNA to achieve reliable mutation detection. The authors concluded that (1) HRM samples with abnormal denaturation points should be sequenced to confirm the presence of mutation (making testing cumbersome), (2) DNA sequencing sensitivity may be suboptimal for clinical testing, and (3) ARMS is the most sensitive and rapid of these techniques and probably the most clinically useful technique. Other studies have found similar results with real-time PCR-based assay techniques having greater sensitivity than DNA sequencing [73]. Additionally, many of these techniques, such as ARMS, do not test for the rare KRAS exon three codons 59 and 61 mutations or uncommon codon 13 mutations [32, 70–73]. While these mutations are rare, not testing for them may result in a low number of patients receiving cetuximab or panitumumab inappropriately. For example, individuals with exon 3 codon 61 mutations do not respond to cetuximab therapy, despite having unmutated codons 12 and 13 [74]. Last, differences exist within different sequencing methods. For example, Sanger sequencing requires a ~20 % mutant DNA concentration for mutation detection, while pyrosequencing requires 5 %. Sanger sequencing also yielded 11.1 % and 6.1 % false positive and negatives, respectively, while pyrosequencing gave no false positives and negatives [67, 70]. Interestingly, Tsiatis et al. [67] demonstrated that the same tumor can have different activating KRAS mutations.

5.6 Other Mutations in De Novo CRC

While KRAS is most frequently mutated in cetuximab/panitumumab resistant CRC, other mutations in proteins downstream of the EGFR also confer resistance [48, 74].

5.6.1 Braf

Braf, also known as V-raf murine sarcoma viral oncogene homolog B1 (B-raf-1), is a serine/threonine kinase downstream of KRAS. Activated KRAS phosphorylates and activates Braf, increasing cyclins D1-3, mdm2, and c-myc expression, promoting cell cycle entrance, increasing cell growth potential, and inhibiting apoptosis [48, 74, 75]. Braf is mutated and constitutively activated in several human malignancies, including de novo CRC, malignant melanoma, papillary thyroid cancer, and low-grade ovarian serous carcinomas [48, 74–78]. In CRC, Braf mutation is often associated with MSI [74]. Approximately 8.7–40 % of CRCs carry activating Braf mutations that confer cetuximab/panitumumab resistance [23, 48, 74, 75, 79, 80]. Braf mutations are frequently identified in sessile serrated adenomas, mixed polyps, high-level MSI CRC, and high CpG island methylator phenotype CRC and serrated adenomas. Braf mutations are less common in low CpG island methylator phenotype low and negative CRC, hereditary non-polyposis CRCs, hyperplastic polyps, conventional adenomas, and sporadic non-MSI-high CRCs [81]. Although not yet common, Braf mutation testing is done as reflex testing in some labs, following the determination of unmutated KRAS status. The exact role of Braf mutation testing for determining EGFR inhibitor sensitivity remains somewhat inconclusive. Currently, in the 2012 NCCN guidelines, Braf genotyping remains optional in the setting of Kras wild-type tumors [60].

5.6.2 Molecular Testing for Braf Mutations

Braf is found on 7q34 and consists of 19 exons. Activating mutations occur in exons 11 and 15, with over 90 % of mutations involving a T → A transversion at position 1,779, causing a valine → glutamate substitution at residue 600 (V600E), resulting in 500-fold increased kinase activity compared to wild-type Braf [82]. Braf mutation testing has been performed by several different techniques, including direct sequencing, ARMS, single strand conformation analysis, and restriction fragment length polymorphism analysis [83–85]. While direct automated sequencing is widely accepted as standard, Benlloch et al. [83] compared V600E mutation detection via ARMS vs. automated sequencing and found ARMS to be less costly, labor intensive, require a shorter assay time, and have 100 % sensitivity and specificity, demonstrating that this technique has value for clinical testing. Molecular testing for Braf mutation is complicated by the Braf pseudogene (B-raf-2) located at Xq13, necessitating careful primer design to avoid pseudogene amplification [83, 86]. Interestingly, B-raf-2 is often expressed in B-raf-1 negative papillary thyroid carcinomas. Additionally, B-raf-2 expression is tumorigenic in nude mice, activates the MAP kinase, and can transform NIH3T3 cells, demonstrating oncogenic potential [87]. Presently, there is no evidence for a role in B-raf-2 expression or mutation in CRC.

5.6.3 NRAS

NRAS mutations are found in ~3 % of CRC [88]. *NRAS* functions in a pathway similar to *KRAS*, but exerts apoptosis suppressive effects and its mutations arise much later in CRC genesis than *KRAS* mutations [53]. *NRAS* is commonly mutated at codons 2, 3, 12, 13, and 61, conferring cetuximab therapy resistance [53, 89, 90]. Multiplex PCR has been used to identify NRAS codon 2 and 3 mutations [88]. Presently, reflex *NRAS* testing is offered by Quest Diagnostics following identification of unmutated *KRAS* and *Braf* status.

5.6.4 PIK3CA and PTEN

PIK3CA, a member of the phosphatidylinositol 3-kinase family, is mutated in 9.9–32 % of CRCs [23, 86]. Activated PIK3CA promotes cell proliferation, motility, and cell invasion, via AKT and PDK1 activation [91–94]. PIK3CA is mutated in CRC; however, the significance of these mutations in anti-EGFR therapy is presently controversial [91, 95, 96].

PTEN, a phosphatidylinosital trisphosphate phosphatase that antagonizes *PIK3CA* activity, is lost in 42 % of CRCs [23]. PTEN loss and *PIK3CA* mutation are likely to contribute to malignant progression [23, 91–94, 97]. However, Tol et al. [23] demonstrated that PTEN loss has no predictive value for cetuximab response.

5.6.5 Future Directions

Only 10 % of EGFR-positive mCRCs respond to cetuximab or panitumumab therapy, while those with indentified unmutated *KRAS* show a ~22 % response [49]. Mutations in *KRAS*, *BRAF*, or *NRAS* are largely mutually exclusive of each other, while *PIK3CA* mutation may coexist with *KRAS*, *BRAF*, or *NRAS* mutations and PTEN loss may coexist with *KRAS* or *BRAF* mutations [23, 48, 74, 97–99]. *KRAS*, *BRAF*, and *NRAS* mutation may all result in resistance to anti-EGFR therapy and since they are largely mutually exclusive, molecular testing for mutations of all three may help better identify patients who can benefit from anti-EGFR therapy.

Presently *KRAS* testing followed by reflex *Braf* testing for unmutated *KRAS* status is recommended [59, 81, 100]. *PIK3CA* and PTEN testing is not presently useful in the evaluation of anti-EGFR therapy use.

5.7 Hereditary Colorectal Cancer Syndromes and Molecular-Genetic Testing

Although 15–35 % of CRCs have a statistically significant genetic component, only 3–10 % of these malignancies result from highly penetrant germline mutations identified as hereditary CRC syndromes [5–8]. The first hereditary CRC was described in 1861 and was probably Familial Adenomatous Polyposis (FAP) [101]. Since then, several hereditable CRC syndromes have been described in detail, including FAP, Attenuated Familial Adenomatous (AFAP), Polyposis Hereditary Nonpolyposis Colon Cancer (HNPCC) or Lynch Syndrome, MYH-Associated Polyposis (MAP), and the *I1307K* adenomatous polyposis (APC) mutation in the Ashkenazi Jewish population. In general, most hereditary CRC results from either *APC* gene loss resulting in chromosomal instability or MSI with loss of mismatch repair gene function [5–8]. Molecular testing plays an important role in the diagnosis and management of these syndromes, providing information for genetic counseling. Failure to detect a mutation does not invalidate a clinically definite hereditary CRC syndrome diagnosis, but identification of a mutation is required to perform predictive at-risk testing for relatives presently without symptoms. In general, the more the clinical picture fits a specific hereditary CRC syndrome, the more likely a positive molecular testing result [102, 103].

5.7.1 Sample Preparation

For hereditary CRC syndrome testing, genomic DNA can be obtained from peripheral blood, formalin-fixed, or formalin-fixed, paraffin-embedded tissue. In general peripheral blood is a better DNA source as it is easier to process, less fragmented/cross-linked, and contains the possible germline mutation.

5.8 FAP

FAP is an autosomal dominant hereditary CRC syndrome, which accounts for slightly less than 1 % of all CRCs with an incidence of 1:7,000–10,000 [9, 104]. FAP is the second most common hereditary CRC and characterized by the development of hundreds to thousand of colorectal adenomas of different sizes. It typically has few symptoms until the mid-to-late teens (average age of 16 years), when the adenomas grow large enough to cause adenoma-related symptoms, such as rectal bleeding, anemia, palpable abdominal masses, weight loss, constipation, and diarrhea.

In FAP, CRC usually develops ~10 years following the clinical appearance of adenomatous colonic polyps, resulting in nearly 100 % of FAP individuals having CRC by their early 1940s, with a mean age of 39 years in untreated individuals and a range of 34–43 years. Other gastrointestinal manifestations include gastric fundic gland polyps and adenomatous polyps in the 2nd and 3rd portion of the duodenum and periampullary region [105]. Interestingly, 40 % of the fundic gland polyps show adenomatous changes, although an increased risk for gastric cancer is none to slight in Western populations, but significantly higher in Asian populations [106, 107]. FAP confers a 100–330-fold higher risk for duodenal cancer, compared with the general population, resulting in a life-time risk for duodenal and periampullary cancers of 10 % and 5 %, respectively [108, 109].

Extraintestinal FAP manifestations include osteomas, desmoid tumors, congenital hypertrophy of the retinal pigmented epithelium (CHRPE), nasopharengyeal angiofibromas, pancreatic mucinous adenocarcinomas, hepatoblastomas, sebaceous and epidermal cysts, and brain tumors, including medulloblastomas and glioblastomas [110]. The clinical diagnosis of FAP rests upon endoscopic identification of more than 100 adenomatous colonic polyps, extraintestinal manifestations of FAP, and a family history of an autosomal dominant inheritance pattern [105].

The genes mutated in FAP and APAP are *APC* located at 5q21-22 and *MUTYH* located at 1p34.3-p32.1. *APC* mutations account for 70–95 % of FAP and 20–30 % of AFAP, while *MUTYH* mutations account for ~6.6 % of FAP and ~18 % of AFAP cases [105, 111–114]. In general, the more severe the FAP symptoms are, the more likely molecular testing will locate a specific *APC* mutation [104, 111–115]. *APC* spans 108,353 bp consisting of 16 exons of which exons 2–16 are coding. Interestingly, exons 2–15 code for 653 amino acids, whereas exon 16 codes for 2,190 [105, 111–115]. APC function is lost in de novo CRC genesis and some cancers of the stomach, pancreas, thyroid, and ovary [116]. It is also, among the early genes, lost in the Vogelstein model of CRC genesis [117–121]. The APC gene product has a molecular weight of 310 kDa and is localized in the cytoplasm and nucleus [122–125]. APC exerts numerous functions, including acting as a negative regulator of β-catenin function, indirectly suppressing *c-myc* levels, maintaining cytoskeletal integrity, cellular adhesion, functioning in Wnt signaling, and regulating the $G_0 \rightarrow G_1$ transition in part via regulating cyclin D1 expression [126–130]. APC also binds the ends of microtubules embedded within kinetochores, forming a complex with the checkpoint Bub1 and Bub3 proteins, with APC being a high-affinity substrate for the Bub kinases. Truncating APC mutations, common in FAP, may alter normal chromosome-spindle attachment, disrupting the mitotic spindle cell checkpoint, causing genomic instability [131].

5.9 *APC* Molecular Testing Methods

Over 700 different *APC* have been reported, with greater than 98 % either being frameshift (68 %) or nonsense mutations (30 %) [111, 131]. Most individuals with FAP will have a family history of FAP with accompanying *APC* mutations;

however, 25–30 % will have de novo *APC* mutations and lack a family history of FAP [132, 133]. The specific mutation patterns show variation, with germline mutations common 5′ at codons 1,061 and 1,309 and somatic mutations common at codons 1,309 and 1,450 within the mutation cluster region [116]. Interestingly, there is a strong, but not complete correlation between the specific *APC* gene region mutated and the FAP phenotype. For example, congenital hypertrophy of the retinal pigment usually only appear with mutations 3′ to exon 9, while individuals with profuse FAP (more than 5,000 polyps) commonly show frameshift mutations between codons 1,255 and 1,467 [134, 135]. The number of mutations and relatively large size of the APC gene make molecular testing complex. Several protocols are currently employed in testing:

5.9.1 APC Protein Truncation Test

Over 98 % of FAP *APC* mutations result in truncated APC protein expression [116]. Based on this, a molecular assay has been developed, the protein truncation test (PTT), which measures disease-inducing *APC* mutations via analyzing protein truncation. The assay involves three steps:

1. Patient nucleic acid is isolated, usually from peripheral leukocytes. Either RNA or genomic DNA is isolated, with RNA transcribed into DNA via reverse transcription PCR. The resulting DNA is amplified via PCR into one or several DNA templates, depending on the size of the original.
2. The templates are transcribed in vitro into RNA, which is subsequently translated into protein, in a reticulocytelysate system.
3. The translated proteins are analyzed with gel electrophoresis, and any changes in the molecular weight of the APC protein are detected by comparison to a wild-type control.

The PCR primers employed introduce a promoter sequence allowing the DNA template to be transcribed into RNA, and subsequently translated into protein in a coupled reaction. Often a T7 promoter sequence is employed for transcription by T7 RNA polymerase, as well as a consensus sequence for the initiation of translation [136, 137]. The protein is visualized by several techniques, such as radiolabeling with ^{35}S-cysteine, ^{35}S-methionine, or ^{3}H-leucine in the reticulocytelysate system. An example of a PTT gel is shown in Fig. 5.1 [136].

PTT has good sensitivity, a low-false-positive rate, and detects disease-inducing APC protein truncations, but not silent mutations, or the more than 20 *APC* gene polymorphisms, none of which cause disease [116, 136, 137]. PTT can also detect promoter mutations that lower *APC* mRNA expression and mutations, which create unstable mRNA (for those assays that amplify *APC* RNA). Disadvantages of the PTT are that it does not identify all *APC* gene mutations and does not identify the specific *APC* gene mutation, which is useful for directed mutation testing within effected kindreds. Last, PTT is superior to Western blotting, having a significantly higher

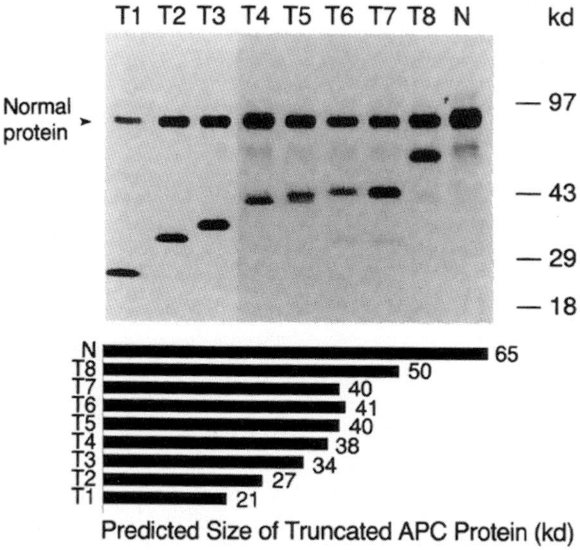

Fig. 5.1 An example of a PTT from Ref. [136]. Eight representative samples from de novo CRCs (T1→T8), with truncating mutations identified by sequencing analysis. A substantial amount of normal full-length APC protein is seen from remaining normal alleles. The proteins were transcribed and translated in a reticulocytelysate system with ^{35}S-methionine as a label. The kDa of the truncated proteins is predicted of the right

APC protein detection rate [134]. Using this assay, Powell et al. [136] successfully identified APC mutations in 87 % 62 individuals with FAP tested. The PTT test is also used to identify mutations in other genes, such as *BRCA1* and *dystrophin* [126, 138].

5.9.2 Direct APC Gene Sequencing and Multiplex Ligation-Dependent Probe Amplification

Direct DNA sequencing of the *APC* gene is considered the gold standard and detects *APC* gene mutations in ~70 % of individuals with FAP. The advantage of this technique is that all amplified bps are analyzed. However, the length of the APC coding region requires that many primers (~30) be used, making sequencing expensive, labor intensive, and time consuming [139]. Additionally, submicroscopic deletions have been detected in 6–55 % of *APC* kindreds, with larger deletions seen in 2 % and insertions seen in 6 % [115, 139, 140]. Since primer-dependent DNA sequencing is poor at detecting deletions/insertions, techniques such as multiplex ligation-dependent probe amplification (MLPA) have been employed to detect these *APC* mutations [140–142]. In MLPA, genomic DNA is interrogated with two probes that

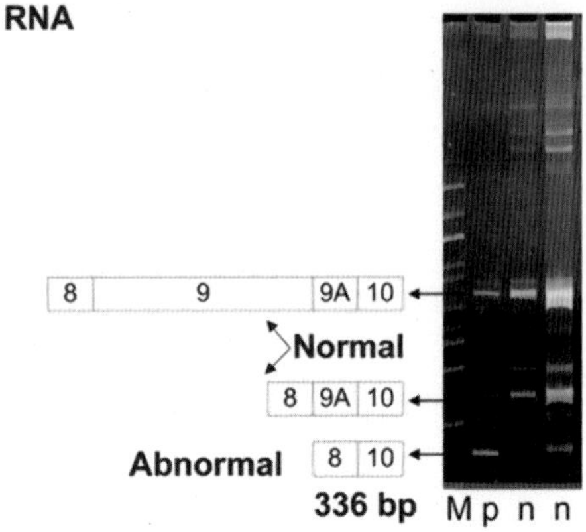

Fig. 5.2 An example of an MLPA analysis run on 6 % PAGE. **M** is a 100 bp ladder. The two **n**'s are normal splice variants of the APC gene; exons 8-9-9A-10 and 8-9A-10. **p** is from an individual with FAP showing a deletion resulting in a shorter 336 bp amplicon. The patient's RNA was amplified by reverse transcription PCR and visualized with ethidium bromide staining

bind adjacent to each other. Each probe has one primer sequence that will amplify the two probes and intervening sequences only if the two probes are ligated. Once the two probes are hybridized to the genomic DNA, a ligation step is performed. If the two probes are hybridized and near enough to each other, the ligation step will produce one probe with an intervening sequence possibly revealing an insertion or deletion. Additionally, the probe will now have two primer sites allowing PCR amplification. The molecular weight of the amplified/ligated region is often measured via gel electrophoresis or by automated systems that measure a labeled and incorporated primer [140–144]. An example of MLPA is shown in Fig. 5.2.

5.9.3 Conformation Strand Gel Electrophoresis and Single Strand Conformation Polymorphism Testing

Conformation strand gel electrophoresis and single strand conformation polymorphism testing (CSGE and SSCP, respectively) have both been used to detect *APC* gene mutations [105, 145]. In CSGE, control homoduplex wild-type dsDNA is compared to dsDNA, which may carry a point mutation. The two DNA duplexes are subjected to electrophoresis under mildly denaturing conditions. Under such conditions, heteroduplexes will often adopt a more complex three-dimensional conformation than homoduplexes and as a result migrate more slowly. In SSCP, wild-type and possibly mutant ssDNAs are compared. The two DNAs are denatured, rapidly renatured, and subjected to electrophoresis. A ssDNA segment with a point mutation will assume a different secondary and tertiary structure, resulting in a different migration pattern compared to the wild-type control. In general, CSGE and SSCP are less efficient and accurate than DNA sequencing; hence, sequencing has largely supplanted these testing methods. However, both still have value and have been used to screen for mutations that are then further analyzed via PTT or DNA sequencing [105]. Some data indicate that CSGE is more sensitive than SSCP [145].

5.10 FAP Management

FAP has an autosomal dominant inheritance pattern, and affected individuals have a virtually 100 % chance of developing CRC by their 1940s, making FAP detection and kindred analysis important in the management and prevention of FAP-associated CRC [105, 146, 147]. Once diagnosed, individuals with FAP should undergo annual lower endoscopy and have as many polys removed as possible. Upper endoscopy should be performed every 6 months to 3–4 years to detect duodenal, gastric, and periampullary adenomas, with the frequency determined by the polyp burden [146, 147]. Prophylactic colectomy is recommended by the end of the second decade, when there is usually a large polyp burden. A total protocolectomy with ileoanal J-pouch is recommended, although an ileorectal anastomosis can be performed on individuals with low rectal polyp numbers. With the latter procedure, yearly endoscopic rectal surveillance is still required [146–149]. Known individuals with FAP while under the age of 10 years should have annual α-fetoprotein levels and abdominal ultrasound to monitor for hepatoblastoma, 1 in 20 of which occur due to FAP [150].

Individuals with FAP given 400 mg/day celecoxib for 6 months showed a 28 % reduction in colorectal adenomas compared to a 4.5 % reduction in the control placebo group. Similarly, 400 mg celecoxib twice per day for 6 months reduced duodenal polyps 14.5 % compared to 1.4 % in placebo controls and 31 % in individuals with a high polyp burden [151, 152]. The US Food and Drug Administration Oncologic Drug Advisory Committee recommends celecoxib as an adjunctive treatment to endoscopic surveillance and colectomy in FAP treatment (New Drug Application Number 21,156).

Following a clinical FAP diagnosis, *APC* mutation testing should be performed. Standard APC mutation testing via DNA sequencing will identify mutations in 70–80 % of individuals clinically diagnosed with FAP [105]. MLPA and other methods will identify a further 2–5 % of mutations involving *APC* insertions/deletions, while *MUTHY* mutations will account for ~6.6 % of cases [105, 111, 141–144]. The remaining ~20 % of FAP have a more severe phenotype and appear to be due to *APC* mutations not identifiable by standard testing [111, 113]. Laken et al. [111] employed monoallelic mutation analysis to independently examine the status of each of the two *APC* alleles without mutations by standard testing. 78 % of the "unmutated" samples tested were found to have significantly reduced expression from one of their two *APC* alleles. Thus ~95 % of FAP is due to APC mutation. Monoallelic mutation analysis is complex and cumbersome, making it difficult to apply to molecular diagnostics.

Once a proband *APC* mutation is identified, all first degree relatives should have genetic counseling and molecular testing for the proband mutation. Individuals with FAP identified by an effected relative have a significantly greater life expectancy than individuals identified by FAP symptoms, warranting presymptomatic testing [153]. Directed mutation testing should be performed to simplify testing and lower costs [154]. Individuals with *APC* mutations should receive endoscopy, celecoxib treatment, and eventual colectomy. Individuals without mutations should receive endoscopic surveillance recommended for the general population.

When no *APC* mutation is detected in the proband, first degree relatives should receive annual lower endoscopic examines until age 35. If no colonic adenomatous polyps are found by age 35, lower endoscopic examines should be performed every 3 years until age 50, where endoscopic surveillance should match the general population. Where first degree relatives have a high burden of colonic adenomatous polyps, they should be managed as having FAP [105]. Presently, *MUTYH*, MLPA, or monoallelic mutation analyses are not routinely done for FAP testing [105, 111].

5.11 Attenuated FAP (AFAP)

AFAP is clinically defined by an autosomal dominant inheritance pattern, 10–99 adenomatous colonic polyps occurring at a later age than in FAP, and an 80–100 % lifetime CRC risk. Often, the colonic polyps are mostly proximal with little rectal involvement, increasing the likelihood of a misdiagnosis of sporadic polyps [105, 155]. Additionally, gastric and duodenal polyps occur and can rarely become malignant. Breast cancer and hepatoblastoma occur, with other extraintestinal manifestations being rare [155]. *APC* mutations are found in 20–30 % of individuals with AFAP and another 18 % have *MUTHY* mutations [105, 112]. *APC* mutations in AFAP are generally found 5′ or at the 3′ end of the gene, proximal to codon 1,517 or distal to codon 1,900 [105, 156–158]. Molecular testing for *APC* mutations in AFAP are done as for FAP. If testing reveals no APC mutation in individuals with AFAP, *MUTHY* testing should also be performed [105]. Due to the very high CRC incidence in AFAP, effected individuals and their first degree relatives should receive the same counseling and treatment as those with FAP [105].

5.12 Turcot and Gardner Syndromes

Turcot and Gardner syndromes are phenotypic variants of FAP. Gardner syndrome is characterized by colonic, gastric, and duodenal polyposis and soft tissue tumor, including osteomas, lipomas, fibromas, epidermal inclusion cysts, and desmoids tumors [159, 160]. *APC* mutations associated with Gardner syndrome are usually truncating mutations between codons 1,403 and 1,578 [160]. Molecular testing is the same as for other FAP variants [160].

Turcot syndrome is characterized by primary brain tumors accompanied by colorectal adenomas and/or CRC [161, 162]. Interestingly, Turcot syndrome shows molecular heterogeneity, with one form caused by *APC* mutations and the other resulting from HNPCC with mutations in one of the DNA mismatch repair genes

MSH2, MLH1, PMS1, or *PMS2* (see below, [162, 163]). In general, individuals with Turcot syndrome with *APC* mutations will have medulloblastomas, while those with HNPCC will have gliomas [162, 163]. Molecular testing for Turcot syndrome involves *APC* mutation analysis or DNA mismatch repair gene (MMR) analysis (see below).

5.13 I1307K *APC* Mutation in Ashkenazi Jews

Ashkenazi Jews carry a number of ancestral mutations conferring predisposition to several diseases, including CRC. One mutation found in 6–12 % of this population is the *APC:I1307K* mutation, involving a T→A transversion at nucleotide 3,920 converting AAATAAAA to an extended mononucleotide tract (A_8), resulting in a lysine replacing isoleucine at codon 1,307 [164, 165]. While this amino acid substitution does not alter *APC* gene function, the A_8 polymorphism is ~32 times more mutatable than the most mutatable wild-type *APC* sequences and often results in somatic biallelic *APC* inactivation and CRC tumorigenesis [164–166]. Interestingly, Gryfe et al. [166] found that, of the CRCs in *APC:I1307K* mutation carriers, only 42 % had *APC*-specific mutations that could be linked to the CRCs, a very modest mutation rate compared with HNPCC. Additionally, unlike in FAP, *APC:I1307K* must undergo somatic biallelic *APC* inactivation, resulting in only a 1.5–2-fold increased CRC incidence [164]. After adjustment for age, *APC:I1307K* carriers are more likely than noncarriers to have colorectal polyps, with either tubular adenomas or tubulovillous adenomas, but not villous adenomas, significantly more frequent among carriers (37.2 % vs. 23.6 %, P=0.005) [166].

APC:I1307K mutation testing is limited to measuring a T→A transversion, making analysis via allele-specific oligonucleotide hybridization PCR a logical choice. For example, Niell et al. [167], employed a common reverse primer and two forward primers: one wild-type (5′-CTTTTCTTTTATTCTGC-3′) and one *APC:I1307K* (5′-CTTTTCTTTTTTTCTGC-3′) specific primer. The 1 bp difference allowed the identification of the *APC:I1307K* transversion incidence in different populations. Other investigators have used PCR to amplify the genomic region around the *APC:I1307K* transversion and employed SSCP analysis, with transversion positive samples confirmed via DNA sequencing [168]. Not surprisingly, PCR has also been used to amplify the genomic region around the *APC:I1307K* transversion followed by direct amplicon sequencing [165].

Individuals with a positive *APC:I1307K* mutation test should undergo colonoscopic surveillance, as they may benefit from the early eradication of pre-cancerous polyps [169]. There is some evidence that smoking may increase CRC in *APC:I1307K* carriers, so smoking cessation should be encouraged [165]. The Ashkenazim population also have a low (0.7 %) carrier incidence of *MSH21906G>C* mutation, which is highly penetrant and causes CRC at an early age [164]. Last, although this population has a low (0.9 %) incidence of a *BLM* exon 10 frameshift mutation; BLM^{ASH}. BLM^{ASH} carriers do not have an elevated CRC incidence [165, 170].

5.14 MYH-Associated Polyposis

5.14.1 *MUTYH and the MAP Phenotype*

Reactive oxygen species derived from normal aerobic metabolism and exogenous sources readily damage DNA forming a wide variety of lesions, including oxidized bases [171–174]. One well-studied and common oxidized base is 7,8-dihydro-8-oxo-deoxyguanosine (8-oxo-G). 8-oxo-G readily pairs with adenine, leading to G:C→T:A transversion mutations following DNA replication [172–174]. MYH, the *MUTYH* gene product, is a glycosylase that catalyzes the cleavage of adenine mismatched to 8-oxo-G via base excision repair, preventing G:C→T:A transversions [175, 176]. Biallelic *MUTYH* mutation results in glycosylase activity loss and increased G:C→T:A transversions, including in *APC* and *KRAS*, but not *Braf*, leading adenoma development and CRC [177, 178].

MAP is the most important differential diagnosis for FAP and AFAP, occurring in ~1/10,000 individuals, accounting for ~0.6 % of all CRC [179, 180]. Phenotypically, biallelic *MUTYH* mutation (homozygous or compound heterozygous) results in a 93-fold increased CRC risk, with clinical symptoms appearing at 40–60 years, and a variable number of adenomatous colonic polyps, 10–100, rarely up to 1,000 [180]. Extraintestinal manifestations are less common than in FAP, with ~31 % of effected individuals having duodenal adenomas and/or gastric fundic polyps and a 4 % lifetime duodenal cancer risk [180–182]. MAP is autosomal recessive and therefore does not show the strong intergenerational history of FAP [180, 181]. The CRC incidence is high in MAP, with a 100 % lifetime risk and 50 % of effected individuals having CRC at diagnosis [181, 183]. Extraintestinal manifestations of MAP include breast, endometrial, and sebaceous carcinomas [182, 184]. Interesting, neither immunohistochemistry nor histology reveal any significant differences between MAP-associated CRC and sporadic CRC [185].

5.14.2 *Molecular Testing for MAP*

Unlike the 700+ known *APC* mutations, about 23 pathogenic *MUTYH* mutations are known, with two (Y165C and G382D), accounting for ~82 % of inactivating mutations [114, 115, 186]. Thus initial MAP testing is often directed at these two mutations. If one of these mutations is identified, sequencing is performed to identify the inactivating mutation on the opposite allele. If two inactivating mutations are found, the CRC risk will be very high. Failure to initially identify the Y165C or G382D combined with a strong suspicion for *MUTYH* mutation necessitates testing for less common mutations usually by DNA sequencing, which has the highest clinical sensitivity [187].

Numerous studies have demonstrated that in many cases ARMS is useful in MAP testing. For example, Piccioli et al. [188] employed a tetra-primer amplification refractory mutation system PCR (T-ARMS-PCR) to examine six common *MUTYH* mutations, which would identify at least 85 % of all mutations; Y165C, G382D,

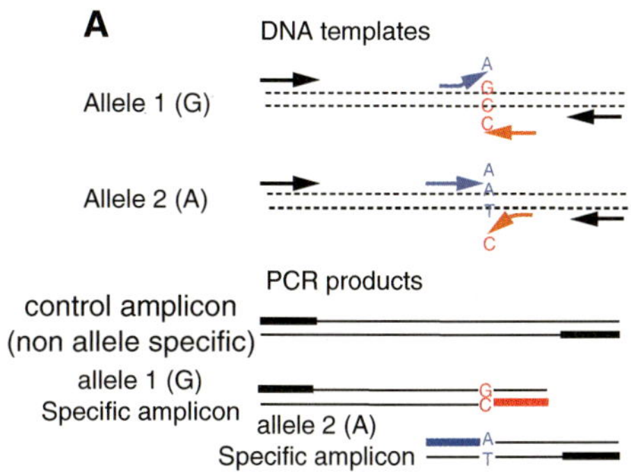

Fig. 5.3 T-ARMS-PCR from Ref. [188]. Two control primers (*black arrows*) which flank the mutation site, amplify one non-allele-specific control fragment, while two allele-specific primers in opposite orientations (*blue and red arrows*) in combination with the control primers, can amplify both smaller wild-type or mutant amplicons. The two allele-specific amplicons have different lengths and can easy be separated and identified via electrophoresis. Thus, the presents of wild-type and/or mutant amplicons can be determined with the longer non-allele-specific control amplicon serving as a positive control

1395_7delGGA, Y90X, 1103delC, and R231H. T-ARMS-PCR amplifies both wild-type and mutant alleles in one PCR reaction. T-ARMS-PCR and ARMS-PCR work well for MAP testing and cover ~85 % of known mutations [188, 189]. It is relatively inexpensive, can identity small deletions, requires no specialized equipment, and importantly is ideal for targeted molecular testing. Thus, once a kindred-specific mutation has been identified, ARMS-PCR and T-ARMS-PCR allow inexpensive, accurate, and rapid molecular analyses. Again ARMS-PCR does not identify ~15 % of known mutations, making DNA sequencing analysis necessary to identify uncommon mutations [187, 189]. The T-ARMS-PCR protocol is described in Fig. 5.3.

5.14.3 MAP Management

For individuals with a significant colonic adenoma burden, *MUTYH* and *APC* mutation testing can be performed simultaneously, particularly if the family history suggests an autosomal recessive inheritance pattern. *MUTYH* testing should also be considered for the 20–30 % and 70–90 % of *APC* mutation negative FAP or AFAP cases, respectively. For FAP, the number due to *MUTYH* mutations is low, accounting for only ~5 % of FAP [111–114]. Once an individual is identified as having inactivating biallelic *MUTYH* mutations, molecular testing of all siblings is recommended as they have a 25 % chance of having the same mutation [112]. Presently, testing the partners of individuals with bilallelic *MUTYH* mutations is controversial, as the risk of MAP for children of an effected parent is ~1 % [181]. However if the partner of a bilallelic mutation carrier has one *MUTYH* mutation, an apparently autosomal dominant CRC inheritance is seen, possibly resulting in a misdiagnosis of FAP. Additionally, the CRC risk for *MUTYH* mutation heterozygotes is low, with a relative risk of 1.5–2.1 to the general population. Presently, the need for increased lower endoscopic surveillance is this population is undetermined [112, 190, 191].

Individuals with biallelic *MUTYH* mutations should undergo annual or biennial lower endoscopic surveillance beginning as teens. Upper endoscopic surveillance for duodenal adenomas/adenocarcinomas should be performed every 2 years [192]. The high rate of progression to CRC often necessitates a prophylactic colectomy [112, 192].

5.15 HNPCC

Lynch Syndrome, also known as HNPCC, is the most common hereditary CRC, accounting for ~2 % of all CRCs [193]. HNPCC was identified in 1996, when two large kindreds in the Midwestern United States showed excess CRC that lacked multiple colonic adenomas with a constellation of associated malignancies, particularly endometrial cancers [194]. Subsequent researchers named the disorder "Lynch Syndrome" or HNPCC. HNPCC is characterized by an autosomal dominant inheritance, high penetrance (~85 %), early onset CRC (~45 years), proximal CRC predilection, accelerated adenoma→CRC progression, increased survival with CRC, and CRC, which is histologically poorly differentiated, having increased mucinous and signet ring cell-features, and an excess of tumor-infiltrating lymphocytes. HNPCC associated extracolonic tumors include endometrial, ovarian, sebaceous, gastric, small intestinal, pancreatic, brain, hepatobillary tract, and upper urothelial cancers [193–195].

HNPCC results from activity loss of one or more DNA mismatch repair (MMR) genes, resulting in MSI, a specific form of genomic instability: [194, 195]. DNA polymerase activities collectively have a 10^{-7} error rate/bp synthesized. MMR gene activity locates and removes the substitution mismatches and insertion/deletion mismatches that arise during DNA replication. Additionally, the MMR genes play a role in dsDNA break repair (the most harmful DNA lesion), the initial sensing of DNA damage, and the initiation of apoptosis with severe DNA damage [171, 196, 197]. Overall, MMR gene activity increases genomic stability 50–10^3-fold, making MMR activity loss a powerful mutator phenotype [196]. The MMR genes are described below.

5.15.1 MutL Homolog 1 (MLH1)

MLH1 is located at 3p21.3-23 and consists of 19 exons of 57.36 kb, coding for an 84.6-kDa nuclear protein. MLH1 has two interaction domains, one which interacts with MSH2, MSH3, or MSH6 and the other which interacts with PMS2, MLH3, or PMS1. More than 250 different *MLH1* germline mutations in NHPCC have been identified, consisting of missense, nonsense, splicing errors, and insertion/deletions, many of which truncated protein expression [198, 199]. Germline *MLH1* mutations are seen in ~46 % of HNPCC cases, while 78 % of sporadic CRCs with high MSI (MSI-H) have reduced *MLH1* expression secondary to promoter methylation and *BRAF* mutation. Thus *MLH1* inactivation appears to occur by separate molecular pathways in HNPCC vs. sporadic CRC [200].

5.15.2 MutS Homolog 2 (MSH2)

MSH2 is located at 2p22-p21 and consists of 16 exons of 80.10 kb, coding for a 104.7 kDa nuclear protein. MSH2 has DNA, MSH3/MSH6, and MLH1/PMS2 binding domains. More than 300 different *MLH2* germline mutations in HNPCC have been identified, consisting of mutation types similar to those seen in *MHL1*. *MLH2* mutations are seen in ~40 % of HNPCC cases, thus ~90 % of HNPCC CRCs result from *MHL1* or *MLH2* mutations [198–202].

5.15.3 MutS Homolog 6 (MSH6)

MSH6 is located at 2p16 and consists of 10 exons of 23.8 kb, coding for a 160 kDa nuclear protein. *MSH6* mutations account for 7–10 % of HNPCC [202–204]. 73 % of female *MSH6* mutation carriers develop endometrial hyperplasia and carcinoma, compared to 29 % in *MSH2* and 31 % in *MLH1* carriers, making endometrial tumors more common among female *MSH6* mutation carriers than CRC [205]. Most mutations are truncating mutations producing an inactive protein [205]. Interestingly, individuals with *MSH6* mutations have a lower CRC incidence and a later age of onset than those with *MSH2* and *MLH1*mutations [206].

5.15.4 Postmeiotic Segregation Increased 2 (PMS2)

PMS2 is located at 7p22.2 and consists of 15 exons of 63.14 kb, coding for a 96 kDa nuclear protein. *PMS2* mutations account for less than 2 % of HNPCC kindreds and normally function as heterodimers with *MLH1* forming MutLα [198, 202–204]. MSH2, MSH6, MLH1, and PMS2 associate with BRCA1, ATM, RAD50, MRE11, NBS1, and PCNA, forming a complex suggested to regulate DNA replication and maintain genomic integrity [207].

5.15.5 MutS Homolog 3 (MLH3)

Wu et al. [208] examined 39 unrelated HNPCC families who fulfilled the Amsterdam Criteria for HNPCC. Of 288 individuals examined, 12 had 10 different germline *MLH3* variants, including one frameshift, and nine missense mutations. Normal immunostaining for MSH2, MLH1, or MSH6 was detected. The authors concluded that *MLH3* mutation probably played a role in a small subset of HNPCC.

The molecular mechanism underlying CRC carcinogenesis in HNPCC appears to be increased genomic instability in ~32 target genes that have mononucleotide repeats of 7 or more within their coding sequences. Many of these genes, such as *RAD50, BLM,* and *PTEN*, are tumor suppressors; others such as *TGFβ1R2* and *BAX* inhibit epithelial cell growth or exert proapoptotic effects. MSI causes frameshift mutations in these genes, leading to loss of function [209, 210]. Interestingly, *MLH3, MSH3,* and *MSH6* have A_9, A_8, and C_8 tracts, respectively, thus loss of one MMR gene may lead to progressive inactivation of the entire MMR system, possibly explaining the rapid adenoma → CRC progression seen in HNPCC [211].

5.16 HNPCC Diagnosis

Several guidelines have been developed to aid in HNPCC diagnosis: the Amsterdam criteria, the Amsterdam II criteria, and recently the Revised Bethesda Guidelines [212]. The Revised Bethesda Guidelines recommend MSI testing and/or immunohistochemical analysis in the following groups:

- Colorectal cancer diagnosed in a patient less than 50.
- Presence of synchronous, metachronous CRC, or other HNPCC associated tumors, regardless of age.
- CRC with the MSI-H histology diagnosed in a patient less than 60.
- CRC diagnosed in one or more first-degree relatives with an HNPCC-related tumor, with one of the cancers being diagnosed under age 50 years.
- CRC diagnosed in two or more first-or second-degree relatives with HNPCC-related tumors, regardless of age.

Additionally, the following patients should also receive the same testing:

- Patients diagnosed with Muir-Torre syndrome (association of CRC with cutaneous sebaceous neoplasms) or Turcot Syndrome (especially glioblastoma brain tumor).
- Family members of individuals with a known MMR gene mutation.

5.16.1 HNPCC Testing Guidelines

Once HNPCC is suspected, specific testing protocols should be followed to obtain a definitive diagnosis. First, MSI or immunohistochemical analyses of CRC and normal tissue should be performed. Should MSI be present, or MMR protein expression lost in CRC, further analyses are performed to diagnose HNPCC [212, 213].

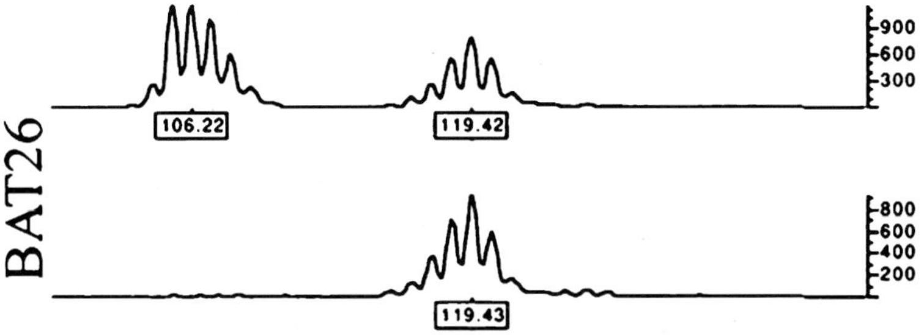

Fig. 5.4 An example of CRC MSI positivity at the BAT26 microsatellite from Ref. [212]. Genomic was PCR-amplified from tumor (*upper*) and normal (*lower*) tissue and run in an ABI PRISM 377 DNA Sequencer. The data were collected automatically and analyzed by GeneScan 3.1 software

5.16.2 MSI Testing for HNPCC

MSI testing involves the analysis of five microsatellite markers standardized by the National Cancer Institute for HNPCC screening: BAT-25, BAT-26, D2S123, D5S346, and D17S250. Typically, both tumor and matching normal patient DNA are compared. MSI testing may be performed without normal patient DNA, but it is recommended that all studies assessing MSI using these markers should use matched normal-tumor DNA pairs [212]. Each microsatellite marker is PCR amplified with primers specific for each marker, and the resulting amplicons are analyzed for length variation via techniques such as gel electrophoresis, automated sizing equipment, or denaturing high-performance liquid chromatography. The primers may be labeled or unlabeled, depending on the requirements of the amplicon detection method [213–215].

MSI is defined as a change of any length due to a deletion/insertion of repeating units within a tumor microsatellite not seen in normal tissue DNA. With five markers, MSI is present and high (MSI-H) when ≥ 2 or more microsatellite markers show MSI. MSI is low (MSI-L) when one marker has MSI, and the tumor is MSI-L or microsatellite stable when one or no markers show MSI. Where more the five markers are analyzed, ≥ 30–40 % with MSI equals MSI-H, < 30–40 % is MSI-L, and no MSI is microsatellite stable [213]. Microsatellite stable or MSI-L tumors are unlikely to result from HNPCC [212]. An example of an MSI analysis is shown in Fig. 5.4.

5.16.3 Immunohistochemical Analysis for HNPCC

Immunohistochemical analysis for the loss of MMR genes is as effective as molecular MSI testing for HNPCC [212, 215, 216]. Immunohistochemical analysis of CRC and adjacent normal colorectal epithelium from individuals with HNPCC will often reveal loss of nuclear MSH2, MLH1, MSH6, or PMS2 protein expression. Following

CRC analysis, if staining for each MMR protein is identified, the individual is unlikely to have HNPCC. If staining for an MMR protein is lost in CRC, but present in adjacent normal colonic epithelium, HNPCC is likely to be present [212, 215, 216]. The correlation between immunohistochemical MMR protein loss in CRC and MSI is high, with some studies showing MLH1 or MSH2 loss having 100 % specificity and 92.3 % sensitivity for predicting CRC with MSI-H [216]. Although both MSI and immunohistochemistry will work for initial testing, ideally both should be performed [212, 215]. Interestingly, both MSI-H and loss of MMR protein expression has been identified in a significant portion of colonic adenomas from individuals with HNPCC, demonstrating that these events occur early in CRC genesis [215]. Immunohistochemical testing has the advantage of being both cheaper and faster than MSI testing, with costs estimated to be 14–28 % of MSI testing [217]. There is growing interest in the application of reflex testing for MMR and/or MSI for all patients diagnosed with CRC. In particular, the Evaluation of Genomic application in Practice and Prevention (EGAPP) Working Group has provided genetic testing strategies in newly diagnosed individuals with colorectal cancer aimed at reducing morbidity and mortality from Lynch Syndrome in relative.

5.16.4 Molecular MMR and BRAF V600E Mutation Testing in HNPCC

With no loss of MMR protein immunopositivity, or MSI testing showing MSI-L/MMS, HNPCC is unlikely and no further testing is required [212]. Should MSI-H and/or MMR protein loss be identified, molecular testing should be performed for MMR gene mutations. Most protocols recommend *MLH1* and *MSH2* molecular testing, as these make up ~90 % of MMR gene HNPCC mutations [198–202, 212, 215, 216]. If immunohistochemistry detected loss of a specific MMR protein, molecular testing should be directed to the encoding gene [212, 215, 216].

Ten to fifteen percent of sporadic CRCs are MSI-H, have MLH1 protein loss, and have the specific *BRAF-V600E* mutation [82–86, 218, 219]. In these tumors, the *MLH1* promoter is hypermethylated, leading to loss of protein expression, while the *MLH1* sequence is unmutated [84, 85, 218, 219]. *BRAF-V600E* occurs only in sporadic CRCs and is not seen in HNPCC-associated CRCs [84, 85, 220, 221]. Therefore, *MLH1* molecular testing is unnecessary where a *BRAF-V600E* mutation has been identified, unless there remains a high clinical suspicion for HNPCC [84, 85, 195, 220, 221]. Thus *BRAF-V600E* testing can rule out HNPCC, saving time and avoiding costly MMR gene molecular analysis [82, 84, 85, 220].

Molecular testing for *BRAF-V600E* is described above. Testing typically follows two approaches:

1. With MSI testing, *BRAF-V600E* mutation testing should be performed. With no identified *BRAF-V600E* mutation, *MLH1* and *MLH2* mutation testing should be performed. If no *MLH1* and *MLH2* mutations are identified, *MSH6* and *PMS2* testing can be performed.

2. Where immunohistochemistry for MMR protein expression is employed, the specifically lost MMR gene should be tested for mutations. If the lost MMR protein is MLH1, *BRAF-V600E* mutation testing should be done first and followed by *MLH1* gene analysis if *Braf* is unmutated.

Failure to identify an MMR gene mutation usually rules out HNPCC, while identification of an MMR gene allows an HNPCC diagnosis. In some cases, a gene variation of unknown significance is identified. In other cases, no MMR gene mutation is identified, but the family history and/or individual's presentation still strongly indicate HNPCC. Genetic testing will not identify all mutations leading to a HNPCC phenotype. Where an MMR gene mutation is identified, directed testing should be performed on the probands at-risk relatives and genetic counseling should be offered [195].

MMR gene analysis has been performed in a variety of ways, including Southern blotting, SSCP, DNA sequencing, MLPA, denaturing gradient gel-electrophoresis, quantitative PCR, and combinations of these methods [222–225]. Many germline *MLH1* and *MSH2* mutations are missense, nonsense, and frameshift mutations and are readily detected by these techniques. However, other mutations include large deletions and duplications [225–227]. While Southern analysis will detect large genomic rearrangements, it is also cumbersome, expensive, and time-consuming compared to other methods [222]. Charbonnier et al. [225] employed short fluorescent fragments to analyze *MLH1* and *MSH2* mutations, detecting deletions and duplications. 19 and 16 labeled primer sets were required for *MLH1* and *MSH2* analysis, respectively, with the reactions multiplexed and analyzed on a Gene scanner model 672 fluorescent fragment Analyzer. Control and patient electropherograms were superimposed and amplifications/deletions were detected by observing changes between superimposed control DNA and control and patient DNA. Most *MLH1* and *MSH2* mutations are unique with only a few common and recurring mutations identified, thus ARMS would be an extremely inefficient approach to MMR gene mutation analysis [226]. An example of the technique employed in Vasen et al. [228] is shown in Fig. 5.5.

5.16.5 HNPCC Management

Järvinen et al. [229] compared two at-risk HNPCC cohorts over a 15-year period. Colonoscopic screening reduced the CRC incidence 62 %. Additionally, the CRCs in the screened cohort were localized and caused no deaths, compared to 9 CRC-related deaths in individuals who declined colonoscopy. Interestingly, Vasen et al. [228] found several HNPCC patients with CRC 3.5 years following a negative colonoscopy, demonstrating a need for short screening intervals. Currently, individuals with HNPCC should receive colonoscopy every 1–2 years, beginning at age 20–25 (age 30 years with *MSH6* mutation), or 10 years before the first effected family member presented with CRC.

In HNPCC, an increased incidence of CRC is found arising in flat and diminutive adenomas proximal to the splenic flexure. Interestingly, pan-colonic chromoscopic

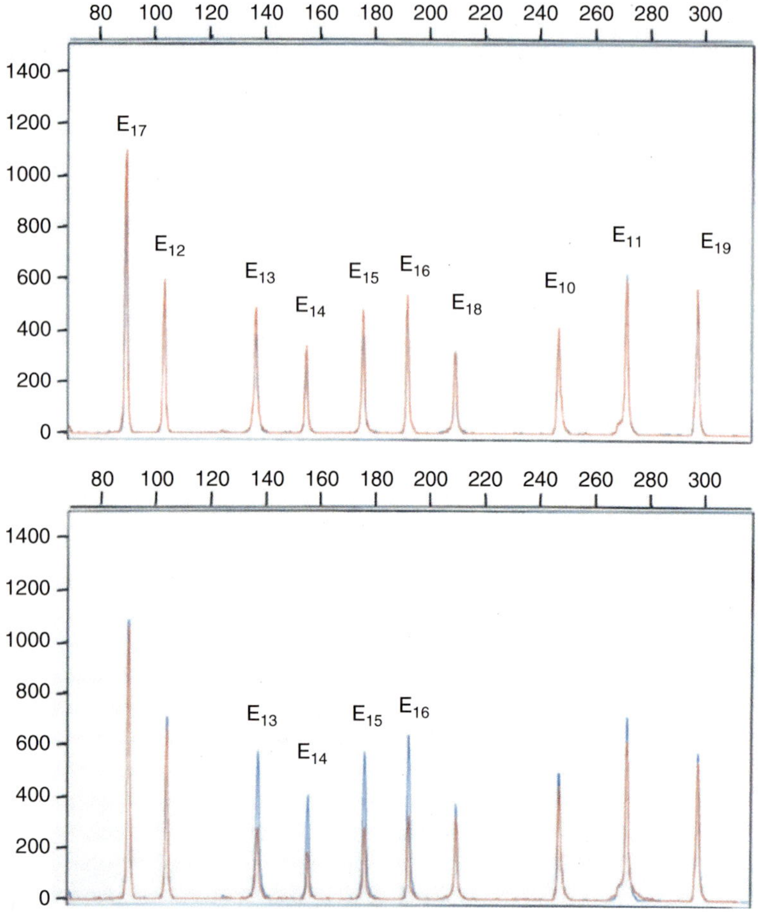

Fig. 5.5 The technique employed by Charbonnier et al. [226] to analyze exon deletions and duplications of the MMR genes in HNPCC CRC families, using multiplex polymerase chain reaction of short fluorescent fragments. Electropherograms from two individuals were superimposed. The *Y* axis displays fluorescence in arbitrary units, and the *X* axis indicates the size in bp. The upper diagram is a multiplex PCR of 10 *MLH1* exons in two controls (*in blue and red*). The lower diagram shows detection of a genomic *MLH1* deletion (*in red*) involving exons 13–16

colonoscopy significantly increased flat and pedunculated adenoma detection in HNPCC. Presently however, pan-colonic chromoscopic colonoscopy is not routinely employed in the endoscopic surveillance of individuals with HNPCC, although it may allow a longer surveillance period prior to colectomy [230]. If endoscopic surveillance cannot be performed, a subtotal colectomy should be considered [231]. Prophylactic colectomy, whether subtotal or complete proctocolectomy, is not recommended if annual endoscopic surveillance can be carried out [231]. When unresectable adenomas or CRC are found, subtotal colectomy may be performed due the increased rate of secondary tumors [231].

Women with HNPCC have a 20–60 % lifetime risk for endometrial cancer and should undergo annual endometrial biopsy beginning at age 30–35 years. Transvaginal ultrasound has little value in screening for endometrial cancer, but can be used for annual ovarian screening [231–233]. Prophylactic hysterectomy/oophorectomy can be performed once the childbearing years are completed, as it results in a significant reduction in endometrial and ovarian cancer [234]. Screening for the more common Lynch Syndrome-associated malignancies, such as gastric cancer and urothelial cancer, is also recommended with frequency dictated by individual and family history (NCCN CRC screening guidelines). Screening for rarer malignancies is not defined by guidelines but is determined by individual and family history.

Most studies on NSAID use and chemoprevention in hereditary CRC have focused on FAP. There are no data on the effects of NSAIDS on chemoprevention in HNPCC, and they are currently not recommended. Additionally, although oral contraceptives are known to lower the incidence of endometrial and ovarian cancer in the general population, no data have demonstrated a chemopreventative effect in HNPCC. Last, individuals with HNPCC show an increased CRC with smoking and should be encouraged not to smoke [231].

5.17 Hamartomatous Polyposis Syndromes

Several heritable CRC syndromes are characterized by a specific constellation of extracolonic manifestations and increased hamartomatous rather than adenomatous polyps. Hamartomatous polyposis syndromes were first described in 1957 when investigators [232] reviewed the literature on pediatric on colorectal polyps and found that most contained mucous-filed glands with retention cysts, abundant connective tissue, and a high number of eosinophils. Presently, two hamartomatous polyposis syndromes with increased CRC are recognized: Juvenile polyposis syndrome (JPS) and Peutz-Jeghers syndrome (PJS). Although both are diagnosed based on clinical manifestations, molecular tests are used to aid diagnosis.

5.17.1 JPS

JPS was first reported by Diamond et al. [235] who described a 30-month-old girl with a prolapsed polyp, accompanied by constipation, hematochezia, and a pedunculated sessile polyp on proctoscopy. In 1975, Stemper et al. [236] described a family with 10 affected members; juvenile polyps were identified in the stomach, small and large intestines, and rectum. Several developed gastric and CRC. Since that time, many studies have found increased gastrointestinal malignancies in kindreds affected by JPS, including gastric, colon, pancreatic, and small intestinal cancers [236–240]. The lifetime risk for malignancy in JPS is estimated to be 9–50 % [241, 242]. Histologically juvenile polyps are characterized by a smooth appearance, with cystically dilated glands embedded in a hyperplasic stroma which has an inflammatory infiltrate.

JPS is presently defined by any of three manifestations: (1) more than 5 juvenile polyps in the colorectum, (2) multiple juvenile polyps throughout the GI tract, and (3) any number of juvenile polyps and a family history of JPS [243]. JPS has been divided into three distinct categories: (1) JPS where the disease is limited to the colon, (2) JPS of infancy characterized by early onset, failure to thrive, hypoalbuminemia, and a poor prognosis, and (3) generalized JPS, where juvenile polyps are seen in the upper and lower gastrointestinal tract [244]. JPS is rare, occurring in ~1 in 10^5 individuals and shows an autosomal dominant inheritance pattern, with approximately 75 % of individuals having an affected parent and 25 % of cases arising de novo [245, 246]. The diagnosis of JPS is largely clinical, with molecular testing employed for prenatal diagnosis, kindred testing, and clinical diagnosis confirmation.

5.17.2 BMPR1A and SMAD4

Two genes are mutated in PJS: *BMPR1A* and *SMAD4*, both accounting for ~20 % of JPS cases [247].

SMAD4 or mothers against decapentaplegic homolog 4, is located at 18q21.1 and consists of 13 exons, which encode a 60.4-kDa protein of 552 residues. *SMAD4* encodes an intracellular mediator of the TGF-β family and activin type 1 receptor signaling. Ligation of the TGF-β family receptor leads to SMAD1,–5 and–8 phosphorylation and activation, forming a complex with Smad4, activating pathways that mediate growth inhibitory signals [247–249]. Over 60 *SMAD4* mutations have been identified in JPS. Interestingly, one mutation identified in multiple kindreds deletes 4 nucleotides (1244_1247delACAG), creating a truncated protein of 433 residues lacking regions critical for normal protein activity [249, 250].

BMPR1A or bone morphogenetic protein receptor, type IA, is located at 10q22.3, and consists of 13 exons that encode a 60.2 kDA protein of 532 residues. BMPR1A is a serine-threonine kinase, which upon binding TGF-β, phosphorylates and activates SMAD1,–5, and–8. These SMADs bind SMAD4, creating a complex that inhibits cell growth and division [247–249]. Thus loss of either BMPR1A or SMAD4 activity results in cellular release from the TGF-β growth-inhibitory pathway, increasing malignant transformation risk [247, 248]. More than 60 *BMPR1A* have been identified, most of which produce a truncated, nonfunctional protein [247–250]. Together, *BMPR1A* or *SMAD4* mutations account for ~45 % of all JPS cases [250]. Patients lacking *BMPR1A* or *SMAD4* mutations are likely to have undiscovered gene mutations. Therefore, failure to identity *BMPR1A* or *SMAD4* mutations does not exclude a JPS diagnosis. The identities of other genes mutated in JPS are currently unknown, although some data implicate endoglin (*Eng*) gene mutation [251].

5.17.3 Molecular Testing for JPS

Due to the large number of *BMPR1A* or *SMAD4* mutations, DNA sequencing is most often employed in mutation analysis of these genes, although techniques such as PCR based denaturing gradient gel electrophoresis have been employed [249–251]. As for other genes analyzed, a set of specific forward and reverse primers first amplify the genomic DNA, which is purified, analyzed in a commercial sequencer, and compared to the wild-type sequence. Where a mutation is identified, it is often confirmed by sequencing in the opposite direction [249]. Such approaches have been able to identity 18 % and 21 % of *BMPR1A* and *SMAD4* JPS mutations, respectively [249, 250]. As with most direct sequencing techniques, a number of deletions/insertions are missed; hence, techniques such as MLPA have been used to identify 6 % and 7 % more *BMPR1A* and *SMAD4* JPS mutations, respectively [250]. Once identified, directed mutational testing can be performed on individuals related to the proband, who may be at risk for JPS.

5.17.4 JPS Management

Once an individual is identified as having JPS, a thorough history and physical examination should be performed, with particular emphasis on the present or absence of rectal bleeding/prolapse, anemia, constipation, obstruction, diarrhea, and abdominal discomfort. Symptomatic individuals should have upper and lower endoscopies, while asymptomatic individuals should have endoscopic screenings beginning at age 15, with all polyps removed. If the initial endoscopic examinations reveal no polyps, they should be repeated in 3 years. If polyps are found, endoscopies should be repeated every year, with all polyps removed. Once no more polyps are identified, endoscopic screening should performed once every 3 years. Individuals related to the proband without an identified mutation should been screened at age 15 and if no polyps are identified screening should be done 10 years to age 45 and then as the general population if no polyps are found [252].

Children with severe bleeding, iron-deficiency anemia, hypoproteinemia, failure to thrive, and/or a non-reducible intussusception should receive an ileorectal anastomosis [253]. Individuals without these severe symptoms should receive an ileorectal anastomosis by age 20–25, when the cancer risk becomes greater than risks associated with surgery. Individuals receiving an ileorectal anastomosis should undergo flexible sigmoidoscopy every 1–3 years for polyp formation in the rectal remnant [254]. Last, individuals with generalized JPS should undergo upper endoscopy every 3 years or annually if polyps are present, beginning at age 15, due to the increased upper gastrointestinal malignancies seen in generalized JPS [241, 242, 254]. Gastric polyps tend to be diffuse and difficult to endoscopically remove, hence a total of subtotal gastrectomy should be performed where gastric outlet obstruction, adenomatous changes, or adenocarcinoma are identified [254].

5.17.5 PJS

PJS is inherited in an autosomal dominant pattern occurring in ~1 in 60,000 and is characterized by pigmented mucocutaneous lesions, especially on the lips, buccal mucosa, and digits, as well as hamartomatous polyps mainly seen in the small intestine. The first detailed description of PJS was given by Peutz in 1921, who described a Dutch family with familial gastrointestinal polyposis, mucocutaneous lesions, and increased cancer [255]. Individuals with PJS have a ~15-fold increased risk for developing intestinal malignancies compared to the general population, with 50 % of PJS individuals dying of cancer by age 57 [255]. The increased malignancies include small intestinal, colonic, esophageal, gastric, breast, lung, pancreatic, uterine, ovarian, testicular, and cervical cancers. Other manifestations of PJS include intussusception, abdominal pain, intestinal polyp prolapse, and hematochezia [255–258]. Interestingly, women with PJS have a high incidence of cervical adenoma malignum and ovarian sex cord tumors with annular tubules, two very rare, well-differentiated neoplasms [255–258].

PJS polyps are characterized by bundles of smooth muscle between non-neoplastic epithelium, typically having an elongated arborizing, Christmas tree-like pattern. Endoscopically PJS polyps do not have specific features and their identification requires histological examination [255–258]. The diagnosis of PJS is based on clinical findings, although molecular-genetic testing is commonly performed for prenatal diagnosis, mutation-specific kindred testing, and clinical diagnosis confirmation. The syndrome is present when any of these conditions are met: (1) presenting with 2 or more PJS polyps, (2) having one polyp and typical PJS pigmented lesions, and (3) having one PJS polyp and a family history of PJS [259].

5.17.6 STK11/LKB1

PJS is caused by mutation of *LKB1* or *STK11* (*serine/threonine kinase 11*), found at 19p13.3. *STK11* consists of 10 exons spanning 23 kb encoding a nuclear 48.6-kDa protein. STK11 is likely regulated by phosphorylation by cAMP-dependent protein kinase A and prenylation [260]. It functions as a tumor suppressor protein, with roles in the G_1 checkpoint, p53-initiated apoptosis, and regulation of Wnt-β catenin-, vascular endothelial growth factor-, and mammalian target of rapamycin (mTOR) signaling pathways [261–265]. More than 140 different *STK11* mutations have been identified in individuals with PJS, with many resulting in inactive truncated kinases. Germline *STK11* mutations have been found in 50–70 % of PJS kindreds and 12–50 % of sporadic PJS cases [266–269]. The reason for the relatively low detection rate is likely due to genes other than *STK11* being mutated in PJS and *STK11* mutations being missed due to the limitations of specific molecular tests [270, 271].

5.17.7 Molecular Testing for PJS

STK11 mutation testing has been performed with a variety of techniques, including DNA sequencing (often limited to exons), CSGE, SSCP, Southern blotting, real-time PCR, quantitative fluorescent PCR, denaturing gradient gel electrophoresis, long range PCR, and MLPA [272]. Volikos et al. [273] analyzed *STK11* mutations via MLPA and found 39 % (11 of 28 individuals with PJS) had large *STK11* deletions ranging from loss of one exon to whole gene deletions. Taken together, ~59 % of *STK11* mutations (range 10–100 %) are detectable by standard methods such as SSCP, CSGE, and DNA sequencing [269, 273–280]. Another 10 % of PJS cases are detectable by RNA based methods only and ~30 % of cases require MLPA testing to detect larger deletions [273, 274, 279, 280]. Thus, current molecular diagnostics allows 80–85 % *STK11* mutation identification in PJS. Currently, most clinical testing employs sequencing of the 10 *STK11* exons and/or MLPA, with the later technique most being effective at detecting larger deletions [272, 274].

5.17.8 Management of PJS

Due to their high risk for carcinomas, all individuals with PJS must be enrolled in lifelong cancer screening programs. While many individuals with PJS develop clinically apparent gastrointestinal lesions as early as their second decade, there are examples of malignancies in young patients and children [281, 282]. Presently there are no organization-approved guidelines for cancer surveillance in PJS patients and different institutions use different protocols [282]. The protocol used at the Johns Hopkins Hospital includes an initial baseline upper endoscopy and small bowel series at 8 years. If polyps are detected, upper endoscopy and small bowel series should be performed every 2–3 years. Upper endoscopy and small bowel series should be done annually from age 18. Colonic endoscopy should be performed every 2–3 years from age 18. At age 25–30, pancreatic endoscopic ultrasound should be done every 1–2 years. CT scanning and CA19-9 levels are offered as options. For women, a pelvic exam with a Pap smear should be performed annually from age 25. At this age, an annual transvaginal ultrasound and serum CA-125 should be done to screen for ovarian cancer. Last, at age 18, monthly breast exams should be done and at 25 semiannual clinical breast exams and annual mammography should be performed. Prophylactic mastectomy should be discussed with the patient. Males should have testicular exams and/or ultrasound of the testicles every 2 years until age 12 [283]. Recently, double balloon enteroscopy and intra-operative enteroscopy have been used to both facilitate better removal of upper gastrointestinal polyps and improve small bowel surveillance [282].

The macrolide compound rapamycin is an effective inhibitor of mammalian target of rapamycin, a cell growth-promoting kinase hyperactivated in PJS [265].

Rapamycin decreases polyp formation in PJS *lkb1* +/– mice [284]. Currently, there are several clinical trials examining the effect of rapamycin on polyp formation in PJS patients [282]. Similarly, PJS *lkb1* +/– mice treated with the COX-2 inhibitor celecoxib show reduced new polyp formation and a decreased size of preexisting polyps [285]. Two of 6 PJS patients given 200 mg celecoxib twice daily for 6 months showed a significant reduction in gastric polyps, suggesting that COX-2 inhibition may have some value in treating PJS [285].

5.18 Chemotherapy Testing for CRC

Irinotecan is a standard chemotherapeutic agent for mCRC treatment, often used in the FOLFIRI regimen: infused 5-fluorouracil, leucovorin, and irinotecan [14, 15]. The effective irinotecan dose depends on the initial amount of drug infused and rate of drug elimination by uridine diphosphate glucuronosyltransferase [*UGT1A1*, 286]. Patient response to irinotecan has been difficult to predict, and toxic reactions are relatively common [287]. For example, fatal events of up to 5.3 % during single-agents irinotecan treatment have been reported [288]. Recently, molecular diagnostics have been used to prospectively identify patients who may be at risk for toxic irinotecan reactions.

5.18.1 UGT1A1

Irinotecan is a topoisomerase 1 inhibitor approved by the FDA in 1994 [14, 15]. Irinotecan stabilizes the complex between topoisomerase 1 and DNA, causing DNA breaks, DNA synthesis inhibition, and apoptosis [289]. Irinotecan is itself relatively inactive, but is converted to the 100–1,000-fold more active metabolite 7-ethyl-10-hydroxy-camptothecin (SN-38) by tissue and serum carboxylesterase-converting enzymes [286, 290]. SN-38 is glucuronidated and inactivated by hepatic *UGT1A1* [286]. The dose-limiting toxicities of irinotecan are severe diarrhea and myelosuppression [287, 288, 291]. The relative activity of UGT1A1 determines the effective in vivo concentration and exposure time to SN-38 [292]. Thus, decreased UGT1A1 expression may lead to a toxic reaction secondary to increased SN-38 levels and longer exposure time [287, 288, 291, 292].

UGT1A1 is located at 2p37, spans ~160 kb, and has at least 9 promoters and first exons that can be spliced to four common expressed exons, resulting in 9 different UGT1A1 enzymes, with the most common "wild-type" gene/protein designated UGT1A1*1 [293, 294]. More than 60 *UGT1A1* coding and promoter variations have been identified, which lessen UGT1A1 enzyme activity [295]. The most common polymorphism, *UGT1A1*28*, contains 7, rather than 6, TA promoter repeats resulting in 70 % lower UGT1A1 expression [296, 297]. TA_7 homozygotes are relatively slow to glucuronidate/inactivate SN-38, TA_6 homozygotes are more efficient, and TA_7/TA_6 heterozygotes show intermediate activity. As expected, individuals with TA_7 homozygotes are more likely to have severe diarrhea and neutropenia following irinotecan therapy, compared to TA_6/TA_6 and TA_7/TA_6 individuals [298]. Interestingly, individuals homozygous for TA_5 and TA_8 promoter repeats occur in African populations, with TA_8 associated with Gilbert syndrome and lower in vitro glucuronidation rates [299].

Other polymorphisms, such as variants at codons 71, 486, 229, and 233, have amino acid substitutions that significantly reduce enzymatic activity and SN-38 clearance. For example, a T → G transversion at codon 486 (*UGT1A1*7*) substitutes a tyrosine moiety for an aspartic acid, resulting in 93 % reduce enzyme activity [300, 301]. Following irinotecan therapy, UGT1A1*28 homozygotes show an increased incidence of irinotecan toxicity compared to *UGT1A1*1* homozygotes, with other variants such as $G^{71}R$ (*UGT1A1*6*) predictive of severe irinotecan-induced neutropenia and poor chemotherapeutic response in Asian populations [302–304]. Many other polymorphisms exist that alter irinotecan therapy responses, often showing population-related distribution [303, 304]. Not surprisingly, individuals heterozygous for two low-activity *UGT1A1* alleles often exhibit irinotecan toxicity. For example, Takane et al. [305] reported severe irinotecan toxicity in a UGT1A1*6/*28 patient.

5.18.2 UGT1A1 Molecular Testing

UGT1A1 allelic variations have been detected through a variety of techniques, including analysis of single base extension of PCR-amplified products, DNA sequencing, HRM, radioactive PCR, denaturing high performance liquid chromatography, and Invader technology. Currently, Invader technology is FDA-approved for *UGT1A1* molecular testing and is commonly used [297, 302, 306–309].

Invader technology typically distinguishes between two different alleles within one non-PCR-based reaction. The reaction involves two steps. First, two allele-specific oligonucelotides, termed Invader oligonucleotides, bind to an unlabeled primary probe. The two Invader oligonucleotides hybridize in tandem with the primary probe forming a specific overlap structure. The 5′-end of the primary probe contains a non-complementary sequence that does not hybridize with either Invader oligonucleotide. The 3′-end of the Invader oligonucleotides are designed to overlap the primary probe such that one of the Invader oligonucleotides will form a complementary base pair with the primary probe. This bp (or pairs for the *28 TA_7) correspond to the wild-type and polymorphism being tested. The complementary base pairing does occur, the resulting structure is recognized and cleaved by the Cleavace® enzyme (Flap endonuclease), releasing the 5′ portion of the primary probe. Should the 3′ portion of the Invader oligonucleotide not be complementary, the Cleavace® enzyme will not cut the structure.

In the second reaction, a second probe binds to the cleaved 5′primary probe sequence, forming a similar structure that is cleaved by the Cleavace® enzyme.

The second probe is designed such that the second cleaving reaction separates a fluorophore from a quencher, creating an easily measured signal. This system can incorporate two primary probes that will eventually cleave either one of two secondary probes, each labeled with a spectrally distinct fluorophore corresponding to a specific allele. The ratio of one fluorophore to the other allows allele identification.

The accuracy of assay comes from the extreme specificity of the Cleavace® enzyme and the sequence specificity of the oligonucleotide hybridization. Purified genomic DNA may be used without PCR amplification and the system has the advantage of being completely closed once the assay has begun. Invader technology is a medium through-put, relatively low-cost technology that commonly allows up to 96 patient samples and controls to be simultaneously interrogated [308, 309].

Despite the large number of different techniques employed in *UGT1A1* genotyping, the analytic sensitivity was 100 % for the *UGT1A1*28* and 98–100 % for the **6* allele, where the referent test was DNA sequencing [310]. The reproducibility of Invader technology was 98.8 % [309]. Additionally, estimates of the first run failure *UGT1A1*1* and *UGT1A1*28* analysis was 5.0 % for sequencing, 1.7 % for PCR/capillary electrophoresis, and 6.7 % for Invader® technology, with most discrepancies solved by repeat testing [309].

5.18.3 UGT1A1 Polymorphism Management

The risk of a toxic irinotecan reaction is roughly 50, 12.5, and 0 % for **28/*28*, **28/*1*, and **1/*1* individuals, respectively [297]. However, there is significant overlap between these groups, and despite a large number of studies, the association between the **28* homozygotic genotype and irinotecan toxicity is not statistically significant [309]. Additionally, at standard irinotecan doses, the tumor response rate is 41 % for wild-type, 45 % for **28* heterozygotes, and 70 % for **28* heterozygotes [309]. Thus the wild-type individuals may be under dosed, while the **28* heterozygotes show a better response. Based on this, The Evaluation of Genomic Applications in Practice and Prevention Working Group found insufficient evidence to recommend for or against *UGT1A1* genotyping guiding irinotecan treatment protocols [309].

Recently however, one Phase I study was performed on 27 patients with mCRC, examining irinotecan toxicity and the **28* polymorphism: 18 patients were **1/*1* and 9 were **1/*28*. A maximum tolerated dose was not observed up to a 150 mg/m^2 dose in the **1/*1* patients, while the **1/*28* patients showed toxicity at a 100 mg/m^2 irinotecan dose [310]. The study concluded that **1/*1* individuals should receive 150 mg/m^2 dose irinotecan, while **1/*28* individuals should receive 70 mg/m^2. The study was limited to 27 patients and included no **28/*28* individuals. Most likely, further studies will be performed and may demonstrate clinical utility for *UGT1A1* genotyping [310].

5.19 Future Directions

Molecular diagnostic testing in CRC is becoming increasingly important in the diagnosis and management of de novo and hereditary CRC, a trend that will probably continue [14–17, 60]. Several trends are readily apparent.

5.19.1 Increased Molecular Diagnostic Testing

Murff et al. [311] found that only 17 % of individuals who met the criteria for early-onset breast cancer testing were actually referred for genetic testing. Presently, many individuals who would benefit from molecular testing do not receive it. As the clinical utility of molecular testing becomes more apparent and testing costs fall, this diagnostic modality will be increasingly employed.

5.19.2 Expansion of the Number of Genes Tested in CRC

Presently, *UGT1A1* genotyping to guide irinotecan use is not routinely performed, although an initial study suggests that it might have use in determining the optimal irinotecan dose [310]. Additionally, Bedoya et al. [312] found that Dukes stage C and D patients were significantly more likely ($P=0.05$) to have a position 1,359 G→A nucleotide change in the cannabinoid receptor-1. They also had a shorter survival time and increased lymph node metastasis. While not currently a part of molecular diagnostics, increased understanding of mutations/polymorphisms in other genes effecting CRC genesis and progression, such as the cannabinoid receptor-1, will likely become important in the molecular diagnostics of this malignancy [14–17, 311].

5.19.3 Specific Molecular Techniques in CRC Testing and Analysis

Several molecular techniques, while not often employed in clinical testing, have proven to be very useful in the analyses of CRC and are very likely to significantly contribute to the molecular diagnostics of CRC in the near future.

Microarray. Micoarray consists of a solid support, often a glass slide, to which DNA probes of known sequence are fixed in an orderly arrangement. The slides are hybridized under high-stringency conditions with labeled nucleic acids (often cDNAs derived from RNAs), extensively washed, and the relative amount of probe-bound target sequence is measured via label detection. The number of gene/nucleic acid sequences that can be simultaneously measured can range from 10 to 1 million.

Comparisons of normal colonic mucosa and CRC have shown a large number of gene products over-or under-expressed in CRC compared to normal colonic tissue [313]. Microarray has allowed the development of specific gene expression panels with diagnostic (Pathwork test for tissue of origin) or prognostic (OncotypeDX) abilities. For CRC, specific gene products have proven useful in predicting clinical behavior. For example, osteopontin RNA expression is a well-documented biomarker of CRC progression [314].

Proteomics. Proteomics involves the analysis and identification of proteins produced by cells in normal and pathologic conditions. Often these analyses examine protein modifications, such as phosphorylation and protein-protein interactions. The specific techniques used ranges from antibody-based protein chips resembling microarray techniques, to yeast two-hybrid systems to identify protein-protein interactions, high throughput crystallography screens for structural analyses, two-dimensional electrophoresis, and mass spectrometry. Although preliminary, these analyses have proven very useful in identifying proteins, whose expression correlates with chemotherapy response, metastatic potential, and degree of clinical aggressiveness. With time, specific proeomic profiles can be developed to predict the clinical behavior of specific CRC cases [313].

Metabolomics. Metabolomics is the study of the chemical footprints unique to specific fluids or tissues and comparing these chemical footprints to others that have been treated in some way or are involved by a pathologic process. Typically, small molecules are analyzed, such as lipids, sugars, and amino acids. Most often, metabolomic analyses are performed with various forms of mass spectrometry following initial separation by techniques such as high-performance liquid chromatography or by nuclear magnetic resonance spectroscopy (NMR). Although preliminary, encouraging results have been obtained. For example, Bezabeh et al. [315] used NMR to analyze the metobolomic profile of fecal samples diluted in a phosphate-buffered saline/D_2O buffer. 412 controls without and 111 with CRC were analyzed. The fecal samples from individuals with CRC showed a unique NMR profile with an 87 % sensitivity and specificity. Interestingly, the cost of this analysis was about $50/sample, significantly lower than many other molecular techniques. Although not yet employed clinically, metabolomic analysis may prove useful in detecting de novo and recurrent CRC and in predicting clinical behavior.

Whole Genome Sequencing. Since 2005 "next generation" DNA sequencing platforms have become increasingly available. Many of these newer sequencing platforms have reduced the cost of sequencing roughly fourfold, compared to standard Sanger sequencing techniques. With time, our rapidly expanding ability to sequence large DNA sequences at lower costs is likely to allow the molecular analysis of an individual's entire genome and/or tumor genome for molecular diagnostics [316, 317]. Obviously such technology would give a vastly increased amount of molecular data for clinical analysis and be a significant tool in the era of personalized medicine.

One interesting new approach that is currently available is "exome sequencing", also known as "targeted exome capture" In this technique genomic DNA is randomly sheared and the resulting DNA fragments are enriched for exomic DNA by aqueous phase hybridization to short labeled (magnetic beads or biotin) DNA or RNA oligonucleotides that correspond to exonic sequences. The labeled hybrids are captured and washed, removing all unbound DNA, leaving only the exonic portion of the genome—which accounts for less than 2 % of the genome, but carries roughly 85 % of disease-causing mutations [318]. The exomic DNA is then PCR amplified and subjected to massively parallel DNA sequencing methods. The advantage of exomic sequencing is that it reduces the volume of DNA to be analyzed by ~98 %, but still allows analysis of the majority (~85 %) of the DNA containing disease-causing mutations [318]. Presently Agilent, Illumina, and Nimblegen offer kitted reagents for exome capture [317].

MicroRNA (miRNA) Profiling. miRNAs are small (~22 nucleotides) posttranscriptional regulators that function by binding to the 3′ untranslated regions of target mRNAs, repressing their expression. miRNAs in some ways represent "a genome within the genome" as each miRNA commonly regulates multiple mRNA targets, functioning as master controls of gene expression. Bioinformatic analysis has suggested that miRNAs regulate about 30 % of human gene expression [319]. CRCs often show specific patterns of increased and decreased miRNAs, especially those miRNAs known to regulate cellular functions such as metastasis, proliferation, DNA repair, apoptosis, and the epithelial-to-mesenchymal transition. Although in its early stages of analysis, miRNA profiling may eventually have clinical use as a diagnostic marker and as a predictor of clinical outcome [320].

Epigenetics. Epigenetics is the study of heritable changes in gene expression that involve mechanisms other than changes in DNA sequence. These changes can include many different biochemical changes, including aberrant DNA methylation, dysregulated miRNA expression (see above), histone modifications such as acetylation and prenylation, and even such bizarre entities as prions. Analysis of the gene methylation patterns found in CRC has shown that nearly all CRCs carry hundreds to thousands of aberrantly methylated genes [321]. Although too complex to review here, epigenetic changes in CRC are becoming increasingly important in the analysis of this tumor. Additionally, with time pharmacologic treatment modalities involving changing the methylation patterns of the tumor CRC genome to restore non-malignant gene expression patterns may become possible in the near future [321, 322].

5.20 Conclusions

In the future the rapidly increasing ability to sequence large DNA sequences at low cost is likely to lead to molecular analysis by sequencing an individual's genome and/or tumor genome for molecular diagnostics [316]. Obviously such technology would give a vastly increased amount of molecular data for clinical analysis and be a significant tool in the era of personalized medicine.

Acknowledgements We would like to thank Jennifer Burton for her help with proofreading this manuscript.

References

1. Parkin DM, Pisani P, Ferlay J (1999) Global cancer statistics. CA Cancer J Clin 52:33–64
2. van der Voort van Zijp J, Hoekstra HJ, Basson MD (2008) Evolving management of colorectal cancer. World J Gastroenterol 14:3956–3967
3. Markowitz SD, Bertagnolli MM (2009) Molecular origins of cancer: molecular basis of colorectal cancer. N Engl J Med 361:2449–2460
4. Parkin DM, Muir CS, Whelan SL, Gao YT, Ferlay J, Powell J (1992) Cancer incidence in five continents. Vol. 6, vol 120. International Agency for Research on Cancer, Lyon, pp 301–353
5. Lichtenstein P, Holm NV, Verkasalo PK, Iliadou A, Kaprio J, Koskenvuo M, Pukkala E, Skytthe A, Hemminki K (2000) Environmental and heritable factors in the causation of cancer–analyses of cohorts of twins from Sweden, Denmark, and Finland. N Engl J Med 343:78–85
6. Picelli S, Von Holst S, Wessendorf P (2009) The continuing search for predisposing colorectal cancer variants. Cancer Genomics Proteomics 6:305–316
7. Johns LE, Houlston RS (2001) A systematic review and meta-analysis of familial colorectal cancer risk. Am J Gastroenterol 96:2992–3003
8. Cannon-Albright LA, Skolnick MH, Bishop DT, Lee RG, Burt RW (1988) Common inheritance of susceptibility to colonic adenomatous polyps and associated colorectal cancers. N Engl J Med 319:533–537
9. Potter JD (1999) Colorectal cancer: molecules and populations. J Natl Cancer Inst 91:916–932
10. Schernhammer ES, Laden F, Speizer FE, Willett WC, Hunter DJ, Kawachi I, Fuchs CS, Colditz GA (2003) Night-shift work and risk of colorectal cancer in the nurses' health study. J Natl Cancer Inst 95:825–828
11. Giovannucci E (2007) Metabolic syndrome, hyperinsulinemia, and colon cancer: a review. Am J Clin Nutr 86:s836–s842
12. Stallmach A, Bielecki C, Schmidt C (2009) Malignant transformation in inflammatory bowel disease—surveillance guide. Dig Dis 27:584–590
13. Pais R, Silaghi H, Silaghi AC, Rusu ML, Dumitrascu DL (2009) Metabolic syndrome and risk of subsequent colorectal cancer. World J Gastroenterol 15:5141–5148
14. Saltz L (2008) Colorectal cancer treatment: what's next? (or: is there life after EGFR and VEGF?). Gastrointest Cancer Res 2(4 Suppl):S20–S22
15. Sobel ME, Bagg A, Caliendo AM, Ladanyi M, Zehnbauer B (2008) The evolution of molecular genetic pathology: advancing 20th-century diagnostic methods into potent tools for the new millennium. J Mol Diagn 10:480–483
16. Tsongalis GJ, Silverman LM (2006) Molecular diagnostics: a historical perspective. Clin Chim Acta 369:188–192
17. Wang HL, Lopategui J, Amin MB, Patterson SD (2010) KRAS mutation testing in human cancers: the pathologist's role in the era of personalized medicine. Adv Anat Pathol 17:23–32
18. O-charoenrat P, Rhys-Evans P, Eccles S (2000) Expression and regulation of c-ERBB ligands in human head and neck squamous carcinoma cells. Int J Cancer 88:759–765
19. Yarden Y, Sliwkowski MX (2001) Untangling the ErbB signaling network. Nat Rev Mol Cell Biol 2:127–137
20. Mayer A, Takimoto M, Fritz E, Schellander G, Kofler K, Ludwig H (1993) The prognostic significance of proliferating cell nuclear antigen, epidermal growth factor receptor, and mdr gene expression in colorectal cancer. Cancer 71:2454–2460
21. Nicholson RI, Gee JM, Harper ME (2001) EGFR and cancer prognosis. Eur J Cancer 37(Suppl 4):S9–S15
22. Kopp R, Rothbauer E, Mueller E, Schildberg FW, Jauch KW, Pfeiffer A (2003) Reduced survival of rectal cancer patients with increased tumor epidermal growth factor receptor levels. Dis Colon Rectum 46:1391–1399

23. Tol J, Dijkstra JR, Klomp M, Teerenstra S, Dommerholt M, Vink-Börger ME, van Cleef PH, van Krieken JH, Punt CJ, Nagtegaal ID (2010) Markers for EGFR pathway activation as predictor of outcome in metastatic colorectal cancer patients treated with or without cetuximab. Eur J Cancer 46:1997–2009
24. Ziober BL, Willson JK, Hymphrey LE, Childress-Fields K, Brattain MG (1993) Autocrine transforming growth factor-alpha is associated with progression of transformed properties in human colon cancer cells. J Biol Chem 268:691–698
25. Untawale S, Zorbas MA, Hodgson CP, Coffey RJ, Gallick GE, North SM, Wildrick DM, Olive M, Blick M, Yeoman LC et al (1993) Transforming growth factor-alpha production and autoinduction in a colorectal carcinoma cell line (DiFi) with an amplified epidermal growth factor receptor gene. Cancer Res 53:1630–1636
26. Tsushima H, Kawata S, Tamura S, Ito N, Shirai Y, Kiso S, Imai Y, Shimomukai H, Nomura Y, Matsuda Y, Matsuzawa Y (1996) High levels of transforming growth factor beta 1 in patients with colorectal cancer: association with disease progression. Gastroenterology 110:375–382
27. Pennell NA, Lynch TJ Jr (2009) Combined inhibition of the VEGFR and EGFR signaling pathways in the treatment of NSCLC. Oncologist 14:399–411
28. Malumbres M, Barbacid M (2003) RAS oncogenes: the first 30 years. Nat Rev Cancer 3:459–465
29. Der CJ, Krontiris TG, Cooper GM (1982) Transforming genes of human bladder and lung carcinoma cell lines are homologous to the ras genes of Harvey and Kirsten sarcoma viruses. Proc Natl Acad Sci USA 79:3637–3640
30. Graziani A, Gramaglia D, Zonca PD, Comoglio PM (1993) Hepatocyte growth factor/scatter factor stimulates the Ras-guanine nucleotide exchanger. J Biol Chem 268:9165–9168
31. Hu YP, Patil SB, Panasiewicz M, Li W, Hauser J, Humphrey LE, Brattain MG (2008) Heterogeneity of receptor function in colon carcinoma cells determined by cross-talk between type I insulin-like growth factor receptor and epidermal growth factor receptor. Cancer Res 68:8004–8013
32. Bos JL (1989) Ras oncogenes in human cancer: a review. Cancer Res 49:4682–4689
33. McCormick F (1989) Ras GTPase activating protein: signal transmitter and signal terminator. Cell 56:5–8
34. Bourne HR, Sanders DA, McCormick F (1990) The GTPase superfamily: a conserved switch for diverse cell functions. Nature 348:125–132
35. Cunningham D, Humblet Y, Siena S et al (2004) Cetuximab monotherapy and cetuximab plus irinotecan in irinotecan-refractory metastatic colorectal cancer. N Engl J Med 351:337–345
36. Bonner JA, Harari PM, Giralt J et al (2006) Radiotherapy plus cetuximab for squamous-cell carcinoma of the head and neck. N Engl J Med 354:567–578
37. Vermorken JB, Trigo J, Hitt R et al (2007) Open-label, uncontrolled, multicenter phase II study to evaluate the efficacy and toxicity of cetuximab as a single agent in patients with recurrent and/or metastatic squamous cell carcinoma of the head and neck who failed to respond to platinum based therapy. J Clin Oncol 25:2171–2177
38. Goldstein NI, Prewett M, Zuklys K, Rockwell P, Mendelsohn J (1995) Biological efficacy of a chimeric antibody to the epidermal growth factor receptor in a human tumor xenograft model. Clin Cancer Res 1:1311–1318
39. Li S, Schmitz KR, Jeffrey PD et al (2005) Structural basis for inhibition of the epidermal growth factor receptor by cetuximab. Cancer Cell 7:301–311
40. Gill GN, Kawamoto T, Cochet C et al (1984) Monoclonal anti-epidermal growth factor receptor antibodies which are inhibitors of epidermal growth factor binding and antagonists of epidermal growth factor binding and antagonists of epidermal growth factor-stimulated tyrosine protein kinase activity. J Biol Chem 259:7755–7760
41. Peng D, Fan Z, Lu Y et al (1996) Anti-epidermal growth factor receptor monoclonal antibody 225 up-regulates p27KIP1 and induces G1 arrest in prostatic cancer cell line DU145. Cancer Res 56:3666–3669
42. Roda JM, Joshi T, Butchar JP, McAlees JW, Lehman A, Tridandapani S, Carson WE 3rd (2007) The activation of natural killer cell effector functions by cetuximab-coated, epidermal

growth factor receptor positive tumor cells is enhanced by cytokines. Clin Cancer Res 13:6419–6428
43. Yang XD, Jia XC, Corvalan JR et al (2001) Development of ABX-EGF, a fully human anti-EGF receptor monoclonal antibody for cancer therapy. Crit Rev Oncol Hematol 38:17–23
44. Foon KA, Yang XD, Weiner LM, Belldegrun AS, Figlin RA, Crawford J, Rowinsky EK, Dutcher JP, Vogelzang NJ, Gollub J, Thompson JA, Schwartz G, Bukowski RM, Roskos LK, Schwab GM (2004) Preclinical and clinical evaluations of ABX-EGF, a fully human anti-epidermal growth factor receptor antibody. Int J Radiat Oncol Biol Phys 58:984–990
45. Van Cutsem E, Peeters M, Siena S, Humblet Y, Hendlisz A, Neyns B, Canon JL, Van Laethem JL, Maurel J, Richardson G, Wolf M, Amado RG (2007) Open-label phase III trial of panitumumab plus best supportive care compared with best supportive care alone in patients with chemotherapy-refractory metastatic colorectal cancer. J Clin Oncol 25:1658–1664
46. Chung KY, Shia J, Kemeny NE, Shah M, Schwartz GK, Tse A, Hamilton A, Pan D, Schrag D, Schwartz L, Klimstra DS, Fridman D, Kelsen DP, Saltz LB (2005) Cetuximab shows activity in colorectal cancer patients with tumors that do not express the epidermal growth factor receptor by immunohistochemistry. J Clin Oncol 23:1803–1810
47. Lièvre A, Bachet JB, Boige V, Cayre A, Le Corre D, Buc E, Ychou M, Bouché O, Landi B, Louvet C, André T, Bibeau F, Diebold MD, Rougier P, Ducreux M, Tomasic G, Emile JF, Penault-Llorca F, Laurent-Puig P (2008) KRAS mutations as an independent prognostic factor in patients with advanced colorectal cancer treated with cetuximab. J Clin Oncol 26:374–379
48. Barault L, Veyrie N, Jooste V, Lecorre D, Chapusot C, Ferraz JM, Lièvre A, Cortet M, Bouvier AM, Rat P, Roignot P, Faivre J, Laurent-Puig P, Piard F (2008) Mutations in the RAS-MAPK, PI(3)K (phosphatidylinositol-3-OH kinase) signaling network correlate with poor survival in a population-based series of colon cancers. Int J Cancer 122:2255–2259
49. Amado RG, Wolf M, Peeters M, Van Cutsem E, Siena S, Freeman DJ, Juan T, Sikorski R, Suggs S, Radinsky R, Patterson SD, Chang DD (2008) Wild-type KRAS is required for panitumumab efficacy in patients with metastatic colorectal cancer. J Clin Oncol 26:1626–1634
50. Zavodna K, Konecny M, Krivulcik T, Spanik S, Behulova R, Vizvaryova M, Weismanova E, Galbavy S, Kausitz J (2009) Genetic analysis of KRAS mutation status in metastatic colorectal cancer patients. Neoplasma 56:275–278
51. Kislitsin D, Lerner A, Rennert G, Lev Z (2002) K-ras mutations in sporadic colorectal tumors in Israel: unusual high frequency of codon 13 mutations and evidence for nonhomogeneous representation of mutation subtypes. Dig Dis Sci 47:1073–1079
52. Breivik J, Meling GI, Spurkland A, Rognum TO, Gaudernack G (1994) K-ras mutation in colorectal cancer: relations to patient age, sex and tumour location. Br J Cancer 69:367–371
53. Vogelstein B, Fearon ER, Hamilton SR, Kern SE, Preisinger AC, Leppert M, Nakamura Y, White R, Smits AM, Bos JL (1988) Genetic alterations during colorectal-tumor development. N Engl J Med 319:525–532
54. Zlobec I, Kovac M, Erzberger P, Molinari F, Bihl MP, Rufle A, Foerster A, Frattini M, Terracciano L, Heinimann K, Lugli A (2010) Combined analysis of specific KRAS mutation, BRAF and microsatellite instability identifies prognostic subgroups of sporadic and hereditary colorectal cancer. Int J Cancer 127:2569–2575
55. De Roock W, Jonker DJ, Di Nicolantonio F, Sartore-Bianchi A, Tu D, Siena S, Lamba S, Arena S, Frattini M, Piessevaux H, Van Cutsem E, O'Callaghan CJ, Khambata-Ford S, Zalcberg JR, Simes J, Karapetis CS, Bardelli A, Tejpar S (2010) Association of KRAS p. G13D mutation with outcome in patients with chemotherapy-refractory metastatic colorectal cancer treated with cetuximab. JAMA 304:1812–1820
56. Lièvre A, Bachet JB, Le Corre D, Boige V, Landi B, Emile JF, Côté JF, Tomasic G, Penna C, Ducreux M, Rougier P, Penault-Llorca F, Laurent-Puig P (2006) KRAS mutation status is predictive of response to cetuximab therapy in colorectal cancer. Cancer Res 66: 3992–3995

57. Karapetis CS, Khambata-Ford S, Jonker DJ, O'Callaghan CJ, Tu D, Tebbutt NC, Simes RJ, Chalchal H, Shapiro JD, Robitaille S, Price TJ, Shepherd L, Au HJ, Langer C, Moore MJ, Zalcberg JR (2008) K-ras mutations and benefit from cetuximab in advanced colorectal cancer. N Engl J Med 359:1757–1765
58. De Roock W, Piessevaux H, De Schutter J, Janssens M, De Hertogh G, Personeni N, Biesmans B, Van Laethem JL, Peeters M, Humblet Y, Van Cutsem E, Tejpar S (2008) KRAS wild-type state predicts survival and is associated to early radiological response in metastatic colorectal cancer treated with cetuximab. Ann Oncol 19:508–515
59. Bokemeyer C, Bondarenko I, Makhson A, Hartmann JT, Aparicio J, de Braud F, Donea S, Ludwig H, Schuch G, Stroh C, Loos AH, Zubel A, Koralewski P (2009) Fluorouracil, leucovorin, and oxaliplatin with and without cetuximab in the first-line treatment of metastatic colorectal cancer. J Clin Oncol 27:663–671
60. National Comprehensive Cancer Network (2012) NCCI clinical practice guidelines in oncology. Non Small Cell Lung Cancer (Version 2.2009) and Colon Cancer (Version 3.2009). http://www.nccn.org/professionals/physician_gls/PDF/colon.ncl.pdf, http://www.nccn.org/professionals/physician_gls/PDF/colon.pdf
61. Gilbert MT, Haselkorn T, Bunce M, Sanchez JJ, Lucas SB, Jewell LD, Van Marck E, Worobey M (2007) The isolation of nucleic acids from fixed, paraffin-embedded tissues-which methods are useful when? PLoS One 2:e537
62. Williams C, Pontén F, Moberg C, Söderkvist P, Uhlén M, Pontén J, Sitbon G, Lundeberg J (1999) A high frequency of sequence alterations is due to formalin fixation of archival specimens. Am J Pathol 155:1467–1471
63. Esposito G (2007) Complementary techniques: laser capture microdissection–increasing specificity of gene expression profiling of cancer specimens. Adv Exp Med Biol 593:54–65
64. Chien CC, Chen SH, Liu CC, Lee CL, Yang RN, Yang SH, Huang CJ (2007) Correlation of K-ras codon 12 mutations in human feces and ages of patients with colorectal cancer (CRC). Transl Res 149:96–102
65. Brink M, de Goeij AF, Weijenberg MP, Roemen GM, Lentjes MH, Pachen MM, Smits KM, de Bruïne AP, Goldbohm RA, van den Brandt PA (2003) K-ras oncogene mutations in sporadic colorectal cancer in The Netherlands cohort study. Carcinogenesis 24:703–710
66. Do H, Krypuy M, Mitchell PL, Fox SB, Dobrovic A (2008) High resolution melting analysis for rapid and sensitive EGFR and KRAS mutation detection in formalin fixed paraffin embedded biopsies. BMC Cancer 8:142
67. Tsiatis AC, Norris-Kirby A, Rich RG, Hafez MJ, Gocke CD, Eshleman JR, Murphy KM (2010) Comparison of Sanger sequencing, pyrosequencing, and melting curve analysis for the detection of KRAS mutations. Diagnostic and clinical implications. J Mol Diagn 12:425–432
68. Huang MM, Arnheim N, Goodman MF (1992) Extension of base mispairs by Taq DNA polymerase: implications for single nucleotide discrimination in PCR. Nucleic Acids Res 20:4567–4573
69. Clayton SJ, Scott FM, Walker J, Callaghan K, Haque K, Liloglou T, Xinarianos G, Shawcross S, Ceuppens P, Field JK, Fox JC (2000) K-ras point mutation detection in lung cancer: comparison of two approaches to somatic mutation detection using ARMS allele-specific amplification. Clin Chem 46:1929–1938
70. Franklin WA, Haney J, Sugita M, Bemis L, Jimeno A, Messersmith WA (2010) KRAS mutation: comparison of testing methods and tissue sampling techniques in colon cancer. J Mol Diagn 12:43–50
71. Kimura H, Kasahara K, Kawaishi M, Kunitoh H, Tamura T, Holloway B, Nishio K (2006) Detection of epidermal growth factor receptor mutations in serum as a predictor of the response to gefitinib in patients with non-small-cell lung cancer. Clin Cancer Res 12:3915–3921
72. Weichert W, Schewe C, Lehmann A, Sers C, Denkert C, Budczies J, Stenzinger A, Joos H, Landt O, Heiser V, Röcken C, Dietel M (2010) KRAS genotyping of paraffin-embedded colorectal cancer tissue in routine diagnostics: comparison of methods and impact of histology. J Mol Diagn 12:35–42

73. Kobunai T, Watanabe T, Yamamoto Y, Eshima K (2010) The frequency of KRAS mutation detection in human colon carcinoma is influenced by the sensitivity of assay methodology: a comparison between direct sequencing and real-time PCR. Biochem Biophys Res Commun 395:158–162
74. Loupakis F, Ruzzo A, Cremolini C, Vincenzi B, Salvatore L, Santini D, Masi G, Stasi I, Canestrari E, Rulli E, Floriani I, Bencardino K, Galluccio N, Catalano V, Tonini G, Magnani M, Fontanini G, Basolo F, Falcone A, Graziano F (2009) KRAS codon 61, 146 and BRAF mutations predict resistance to cetuximab plus irinotecan in KRAS codon 12 and 13 wild-type metastatic colorectal cancer. Br J Cancer 101:715–721
75. Benvenuti S, Sartore-Bianchi A, Di Nicolantonio F, Zanon C, Moroni M, Veronese S, Siena S, Bardelli A (2007) Oncogenic activation of the RAS/RAF signaling pathway impairs the response of metastatic colorectal cancers to anti-epidermal growth factor receptor antibody therapies. Cancer Res 67:2643–2648
76. Tang KT, Lee CH (2010) BRAF mutation in papillary thyroid carcinoma: pathogenic role and clinical implications. J Chin Med Assoc 73:113–128
77. Shepherd C, Puzanov I, Sosman JA (2010) B-RAF inhibitors: an evolving role in the therapy of malignant melanoma. Curr Oncol Rep 12:146–152
78. Vang R, IeM S, Kurman RJ (2009) Ovarian low-grade and high-grade serous carcinoma: pathogenesis, clinicopathologic and molecular biologic features, and diagnostic problems. Adv Anat Pathol 16:267–282
79. Fransén K, Klintenäs M, Osterström A, Dimberg J, Monstein HJ, Söderkvist P (2004) Mutation analysis of the BRAF, ARAF and RAF-1 genes in human colorectal adenocarcinomas. Carcinogenesis 25:527–533
80. Domingo E, Espín E, Armengol M, Oliveira C, Pinto M, Duval A, Brennetot C, Seruca R, Hamelin R, Yamamoto H, Schwartz S Jr (2004) Activated BRAF targets proximal colon tumors with mismatch repair deficiency and MLH1 inactivation. Genes Chromosomes Cancer 39:138–142
81. Kumara T, Simms LA, Whitehall VL, Spring KJ, Wynter CV, Walsh MD, Barker MA, Arnold S, McGivern A, Matsubara N, Tanaka N, Higuchi T, Young J, Jass JR, Leggett BA (2004) BRAF mutation is associated with DNA methylation in serrated polyps and cancers of the colorectum. Gut 53:1137–1144
82. Wan PT, Garnett MJ, Roe SM, Lee S, Niculescu-Duvaz D, Good VM, Jones CM, Marshall CJ, Springer CJ, Barford D, Marais R (2004) Mechanism of activation of the RAF-ERK signaling pathway by oncogenic mutations of B-RAF. Cell 116:855–867
83. Benlloch S, Payá A, Alenda C, Bessa X, Andreu M, Jover R, Castells A, Llor X, Aranda FI, Massutí B (2006) Detection of BRAF V600E mutation in colorectal cancer: comparison of automatic sequencing and real-time chemistry methodology. J Mol Diagn 8:540–543
84. McGivern A, Wynter CV, Whitehall VL, Kambara T, Spring KJ, Walsh MD, Barker MA, Arnold S, Simms LA, Leggett BA, Young J, Jass JR (2004) Promoter hypermethylation frequency and BRAF mutations distinguish hereditary non-polyposis colon cancer from sporadic MSI-H colon cancer. Fam Cancer 3:101–107
85. Kadiyska TK, Konstantinova DV, Atanasov VR, Kremensky IM, Mitev VI (2007) Frequency and application of the hot spot BRAF gene mutation (p.V600E) in the diagnostic strategy for hereditary nonpolyposis colorectal cancer. Cancer Detect Prev 31:254–256
86. Eychene A, Barnier JV, Apiou F, Dutrillaux B, Calothy G (1992) Chromosomal assignment of two human B-raf (Rmil) proto-oncogene loci: B-raf-1 encoding the p94Braf/Rmil and B-raf-2, a processed pseudogene. Oncogene 7:1657–1660
87. Zou M, Baitei EY, Alzahrani AS, Al-Mohanna F, Farid NR, Meyer B, Shi Y (2009) Oncogenic activation of MAP kinase by BRAF pseudogene in thyroid tumors. Neoplasia 11:57–65
88. Lurkin I, Stoehr R, Hurst CD, van Tilborg AA, Knowles MA, Hartmann A, Zwarthoff EC (2010) Two multiplex assays that simultaneously identify 22 possible mutation sites in the KRAS, BRAF, NRAS and PIK3CA genes. PLoS One 5:e8802
89. Albitar M, Yeh C, Ma W (2009) K-ras mutations and cetuximab in colorectal cancer. N Engl J Med 360:834

90. De Roock W, Lambrechts D, Tejpar S (2009) K-ras mutations and cetuximab in colorectal cancer [letter to editor]. N Engl J Med 360:834
91. Samuels Y, Velculescu VE (2004) Oncogenic mutations of PIK3CA in human cancers. Cell Cycle 3:1221–1224
92. Wong KK, Engelman JA, Cantley LC (2010) Targeting the PI3K signaling pathway in cancer. Curr Opin Genet Dev 20:87–90
93. Liu P, Cheng H, Roberts TM, Zhao JJ (2009) Targeting the phosphoinositide 3-kinase pathway in cancer. Nat Rev Drug Discov 8:627–644
94. Cantley LC (2002) The phosphoinositide 3-kinase pathway. Science 296:1655–1657
95. Jhawer M, Goel S, Wilson AJ, Montagna C, Ling YH et al (2008) PIK3CA mutation/PTEN expression status predicts response of colon cancer cells to the epidermal growth factor receptor inhibitor cetuximab. Cancer Res 68:1953–1961
96. Prenen H, De Schutter J, Jacobs B, De Roock W, Biesmans B et al (2009) PIK3CA mutations are not a major determinant of resistance to the epidermal growth factor receptor inhibitor cetuximab in metastatic colorectal cancer. Clin Cancer Res 15:3184–3188
97. Perrone F, Lampis A, Orsenigo M, Di Bartolomeo M, Gevorgyan A, Losa M, Frattini M, Riva C, Andreola S, Bajetta E, Bertario L, Leo E, Pierotti MA, Pilotti S (2009) PI3KCA/PTEN deregulation contributes to impaired responses to cetuximab in metastatic colorectal cancer patients. Ann Oncol 20:84–90
98. Velho S, Oliveira C, Ferreira A, Ferreira AC, Suriano G, Schwartz S Jr, Duval A, Carneiro F, Machado JC, Hamelin R, Seruca R (2005) The prevalence of PIK3CA mutations in gastric and colon cancer. Eur J Cancer 41:1649–1654
99. Lambrechts D, De Roock W, Prenen H, De Schutter J, Jacobs B, Biesmans B, Claes B, De Hertogh G, Van Cutsem E, Tejpar S (2009) The role of KRAS, BRAF, NRAS, and PIK3CA mutations as markers of resistance to cetuximab in chemorefractory metastatic colorectal cancer. J Clin Oncol 27:4020
100. Russo A, Rizzo S, Bronte G, Silvestris N, Colucci G, Gebbia N, Bazan V, Fulfaro F (2009) The long and winding road to useful predictive factors for anti-EGFR therapy in metastatic colorectal carcinoma: the KRAS/BRAF pathway. Oncology 77(Suppl 1):57–68
101. Luschka H (1861) Ueber polypose Vegetationen der gesammten Dickdarmschleimhaut. Arch Pathol Anat Physiol Klin Med 20:133–142
102. Aretz S, Stienen D, Uhlhaas S, Loff S, Back W, Pagenstecher C, McLeod DR, Graham GE, Mangold E, Santer R, Propping P, Friedl W (2005) High proportion of large genomic STK11 deletions in Peutz-Jeghers syndrome. Hum Mutat 26:513–519
103. Aretz S, Stienen D, Uhlhaas S, Stolte M, Entius MM, Loff S, Back W, Kaufmann A, Keller KM, Blaas SH, Siebert R, Vogt S, Spranger S, Holinski-Feder E, Sunde L, Propping P, Friedl W (2007) High proportion of large genomic deletions and a genotype phenotype update in 80 unrelated families with juvenile polyposis syndrome. J Med Genet 44:702–709
104. Kinzler KW, Vogelstein B (1996) Lessons from hereditary colorectal cancer. Cell 87:159–170
105. Half E, Bercovich D, Rozen P (2009) Familial adenomatous polyposis. Orphanet J Rare Dis 4:22
106. Offerhaus GJ, Giardiello FM, Krush AJ et al (1992) The risk of upper gastrointestinal cancer in familial adenomatous polyposis. Gastroenterology 102:1980–1982
107. Park JG, Park KJ, Ahn YO et al (1992) Risk of gastric cancer among Korean familial adenomatous polyposis patients. Report of three cases. Dis Colon Rectum 35:996–998
108. Brosens LA, Keller JJ, Offerhaus GJ, Goggins M, Giardiello FM (2005) Prevention and management of duodenal polyps in familial adenomatous polyposis. Gut 54:1034–1043
109. Johnson JC, DiSario JA, Grady WM (2004) Surveillance and treatment of periampullary and duodenal adenomas in familial adenomatous polyposis. Curr Treat Options Gastroenterol 7:79–89
110. Anaya DA, Chang GJ, Rodriguez-Bigas MA (2008) Extracolonic manifestations of hereditary colorectal cancer syndromes. Clin Colon Rectal Surg 21:263–272
111. Laken SJ, Papadopoulos N, Petersen GM, Gruber SB, Hamilton SR, Giardiello FM, Brensinger JD, Vogelstein B, Kinzler KW (1999) Analysis of masked mutations in familial adenomatous polyposis. Proc Natl Acad Sci USA 96:2322–2326

112. Sampson JR, Jones S, Dolwani S, Cheadle JP (2005) MutYH (MYH) and colorectal cancer. Biochem Soc Trans 33:679–683
113. Bisgaard ML, Ripa R, Knudsen AL, Bülow S (2004) Familial adenomatous polyposis patients without an identified APC germline mutation have a severe phenotype. Gut 53: 266–270
114. Jones S, Emmerson P, Maynard J et al (2002) Biallelic germline mutations in MYH predispose to multiple colorectal adenoma and somatic G:CRT:a mutations. Hum Mol Genet 11: 2961–2967
115. Sieber OM, Lipton L, Crabtree M et al (2003) Multiple colorectal adenomas, classic adenomatous polyposis, and germ-line mutations in MYH. N Engl J Med 348:791–799
116. Béroud C, Soussi T (1996) APC gene: database of germline and somatic mutations in human tumors and cell lines. Nucleic Acids Res 24:121–124
117. Bos JL, Fearon ER, Hamilton SR, de Veerlan v M, van Boom JH, Vogelstein B (1987) Presence of ras gene mutations in human colorectal cancers. Nature 327:293–297
118. Kinzler KW, Nilbert MC, Su LK, Vogelstein B, Bryan TM, Levy DB, Smith KJ, Preisinger AC, Hedge P, McKechnie D, Finniear R, Markham A, Groffen J, Boguski MS, Altschul SF, Horii A, Ando H, Miyoshi Y, Miki Y, Nishisho I, Nakamura Y (1991) Identification of FAP locus genes from chromosome 5q21. Science 253:661–665
119. Fearon ER, Cho KR, Nigro JM, Kern SE, Simons JW, Ruppert JM, Hamilton SR, Preisinger AC, Thomas G, Kinzler KW, Vogelstein B (1990) Identification of a chromosome 18q gene that is altered in colorectal cancers. Science 247:49–56
120. Baker SJ, Fearon ER, Nigro JM, Hamilton SR, Preisinger AC, Jessup JM, van Tuinen P, Ledbetter DH, Barker DF, Nakamura Y, White R, Vogelstein B (1989) Chromosome 17 deletions and p53 gene mutations in colorectal carcinomas. Science 244:217–221
121. Fearon ER, Vogelstein B (1990) A genetic model for colorectal tumorigenesis. Cell 61:759–767
122. Neufeld KL, White RL (1997) Nuclear and cytoplasmic localizations of the adenomatous polyposis coli protein. Proc Natl Acad Sci USA 94:3034–3039
123. Henderson BR (2000) Nuclear-cytoplasmic shuttling of APC regulates beta-catenin subcellular localization and turnover. Nat Cell Biol 2:653–660
124. Rosin-Arbesfeld R, Townsley F, Bienz M (2000) The APC tumour suppressor has a nuclear export function. Nature 406:1009–1012
125. Smith KJ, Levy DB, Maupin P, Pollard TD, Vogelstein B, Kinzler KW (1994) Wild-type but not mutant APC associates with the microtubule cytoskeleton. Cancer Res 54:3672–3675
126. Kennell J, Cadigan KM (2009) APC and beta-catenin degradation. Adv Exp Med Biol 656:1–12
127. Zhang T, Nanney LB, Luongo C, Lamps L, Heppner KJ, DuBois RN, Beauchamp RD (1997) Concurrent overexpression of cyclin D1 and cyclin-dependent kinase 4 (Cdk4) in intestinal adenomas from multiple intestinal neoplasia (Min) mice and human familial adenomatous polyposis patients. Cancer Res 57:169–175
128. Wilding J, Straub J, Bee J, Churchman M, Bodmer W, Dickson C, Tomlinson I, Ilyas M (2002) Cyclin D1 is not an essential target of beta-catenin signaling during intestinal tumorigenesis, but it may act as a modifier of disease severity in multiple intestinal neoplasia (Min) mice. Cancer Res 62:4562–4565
129. Venesio T, Balsamo A, Scordamaglia A, Bertolaso M, Arrigoni A, Sprujevnik T, Rossini FP, Risio M (2003) Germline APC mutation on the beta-catenin binding site is associated with a decreased apoptotic level in colorectal adenomas. Mod Pathol 16:57–65
130. Shinozaki H, Yang K, Fan K, Edelmann W, Kucherlapati R, Weinstein IB, Lipkin M (2003) Cyclin D1 expression in the intestinal mucosa and tumors of Apc1638N mice. Anticancer Res 23:2217–2226
131. Kaplan KB, Burds AA, Swedlow JR, Bekir SS, Sorger PK, Näthke IS (2001) A role for the adenomatous polyposis coli protein in chromosome segregation. Nat Cell Biol 3:429–432
132. Bisgaard ML, Fenger K, Bülow S, Niebuhr E, Mohr J (2003) Familial adenomatous polyposis (FAP): frequency, penetrance, and mutation rate. Hum Mutat 3:121–125

133. Rozen P, Samuel Z, Rabau M, Goldman G, Shomrat R, Legum C, Orr-Urtreger A (2001) Familial adenomatous polyposis at the Tel Aviv Medical Center: demographic and clinical features. Fam Cancer 1:75–82
134. Olschwang S, Tiret A, Laurent-Puig P, Muleris M, Parc R, Thomas G (1993) Restriction of ocular fundus lesions to a specific subgroup of APC mutations in adenomatous polyposis coli patients. Cell 75:959–968
135. Nagase H, Miyoshi Y, Horii A, Aoki T, Ogawa M, Utsunomiya J, Baba S, Sasazuki T, Nakamura Y (1992) Correlation between the location of germ-line mutations in the APC gene and the number of colorectal polyps in familial adenomatous polyposis patients. Cancer Res 52:4055–4057
136. Powell SM, Petersen GM, Krush AJ, Booker S, Jen J, Giardiello FM, Hamilton SR, Vogelstein B, Kinzler KW (1993) Molecular diagnosis of familial adenomatous polyposis. N Engl J Med 329:1982–1987
137. Hogervorst FB, Cornelis RS, Bout M, van Vliet M, Oosterwijk JC, Olmer R, Bakker B, Klijn JG, Vasen HF, Meijers-Heijboer H et al (1995) Rapid detection of BRCA1 mutations by the protein truncation test. Nat Genet 10:208–212
138. Roest PA, Roberts RG, van der Tuijn AC, Heikoop JC, van Ommen GJ, den Dunnen JT (1993) Protein truncation test (PTT) to rapidly screen the DMD gene for translation terminating mutations. Neuromuscul Disord 3:391–394
139. De Rosa M, Scarano MI, Panariello L, Morelli G, Riegler G, Rossi GB, Tempesta A, Romano G, Renda A, Pettinato G, Izzo P (2003) The mutation spectrum of the APC gene in FAP patients from southern Italy: detection of known and four novel mutations. Hum Mutat 21:655–656
140. Aretz S, Stienen D, Uhlhaas S, Pagenstecher C, Mangold E, Caspari R et al (2005) Large submicroscopic genomic APC deletions are a common cause of typical familial adenomatous polyposis. J Med Genet 42:185–192
141. Gismondi V, Bafico A, Biticchi R et al (1998) 310 Basepair APC deletion with duplication of breakpoint (4394ins15del310) in an Italian polyposis patient. Hum Mutat 1:S220–S222
142. Mihalatos M, Apessos A, Dauwerse H, Velissariou V, Psychias A, Koliopanos A, Petropoulos K, Triantafillidis JK, Danielidis I, Fountzilas G, Agnantis NJ, Nasioulas G (2005) Rare mutations predisposing to familial adenomatous polyposis in Greek FAP patients. BMC Cancer 5:40
143. Pagenstecher C, Gadzicki D, Stienen D, Uhlhaas S, Mangold E, Rahner N, Arslan-Kirchner M, Propping P, Friedl W, Aretz S (2007) A complex rearrangement in the APC gene uncovered by multiplex ligation-dependent probe amplification. J Mol Diagn 9:122–126
144. Castellsagué E, González S, Nadal M, Campos O, Guinó E, Urioste M, Blanco I, Frebourg T, Capellá G (2008) Detection of APC gene deletions using quantitative multiplex PCR of short fluorescent fragments. Clin Chem 54:1132–1140
145. Varesco L, Gismondi V, James R, Robertson M, Grammatico P, Groden J, Casarino L, De Benedetti L, Bafico A, Bertario L et al (1993) Identification of APC gene mutations in Italian adenomatous polyposis coli patients by PCR-SSCP analysis. Am J Hum Genet 52:280–285
146. Trimbath JD, Griffin C, Romans K, Giardiello FM (2003) Attenuated familial adenomatous polyposis presenting as ampullary adenocarcinoma. Gut 52:903–904
147. Watson P, Lynch HT (1993) Extracolonic cancer in hereditary nonpolyposis colorectal cancer. Cancer 71:677–685
148. Aziz O, Athanasiou T, Fazio VW, Nicholls RJ, Darzi AW, Church J, Phillips RK, Tekkis PP (2006) Meta-analysis of observational studies of ileorectal versus ileal pouch-anal anastomosis for familial adenomatous polyposis. Br J Surg 93:407–417
149. Kartheuser AH, Parc R, Penna CP, Tiret E, Frileux P, Hannoun L, Nordlinger B, Loygue J (1996) Ileal pouch-anal anastomosis as the first choice operation in patients with familial adenomatous polyposis: a ten-year experience. Surgery 119:615–623
150. Hirschman BA, Pollock BH, Tomlinson GE (2005) The spectrum of APC mutations in children with hepatoblastoma from familial adenomatous polyposis kindreds. J Pediatr 147:263–266

151. Steinbach G, Lynch PM, Phillips RK, Wallace MH, Hawk E, Gordon GB, Wakabayashi N, Saunders B, Shen Y, Fujimura T, Su LK, Levin B (2000) The effect of celecoxib, a cyclooxygenase-2 inhibitor, in familial adenomatous polyposis. N Engl J Med 342:1946–1952
152. Phillips RK, Wallace MH, Lynch PM, Hawk E, Gordon GB, Saunders BP, Wakabayashi N, Shen Y, Zimmerman S, Godio L, Rodrigues-Bigas M, Su LK, Sherman J, Kelloff G, Levin B, Steinbach G, FAP Study Group (2002) A randomised, double blind, placebo controlled study of celecoxib, a selective cyclooxygenase 2 inhibitor, on duodenal polyposis in familial adenomatous polyposis. Gut 50:857–860
153. Heiskanen I, Luostarinen T, Järvinen HJ (2000) Impact of screening examinations on survival in familial adenomatous polyposis. Scand J Gastroenterol 35:1284–1287
154. Dowton SB, Slaugh RA (1995) Diagnosis of human heritable diseases–laboratory approaches and outcomes. Clin Chem 41:785–794
155. Knudsen AL, Bisgaard ML, Bülow S (2003) Attenuated familial adenomatous polyposis (AFAP). A review of the literature. Fam Cancer 2:43–55
156. Grady WM (2003) Genetic testing for high-risk colon cancer patients. Gastroenterology 124:1574–1594
157. Nishisho I, Nakamura Y, Miyoshi Y, Miki Y, Ando H, Horii A, Koyama K, Utsunomiya J, Baba S, Hedge P (1991) Mutations of chromosome 5q21 genes in FAP and colorectal cancer patients. Science 253:665–669
158. Rowley PT (2004) Screening for an inherited susceptibility to colorectal cancer. Genet Test 8:421–430
159. Gardner EJ (1962) Follow-up study of a family group exhibiting dominant inheritance for a syndrome including intestinal polyps, osteomas, fibromas and epidermal cysts. Am J Hum Genet 14:376
160. Fotiadis C, Tsekouras DK, Antonakis P, Sfiniadakis J, Genetzakis M, Zografos GC (2005) Gardner's syndrome: a case report and review of the literature. World J Gastroenterol 11:5408–5411
161. Turcot J, Després J-P, St Pierre F (1959) Malignant tumors of the central nervous system associated with familial polyposis of the colon: report of two cases. Dis Colon Rectum 2:465–468
162. Hamilton SR, Liu B, Parsons RE, Papadopoulos N, Jen J, Powell SM, Krush AJ, Berk T, Cohen Z, Tetu B et al (1995) The molecular basis of Turcot's syndrome. N Engl J Med 332:839–847
163. Paraf F, Jothy S, Van Meir EG (1997) Brain tumor-polyposis syndrome: two genetic diseases? J Clin Oncol 15:2744–2758
164. Laken SJ, Petersen GM, Gruber SB, Oddoux C, Ostrer H, Giardiello FM, Hamilton SR, Hampel H, Markowitz A, Klimstra D, Jhanwar S, Winawer S, Offit K, Luce MC, Kinzler KW, Vogelstein B (1997) Familial colorectal cancer in Ashkenazim due to a hypermutable tract in APC. Nat Genet 17:79–83
165. Zauber NP, Sabbath-Solitare M, Marotta S, Zauber AG, Foulkes W, Chan M, Turner F, Bishop DT (2005) Clinical and genetic findings in an Ashkenazi Jewish population with colorectal neoplasms. Cancer 104:719–729
166. Gryfe R, Di Nicola N, Gallinger S, Redston M (1998) Somatic instability of the APC I1307K allele in colorectal neoplasia. Cancer Res 58:4040–4043
167. Niell BL, Long JC, Rennert G, Gruber SB (2003) Genetic anthropology of the colorectal cancer-susceptibility allele APC I1307K: evidence of genetic drift within the Ashkenazim. Am J Hum Genet 73:1250–1260
168. Gryfe R, Di Nicola N, Lal G, Gallinger S, Redston M (1999) Inherited colorectal polyposis and cancer risk of the APC I1307K polymorphism. Am J Hum Genet 64:378–384
169. Rennert G, Almog R, Tomsho LP, Low M, Pinchev M, Chaiter Y, Bonner JD, Rennert HS, Greenson JK, Gruber SB (2005) Colorectal polyps in carriers of the APC I1307K polymorphism. Dis Colon Rectum 48:2317–2321

170. Baris HN, Kedar I, Halpern GJ, Shohat T, Magal N, Ludman MD, Shohat M (2007) Prevalence of breast and colorectal cancer in Ashkenazi Jewish carriers of Fanconi anemia and bloom syndrome. Isr Med Assoc J 9:847–850
171. Shackelford RE, Kaufmann WK, Paules RS (2000) Oxidative stress and cell cycle checkpoint function. Free Radic Biol Med 28:1387–1404
172. Lee SH, Blair IA (2001) Oxidative DNA damage and cardiovascular disease. Trends Cardiovasc Med 11:148–155
173. Cooke MS, Olinski R, Evans MD (2006) Does measurement of oxidative damage to DNA have clinical significance? Clin Chim Acta 365:30–49
174. Marnett LJ (2000) Oxyradicals and DNA damage. Carcinogenesis 21:361–370
175. Slupska MM, Luther WM, Chiang JH, Yang H, Miller JH (1999) Functional expression of hMYH, a human homolog of the Escherichia coli MutY protein. J Bacteriol 181:6210–6213
176. Yang H, Clendenin WM, Wong D, Demple B, Slupska MM, Chiang JH, Miller JH (2001) Enhanced activity of adenine-DNA glycosylase (Myh) by apurinic/apyrimidinic endonuclease (Ape1) in mammalian base excision repair of an A/GO mismatch. Nucleic Acids Res 29:743–752
177. Lipton L, Halford SE, Johnson V, Novelli MR, Jones A, Cummings C, Barclay E, Sieber O, Sadat A, Bisgaard ML, Hodgson SV, Aaltonen LA, Thomas HJ, Tomlinson IP (2003) Carcinogenesis in MYH-associated polyposis follows a distinct genetic pathway. Cancer Res 63:7595–7599
178. Al-Tassan N, Chmiel NH, Maynard J, Fleming N, Livingston AL, Williams GT, Hodges AK, Davies DR, David SS, Sampson JR, Cheadle JP (2002) Inherited variants of MYH associated with somatic G:C → T: a mutations in colorectal tumors. Nat Genet 30:227–232
179. Fleischmann C, Peto J, Cheadle J, Shah B, Sampson J, Houlston RS (2004) Comprehensive analysis of the contribution of germline MYH variation to early-onset colorectal cancer. Int J Cancer 109:554–558
180. Farrington SM, Tenesa A, Barnetson R, Wiltshire A, Prendergast J, Porteous M, Campbell H, Dunlop MG (2005) Germline susceptibility to colorectal cancer due to base-excision repair gene defects. Am J Hum Genet 77:112–119
181. Vogt S, Jones N, Christian D et al (2009) Expanded extracolonic tumor spectrum in MUTYH-associated polyposis. Gastroenterology 137:1976–1985
182. Nielsen M, Franken PF, Reinards TH, Weiss MM, Wagner A, van der Klift H et al (2005) Multiplicity in polyp count and extracolonic manifestations in 40 Dutch patients with MYH associated polyposis coli (MAP). J Med Genet 42:e54
183. Sampson JR, Dolwani S, Jones S, Eccles D, Ellis A, Evans DG, Frayling I, Jordan S, Maher ER, Mak T, Maynard J, Pigatto F, Shaw J, Cheadle JP (2003) Autosomal recessive colorectal adenomatous polyposis due to inherited mutations of MYH. Lancet 362:39–41
184. Barnetson RA, Devlin L, Miller J, Farrington SM, Slater S, Drake AC, Campbell H, Dunlop MG, Porteous ME (2007) Germline mutation prevalence in the base excision repair gene, MYH, in patients with endometrial cancer. Clin Genet 72:551–555
185. O'Shea AM, Cleary SP, Croitoru MA, Kim H, Berk T, Monga N, Riddell RH, Pollett A, Gallinger S (2008) Pathological features of colorectal carcinomas in MYH-associated polyposis. Histopathology 53:184–194
186. Chow E, Thirlwell C, Macrae F, Lipton L (2004) Colorectal cancer and inherited mutations in base-excision repair. Lancet Oncol 5:600–606
187. Prior TW, Bridgeman SJ (2010) Identifying mutations for MYH-associated polyposis. Curr Protoc Hum Genet, Chapter 10:Unit 10.13
188. Piccioli P, Serra M, Gismondi V, Pedemonte S, Loiacono F, Lastraioli S, Bertario L, De Angioletti M, Varesco L, Notaro R (2006) Multiplex tetra-primer amplification refractory mutation system PCR to detect 6 common germline mutations of the MUTYH gene associated with polyposis and colorectal cancer. Clin Chem 52:739–743
189. Gismondi V, Meta M, Bonelli L, Radice P, Sala P, Bertario L, Viel A, Fornasarig M, Arrigoni A, Gentile M, Ponz de Leon M, Anselmi L, Mareni C, Bruzzi P, Varesco L (2004) Prevalence

of the Y165C, G382D and 1395delGGA germline mutations of the MYH gene in Italian patients with adenomatous polyposis coli and colorectal adenomas. Int J Cancer 109: 680–684
190. Cleary SP, Cotterchio M, Jenkins MA et al (2009) Germline MutY human homologue mutations and colorectal cancer: a multisite case–control study. Gastroenterology 136: 1251–1260
191. Jones N, Vogt S, Nielsen M et al (2009) Cancer risks in MUTYH heterozygotes: increased colorectal cancer incidence in obligate carriers of heterozygous mutations in MUTYH. Gastroenterology 137:489–494
192. Olschwang S, Blanché H, de Moncuit C, Thomas G (2007) Similar colorectal cancer risk in patients with monoallelic and biallelic mutations in the MYH gene identified in a population with adenomatous polyposis. Genet Test 11:315–320
193. Hampel H, Frankel WL, Martin E, Arnold M, Khanduja K, Kuebler P, Clendenning M, Sotamaa K, Prior T, Westman JA, Panescu J, Fix D, Lockman J, LaJeunesse J, Comeras I, de la Chapelle A (2008) Feasibility of screening for Lynch syndrome among patients with colorectal cancer. J Clin Oncol 26:5783–5788
194. Lynch HT, Shaw MW, Magnuson CW, Larsen AL, Krush AJ (1966) Hereditary factors in cancer. Study of two large midwestern kindreds. Arch Intern Med 117:206–212
195. Umar A, Boland CR, Terdiman JP et al (2004) Revised Bethesda guidelines for hereditary nonpolyposis colorectal cancer (Lynch syndrome) and microsatellite instability. J Natl Cancer Inst 96:261–268
196. Hsieh P, Yamane K (2008) DNA mismatch repair: molecular mechanism, cancer, and ageing. Mech Ageing Dev 129:391–407
197. Zhang Y, Rohde LH, Wu H (2009) Involvement of nucleotide excision and mismatch repair mechanisms in double strand break repair. Curr Genomics 10:250–258
198. Bronner CE, Baker SM, Morrison PT, Warren G, Smith LG, Lescoe MK, Kane M, Earabino C, Lipford J, Lindblom A et al (1994) Mutation in the DNA mismatch repair gene homologue hMLH1 is associated with hereditary non-polyposis colon cancer. Nature 368:258–261
199. Mitchell RJ, Farrington SM, Dunlop MG, Campbell H (2002) Mismatch repair genes hMLH1 and hMSH2 and colorectal cancer: a HuGE review. Am J Epidemiol 156:885–902
200. Kuismanen SA, Holmberg MT, Salovaara R, de la Chapelle A, Peltomäki P (2000) Genetic and epigenetic modification of MLH1 accounts for a major share of microsatellite-unstable colorectal cancers. Am J Pathol 156:1773–1779
201. Wijnen J, Khan PM, Vasen H, van der Klift H, Mulder A, van Leeuwen-Cornelisse I, Bakker B, Losekoot M, Møller P, Fodde R (1997) Hereditary nonpolyposis colorectal cancer families not complying with the Amsterdam criteria show extremely low frequency of mismatch-repair-gene mutations. Am J Hum Genet 61:329–335
202. Peltomaki P (2003) Role of DNA mismatch repair defects in the pathogenesis of human cancer. J Clin Oncol 21:1174–1179
203. Miyaki M, Konishi M, Tanaka K, Kikuchi-Yanoshita R, Muraoka M, Yasuno M, Igari T, Koike M, Chiba M, Mori T (1997) Germline mutation of MSH6 as the cause of hereditary nonpolyposis colorectal cancer. Nat Genet 17:271–272
204. Berends MJ, Wu Y, Sijmons RH, Mensink RG, van der Sluis T, Hordijk-Hos JM, de Vries EG, Hollema H, Karrenbeld A, Buys CH, van der Zee AG, Hofstra RM, Kleibeuker JH (2002) Molecular and clinical characteristics of MSH6 variants: an analysis of 25 index carriers of a germline variant. Am J Hum Genet 70:26–37
205. Wijnen J, de Leeuw W, Vasen H, van der Klift H, Moller P, Stormorken A, Meijers-Heijboer H, Lindhout D, Menko F, Vossen S, Moslein G, Tops C, Brocker-Vriends A, Wu Y, Hofstra R, Sijmons R, Cornelisse C, Morreau H, Fodde R (1999) Familial endometrial cancer in female carriers of MSH6 germline mutations. Nat Genet 23:142–144
206. Plaschke J, Engel C, Krüger S, Holinski-Feder E, Pagenstecher C, Mangold E, Moeslein G, Schulmann K, Gebert J, von Knebel DM, Rüschoff J, Loeffler M, Schackert HK (2004) Lower incidence of colorectal cancer and later age of disease onset in 27 families with

pathogenic MSH6 germline mutations compared with families with MLH1 or MSH2 mutations: the German hereditary nonpolyposis colorectal cancer consortium. J Clin Oncol 22:4486–4494

207. Wang Y, Cortez D, Yazdi P, Neff N, Elledge SJ, Qin J (2000) BASC, a super complex of BRCA1-associated proteins involved in the recognition and repair of aberrant DNA structures. Genes Dev 14:927–939
208. Wu Y, Berends MJ, Sijmons RH, Mensink RG, Verlind E, Kooi KA, van der Sluis T, Kempinga C, van dDer Zee AG, Hollema H, Buys CH, Kleibeuker JH, Hofstra RM (2001) A role for MLH3 in hereditary nonpolyposis colorectal cancer. Nat Genet 29:137–138
209. Duval A, Hamelin R (2002) Mutations at coding repeat sequences in mismatch repair-deficient human cancers: toward a new concept of target genes for instability. Cancer Res 62:2447–2454
210. Markowitz S, Wang J, Myeroff L, Parsons R, Sun L, Lutterbaugh J, Fan RS, Zborowska E, Kinzler KW, Vogelstein B, Brattain M, Willson JKV (1995) Inactivation of the type II TGF-β receptor in colon cancer cells with microsatellite instability. Science 268:1336–1338
211. Perucho M (1996) Microsatellite instability: the mutator that mutates the other mutator. Nat Med 2:630–631
212. Loukola A, Eklin K, Laiho P, Salovaara R, Kristo P, Jarvinen H, Mecklin JP, Launonen V, Aaltonen LA (2001) Microsatellite marker analysis in screening for hereditary nonpolyposis colorectal cancer (HNPCC). Cancer Res 61:4545–4549
213. Yuan ZQ, Legendre B, Cai DQ, Cao J, Zhu J, Weber TK (2009) High throughput detection of microsatellite instability (MSI) in sporadic colorectal cancer by MSI COPPER denaturing high performance liquid chromatography. Pathology 41:393–394
214. Chialina SG, Fornes C, Landi C, de la Vega Elena CD, Nicolorich MV, Dourisboure RJ, Solano A, Solis EA (2006) Microsatellite instability analysis in hereditary non-polyposis colon cancer using the Bethesda consensus panel of microsatellite markers in the absence of proband normal tissue. BMC Med Genet 7:5
215. Piñol V, Castells A, Andreu M, Castellví-Bel S, Alenda C, Llor X, Xicola RM, Rodríguez-Moranta F, Payá A, Jover R, Bessa X (2005) Accuracy of revised Bethesda guidelines, microsatellite instability, and immunohistochemistry for the identification of patients with hereditary nonpolyposis colorectal cancer. JAMA 293:1986–1994
216. Lindor NM, Burgart LJ, Leontovich O, Goldberg RM, Cunningham JM, Sargent DJ, Walsh-Vockley C, Petersen GM, Walsh MD, Leggett BA, Young JP, Barker MA, Jass JR, Hopper J, Gallinger S, Bapat B, Redston M, Thibodeau SN (2002) Immunohistochemistry versus microsatellite instability testing in phenotyping colorectal tumors. J Clin Oncol 20:1043–1048
217. Debniak T, Kurzawski G, Gorski B et al (2000) Value of pedigree/clinical data, immunohistochemistry and microsatellite instability analyses in reducing the cost of determining hMLH1 and hMSH2 gene mutations in patients with colorectal cancer. Eur J Cancer 36:49–54
218. Ionov Y, Peinado MA, Malkhosyan S, Shibata D, Perucho M (1993) Ubiquitous somatic mutations in simple repeated sequences reveal a new mechanism for colonic carcinogenesis. Nature 363:558–561
219. Thibodeau SN, Bren G, Schaid D (1993) Microsatellite instability in cancer of the proximal colon. Science 260:816–819
220. Domingo E, Laiho P, Ollikainen M, Pinto M, Wang L, French AJ, Westra J, Frebourg T, Espín E, Armengol M, Hamelin R, Yamamoto H, Hofstra RM, Seruca R, Lindblom A, Peltomäki P, Thibodeau SN, Aaltonen LA, Schwartz S Jr (2004) BRAF screening as a low-cost effective strategy for simplifying HNPCC genetic testing. J Med Genet 41:664–668
221. Domingo E, Niessen RC, Oliveira C, Alhopuro P, Moutinho C, Espín E, Armengol M, Sijmons RH, Kleibeuker JH, Seruca R, Aaltonen LA, Imai K, Yamamoto H, Schwartz S Jr, Hofstra RM (2005) BRAF-V600E is not involved in the colorectal tumorigenesis of HNPCC in patients with functional MLH1 and MSH2 genes. Oncogene 24:3995–3998

222. Baudhuin LM, Mai M, French AJ, Kruckeberg KE, Swanson RL, Winters JL, Courteau LK, Thibodeau SN (2005) Analysis of hMLH1 and hMSH2 gene dosage alterations in hereditary nonpolyposis colorectal cancer patients by novel methods. J Mol Diagn 7:226–235
223. Miyaki M, Konishi M, Muraoka M, Kikuchi-Yanoshita R, Tanaka K, Iwama T, Mori T, Koike M, Ushio K, Chiba M et al (1995) Germ line mutations of hMSH2 and hMLH1 genes in Japanese families with hereditary nonpolyposis colorectal cancer (HNPCC): usefulness of DNA analysis for screening and diagnosis of HNPCC patients. J Mol Med 73:515–520
224. Wijnen J, Vasen H, Khan PM, Menko FH, van der Klift H, van Leeuwen C, van den Broek M, van Leeuwen-Cornelisse I, Nagengast F, Meijers-Heijboer A et al (1995) Seven new mutations in hMSH2, an HNPCC gene, identified by denaturing gradient-gel electrophoresis. Am J Hum Genet 56:1060–1066
225. Charbonnier F, Raux G, Wang Q, Drouot N, Cordier F, Limacher JM, Saurin JC, Puisieux A, Olschwang S, Frebourg T (2000) Detection of exon deletions and duplications of the mismatch repair genes in hereditary nonpolyposis colorectal cancer families using multiplex polymerase chain reaction of short fluorescent fragments. Cancer Res 60:2760–2763
226. Peltoma¨ki P, Vasen H (1997) The international collaborative group on hereditary nonpolyposis colorectal cancer. Mutations predisposing to hereditary nonpolyposis colorectal cancer: database and results of a collaborative study. Gastroenterology 113:1146–1158
227. Mauillon J, Michel P, Limacher JM, Dechelotte P, Charbonnier F, Martin C, Moreau V, Metayer J, Paillot B, Frebourg T (1996) Identification of novel germline hMLH1 mutations including a 22-kb Alu-mediated deletion in patients with familial colorectal cancer. Cancer Res 56:5728–5733
228. Vasen HFA, Nagengast FM, Khan PM (1995) Interval cancers in hereditary non-polyposis colorectal cancer (Lynch syndrome). Lancet 345:1183–1184
229. Järvinen HJ, Aarnio M, Mustonen H et al (2000) Controlled 15-year trial on screening for colorectal cancer in families with hereditary nonpolyposis colorectal cancer. Gastroenterology 118:829–834
230. Hurlstone DP, Cross SS, Slater R, Sanders DS, Brown S (2004) Detecting diminutive colorectal lesions at colonoscopy: a randomized controlled trial of pan-colonic versus targeted chromoscopy. Gut 53:376–380
231. Lindor NM, Petersen GM, Hadley DW, Kinney AY, Miesfeldt S, Lu KH, Lynch P, Burke W, Press N (2006) Recommendations for the care of individuals with an inherited predisposition to Lynch syndrome: a systematic review. JAMA 296:1507–1517
232. Dunlop MG, Farrington SM, Carothers AD, Wyllie AH, Sharp L, Burn J, Liu B, Kinzler KW, Vogelstein B (1997) Cancer risk associated with germline DNA mismatch repair gene mutations. Hum Mol Genet 6:105–110
233. Vasen HF, Wijnen JT, Menko FH, Kleibeuker JH, Taal BG, Griffioen G, Nagengast FM, Meijers-Heijboer EH, Bertario L, Varesco L, Bisgaard ML, Mohr J, Fodde R, Khan PM (1996) Cancer risk in families with hereditary nonpolyposis colorectal cancer diagnosed by mutation analysis. Gastroenterology 110:1020–1027
234. Schmeler KM, Lynch HT, Chen L-M et al (2006) Prophylactic surgery to reduce the risk of gynecologic cancers in the Lynch syndrome. N Engl J Med 354:261–269
235. Diamond M (1939) Adenoma of the rectum in children: report of a case in a thirty month old girl. Am J Dis Children 57:360
236. Stemper TJ, Kent TH, Summers RW (1975) Juvenile polyposis and gastrointestinal carcinoma. Ann Intern Med 83:639–646
237. Goodman ZD, Yardley JH, Milligan FD (1979) Pathogenesis of colonic polyps in multiple juvenile polyposis. Cancer 43:1906–1913
238. Yoshida T, Haraguchi Y, Tanaka A, Higa A, Daimon Y, Mizuta Y, Tamaki M et al (1988) A case of generalized juvenile gastrointestinal polyposis associated with gastric carcinoma. Endoscopy 20:33–35
239. Walpole IR, Cullity G (1989) Juvenile polyposis: a case with early presentation and death attributable to adenocarcinoma of the pancreas. Am J Med Genet 32:1–8

240. Bentley E, Chandrasoma P, Radin R, Cohen H (1989) Generalized juvenile polyposis with carcinoma. Am J Gastroenterol 84:1456–1459
241. Jarvinen HJ, Franssila KO (1984) Familial juvenile polyposis coli: increased risk of colorectal cancer. Gut 25:792–800
242. Jass JR (1990) Pathology of polyposis syndromes with special reference to juvenile polyposis. In: Utsunomiya J, Lynch HT (eds) Hereditary colorectal cancer. Springer, Tokyo, pp 343–350
243. Jass JR, Williams CB, Bussey HJ, Morson BC (1988) Juvenile polyposis–a precancerous condition. Histopathology 13:619–630
244. Sachatello CR (1972) Polypoid diseases of the gastrointestinal tract. J Ky Med Assoc 70:540
245. Bussey HJ, Veale AM, Morson BC (1978) Genetics of gastrointestinal polyposis. Gastroenterology 74:1325
246. Burt RW, Bishop DT, Lynch HT, Rozen P, Winawer SJ (1990) Risk and surveillance of individuals with heritable factors for colorectal cancer. WHO collaborating centre for the prevention of colorectal cancer. Bull World Health Organ 68:655–665
247. Howe JR, Sayed MG, Ahmed AF, Ringold J, Larsen-Haidle J, Merg A, Mitros FA, Vaccaro CA, Petersen GM, Giardiello FM, Tinley ST, Aaltonen LA, Lynch HT (2004) The prevalence of MADH4 and BMPR1A mutations in juvenile polyposis and absence of BMPR2, BMPR1B, and ACVR1 mutations. J Med Genet 41:484–491
248. Mishina Y (2003) Function of bone morphogenetic protein signaling during mouse development. Front Biosci 8:d855–d869
249. Howe JR, Roth S, Ringold JC, Summers RW, Järvinen HJ, Sistonen P, Tomlinson IP, Houlston RS, Bevan S, Mitros FA, Stone EM, Aaltonen LA (1998) Mutations in the SMAD4/DPC4 gene in juvenile polyposis. Science 280:1086–1088
250. Calva-Cerqueira D, Chinnathambi S, Pechman B, Bair J, Larsen-Haidle J, Howe JR (2009) The rate of germline mutations and large deletions of SMAD4 and BMPR1A in juvenile polyposis. Clin Genet 75:79–85
251. Sweet K, Willis J, Zhou XP, Gallione C, Sawada T, Alhopuro P, Khoo SK, Patocs A, Martin C, Bridgeman S, Heinz J, Pilarski R, Lehtonen R, Prior TW, Frebourg T, Teh BT, Marchuk DA, Aaltonen LA, Eng C (2005) Molecular classification of patients with unexplained hamartomatous and hyperplastic polyposis. JAMA 294:2465–2473
252. Calva D, Howe JR (2008) Hamartomatous polyposis syndromes. Surg Clin North Am 88:779–817
253. Grosfeld JL, West KW (1986) Generalized juvenile polyposis coli. Arch Surg 121:530
254. Järvinen H (1993) Juvenile gastrointestinal polyposis. Probl Gen Surg 10:749–757
255. Peutz JL (1921) Over een zeer merkwaardige, gecombineerde familiaire pollyposis van de sligmliezen van den tractus intestinalis met die van de neuskeelholte en gepaard met eigenaardige pigmentaties van huid-en slijmvliezen. Ned Maandschr v Gen 10:134
256. Brosens LA, van Hattem WA, Jansen M, de Leng WW, Giardiello FM, Offerhaus GJ (2007) Gastrointestinal polyposis syndromes. Curr Mol Med 7:29–46
257. Boardman LA, Thibodeau SN, Schaid DJ, Lindor NM, McDonnell SK, Burgart LJ, Ahlquist DA, Podratz KC, Pittelkow M, Hartmann LC (1998) Increased risk for cancer in patients with the Peutz-Jeghers syndrome. Ann Intern Med 128:896–899
258. Giardiello FM, Welsh SB, Hamilton SR, Offerhaus GJ, Gittelsohn AM, Booker SV, Krush AJ, Yardley JH, Luk GD (1987) Increased risk of cancer in the Peutz-Jeghers syndrome. N Engl J Med 316:1511–1514
259. Zbuk KM, Eng C (2007) Hamartomatous polyposis syndromes. Nat Clin Pract Gastroenterol Hepatol 4:492–502
260. Collins SP, Reoma JL, Gamm DM, Uhler MD (2000) LKB1, a novel serine/threonine protein kinase and potential tumour suppressor, is phosphorylated by cAMP-dependent protein kinase (PKA) and prenylated in vivo. Biochem J 345:673–680
261. Tiainen M, Ylikorkala A, Makela TP (1999) Growth suppression by Lkb1 is mediated by a G(1) cell cycle arrest. Proc Natl Acad Sci USA 96:9248–9251

262. Karuman P, Gozani O, Odze RD et al (2001) The Peutz–Jegher gene product LKB1 is a mediator of p53-dependent cell death. Mol Cell 7:1307–1319
263. Ylikorkala A, Rossi DJ, Korsisaari N et al (2001) Vascular abnormalities and deregulation of VEGF in Lkb1-deficient mice. Science 293:1323–1326
264. Spicer J, Rayter S, Young N, Elliott R, Ashworth A, Smith D (2003) Regulation of the Wnt signalling component PAR1A by the Peutz–Jeghers syndrome kinase LKB1. Oncogene 22:4752–4756
265. Rosner M, Hanneder M, Siegel N, Valli A, Fuchs C, Hengstschlager M (2008) The mTOR pathway and its role in human genetic diseases. Mutat Res 659:284–292
266. Scott RJ, Crooks R, Meldrum CJ, Thomas L, Smith CJ, Mowat D, McPhillips M, Spigelman AD (2002) Mutation analysis of the STK11/LKB1 gene and clinical characteristics of an Australian series of Peutz-Jeghers syndrome patients. Clin Genet 62:282–287
267. Ylikorkala A, Avizienyte E, Tomlinson IP et al (1999) Mutations and impaired function of LKB1 in familial and non-familial Peutz–Jeghers syndrome and a sporadic testicular cancer. Hum Mol Genet 8:45–51
268. Lim W, Hearle N, Shah B et al (2003) Further observations on LKB1/STK11 status and cancer risk in Peutz–Jeghers syndrome. Br J Cancer 89:308–313
269. Olschwang S, Boisson C, Thomas G (2001) Peutz–Jeghers families unlinked to STK11/LKB1 gene mutations are highly predisposed to primitive biliary adenocarcinoma. J Med Genet 38:356–360
270. Mehenni H, Blouin JL, Radhakrishna U, Bhardwaj SS, Bhardwaj K, Dixit VB, Richards KF, Bermejo-Fenoll A, Leal AS, Raval RC, Antonarakis SE (1997) Peutz-Jeghers syndrome: confirmation of linkage to chromosome 19p13.3 and identification of a potential second locus, on 19q13.4. Am J Hum Genet 61:1327–1334
271. Olschwang S, Markie D, Seal S, Neale K, Phillips R, Cottrell S, Ellis I, Hodgson S, Zauber P, Spigelman A, Iwama T, Loff S, McKeown C, Marchese C, Sampson J, Davies S, Talbot I, Wyke J, Thomas G, Bodmer W, Hemminki A, Avizienyte E, de la Chapelle A, Aaltonen L, Stratton M, Houlston R, Tomlinson I (1998) Peutz-Jeghers disease: most, but not all, families are compatible with linkage to 19p13.3. J Med Genet 35:42–44
272. Hearle N, Schumacher V, Menko FH, Olschwang S, Boardman LA, Gille JJ, Keller JJ, Westerman AM, Scott RJ, Lim W, Trimbath JD, Giardiello FM, Gruber SB, Offerhaus GJ, Rooij FW, Wilson JH, Hansmann A, Möslein G, Royer-Pokora B, Vogel T, Phillips RK, Spigelman AD, Houlston RS (2006) STK11 status and intussusception risk in Peutz-Jeghers syndrome. J Med Genet 43:e41
273. Volikos E, Robinson J, Aittomäki K, Mecklin JP, Järvinen H, Westerman AM, de Rooji FW, Vogel T, Moeslein G, Launonen V, Tomlinson IP, Silver AR, Aaltonen LA (2006) LKB1 exonic and whole gene deletions are a common cause of Peutz-Jeghers syndrome. J Med Genet 43:e18
274. Hemminki A, Markie D, Tomlinson I, Avizienyte E, Roth S, Loukola A, Bignell G, Warren W, Aminoff M, Höglund P, Järvinen H, Kristo P, Pelin K, Ridanpää M, Salovaara R, Toro T, Bodmer W, Olschwang S, Olsen AS, Stratton MR, de la Chapelle A, Aaltonen LA (1998) A serine/threonine kinase gene defective in Peutz-Jeghers syndrome. Nature 391(6663): 184–187
275. Jiang CY, Esufali S, Berk T, Gallinger S, Cohen Z, Tobi M, Redston M, Bapat B (1999) STK11/LKB1 germline mutations are not identified in most Peutz-Jeghers syndrome patients. Clin Genet 56:136–141
276. Boardman LA, Couch FJ, Burgart LJ, Schwartz D, Berry R, McDonnell SK, Schaid DJ, Hartmann LC, Schroeder JJ, Stratakis CA, Thibodeau SN (2000) Genetic heterogeneity in Peutz-Jeghers syndrome. Hum Mutat 16:23–30
277. Mehenni H, Gehrig C, Nezu J, Oku A, Shimane M, Rossier C, Guex N, Blouin JL, Scott HS, Antonarakis SE (1998) Loss of LKB1 kinase activity in Peutz-Jeghers syndrome, and evidence for allelic and locus heterogeneity. Am J Hum Genet 63:1641–1650
278. Wang ZJ, Churchman M, Avizienyte E, McKeown C, Davies S, Evans DG, Ferguson A, Ellis I, Xu WH, Yan ZY, Aaltonen LA, Tomlinson IP (1999) Germline mutations of the LKB1 (STK11) gene in Peutz-Jeghers patients. J Med Genet 36:365–368

279. Abed AA, Günther K, Kraus C, Hohenberger W, Ballhausen WG (2001) Mutation screening at the RNA level of the STK11/LKB1 gene in Peutz-Jeghers syndrome reveals complex splicing abnormalities and a novel mRNA isoform (STK11 c.597(insertion mark)598insIVS4). Hum Mutat 18:397–410
280. Yoon KA, Ku JL, Choi HS, Heo SC, Jeong SY, Park YJ, Kim NK, Kim JC, Jung PM, Park JG (2000) Germline mutations of the STK11 gene in Korean Peutz-Jeghers syndrome patients. Br J Cancer 82:1403–1406
281. Saranrittichai S (2008) Peutz-jeghers syndrome and colon cancer in a 10-year-old girl: implications for when and how to start screening? Asian Pac J Cancer Prev 9:159–161
282. Kopacova M, Tacheci I, Rejchrt S, Bures J (2009) Peutz-Jeghers syndrome: diagnostic and therapeutic approach. World J Gastroenterol 15:5397–5408
283. Giardiello FM, Trimbath JD (2006) Peutz-Jeghers syndrome and management recommendations. Clin Gastroenterol Hepatol 4:408–415
284. Wei C, Amos CI, Zhang N, Wang X, Rashid A, Walker CL, Behringer RR, Frazier ML (2008) Suppression of Peutz-Jeghers polyposis by targeting mammalian target of rapamycin signaling. Clin Cancer Res 14:1167–1171
285. Udd L, Katajisto P, Rossi DJ, Lepistö A, Lahesmaa AM, Ylikorkala A, Järvinen HJ, Ristimäki AP, Mäkelä TP (2004) Suppression of Peutz-Jeghers polyposis by inhibition of cyclooxygenase-2. Gastroenterology 127:1030–1037
286. Kawato Y, Aonuma M, Matsumoto K, Sato K (1991) Production of SN-38, a main metabolite of the camptothecin derivative CPT-11, and its species and tissue specificities. Yakubutsu Dotai 6:899–907
287. Ratain MJ (2002) Irinotecan dosing: does the CPT in CPT-11 stand for "can't predict toxicity"? J Clin Oncol 20:7–8
288. Fuchs CS, Moore MR, Harker G, Villa L, Rinaldi D, Hecht JR (2003) Phase III comparison of two irinotecan dosing regimens in second-line therapy of metastatic colorectal cancer. J Clin Oncol 21:807–814
289. Kunimoto T, Nitta K, Tanaka T, Uehara N, Baba H, Takeuchi M, Yokokura T, Sawada S, Miyasaka T, Mutai M (1987) Antitumor activity of inhibitor 7-ethyl-10-[4-(1-piperidino)-1-piperidino]-carbonyloxy-camptothecin, a novel water-soluble derivative of camptothecin against murine tumors. Cancer Res 47:5944–5947
290. Kawato Y, Nagata H, Furuta T, Yokokura T (1991) Intracellular roles of SN-38, a metabolite of the camptothecin derivative CPT-11, in the antitumor effect of CPT-11. Cancer Res 51:4187–4191
291. Takasuna K, Kasai Y, Kitano Y, Mori K, Kakihata K, Hirohashi M, Nomura M (1995) Study of mechanisms of diarrhea induced by the new anticancer agent drug irinotecan hydrochloride (CPT-11). Folia Pharmacol Jpn 105:447–460
292. Iyer L, King CD, Whitington PF, Green MD, Roy SK, Tephly TR, Coffman BL, Ratain MJ (1998) Genetic predisposition to the metabolism of irinotecan (CPT-11). Role of uridine diphosphate glucuronosyltransferase isoform 1A1 in the glucuronidation of its active metabolite (SN-38) in human liver microsomes. J Clin Invest 101:847–854
293. Ritter JK, Chen F, Sheen YY, Tran HM, Kimura S, Yeatman MT, Owens IS (1992) A novel complex locus UGT1 encodes human bilirubin, phenol and other UDP-glucuronosyltransferase isozymes with identical carboxyl termini. J Biol Chem 267:3257–3261
294. Owens IS, Ritter JK (1995) Gene structure at the human UGT1 locus creates diversity in isozyme structure, structure specificity and regulation. Prog Nucleic Acid Res 51:306–308
295. Hasegawa Y, Ando Y, Ando M, Hashimoto N, Imaizumi K, Shimokata K (2006) Pharmacogenetic approach for cancer treatment-tailored medicine in practice. Ann N Y Acad Sci 1086:223–232
296. Ando Y, Saka H, Ando M, Sawa T, Muro K, Ueoka H, Yokohama A, Saitoh S, Shimokata K, Hasegawa Y (2000) Polymorphisms of UDP-glucuronosyltransferase gene and irinotecan toxicity: a pharmacogenetic analysis. Cancer Res 60:6921–6926
297. Innocenti F, Undevia SD, Iyer L, Chen PX, Das S, Kocherginsky M, Karrison T, Janisch L, Ramírez J, Rudin CM, Vokes EE, Ratain MJ (2004) Genetic variants in the UDP-glucuronosyltransferase 1A1 gene predict the risk of severe neutropenia of irinotecan. J Clin Oncol 22:1382–1388

298. Iyer L, Das S, Janisch L, Wen M, Ramírez J, Karrison T, Fleming GF, Vokes EE, Schilsky RL, Ratain MJ (2002) UGT1A1*28 polymorphism as a determinant of irinotecan disposition and toxicity. Pharmacogenomics J 2:43–47
299. Beutler E, Gelbart T, Demina A (1998) Racial variability in the UDP-glucuronosyltransferase 1 (UGT1A1) promoter: a balanced polymorphism for regulation of bilirubin metabolism? Proc Natl Acad Sci USA 95:8170–8174
300. Gagné JF, Montminy V, Belanger P, Journault K, Gaucher G, Guillemette C (2002) Common human UGT1A polymorphisms and the altered metabolism of irinotecan active metabolite 7-ethyl-10-hydroxycamptothecin (SN-38). Mol Pharmacol 62:608–617
301. Yamamoto K, Sato H, Fujiyama Y, Doida Y, Bamba T (1998) Contribution of two missense mutations (G71R and Y486D) of the bilirubin UDP glycosyltransferase (UGT1A1) gene to phenotypes of Gilbert's syndrome and Crigler-Najjar syndrome type II. Biochim Biophys Acta 1406:267–273
302. Marcuello E, Altés A, Menoyo A, Del Rio E, Gómez-Pardo M, Baiget M (2004) UGT1A1 gene variations and irinotecan treatment in patients with metastatic colorectal cancer. Br J Cancer 91:678–682
303. Onoue M, Terada T, Kobayashi M, Katsura T, Matsumoto S, Yanagihara K, Nishimura T, Kanai M, Teramukai S, Shimizu A, Fukushima M, Inui K (2009) UGT1A1*6 polymorphism is most predictive of severe neutropenia induced by irinotecan in Japanese cancer patients. Int J Clin Oncol 14:136–142
304. Han JY, Lim HS, Shin ES, Yoo YK, Park YH, Lee JE, Jang IJ, Lee DH, Lee JS (2006) Comprehensive analysis of UGT1A polymorphisms predictive for pharmacokinetics and treatment outcome in patients with non-small-cell lung cancer treated with irinotecan and cisplatin. J Clin Oncol 24:2237–2244
305. Takane H, Kawamoto K, Sasaki T, Moriki K, Moriki K, Kitano H, Higuchi S, Otsubo K, Ieiri I (2009) Life-threatening toxicities in a patient with UGT1A1*6/*28 and SLCO1B1*15/*15 genotypes after irinotecan-based chemotherapy. Cancer Chemother Pharmacol 63:1165–1169
306. Monaghan G, Ryan M, Seddon R, Hume R, Burchell B (1996) Genetic variation in bilirubin UPD-glucuronosyltransferase gene promoter and Gilbert's syndrome. Lancet 347:578–581
307. Pirulli D, Giordano M, Puzzer D, Crovella S, Rigato I, Tiribelli C, Momigliano-Richiardi P, Amoroso A (2000) Rapid method for detection of extra (TA) in the promoter of the bilirubin-UDP-glucuronosyl transferase 1 gene associated with Gilbert syndrome. Clin Chem 46:129–131
308. Hasegawa Y, Sarashina T, Ando M, Kitagawa C, Mori A, Yoneyama M, Ando Y, Shimokata K (2004) Rapid detection of UGT1A1 gene polymorphisms by newly developed invader assay. Clin Chem 50:1479–1480
309. Recommendations from the EGAPP Working Group (2009) Can UGT1A1 genotyping reduce morbidity and mortality in patients with metastatic colorectal cancer treated with irinotecan? Genet Med 11:15–20
310. Hazama S, Nagashima A, Kondo H, Yoshida S, Shimizu R, Araki A, Yoshino S, Okayama N, Hinoda Y, Oka M (2010) Phase I study of irinotecan and doxifluridine for metastatic colorectal cancer focusing on the UGT1A1*28 polymorphism. Cancer Sci 101:722–727
311. Murff HJ, Byrne D, Syngal S (2004) Cancer risk assessment: quality and impact of the family history interview. Am J Prev Med 27:239–245
312. Bedoya F, Rubio JC, Morales-Gutierrez C, Abad-Barahona A, Lora Pablos D, Meneu JC, Moreno-Gonzalez E, Enriquez de Salamanca R, Vegh I (2009) Single nucleotide change in the cannabinoid receptor-1 (CNR1) gene in colorectal cancer outcome. Oncology 76:435–441
313. McHugh SM, O'Donnell J, Gillen P (2009) Genomic and oncoproteomic advances in detection and treatment of colorectal cancer. World J Surg Oncol 7:36
314. Likui W, Hong W, Shuwen Z (2010) Clinical significance of the upregulated osteopontin mRNA expression in human colorectal cancer. J Gastrointest Surg 14:74–81

315. Bezabeh T, Somorjai R, Dolenko B, Bryskina N, Levin B, Bernstein CN, Jeyarajah E, Steinhart AH, Rubin DT, Smith IC (2009) Detecting colorectal cancer by 1H magnetic resonance spectroscopy of fecal extracts. NMR Biomed 22:593–600
316. Snyder M, Du J, Gerstein M (2010) Personal genome sequencing: current approaches and challenges. Genes Dev 24:423–431
317. Bamshad MJ, Ng SB, Bigham AW, Tabor HK, Emond MJ, Nickerson DA, Shendure J (2011) Exome sequencing as a tool for mendelian disease gene discovery. Nat Rev Genet 12:745–755
318. Choi M, Scholl UI, Ji W, Liu T, Tikhonova IR, Zumbo P, Nayir A, Bakkaloğlu A, Ozen S, Sanjad S, Nelson-Williams C, Farhi A, Mane S, Lifton RP (2009) Genetic diagnosis by whole exome capture and massively parallel DNA sequencing. Proc Natl Acad Sci USA 106:19096–19101
319. Carthew RW, Sontheimer EJ (2009) Origins and mechanisms of miRNAs and siRNAs. Cell 136:642–655
320. Wu WK, Law PT, Lee CW, Cho CH, Fan D, Wu K, Yu J, Sung JJ (2011) MicroRNA in colorectal cancer: from benchtop to bedside. Carcinogenesis 32:247–253
321. Lao VV, Grady WM (2011) Epigenetics and colorectal cancer. Nat Rev Gastroenterol Hepatol 8:686–700
322. Khare S, Verma M (2012) Epigenetics of colon cancer. Methods Mol Biol 863:177–185

Chapter 6
Molecular Pathology and Diagnostics in Esophago-gastric Cancer

Rodney E. Shackelford, Maisoun Qassim Abdelbaqi, Khaldoon Almhanna, Kenneth Meredith, and Domenico Coppola

Contents

R.E. Shackelford, DO, Ph.D.
Department of Pathology and Laboratory Medicine, Tulane University School of Medicine, 1430 Tulane Avenue, SL-79, New Orleans, LA 70112, United States

M.Q. Abdelbaqi
Department of Pathology, LSU Health Sciences Center Shreveport, 1501 Kings Highway, Shreveport, LA 71130, USA

K. Almhanna, M.D. • K. Meredith, M.D.
Department of GI Oncology, H. Lee Moffitt Cancer Center & Research Institute, 12902 Magnolia Drive, Tampa, FL 33612, United States

D. Coppola, M.D. (✉)
Department of Pathology, H. Lee Moffitt Cancer Center & Research Institute, 12902 Magnolia Drive, Tampa, FL 33612, United States
e-mail: Domenico.Coppola@moffitt.org

D. Coppola (ed.), *Molecular Pathology and Diagnostics of Cancer*, Cancer Growth and Progression 16, DOI 10.1007/978-94-007-7192-5_6,

Abstract Esophageal and gastric cancers are the eighth and fourth most common cancers worldwide, respectively. Because of their often-aggressive clinical courses and high fatality rates, they represent the sixth and second most common causes of cancer deaths worldwide. The diagnosis of these malignancies is mainly established by their clinical presentation, combined with biopsy and subsequent histologic analysis of hematoxylin-eosin-stained tissue sections. Recently, however, molecular studies have become increasingly important in establishing a diagnosis and prognosis and guiding the clinical management of these malignancies. For some subtypes of these malignancies, such as hereditary diffuse gastric cancer, molecular diagnostics is central in establishing a diagnosis and in determining appropriate clinical management. Here, we review current methods and recommendations for molecular-genetic testing for esophageal and gastric cancers and briefly discuss future possible applications of this technology to these malignancies.

Keywords Esophageal cancer • Gastric cancer • Gastrointestinal stromal tumor • CDX2 • miRNA • Microarray • *H. pylori* • Diffuse gastric carcinoma

Abbreviations

BE	Barrett's esophagitis
DHPLC	Denaturing high-performance liquid chromatography
EAC	Esophageal adenocarcinoma
ESCC	Esophageal squamous cell carcinoma
ESD	Esophageal squamous dysplasia

GIST	Gastrointestinal stromal tumors
miRNA	MicroRNA
NSAIDS	Non-steroidal anti-inflammatory drugs
POD	Days post-operatively

6.1 Esophageal Cancer

Esophageal cancer is the eighth most common malignancy worldwide and the sixth leading cause of cancer-related deaths due to its often-aggressive clinical course and fatal outcome. Overall, esophageal cancer has a poor survival rate, with 16 % and 10 % 5-year survival rates seen in the United States and Europe, respectively. Like colorectal carcinoma, esophageal cancer shows a striking geographical variation, with its incidence varying by over 20-fold in areas such as China, with an incidence of 27.4 cases/100,000 in Chinese men compared to 1.3/100,000 seen in Western African men. In general, the sex ratio of esophageal cancer is skewed strongly toward men, with the male-to-female ratio in Eastern Europe being 7:1 for example. In places where the esophageal cancer incidence is lower, such as Western Africa, the sex ratio is much closer to one [1]. Although genetic factors play a role in the incidence of esophageal cancer [2], much of the variation seen in esophageal cancer rates is due to differential carcinogen exposure, particularly as related to tobacco and alcohol use [3].

6.2 Esophageal Cancer Types

Although esophageal anatomy is relatively simple, the esophagus is host to many different malignancies, including salivary gland tumors (such as adenoid cystic and mucoepidermoid carcinomas), stromal tumors (such as gastrointestinal stromal tumors, leiomyosarcoma, and liposarcomas), signet ring cell esophageal adenocarcinomas, hematopoietic malignancies, melanoma, and small cell and lymphoepithelioma-like carcinomas. However, most of these esophageal malignancies are relatively rare. The most common esophageal malignancies are esophageal squamous cell carcinoma (ESCC) and esophageal adenocarcinoma (EAC), which together account for more than 90 % of all esophageal cancers [4]. These malignancies differ significantly in their histology, precursor lesions and development, epidemiology, clinical behavior, and anatomic origin, with ESCC most commonly arising in the proximal esophagus and EAC arising in the distal esophagus. Unfortunately, both ESCC and EAC are aggressive diseases, typically presenting with early lymphatic and hematogenous dissemination, making their surgical resection difficult and sometimes not an option, particularly for disseminated disease.

Interestingly, the epidemiology of esophageal cancer has been changing. For example, before the 1970s, ESCC constituted over 90 % of all esophageal cancer worldwide [3–6], while in some Western countries EAC presently accounts for ~ 50 % of all esophageal cancers [3]. Interestingly, one study demonstrated that in westernized areas, the ratio of adenocarcinomas of the lower esophagus and gastric-esophageal junction to ESCC has changed from 1:4.7 in 1975 to 1:0.43 in 1998; within the last decade, the incidence of lower esophageal adenocarcinoma has exceeded that of ESCC in several Western countries, including the United States [7–9]. In this review, we will mainly focus on esophageal ESCC and EAC.

6.3 Environmental Risk and Protective Factors for Esophageal Cancer

Multiple environmental toxins have shown a strong association with esophageal cancer, with esophageal ESCC and EAC often showing stronger or weaker associations following exposure to specific environmental toxins. Because of the often-aggressive clinical course of esophageal cancer, the association of esophageal cancer with specific exposures has been documented for over a century [10, 11]. Below are some of these toxic agents.

6.3.1 Alcohol Abuse

Alcohol abuse has been identified as a significant risk factor for ESCC since the 1930s [10, 11]. The risk for ESCC is elevated three- to fivefold with excessive alcohol consumption of more than three drinks per day [12–14]. Interestingly, however, alcohol abuse appears to have no effect on the incidence of EAC [4, 12–14]. The mechanism by which alcohol causes ESCC is presently poorly understood; however, several factors are likely involved. First, the initial metabolite of ethyl alcohol is acetaldehyde, a known highly toxic carcinogen [15]. Acetaldehyde binds strongly to DNA, forming adducts and interstrand cross-links, many of which block DNA synthesis, causing replication errors and polymerase errors resulting in mutations, and can eventually activate proto-oncogenes and inactivate tumor suppressor genes leading to malignancy via the accumulation of unrepaired mutations [16]. Additionally, chronic alcohol consumption induces certain gene products involved in alcohol detoxification, some of which actually promote malignancy. For example, Millonig et al. [17] examined 37 patients with a history of alcohol abuse and upper aerodigestive tract cancer and compared this group to 16 control patients without cancer. Patients with cancer and a history of alcohol abuse showed significant induction of cytochrome P-450 2E1 levels, which strongly correlated with the carcinogenic etheno-DNA adducts and cell proliferation. Interestingly, cell proliferation indices were highest in those who both smoked and drank. Non-smokers and drinkers had the lowest levels of cytochrome P-450 2E1, etheno-DNA adducts, and Ki-67. The authors concluded that chronic alcohol abuse leads to increased DNA damage and cell proliferation, thus likely to contribute to cancer. Alcohol may further contribute to carcinogenesis by increasing the solubility of other carcinogens, such as those found in tobacco smoke, and may contribute to nutritional deficiencies, which play a role in carcinogenesis [18].

6.3.2 Tobacco

Approximately 78 % of male and 75 % of female deaths are due to esophageal cancer [19]. Unlike alcohol, tobacco use increases the risk for both ESCC and EAC, about three- to sevenfold for ESCC and twofold for EAC, depending on the amount and duration of tobacco use [13, 19]. Tobacco is largely carcinogenic due to the wide variety of toxic agents produced by the combustion of the tobacco during smoking, including acetylaldehyde, nitrosamines, and polycyclic aromatic hydrocarbons [20]. The mechanisms of tobacco-induced carcinogenesis are complex, although they are partially understood and include the formation of mutagenic DNA adducts, intercalation of polycyclic aromatic hydrocarbons causing frame-shift mutations, and mutagenesis resulting from DNA replication forks stalled by tobacco toxin-induced DNA modifications [20]. Interestingly, some smoking-induced cancers may arise from radioactive agents in tobacco and tobacco smoke, including ^{210}Pb and ^{210}Po. These agents may be preferentially deposited in specific areas of epithelium and cleared slowly, contributing to carcinogenesis [21]. Within the squamous epithelial lining of the esophagus, both smoking and excess of alcohol induce esophageal squamous dysplasia (ESD), the precursor lesion of ESCC. ESD can be mild, moderate, or severe. ESD confers an elevated risk for ESCC of 3-, 10, and 30-fold, depending on whether the dysplasia is mild, moderate, or severe [22]. Together, alcohol abuse and tobacco account for over 90 % of all esophageal cancer cases worldwide and together synergistically increase the risk for esophageal cancer [23]. Several other recognized causes of esophageal cancer include are summarized below.

6.3.3 Mycotoxins

Mycotoxins are found in many sources, such as pickled vegetables and spoiled foods, and include aflatoxins, ochratoxin A, fumonisins, trichothecenes, and zearalenone. They exert a range of effects, including allergic reactions, immune suppression, mutagenesis and taratogenesis, and cancer. The fumonisins were discovered in the 1980s and consist of 20 carbon aliphatic chains with two ester-linked hydrophilic side chains that structurally resemble sphingosine, a common and essential phospholipid found in cell membranes [24, 25]. The toxicity of the fumonisins arises from its inhibition of ceramide synthase, resulting in the accumulation of sphinganine, some of which are metabolized into highly toxic-free sphingoid bases [26]. Fumonisin B_1 is found at relatively high levels in maize, where it is produced by the fungal pest *Fusanum moniliforme* and related species. Fumonisin B_1 is found only on maize and is thought to cause high levels of esophageal cancer in areas of Southern Africa and parts of China [27, 28]. The molecular actions of Fumonisin B_1 are poorly understood, but it appears to cause cancer, in part by altering cellular proliferative and apoptotic responses [29].

6.3.4 *Opium*

By itself, opium is not a mutagen [30, 31]. However, opium is often smoked, a process that produces a large array of mutagenic agents, particularly polycyclic aromatic hydrocarbons that are potent carcinogens [20]. One study in the Golestan Providence of Northeastern Iran, where both opium and tobacco are commonly smoked, showed an odds ratio for esophageal cancer of 1.70 for tobacco use and 2.35 for opium smoking compared to individuals who did not smoke either substance. Three hundred esophageal cancer cases compared to 571 controls were matched on neighborhood of residence and age [32]. Interestingly, 2 % of the individuals studied used alcohol, which was not associated with an increase in esophageal cancer.

6.3.5 *Maté*

Maté, also known as yerba maté, an infusion of the herb *Ilex paraguayensis,* is commonly consumed in relatively large quantities in areas of South America known to have an elevated esophageal cancer incidence [33–35]. Several studies have shown a correlation between maté use and ESCC, showing odds ratios of 3.81 and 1.87 for ESCC among maté drinkers compared to non-maté drinkers [33–35]. The mechanism(s) underlying the carcinogenic activity of maté appears to be the relatively high levels of polycyclic aromatic hydrocarbons found in maté [36–38]. Interestingly, maté use does not appear to increase the risk for EAC [33–35].

6.3.6 Helicobacter pylori

H. pylori is a helical, gram-negative bacterium that infects the stomach, often producing chronic gastritis, which confers an increased risk for MALT lymphomas and gastric adenocarcinoma [39]. Unlike these malignancies, *H. pylori* exerts a protective effect on EAC risk and lowers its incidence ~ 50 %. It does not appear to affect ESCC risk [40, 41]. The mechanism(s) underlying the protective effects of *H. pylori* appears to come from lowered gastric acid secretion and hence lower esophageal irritation, due to *H. pylori*-induced parietal cell apoptosis and lowered H^+-K^+-ATPase parietal cell expression by increased NF-κB activity following exposure to bacterial endotoxins [42, 43].

6.3.7 Non-steroidal Anti-inflammatory Drugs

Non-steroidal anti-inflammatory drugs (NSAIDs) have been demonstrated to reduce multiple cancer types, including EAC but not ESCC [44]. The overall reduction on EAC is ~40 %, although the degree of reduction varied with the frequency of NSAID use; interestingly, as little as 75 mg/day of aspirin significantly reduced the risk for EAC [44, 45]. The mechanism underlying this risk reduction is unknown, although one meta-analysis of 14 studies on aspirin use and EAC did show a protective effect that became evident following appearance of Barrett's esophagitis [46].

6.3.8 Gastro-esophageal Acid Reflux, Obesity, and Barrett's Esophagitis

Barrett's esophagitis (BE) is a metaplastic change in response to reflux of bile and acid across the gastro-esophageal junction, possibly functioning as a protective response to caustic effects of reflux [42, 47]. In BE, the normal lower esophageal squamous epithelium is replaced by intestinalized columnar epithelium. Clinically, this change is significant because BE has a propensity to develop dysplasia that can later progress to EAC. A diagnosis of BE requires that two criteria be met. First, there should be cephalad displacement of the squamocolumnar junction seen via upper endoscopy (Fig. 6.1a). Second, intestinalized epithelium or epithelium containing goblet cells should replace the normal squamous epithelium of the lower esophagus, being histologically identified from areas showing cephalad displacement of the squamocolumnar junction (compare Fig. 6.1b, c) [48].

The definition of BE shows some variation, with goblet cells in the metaplastic epithelium required for a diagnosis of BE in the United States but not in the United Kingdom [48–50]. The risk of EAC with BE is relatively low, conferring a risk of

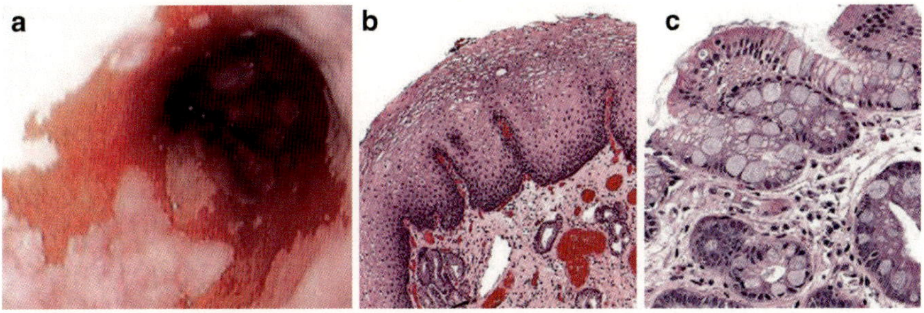

Fig. 6.1 Lower esophageal changes seen in Barrett's esophagitis (BE). Irregular cephalad protrusions of Barrett's esophagitis gastro-esophageal junction (**a**). Normal lower esophageal squamous epithelium compared to Barrett's esophagitis (compare panel **b** to **c**) (From Ref. [48])

about 0.5 % per year, such that most individuals with BE will die with BE and not from EAC. Where EAC does arise in a background of BE, a specific sequence of histologic changes from normal squamous epithelium to BE and from BE to low-grade or high-grade dysplasia and finally invasive EAC has been identified [48]. Not surprisingly, the risk for EAC increases with the dysplastic changes, such that individuals with high-grade dysplasia have an EAC risk of ~ 10 %/year [51]. The risk for BE and EAC is increased by obesity, which increases gastro-esophageal reflux via increasing intra-abdominal pressure, thus weight loss decreases both intra-abdominal pressure and the risk for BE and EAC [52]. Interestingly, specific molecular changes have been identified in the progression from normal lower esophageal epithelium to BE to EAC (discussed below).

6.4 Genetic Risk Factors for Esophageal Cancer and Molecular-Genetic Testing

Although environmental factors are major determinants of esophageal cancer risk, about 30 % of esophageal cancers have a heritable genetic component [53, 54]. Additionally, several genetic factors have been identified as risk factors for esophageal cancer, including enzymes involved in the detoxification of xenobiotics and Tylosis, a rare autosomal dominant characterized by hyperkeratosis of the palms and soles associated with a high incidence of esophageal cancer [55, 56] (also discussed below).

Both ESCC and EAC have defined histologic precursor lesions [3, 4, 48–51]. Recent studies have demonstrated that these precursor lesions are accompanied by specific molecular changes. Although many of these changes are currently studied at the basic research level, they are likely to be incorporated into molecular diagnostic testing in the near future. Others, such as molecular testing for Tylosis, are currently being performed [55]. Here, we will review our understanding of the molecular pathology of esophageal cancer and current molecular diagnostics in this area.

6.4.1 Microarray Studies

Microarray allows the massive, parallel, semiquantitative analysis of the relative gene expression levels between two different cell populations, often comparing different, but related, cell populations such as primary and neoplastic cells or primary and metaplastic cell populations. Anywhere from ten to several hundred thousand expressed RNA species can be simultaneously analyzed, allowing detailed comparisons of global gene expression between two samples. The drawbacks to microarray are its relatively high costs, its high complexity of implementation and validation, its "snapshot" presentation of the transcriptome, the lack of information given on an expressed sequence's ultimate function, and the sometimes poor correlation between mRNA expression and protein expression, which microarray does not measure [57].

One of the earliest microarray analyses of BE and esophageal cancer was performed by Selaru et al. [58]. Thirteen esophageal specimens were compared, consisting of seven BEs, and six esophageal cancers. Eight thousand cDNA clones were analyzed, and hierarchal clusters analysis was performed. The esophageal samples clustered into two predominant groups, each expressing unique gene expression profiles. Comparison to histology revealed that one group consisted of all seven BE samples, whereas the other six were all malignancies. Interestingly, the malignant samples showed sub-clusters consisting of EAC, ESCC, and one signet ring cell esophageal adenocarcinoma. Although the specimen sample size was small, microarray combined with bioinformatics was demonstrated to be able to differentiate malignant and premalignant esophageal disease using small biopsy-sized tissue samples.

Later, Greenawalt et al. [59] employed microarray to examine 128 tissue samples from normal esophageal epithelium, BE, EAC, and ESCC, taken from patients between ages 28 and 86, with a mean age of 63 years. The tumor stage and degree of dysplasia in BE were recorded and incorporated into the analysis. Tissue samples were collected during diagnostic endoscopy and immediately placed in RNAlater solution and stored at −20 °C. Biopsies were divided in half; with one part subjected to independent histologic analysis and the other prepared for RNA extraction. All tumor samples contained 75 % or more tumor. Additionally, biopsies of normal mucosa were taken from greater than 5 cm proximal to any tumor margins and were conformed 100 % normal by histologic examination.

RNA was extracted from each sample via phenol-chloroform followed by column chromatography. Four micrograms of total RNA were amplified with T7 RNA polymerase to linearly amplify the total RNA. The resulting RNA amplicon was annealed to the total RNA, and dsDNA was made in the presence of dNTPs, DNA polymerase, *E. coli* ligase, and RNase H. Transcribed RNA form the dsDNA was purified and labeled with cyanine-5. Reference cDNA was extracted from nucleic acids from a pool of 11 cell lines (MCF7, Hs578T, OVCAR3, HepG2, NTERA2, MOLT4, RPMI-8226, NB41ATRA, UACC-62, SW872, and Colo205) and labeled with cyanine-3. The sample and reference cDNAs were competitively hybridized to cDNA printed microarray slides containing 10,500 elements, representing 9,400 unique cDNA clones. The hybridized slides were scanned with a confocal laser scanner, and the data were processed using GenePix Pro Software 4.1 to calculate the mean intensity of each spot. Hierarchal clustering was done with a Pearson's similarity metric using a Gene Cluster 3.0 and viewed with an R statistical package.

After normalization, 9,386 genes separated the tissue samples into four distinct clusters, ESCC, normal squamous epithelium, BE, and EAC. To qualify as distinct, a fourfold difference in gene expression was required. Consistent with their phenotype, ESCC and normal squamous epithelium clustered closely together and were distinct from EAC and BE, which are columnar lesions. Additionally, the normal and BE samples were clearly distinct, whereas the BE and EAC sample clustered closely together (Fig. 6.2). A large group of cDNA clones were differentially expressed between any two tissues: 2,158 between normal and BE, 2,913 between normal and EAC, and 1,306 between EAC and SCC. Thus a large degree of overlap was identified.

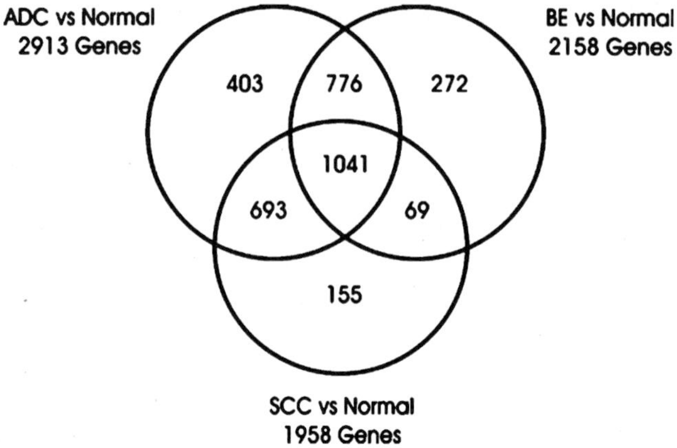

Fig. 6.2 A diagram of differentially expressed genes from the microarray study by Greenawalt et al. [59]. The differentially expressed genes between esophageal *SCC*, *AC*, and *BE* are presented as a Venn diagram. The number of genes expressed in more than one tissue appears in the overlapping regions of the diagram

Several patterns of differential gene expression were identified that correlated with the differentiation state of the esophageal biopsy. For example, genes involved in tissue development, including keratinization, intercellular junction formation, calcium ion binding, and endopeptidase activity, were overexpressed in BE and EAC. EAC overexpressed genes involved in immune and inflammatory responses and those associated with responses to external signaling and collagen metabolism and proteolysis. Interestingly, BE, but not EAC, overexpressed genes involved in digestion and alcohol metabolism. ESCC overexpressed genes involved in cell death and apoptosis, regulation of NF-κB expression metalloprotease activity, and plasminogen activator activity. Last, specific gene expression cluster groups were found to be associated the different malignancies. Malignancy was associated with the expression of genes involved in extracellular matrix formation, collagen binding, immune response, the cell progression and checkpoints, spindle organization, and signal transduction cascades. Thus Greenawalt et al. [59] were able to differentiate EAC and ESCC via molecular profiling and demonstrate both a different cellular origin for each malignancy (squamous vs. columnar), but also show clear molecular differences between benign, premalignant, and malignant esophageal tissues.

In a similar study, Helm et al. [60] employed the Human Hu U133A GeneChip to perform a microarray analysis of ten endoscopic biopsy specimens from nine patients with esophageal adenocarcinoma. Six patients had adenocarcinoma without BE, while three had adenocarcinoma arising in BE. Ten biopsies were taken three patients in which BE cancer had arisen and a further ten biopsies were taken from six additional patients with BE, but with no dysplasia or malignancy. Each biopsy specimen was carefully examined and microdissected by a pathologist to remove stroma, necrotic debris, and normal adjacent tissue in cases of BE or malignancy. Total RNA was prepared by Trizol extraction and analyzed for integrity. Five micrograms RNA were hybridized to the Hu U133A GeneChip, which contained 22,214 probe sets. The RNA was prepared by standard Affymetrix protocols [61].

Analysis of gene expression patterns revealed that even in BE without histologic signs of dysplasia genes associated with cell differentiation were under-expressed. Adenocarcinoma overexpressed genes associated with tissue remodeling and invasion. Interestingly, cancers that arose without an identifiable BE precursor lesion showed higher expression of these genes.

Many other microarray studies have been preformed comparing various common esophageal lesions and a number of candidate genes have been identified which may have value in esophageal cancer staging, recurrence prediction, prognosis, and eventually in the selection of different treatment modalities [62]. Although microarray is presently too costly, time-consuming, and technically difficult for most clinical applications, it has been a very valuable tool for identifying specific genes that may be examined by simpler molecular techniques for esophageal cancer molecular diagnostics.

6.4.2 *Prognostic Significance of Serum mRNAs*

One goal of molecular diagnostics is to predict treatment response and establish a prognosis, optimize the management of a patient with a specific malignancy, and accomplish this with the least invasive procedure possible. For esophageal cancer, the measurement of serum RNA profiles is relatively non-invasive. Although not currently used in esophageal cancer molecular diagnostics, some success has been achieved with serum analysis. For example, Takahashi et al. [63] measured the serum levels of MMP9, CRP, HMGB1, MUC1, EGR1, PBEF1, PDGFA, TGF-β1, TNF-α, Von Willebrand factor, and IL-6 mRNA in 27 patients who underwent radical surgery for esophageal cancer. mRNA was obtained for 14 days post-operatively (POD), with collections taken during surgery and at PODs 1, 3, 5, and 14. mRNA was extracted, and real-time RT-PCR was performed following DNase treatment. RNA from 200 μL of serum was dissolved in 200 μL of H_2O. RT-PCR was performed with 1 μg of the extract and 2 μg SYBT Green I employing a one-step RT-PCR kit. RT-PCR conditions were incubation at 50 °C for 30 min, 12 min at 95 °C, and 50 cycles at 95 °C (0 s), annealing at 50–55 °C (10 s), and 72 °C (15 s), followed by extension at 40 °C (20 s). All primers were optimally designed and shown in Table 6.1. The final concentration of the primers was 1 μmol. β-actin was employed as a relative expression-level control. All reactions were done twice, and IL-6 and CRP protein levels were verified by Western blotting.

mRNA expression profiles over 14 days revealed that MMP9 and NAMPT were both up-regulated at POD 5 and onward. Von Willebrand factor and TGFβ1were both up-regulated from POD 3. MUC1 and PDGFA were up-regulated at POD 3, with levels falling at later dates. IL-6 was up regulated at POD 5 and thereafter fell to basal levels. EGR1 and HMGB1 slowly decreased from intraoperative levels to baseline at POD 14. Increased TNF-α mRNA levels correlated with increased time spent under anesthesia. CRP mRNA expression correlated with the length of the

Table 6.1 Primer sets used for each gene investigated by Takahashi et al. [63]

Gene	GenBank accession no.	Forward primer	Reverse primer
VWF	NM_000552.2	TGA CCA GGT TCT CCG AGG AG	CAC ACG TCG TAG CGG CAG TT
TGFβ1	MN_000660.3	GAC TAC TAC GCC AAG GAG GT	GGA GCT CTG ATG TGT TGA AG
PDGFA	MN_002607.5	GGG AGT GAG GAT TCT TTG GA	AAA TGA CCG TCC TGG TCT TT
NAMPT	MN_005746.2	CTG TTC CTG AGG GCA TTG TC	GGC CAC TGT GAT TGG ATA CC
CRP	MN_000567.2	ACA GTG GGT GGG TCT GAA AT	TAC CCA GAA CTC CAC GAT CC
EGR1	MN_001964.2	TTC TTC GTC CTT TTG GTT TA	CTT AAG GCT AGA GGT GAG CA
HMBG1	MN_002128.4	AAC CAC CCA GAT GCT TCA GT	TCC GCT TTT GCC ATA TCT TC
TNF-α	MN_000594.2	TGC TTG TTC CTC AGC CTC TT	GCA CTC ACC TCT TCC CTC TG
MUC1	MN_001018016.1	CCA TTC CAC TCC ACT CAG GT	CCT CTG AAG GAG GCT GTG AT
MMP9	NM_004994.2	TTG ACA GCG ACA AGA AGT GG	CCC TCA GTC AAG CGC TAC AT
IL-6	MN_000600.3	ATG CAA TAA CCA CCC CTG AC	TAA AGC TGC GCA CAA TGA GA
β-actin	MN_031144.2	ACC TGA CTG ACT ACC TCA TG	GCA GCC GTG GCC ATC TCT TG

ICU stay and was associated with the 6-month mortality. Interestingly, high IL-6 mRNA levels on POD 0 was an independent indicator of a poor prognosis, as were days spent on a ventilator or days spent in the ICU, whereas a high POD three levels predicted the onset of pneumonia. Up-regulation of Von Willebrand factor and TGFβ1 mRNA intraoperatively correlated with mortality (P=0.0021). A worse prognosis was also found with POD 1 up-regulation of PDGFA, ERG1, and HMGB1 mRNAs. At POD 3, NAMPT and MUC1 mRNAs were independent prognostic factors for 1-year mortality. High NAMPT mRNA at POD 14 correlated with mortality at 30 days and 1 year. The authors proposed that profiling serum inflammatory gene expression could have value in stratifying patients according to their relative risk for mortality and the onset of severe inflammatory conditions. Although not presently commonly employed in molecular diagnostics, such serum mRNA profiling could have value in patient care, but requires further validation.

6.4.3 MicroRNA Expression Analysis

MicroRNAs (miRNAs) are endogenous, single-stranded, 20–23 base-pair non-coding RNA species that regulate protein expression at the posttranscriptional level by forming base-pair-specific interaction between the 5′portion of the miRNA and sites within the coding and un-translated regions of mRNAs. Typically, these interactions lower mRNA stability, attenuating mRNA translation and, hence, protein synthesis. miRNAs play an important role in multiple cellular pathways, including embryogenesis, apoptosis, cellular differentiation and proliferation, hematopoiesis, immune function and regulation, and carcinogenesis [64, 65] miRNAs are dysregulated in variety human malignancies, including colorectal, thyroid, breast, prostate, lung, and pancreatic malignancies, and in fact are dysregulated in every tumor type so far examined [66–72], miRNAs regulate ~ 30 % of global protein translation, with some miRNAs functioning as tumor suppressors and other as oncogenes. In human malignancies, the former are suppressed and the latter are overexpressed [64, 73–75]. Interestingly, profiling of miRNA expression patterns provides more accurate tissue and tumor classification than does global mRNA expression profiling [76, 77].

In esophageal cancer miRNA expression is dysregulated in BE, EAC, and ESCC [78–87]. In many cases, the down-stream target gene products of specific miRNAs have been identified. For example, miR-93, miR-25, and miR-106b are coordinately expressed from a polycistron at 7q22.1. During the transition from the normal squamous epithelium to BE to EAC, their expression is increased seven- to ninefold [88–90]. miR-93 and miR-25 down-regulate the cyclin-dependent kinase inhibitor 1 (p21), a potent inhibitor of CDK2 and –4, which together move cells though the G_1 and S phases of the cell cycle, promoting cell division. Additionally, Bcl-2-like protein 11 (Bim) levels are also suppressed, inhibiting apoptosis [89–91]. Thus activation of the 7q22.1 polycistron promotes malignant transformation. Many other miRNAs dysregulated in esophageal cancer suppress tumor suppressor genes and cause over-expression of oncogenes [reviewed in 92]. Interestingly, many miRNA species are expressed from polycistrons, possibly forming a basic regulatory network coordinating mRNA translation patters [78–90, 92].

6.4.4 Molecular Analysis of miRNA Expression

miRNA expression has been analyzed with multiple molecular techniques, with RT-PCR and microarray analyses being commonly employed, with Northern blotting sometimes used to confirm PCR results. For example, Chen et al. [79] employed qRT-PCR to analyze miRNA expression in 107 ESCC cases using normal adjacent esophageal squamous epithelium as control tissue. All tissue samples were snap frozen in liquid nitrogen, and total miRNA was isolated from the frozen tissue using a mirVana miRNA isolation kit. The first strand of cDNA was synthesized with a RevertAid first strand cDNA synthesis kit and later amplified with mirVana qRT-PCR primers sets in a TaqMan gene expression master mix. An Applied Biosystems 7,300 Real-Time PCR system was used for amplification, following the manufacturer's instructions. miR-92a was significantly up-regulated in the ESCC compared to the control normal epithelium. Interestingly, the relative expression of mi-92a was significantly increased in lymph node metastases compared to patients without node metastases ($p = 0.001$). miR-92a expression also correlated with the patients TNM stage ($p = 0.049$), but not with age, gender, differentiation grade, tumor position type, and T classification. Additionally, 65 patients were followed for 5 years. Those with higher mi-92a expression had a shorter survival and higher TNM and N stages than those with low expression.

Last, the CDH1 mRNA (E-cadherin) 3′ un-translated region contains a highly conserved binding region from 499 to 524 for mi-92a. Chen et al. [79] found a strong inverse correlation between E-cadherin expression of mi-92a levels. Further proof for a role in mi-92a-regulating E-cadherin expression was shown in a cell line where removal of the mi-92a binding domain in the CDH1 mRNA abrogated the inhibitory effects of mi-92a on E-cadherin expression. The authors concluded that mi-92a overexpression likely promotes metastasis and a poorer clinical course, in part, via down regulating E-cadherin. The advantages of employing qRT-PCR in miRNA analysis is that the technique is cost effective, lends itself to high-throughput analyses, and readily detects low abundance nucleic acid species [93]. While mi-RNA analyses have been often performed on esophageal cancer tissue samples, qRT-PCR has also been successfully employed in the analysis of circulating serum miRNAs, a technique that is relatively uninvasive and that will eventually have clinical applications (for review, see [94]).

*6.4.5 Acetylaldehyde Dehydrogenase*2*

Ethanol is metabolized by a two-step process, being first converted into acetylaldehyde by alcohol dehydrogenase, and subsequently acetylaldehyde is metabolized to acetate by acetylaldehyde dehydrogenase (ALDH2), which is attached to acetyl coenzyme A and enters the citric acid cycle [95]. Acetylaldehyde is a mutagen and potent carcinogen and, like most carcinogens, a longer exposure at higher concentrations results in increased cellular damage [15–18]. ALDH2 is found at 12q24, is 53 kbp, and consists of 13 exons and 12 intones, which encode a 501 amino acid residue protein [96, 97]. ALDH2 has multiple polymorphisms, one of which profoundly affects the enzymes catalytic efficiency [98, 99]. In the ALDH2*2 polymorphism, a lysine at residue 487 replaces a glutamic acid residue found in the more common ALDH2*1 allele. ALDH2*2 has little ability to metabolize ethanol and has a very low affinity for NAD, a cofactor required for enzymatic function and the metabolism of ethanol [99]. Following alcohol consumption, individuals with ALDH2*2 homozygotes show 18 times higher blood alcohol levels and those with ALDH2*1/ALDH2*2 heterozygotes show a five times higher blood alcohol levels than individuals with the wild-type allele [100]. As a result of the very poor enzymatic activity of the ALDH2*2 polymorphism acetylaldehyde, levels are higher in ALDH2*2 hetero- and homozygotes than in ALDH2*1/ALDH2*1 individuals following alcohol consumption [99–101] (Fig. 6.3). Not surprisingly, ALDH2*2 homozygotes and ALDH2*1/ALDH2*1 individuals exhibit higher levels of acetaldehyde-derived DNA damage following alcohol consumption than ALDH2*1 homozygotes [102].

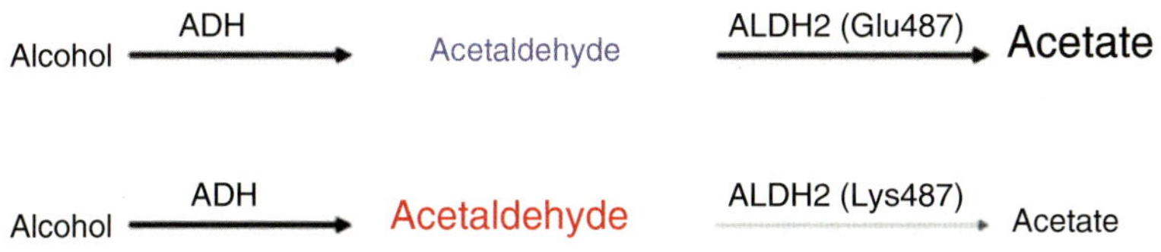

Fig. 6.3 With similar alcohol dehydrogenase (*ADH*) activities, the very poor ability of ALDH2 (Lys487, ALDH2*2) allele results in the accumulation acetylaldehyde that can cause DNA damage [102] (The figure is from Ref. [101])

Lewis et al. [103] performed a meta-analysis of seven articles that reported on ALDH2 polymorphism and esophageal cancer. Compared to ALDH2*1 homozygotes, ALDH2*2 homozygotes had lower rates of esophageal cancer (odds ratio 0.36), while ALDH2*1/ALDH2*1 individuals had elevated esophageal cancer rates (odds ratio 3.19). The reason for the lower esophageal cancer rates seen in the ALDH2*2 homozygotes was attributed to the uncomfortable "alcohol flushing response" seen in ~ 36 % of Asians, where ethanol consumption causes facial flushing, nausea, and tachycardia. These individuals were found to avoid alcohol and therefore have lower esophageal cancer rates than ALDH2*1 homozygotes. The flushing response was largely absent in ALDH2*1/ALDH2*1 individuals who did tend to consume alcohol and show increased esophageal cancer and acetaldehyde-derived DNA damage [101–103]. Interestingly, individuals who show the alcohol flushing response and still consume alcohol show elevated esophageal cancer rates, whereas those who drink everyday, are heavy drinkers, or are alcoholics show an odds ratios of 12.1, 16.4, and 13.5, respectively, compared to control ALDH2*1 homozygotes [102, 104–106].

6.4.6 ALDH2*2 Polymorphism Testing

Many different techniques have been employed in ALDH2 polymorphism testing, including microarray, mass spectrometry, melting curve analysis, sequencing, and conventional fluorescent-based PCR analysis [107, 108]. Itoga et al. [108] compared melting curve analysis, SNaPsnot analysis, denaturing high-performance liquid chromatography (DHPLC), and PCR-SSCP analysis.

Whole blood from 24 healthy men and 74 men with esophageal cancer was collected, and genomic DNA was isolated. The men also answered detailed questionnaires about their alcohol consumption. The portion of the ALDH2 gene surrounding the *2 polymorphism was amplified with the Cy-5 labeled primers Cy5-CAAATTACAGGGTCAACTGCT (forward) and Cy5-CCACACTCACAG TTTTCACTT (reverse) in a 25 μL volume with 100 ng genomic DNA, 0.2 M each primer, 0.2 mM of each dNTP, and 1 U *Taq* polymerase in 10 mM Tris–HCl buffer. The reaction mix was denatured for 3 min at 94 °C and amplified by 30 cycles with annealing at 58 °C for 30 s, extension at 72 °C for 30 s, and denaturation at 94 °C for 30 s. The resulting amplicons were analyzed as described below.

First, amplicons were subjected to *Fluorescent-Based PCR-SSCP Analysis*. One μL of amplicon was diluted in 10 μL of loading buffer solution that contained 99.5 % formamide and 0.5 % blue dextran. The samples were denatured at 94 °C for 3 min; 2 μL of the diluted mix was run into a 10 % native polyacrylamide gel (99:1, acrylamide:bisactymlamide ratio) in 0.5X Tris-borate buffer. Electrophoresis was carried out at 20 W at 18 °C, with data analyzed via Fragment Manager (Amersham Pharmacia Biotech).

Second, samples were subjected to melting curve analysis. One hundred to 500 ng of genomic DNA was mixed in a 20 μL volume with 11.4 μL distilled H_2O, 1.6 μL 25 mM $MgCl_2$, 1 μM of each primer, 1 μL of anchor probe, and 2 μL LightCycler DNA-Master Hybridization Probes. The PCR was carried out with an initial denaturation of 95 °C for 10 min, followed by 40 cycles of 95 °C for 15 s, annealing at 55 °C for 15 s, and extension at 72 °C for 11 s. Following amplification, melting curve analysis was performed with denaturation at 95 °C for 0 s, annealing at 40 °C for 120 s, and analysis carried out with a 0.2 °C/s increase to 80 °C. Emitted fluorescence was measured during the heat ramping step, and the melting curve was plotted as melting peaks.

Third, amplicons were subjected to *SNaPshot Analysis*. Four μL of amplicon that had been subjected to a 7 min extension at 72 °C at the end of the last cycle was used. The amplicon was incubated at 37 °C for 1 h with 2 U exonuclease I and 2 U shrimp alkaline phosphatase. The mix was heated to denature the enzyme, and 1 μL of digested PCR product was mixed with 5 μL of SNaPshot Multiplex Ready Reaction Mix with 1 μM minisequencing primer (5′-CCACACTCACAGTTTTCACTT-3′) and amplified via 25 cycles of 96 °C for 10 s, 50 °C for 5 s, and 60° for 10 s. Upon completion, 0.5 U shrimp alkaline phosphatase was added and the reaction was incubated for 1 h. One μL of the resulting reaction mix was added to 12 μL of HiDi formamide and heated to 95 °C for 5 min. The samples were run in an ABU PRISM 310 Genetic Analyzer, and the results were analyzed with GeneScan 3.0 application software.

6.4.7 Denaturing High-Performance Liquid Chromatography

Denaturing high-performance liquid chromatography (DHPLC) was performed with genomic DNA amplified, prepared as for the SNaPshot procedure. Heteroduplex DNA was produced by mixing ALDH2*1/2*2 by denaturing the PCR products at 94 °C for 3 min and then slowly cooling them. Homoduplex samples were made in the same manner by mixing equal amounts or ALDH2*1 or ALDH2*2 and treating them as per the heteroduplex samples. The DHPLC analysis was carried out using WAVE DNA Fragment Analysis System. The PCR mixture was loaded on a DNASep column and the hetero- and homoduplexes where eluted with a linear acetonitrile gradient formed by mixing two different elution buffers at a constant flow rate of 0.9 mL/min. DNA elution was detected by measuring absorbance at 260 nm at 58 °C.

Interestingly, the study revealed all four techniques to have 100 % concordance. Melting curve analysis required 4 h to complete, PCR-SSCP took 6 h, DHPLC required 21 h, and SNaPshot analysis required 23 h. The costs of each reaction were $4.16, $2.50, $2.50, and $8.33, respectively. Melting curve analysis had the advantage of not requiring opening of the reaction tube, thus eliminating the possibility of contamination. The authors concluded that, for routine 10–20 samples/day molecular diagnostics, melting curve analysis was the best option and PCR-SSCP fluorescent-based genotyping was best applied to large-scale genotyping for epidemiological studies. Interestingly, the study showed that the highest esophageal cancer rates were seen in habitual drinkers with ALDH2*2 homozygosity.

6.5 CDX2 Protein Expression in Barrett's Esophagitis

The molecular events underlying the transition of normal esophageal epithelium to BE is incompletely understood, but recent studies have demonstrated a role for the Caudal homeobox (Cdx) genes in the morphogenesis of BE. Animal studies have shown that CDX expression plays a role in the morphogenesis of normal intestinal epithelium. For example, in normal murine embryogenesis Cdx1 and −2 expression appears at day 12 and continues throughout life, with Cdx protein expression being required for the transformation of endoderm into large and small intestinal columnar epithelium [109]. Mice genetically engineered to express Cdx1 or −2 in their gastric cells develop metaplastic intestinal-type epithelium with goblet cells, enterocytes, and enteroendocrine cells [110–114]. Additionally, while ablation of global *Cdx2* expression is lethal in embryonic mice, causing death before gastrulation [115, 116], conditional ablation of *Cdx2* in the developing gut results in partial foregut like differentiation of the large and small intestines, loss of intestinal villi, and significantly lowered expression of the pro-intestinal transcription factors *Cdx1, Isx, HNF1α*, and *HNF4α*, which together activate the intestinal transcriptome [117].

Cdx1 and −2 is strongly expressed in normal human large and small intestine, but not in the stomach or esophagus [110, 118]. In BE Cdx2 expression is 400 times higher than normal esophageal epithelium and it is 100 % expressed in BE with dysplasia and in EAC [118–120]. Some experiments done on cultured esophageal cells has demonstrated that bile salts and acidic conditions can increase Cdx2 expression, although by itself increased Cdx2 expression is insufficient to cause all the changes seen in BE [121, 122]. Cdx2 is expressed in BE, BE with dysplasia, and EAC, and is a sensitive marker for intestinal dysplasia. However, it cannot differentiate low-grade from high-grade dysplasia, and the expression differences seen in the BE→dysplasia→EAC are not sufficient for immunohistochemistry to be useful [110, 118–124]. Presently the diagnosis of BE, BE with dysplasia, and EAC presently rests almost solely on the examination of histologic sections combined with clinical findings and patient history. Cdx2 immunohistochemistry may become more important in the future as our understanding of its function and down-steam signaling cascades increases.

6.6 Tylosis

Tylosis is an autosomal dominant syndrome first recognized more than 50 years ago. Its common manifestation is palmoplantar keratoderma, an abnormal thickening and callusing of the palms and soles due to abnormal keratinization. Oral leukoplakia and esophageal hyperkeratosis often accompany the palmoplantar keratoderma. Tylosis has a strong association to ESCC, but not EAC, with the ESCC risk reported as 40–95 % by the age of 70 years [125–130]. Initial linkage studies revealed the heritable Tylosis abnormality to be on chromosome 17, with later studies narrowing the region to a 42.5 kb region at 17q25, designated as the TOC gene. This region has also been implicated in some cases of sporadic ESCC [131–139]. One gene within this region, cytoglobin (*CYGB*), has both alleles ~ 70 % down-regulated in Tylosis, while in sporadic esophageal cancer both alleles appear to be suppressed by an epigenetic mechanism. Interestingly, sequencing of the TOC gene in Tylosis and sporadic esophageal cancer failed to show any heritable or somatic mutations, suggesting epigenetic suppression in both disease processes [138, 140]. Tylosis is rare, with only a few known kindreds having the disease. There are few recommendations on how to clinically manage the disease, although at least yearly upper endoscopic screening with intensive biopsies is recommended. Presently, it is not known if upper endoscopic screening will lower the mortality seen in Tylosis [140].

The diagnosis of Tylosis is based on clinical findings, combined with the personal and family history; molecular diagnostic techniques rarely employed [56]. McRonald et al. [140] collected esophageal biopsies during routine upper endoscopy from 18 affected individuals from a Tylosis family, seven biopsies from individuals with gastro-esophageal reflux, and ten individuals without esophageal cancer, gastro-esophageal reflux, or other esophageal pathology. The tissues were collected into RNAlater and stored at −20 °C until the RNA was isolated using RNeasy. Two micrograms of RNA were reverse transcribed with oligo-dT primers. The resulting cDNA was amplified with 0.2 μM of the primers 5′-CTTCGGGGAAGTTGAGTCAG-3′ (forward) and 5′-CAAGGTGGAACCGGTGTACT-3′ (reverse) for 26 cycles with the *TBP* mRNA employed as a control. Twenty-six cycles were chosen as this was determined to be within the exponential phase of the reaction. The resulting amplicons were identified and quantified by agarose gel electrophoresis with the gels scanned with an ABI GeneScanner. As described above, the *CYGB* was ~ 70 % down-regulated in patients with Tylosis compared to normal esophageal epithelium, with both alleles being equally repressed. The authors concluded that the *CYGB* gene was down-regulated by three possible mechanism: (1) there may be an aberrant anti-sense RNA species produced in Tylosis that impairs the function of the *CYGB* gene;

(2) the transcription of the gene is impaired; or (3) the *CYGB* gene may be down-regulated due to the aberrant expression of another gene. Further research will be required to find the mechanism of transcriptional repression.

6.7 Gastric Cancer

Gastric cancer is the fourth most common cancer worldwide with 934,000 new cases each year. In addition, due to its aggressive clinical course, it is also the second most common cause of cancer deaths worldwide, causing an estimated 700,000 deaths each year. The incidence of the cancer varies widely between different geographical locations. Two-thirds occur in the developing countries, with China accounting for 42 % of all cases. High-risk areas included East Asia, Eastern Europe, and parts of Central and South America. Low-risk areas include Southern Asia, North and East Africa, North America, New Zealand, and Australia [1].

6.8 Environmental Versus Genetic Factors for Gastric Cancer

Studies of migrant populations have clearly demonstrated strong environmental factors in the risk for gastric cancer. In particular, studies of populations moving from high-risk to low-risk areas for gastric have highlighted many environmental risks factors, with some studies indicating that the risk factors exert effects beginning in childhood [1, 141, 142]. Many risk factors have been identified several are discussed below:

6.8.1 Helicobacter pylori *(*H. pylori*)*

H. pylori is listed by the international Agency for Research on Cancer as carcinogenic in humans [143]. More than 50 % of the world's population is infected with *H. pylori*, with infection conferring a two to sixfold increased risk for gastric carcinoma [144, 145]. Not surprisingly curing an *H. pylori* infection significantly reduces the risk for gastric cancer in high-risk population [146, 147]. *H. pylori* is a Gram-negative bacterium that synthesizes numerous virulence factors, including urease, arginase, adhesin, vacuolating toxin, and cytotoxin-associated antigen [148, 149]. Evidence indicates that causes gastric cancer via a three-step mechanism; (1) *H. pylori* infection, (2) the development of precancerous including severe gastric atrophy, intestinal metaplasia, and corpus predominant gastritis, and (3) and carcinogenesis [150]. The mechanisms of *H. pylori*–induced carcinogenesis are incompletely understood, however multiple factors appear to promote cancer including increased oxidative stress, chronic inflammation, and impaired host antioxidant defenses and ability to repair DNA damage [151–155]. Presently once found *H. pylori* infections are treated with antibiotics to eradicate the infections [146, 147].

6.8.2 Diet

Extensive data have indicated that diet plays a strong role in gastric cancer risk, that is, a diet high in certain foods such as persevered, salted and or smoked foods, especially meats and pickled vegetables with carcinogenic *N*-nitroso compounds. Animal studies have also demonstrated that ingesting relatively high amount of salt induces gastritis and enhances the potency of carcinogens such as N-methyl-N-nitro-N-nitrosoguanidine and 4-nitroquinoline-1-oxide [156, 157]. Additionally, a diet high in fresh fruits and vegetables exerts a protective effect, lowering the risk for gastric cancer, while the polyphenols found in green tea (*Camellia sinensis*) have anti-inflammatory and anti-oxidant effects, and additionally inhibit nitosation – an event implicated in gastric carcinogenesis [158–164].

6.8.3 Tobacco

Not surprisingly, smoking increases the risk for gastric cancer significantly. Interestingly smoking increases the incidence of distal gastric cancer [165, 166].

6.8.4 Obesity

Obesity is a major risk factor for gastric cardia adenocarcinoma as it promotes gastroesophageal reflux, the development of BE and hence increases the risk of adenocarcinoma of the gastroesophageal junction [48]. One Swedish study revealed that the heaviest quartile of the population had a 2.3fold increased risk for gastric cardia adenocarcinoma compared to the light quartile of the population [167]. Thus weight loss, which reduces reflux, also lowers the risk for gastric cardia adenocarcinoma.

6.9 Genetic Risk Factors for Gastric Carcinoma and Molecular-Genetic Testing

About 90 % of gastric malignancies are sporadic, with the remaining 10 % showing a familial clustering, and 1–3 % representing hereditary gastric cancer syndromes [168]. Molecular diagnostic testing is generally not often performed on gastric malignancies, except for hereditary diffuse gastric carcinoma and mucosa-associated lymphoid tissue lymphomas.

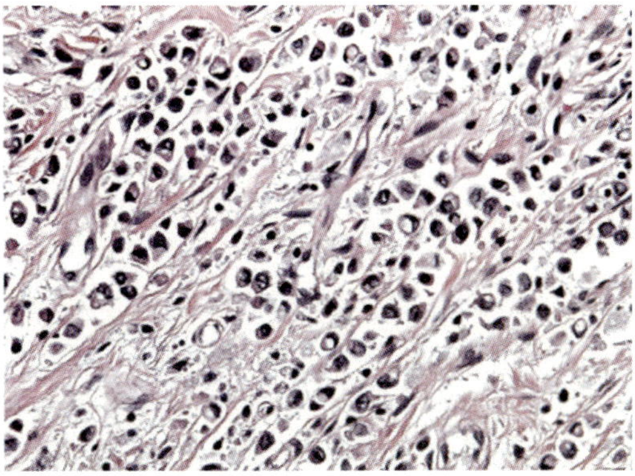

Fig. 6.4 The typical histology of gastric signet ring cell carcinoma (From Ref. [170])

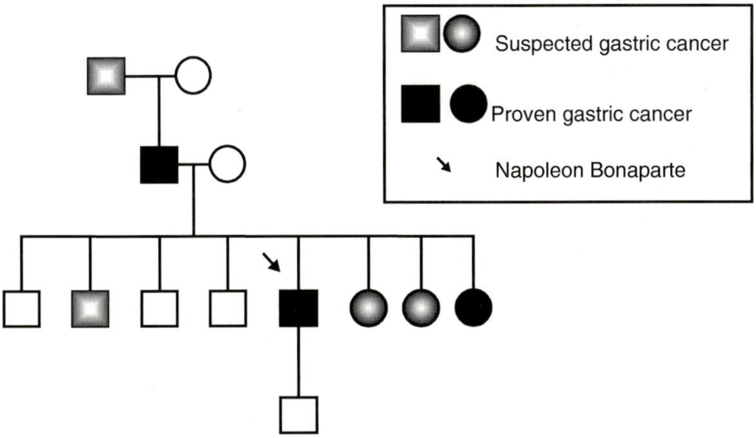

Fig. 6.5 The family pedigree of the Bonaparte family showing a pattern of heredity gastric cancer (From Ref. [56])

6.9.1 Hereditary Diffuse Gastric Carcinoma

Hereditary diffuse gastric carcinoma is an autosomal dominant cancer susceptibility syndrome characterized by an estimated cancer risk of 67 % for men and 83 % for women [169]. Histologically, it is characterized by the development of an aggressive diffusely infiltrating signet ring cell gastric carcinoma that results in linitis plastica once the majority of the stomach is involved (Fig. 6.4). The syndrome was first described in three New Zealand Maori families in 1964, with genetic linkage studies employing microsatellite markers showing that the E-cadherin gene (*CDH1*) at 16q22.1 was involved [171, 172]. Since these early studies, the syndrome has been identified in multiple kindreds in many countries and, interestingly, in the family of Napoleon Bonaparte [56, 173–176] (Fig. 6.5).

Hereditary diffuse gastric carcinoma is defined as follows by the International Gastric Cancer Linkage Consortium [177]:

1. Two or more documented cases of diffuse gastric cancer in first/s degree relatives, with at least one diagnosed before age 50 years; OR
2. Three of more cases of documented diffuse gastric cancer in first/s degree relatives, independently of age of onset.

More recent criteria (also by the International Gastric Cancer Linkage Consortium) are:

1. An individual diagnosed with diffuse gastric cancer before 35 years of age.
2. An individual diagnosed with both diffuse gastric cancer and lobular breast cancer.
3. One family member with diffuse gastric cancer and another with either lobular breast cancer or signet ring colon cancer.

Individuals who meet or exceed these criteria should receive genetic counseling, be tested for germline E-cadherin gene mutations, undergo upper screening endoscopic exams every 6 months with extensive biopsies taken, and undergo prophylatic gastrectomy. The timing of the prophylatic gastrectomy is based on multiple factors, such as patient age, ability to tolerate the operation, and the decision to have children [56, 177].

6.9.2 Molecular-Genetic Testing in Hereditary Diffuse Gastric Carcinoma

Molecular diagnostic testing for hereditary diffuse gastric carcinoma can be performed by several different molecular diagnostic technologies. However, because many of the mutations in this syndrome are missense or inactivating mutations that can occur in different areas of *CDH1,* testing by DNA sequencing of amplified genomic DNA is an efficient method of testing. Suriano et al. [178] employed PCR, DNA sequencing, and DHPLC to examine *CDH1* mutations in 31 previously unreported kindreds with hereditary diffuse gastric carcinoma. Twenty of the families had a positive history of diffuse gastric cancer, ten had early-onset diffuse gastric cancer, and one had lobular breast cancer and diffuse gastric cancer. Genomic DNA was purified from peripheral blood leukocytes using a Puregene DNA Purification Kit. The compete coding sequence of the E-cadherin gene including the splice junctions was PCR amplified using 100 ng genomic template DNA, 0.5 mM/L PCR primers with deoxynucleotide triphosphates, $MgSO_4$, and 1.25 units Optimase polymerase in appropriate buffer conditions. The samples were denatured at 95 °C for 2 min and subjected to 15 touchdown cycles with 0.5 °C annealing temperature decreases at each cycle, and 20–50 s extensions at 72 °C. The end result amplicons were denatured for 4 min at 94 °C and cooled to room temperature at 1 °C/min. Resulting amplicons (3–15 μL) were screened for mutations with high-performance liquid chromatography. The optimal temperatures for resolution of hetero- and homoduplexes were established by analyzing the melting behavior of PCR fragments in temperature ranges corresponding to that calculated on Wavemaker software. PCR amplicons identified as aberrant by chromatography were directly sequenced in both directions using florescent-labeled dye terminators in an ABI 3,700 capillary sequencer. Samples showing a putative pathogenic mutation were confirmed by a second independent PCR and sequencing reaction.

Of the 20 families with a positive history of gastric cancer, 30 % harbored *CDH1* mutations. 20 % of the families with early-onset gastric cancer were mutation positive, and the case with both lobular breast cancer and gastric cancer was mutation positive. Nine different mutations were identified: four nonsense, two deletion, one splice site substitution, one single nucleotide affecting a start condon, and one misssence mutation. With the exception of one previously identified nonsense mutation, 1003C>T, all where novel mutations. All carriers were heterozygotes for their mutations. Although by this assay some *CDH1* mutations, such as deletions, could have been missed due to assay insensitivity, the authors concluded that many of the families probably harbored mutations in other genes that led to gastric cancer.

6.9.3 Other Familial Gastric Cancer Syndromes

An increased risk for gastric cancer is seen in hereditary nonpolyposis colorectal cancer and Peutz-Jeghers syndromes. These cancer-prone syndromes are covered in Chap. 5, which discusses the molecular diagnostics of colorectal carcinoma.

6.10 Gastrointestinal Stromal Tumors

Gastrointestinal stromal tumors (GISTs) are the most common mesenchymal neoplasm of the gastrointestinal tract and can occur anywhere from the esophagus to the anus, with approximately two-thirds occurring in the stomach and less than 5 % occurring in the esophagus. GISTs are submucosal lesions that arise from multipotential stem cells [179]. They are rare; having an incidence of 10–20 per one million people diagnosed every year and show considerable histologic variation, showing spindle, epithelioid, and mixed patterns. Immunohistochemical analyses of GISTs are usually limited to CD117 (c-kit), which the majority of GISTs express, and DOG-1, a cell surface protein of unknown function, expressing roughly 98 % of GISTs regardless of c-kit or PDGFRα gene expression status [180].

GISTs also manifest wide variations in their clinical behavior, ranging from benign neoplasms to very aggressive metastasizing malignancies. The prognosis of a GIST is determined by several factors, including factors such as tumor size at presentation, mitotic index, coagulative necrosis, hypercellular sarcomatous histology, and increased expression of cell cycle progression proteins, such as Ki-67 [181–183]. They typically have activating mutations of either the c-Kit or PDGFRα proto-oncogenes [184]. Most commonly activating c-Kit mutations are found in exon 11 with less common mutations in exons 9, 13, and 17 [185]. The treatment for GISTs, when possibly, is surgical resection. However, for metastatic or recurrent GISTs, imatinib mesylate or other oral tyrosine kinase inhibitors can be employed to slow tumor growth and improve the survival with advanced/aggressive GISTs. The response to tyrosine kinase inhibitors is usually not complete, and most patients eventually develop resistance. Interestingly, the kinase inhibitor response depends on the genomic location of the specific c-Kit mutation [181]. For example, GISTs with c-kit exon 9 mutations show intermediate imatinib sensitivity and better relapse-free survival and overall survival times than those with exon 11 mutations. The exon 11 mutation-bearing GISTs show an increased sensitivity to imatinib and have a worse relapse-free and overall survival time [186].

Molecular diagnostic procedures for the c-Kit mutations found in GISTs have employed FISH, immunohistochemistry, microarrays, and PCR amplification of tumor-derived genomic DNA followed by sequencing [187, 188]. Presently, most c-Kit testing for GISTs involve immunohistochemistry for c-Kit protein expression, as an adjunct to a histology-based diagnoses. Molecular diagnostics is presently rarely preformed to analyze the specific c-Kit mutation [181].

6.11 Conclusion

Presently, molecular diagnostics has limited application in esophageal and gastric pathology, with hereditary diffuse gastric carcinoma testing probably being the best known testing modality. As our knowledge of the growth-promoting signal transduction pathways underlying gastro-esophageal malignancies increases, molecular diagnostics for these organ is likely to become more common and useful in the clinical decision-making and determining treatment options. Additionally, as new molecular diagnostic technologies such as accurate full genome sequencing emerge, our ability to predict an individual's risk for these malignancies may play a role in identifying individuals likely to benefit from periodic screening procedures.

References

1. Parkin DM, Bray F, Ferlay J, Pisani P (2005) Global cancer statistics, 2002. CA Cancer J Clin 55:74–108
2. Miller BA, Kolonel LN, Bernstein L, Young JL, Swanson GM, West D, Key CR, Liff JM, Glover CS, Alexander GA et al (eds) (1996) Racial/Ethnic patterns of cancer in the United States 1988–1992. NIH publication no. 96–4104. National Cancer Institute, Bethesda
3. Kamangar F, Chow WH, Abnet CC, Dawsey SM (2009) Environmental causes of esophageal cancer. Gastroenterol Clin North Am 38:27–57

4. Daly JM, Fry WA, Little AG, Winchester DP, McKee RF, Stewart AK, Fremgen AM (2000) Esophageal cancer: results of an American College of Surgeons Patient Care Evaluation Study. J Am Coll Surg 190:562–572
5. Blot WJ, Devesa SS, Kneller RW, Fraumeni JF (1991) Rising incidence of adenocarcinoma of the esophagus and gastric cardia. JAMA 265:1287–1289
6. Botterweck AA, Schouten LJ, Volovics A, Dorant E, van Den Brandt PA (2000) Trends in incidence of adenocarcinoma of the oesophagus and gastric cardia in ten European countries. Int J Epidemiol 29:645–654
7. Hongo M, Nagasaki Y, Shoji T (2009) Epidemiology of esophageal cancer: orient to occident, effects of chronology, geography and ethnicity. J Gastroenterol Hepatol 24:729–735
8. Devesa SS, Blot WJ, Fraumeni JF Jr (1998) Changing patterns in the incidence of esophageal and gastric carcinoma in the United States. Cancer 83:2049–2053
9. Newnham A, Quinn MJ, Babb P, Kang JY, Majeed A (2003) Trends in the subsite and morphology of oesophageal and gastric cancer in England and Wales 1971–1998. Aliment Pharmacol Ther 17:665–676
10. Craver LF (1932) Clinical study of etiology of gastric and esophageal carcinoma. Am J Cancer 16:68–102
11. Watson WL (1939) Cancer of the esophagus: some etiological considerations. Am J Roentgenol 41:420–424
12. Boffetta P, Garfinkel L (1990) Alcohol drinking and mortality among men enrolled in an American cancer society prospective study. Epidemiology 1:342–348
13. Freedman ND, Abnet CC, Leitzmann MF, Mouw T, Subar AF, Hollenbeck AR, Schatzkin A (2007) A prospective study of tobacco, alcohol, and the risk of esophageal and gastric cancer subtypes. Am J Epidemiol 165:1424–1433
14. Morita M, Kumashiro R, Kubo N, Nakashima Y, Yoshida R, Yoshinaga K, Saeki H, Emi Y, Kakeji Y, Sakaguchi Y, Toh Y, Maehara Y (2010) Alcohol drinking, cigarette smoking, and the development of squamous cell carcinoma of the esophagus: epidemiology, clinical findings, and prevention. Int J Clin Oncol 15:126–134
15. Testino G, Borro P (2010) Alcohol and gastrointestinal oncology. World J Gastrointest Oncol 2:322–325
16. Yu HS, Oyama T, Isse T, Kitagawa K, Pham TT, Tanaka M, Kawamoto T (2010) Formation of acetaldehyde-derived DNA adducts due to alcohol exposure. Chem Biol Interact 188:367–375
17. Millonig G, Wang Y, Homann N, Bernhardt F, Qin H, Mueller S, Bartsch H, Seitz HK (2011) Ethanol-mediated carcinogenesis in the human esophagus implicates CYP2E1 induction and the generation of carcinogenic DNA-lesions. Int J Cancer 128:533–540
18. Boffetta P, Hashibe M (2006) Alcohol and cancer. Lancet Oncol 7:149–156
19. U.S. Department of Health and Human Services (USDHHS) (1989) Reducing the health consequences of smoking: 25 years of progress: a report of the surgeon general. US Government Press Office, Washington, DC
20. Hecht SS (1999) Tobacco smoke carcinogens and lung cancer. J Natl Cancer Inst 91:1194–1210
21. Moeller DW, Sun LS (2010) Chemical and radioactive carcinogens in cigarettes: associated health impacts and responses of the tobacco industry, U.S. congress, and federal regulatory agencies. Health Phys 99:674–679
22. Wang GQ, Abnet CC, Shen Q, Lewin KJ, Sun XD, Roth MJ, Qiao YL, Mark SD, Dong ZW, Taylor PR, Dawsey SM (2005) Histological precursors of oesophageal squamous cell carcinoma: results from a 13 year prospective follow up study in a high risk population. Gut 54:187–192
23. Castellsagué X, Muñoz N, De Stefani E, Victora C, Castelletto R, Rolón P, Quintana M (1999) Independent and joint effects of tobacco smoking and alcohol drinking on the risk of esophageal cancer in men and women. Int J Cancer 82:657–664
24. Pitt JI (2000) Toxigenic fungi and mycotoxins. Br Med Bull 56:184–192

25. Pitt JI, Basílico JC, Abarca ML, López C (2000) Mycotoxins and toxigenic fungi. Med Mycol 38(Suppl 1):41–46
26. Riley RT, Wang E, Schroeder JJ, Smith ER, Plattner RD, Abbas H, Yoo HS, Merrill AH Jr (1996) Evidence for disruption of sphingolipid metabolism as a contributing factor in the toxicity and carcinogenicity of fumonisins. Nat Toxins 4:3–15
27. Sun G, Wang S, Hu X, Su J, Huang T, Yu J, Tang L, Gao W, Wang JS (2007) Fumonisin B1 contamination of home-grown corn in high-risk areas for esophageal and liver cancer in China. Food Addit Contam 24:181–185
28. Marasas WF (2001) Discovery and occurrence of the fumonisins: a historical perspective. Environ Health Perspect 109(Suppl 2):239–243
29. Lim CW, Parker HM, Vesonder RF, Haschek WM (1996) Intravenous fumonisin B1 induces cell proliferation and apoptosis in the rat. Nat Toxins 4:34–41
30. Hewer T, Rose E, Ghadirian P, Castegnaro M, Malaveille C, Bartsch H, Day N (1978) Ingested mutagens from opium and tobacco pyrolysis products and cancer of the oesophagus. Lancet 2:494–496
31. Malaveille C, Friesen M, Camus AM, Garren L, Hautefeuille A, Béréziat JC, Ghadirian P, Day NE, Bartsch H (1982) Mutagens produced by the pyrolysis of opium and its alkaloids as possible risk factors in cancer of the bladder and oesophagus. Carcinogenesis 3:577–585
32. Nasrollahzadeh D, Kamangar F, Aghcheli K, Sotoudeh M, Islami F, Abnet CC, Shakeri R, Pourshams A, Marjani HA, Nouraie M, Khatibian M, Semnani S, Ye W, Boffetta P, Dawsey SM, Malekzadeh R (2008) Opium, tobacco, and alcohol use in relation to oesophageal squamous cell carcinoma in a high-risk area of Iran. Br J Cancer 98:1857–1863
33. Loria D, Barrios E, Zanetti R (2009) Cancer and yerba mate consumption: a review of possible associations. Rev Panam Salud Publica 25:530–539
34. Szymańska K, Matos E, Hung RJ, Wünsch-Filho V, Eluf-Neto J, Menezes A, Daudt AW, Brennan P, Boffetta P (2010) Drinking of maté and the risk of cancers of the upper aerodigestive tract in Latin America: a case–control study. Cancer Causes Control 21:1799–1806
35. Sewram V, De Stefani E, Brennan P, Boffetta P (2003) Maté consumption and the risk of squamous cell esophageal cancer in Uruguay. Cancer Epidemiol Biomarkers Prev 12:508–513
36. Vieira MA, Maraschin M, Rovaris AA, Amboni RD, Pagliosa CM, Xavier JJ, Amante ER (2010) Occurrence of polycyclic aromatic hydrocarbons throughout the processing stages of erva-mate (Ilex paraguariensis). Food Addit Contam Part A Chem Anal Control Expo Risk Assess 27:776–782
37. Kamangar F, Schantz MM, Abnet CC, Fagundes RB, Dawsey SM (2008) High levels of carcinogenic polycyclic aromatic hydrocarbons in mate drinks. Cancer Epidemiol Biomarkers Prev 17:1262–1268
38. Fagundes RB, Abnet CC, Strickland PT, Kamangar F, Roth MJ, Taylor PR, Dawsey SM (2006) Higher urine 1-hydroxy pyrene glucuronide (1-OHPG) is associated with tobacco smoke exposure and drinking maté in healthy subjects from Rio Grande do Sul, Brazil. BMC Cancer 6:139
39. Mbulaiteye SM, Hisada M, El-Omar EM (2009) *Helicobacter pylori* associated global gastric cancer burden. Front Biosci 14:1490–1504
40. Islami F, Kamangar F (2008) *Helicobacter pylori* and esophageal cancer risk – a meta-analysis. Cancer Prev Res 1:329–338
41. Rokkas T, Pistiolas D, Sechopoulos P, Robotis I, Margantinis G (2007) Relationship between *Helicobacter pylori* infection and esophageal neoplasia: a meta-analysis. Clin Gastroenterol Hepatol 5:1413–1417
42. Spechler SJ (2002) Barrett's esophagus. N Engl J Med 346:836–842
43. Schubert ML (2008) Gastric secretion. Curr Opin Gastroenterol 24:659–664
44. Rothwell PM, Fowkes FG, Belch JF, Ogawa H, Warlow CP, Meade TW (2011) Effect of daily aspirin on long-term risk of death due to cancer: analysis of individual patient data from randomised trials. Lancet 377:31–41

45. Corley DA, Kerlikowske K, Verma R, Buffler P (2003) Protective association of aspirin/NSAIDs and esophageal cancer: a systematic review and meta-analysis. Gastroenterology 124:47–56
46. Wang F, Lv ZS, Fu YK (2010) Nonsteroidal anti-inflammatory drugs and esophageal inflammation - Barrett's esophagus - adenocarcinoma sequence: a meta-analysis. Dis Esophagus. doi:10.1111/j.1442-2050.2010.01153.x [Epub ahead of print]
47. Shaheen N, Ransohoff DF (2002) Gastroesophageal reflux, Barrett esophagus, and esophageal cancer: scientific review. JAMA 287:1972–1981
48. Shaheen NJ, Richter JE (2009) Barrett's oesophagus. Lancet 373:850–861
49. Wang KK, Sampliner RE, The Practice Parameters Committee of the American College of Gastroenterology (2008) Updated guidelines 2008 for the diagnosis, surveillance and therapy of Barrett's esophagus. Am J Gastroenterol 103:788–797
50. Playford RJ (2006) New British Society of Gastroenterology (BSG) guidelines for the diagnosis and management of Barrett's oesophagus. Gut 55:442
51. Schnell TG, Sontag SJ, Chejfec G et al (2001) Long-term nonsurgical management of Barrett's esophagus with high-grade dysplasia. Gastroenterology 120:1607–1619
52. Anand G, Katz PO (2010) Gastroesophageal reflux disease and obesity. Gastroenterol Clin North Am 39:39–46
53. Abnet CC, Freedman ND, Hu N, Wang Z, Yu K, Shu XO, Yuan JM, Zheng W, Dawsey SM, Dong LM, Lee MP, Ding T, Qiao YL, Gao YT, Koh WP, Xiang YB, Tang ZZ, Fan JH, Wang C, Wheeler W, Gail MH, Yeager M, Yuenger J, Hutchinson A, Jacobs KB, Giffen CA, Burdett L, Fraumeni JF Jr, Tucker MA, Chow WH, Goldstein AM, Chanock SJ, Taylor PR (2010) A shared susceptibility locus in PLCE1 at 10q23 for gastric adenocarcinoma and esophageal squamous cell carcinoma. Nat Genet 42:764–767
54. Wang LD, Zhou FY, Li XM, Sun LD, Song X, Jin Y, Li JM, Kong GQ, Qi H, Cui J, Zhang LQ, Yang JZ, Li JL, Li XC, Ren JL, Liu ZC, Gao WJ, Yuan L, Wei W, Zhang YR, Wang WP, Sheyhidin I, Li F, Chen BP, Ren SW, Liu B, Li D, Ku JW, Fan ZM, Zhou SL, Guo ZG, Zhao XK, Liu N, Ai YH, Shen FF, Cui WY, Song S, Guo T, Huang J, Yuan C, Huang J, Wu Y, Yue WB, Feng CW, Li HL, Wang Y, Tian JY, Lu Y, Yuan Y, Zhu WL, Liu M, Fu WJ, Yang X, Wang HJ, Han SL, Chen J, Han M, Wang HY, Zhang P, Li XM, Dong JC, Xing GL, Wang R, Guo M, Chang ZW, Liu HL, Guo L, Yuan ZQ, Liu H, Lu Q, Yang LQ, Zhu FG, Yang XF, Feng XS, Wang Z, Li Y, Gao SG, Qige Q, Bai LT, Yang WJ, Lei GY, Shen ZY, Chen LQ, Li EM, Xu LY, Wu ZY, Cao WK, Wang JP, Bao ZQ, Chen JL, Ding GC, Zhuang X, Zhou YF, Zheng HF, Zhang Z, Zuo XB, Dong ZM, Fan DM, He X, Wang J, Zhou Q, Zhang QX, Jiao XY, Lian SY, Ji AF, Lu XM, Wang JS, Chang FB, Lu CD, Chen ZG, Miao JJ, Fan ZL, Lin RB, Liu TJ, Wei JC, Kong QP, Lan Y, Fan YJ, Gao FS, Wang TY, Xie D, Chen SQ, Yang WC, Hong JY, Wang L, Qiu SL, Cai ZM, Zhang XJ (2010) Genome-wide association study of esophageal squamous cell carcinoma in Chinese subjects identifies susceptibility loci at PLCE1 and C20orf54. Nat Genet 42:759–763
55. Lao-Sirieix P, Caldas C, Fitzgerald RC (2010) Genetic predisposition to gastro-oesophageal cancer. Curr Opin Genet Dev 20:210–217
56. Robertson EV, Jankowski JA (2008) Genetics of gastroesophageal cancer: paradigms, paradoxes, and prognostic utility. Am J Gastroenterol 103:443–449
57. Jaluria P, Konstantopoulos K, Betenbaugh M, Shiloach J (2007) A perspective on microarrays: current applications, pitfalls, and potential uses. Microb Cell Fact 6:4
58. Selaru FM, Zou T, Xu Y, Shustova V, Yin J, Mori Y, Sato F, Wang S, Olaru A, Shibata D, Greenwald BD, Krasna MJ, Abraham JM, Meltzer SJ (2002) Global gene expression profiling in Barrett's esophagus and esophageal cancer: a comparative analysis using cDNA microarrays. Oncogene 21:475–478
59. Greenawalt DM, Duong C, Smyth GK, Ciavarella ML, Thompson NJ, Tiang T, Murray WK, Thomas RJ, Phillips WA (2007) Gene expression profiling of esophageal cancer: comparative analysis of Barrett's esophagus, adenocarcinoma, and squamous cell carcinoma. Int J Cancer 120:1914–1921

60. Helm J, Enkemann SA, Coppola D, Barthel JS, Kelley ST, Yeatman TJ (2005) Dedifferentiation precedes invasion in the progression from Barrett's metaplasia to esophageal adenocarcinoma. Clin Cancer Res 11:2478–2485
61. Warrington JA, Nair A, Mahadevappa M et al (2000) Comparison of human adult and fetal expression and identification of 535 housekeeping/maintenance genes. Physiol Genomics 2:143–147
62. Wang XW, Gao HJ, Fang DC (2008) Advances in gene chip technique in Barrett's metaplasia and adenocarcinoma. J Dig Dis 9:68–71
63. Takahashi S, Miura N, Harada T, Wang Z, Wang X, Tsubokura H, Oshima Y, Hasegawa J, Inagaki Y, Shiota G (2010) Prognostic impact of clinical course-specific mRNA expression profiles in the serum of perioperative patients with esophageal cancer in the ICU: a case control study. J Transl Med 8:103
64. Bartel DP (2004) microRNAs: genomics, biogenesis, mechanism, and function. Cell 116:281–297
65. Bartel DP (2009) microRNAs: target recognition and regulatory functions. Cell 136:215–233
66. Farazi TA, Spitzer JI, Morozov P, Tuschl T (2011) miRNAs in human cancer. J Pathol 223:102–115
67. Schee K, Fodstad Ø, Flatmark K (2010) MicroRNAs as biomarkers in colorectal cancer. Am J Pathol 177:1592–1599
68. Nikiforova MN, Chiosea SI, Nikiforov YE (2009) MicroRNA expression profiles in thyroid tumors. Endocr Pathol 20:85–91
69. Li T, Li D, Sha J, Sun P, Huang Y (2009) MicroRNA-21 directly targets MARCKS and promotes apoptosis resistance and invasion in prostate cancer cells. Biochem Biophys Res Commun 383:280–285
70. Bartels CL, Tsongalis GJ (2010) MicroRNAs: novel biomarkers for human cancer. Ann Biol Clin (Paris) 68:263–272
71. Rovira C, Güida MC, Cayota A (2010) MicroRNAs and other small silencing RNAs in cancer. IUBMB Life 62:859–868
72. Visone R, Croce CM (2009) miRNAs and cancer. Am J Pathol 174:1131–1138
73. Xie XH, Lu J, Kulbokas EJ, Golub TR, Mootha V, Lindblad-Toh K, Lander ES (2005) Systematic discovery of regulatory motifs in human promoters and 3′ UTRs by comparison of several mammals. Nature 434:338–345
74. Shyu AB, Wilkinson MF, van Hoof A (2008) Messenger RNA regulation: to translate or to degrade. EMBO J 27:471–481
75. Vrba L, Jensen TJ, Garbe JC, Heimark RL, Cress AE, Dickinson S, Stampfer MR, Futscher BW (2010) Role for DNA methylation in the regulation of miR-200c and miR-141 expression in normal and cancer cells. PLoS One 5:e8697
76. Lu J, Getz G, Miska EA, Alvarez-Saavedra E, Lamb J, Peck D, Sweet-Cordero A, Ebert BL, Mak RH, Ferrando AA, Downing JR, Jacks T, Horvitz HR, Golub TR (2005) MicroRNA expression profiles classify human cancers. Nature 435:834–838
77. Calin GA, Ferracin M, Cimmino A, Di Leva G, Shimizu M, Wojcik SE, Iorio MV, Visone R, Sever NI, Fabbri M, Iuliano R, Palumbo T, Pichiorri F, Roldo C, Garzon R, Sevignani C, Rassenti L, Alder H, Volinia S, Liu CG, Kipps TJ, Negrini M, Croce CM (2005) A microRNA signature associated with prognosis and progression in chronic lymphocytic leukemia. N Engl J Med 353:1793–1801
78. Zhang C, Wang C, Chen X, Yang C, Li K, Wang J, Dai J, Hu Z, Zhou X, Chen L, Zhang Y, Li Y, Qiu H, Xing J, Liang Z, Ren B, Yang C, Zen K, Zhang CY (2010) Expression profile of microRNAs in serum: a fingerprint for esophageal squamous cell carcinoma. Clin Chem 56:1871–1879
79. Chen ZL, Zhao XH, Wang JW, Li BZ, Wang Z, Sun J, Tan FW, Ding DP, Xu XH, Zhou F, Tan XG, Hang J, Shi SS, Feng XL, He J (2011) microRNA-92a promotes lymph node metastasis of human esophageal squamous cell carcinoma via E-cadherin. J Biol Chem 286:10725–10734
80. Fassan M, Volinia S, Palatini J, Pizzi M, Baffa R, De Bernard M, Battaglia G, Parente P, Croce CM, Zaninotto G, Ancona E, Rugge M (2011) MicroRNA expression profiling in human Barrett's carcinogenesis. Int J Cancer 129:1661–1670

81. Matsushima K, Isomoto H, Kohno S, Nakao K (2010) MicroRNAs and esophageal squamous cell carcinoma. Digestion 82:138–144
82. Hu Y, Correa AM, Hoque A, Guan B, Ye F, Huang J, Swisher SG, Wu TT, Ajani JA, Xu XC (2011) Prognostic significance of differentially expressed miRNAs in esophageal cancer. Int J Cancer 128:132–143
83. Kano M, Seki N, Kikkawa N, Fujimura L, Hoshino I, Akutsu Y, Chiyomaru T, Enokida H, Nakagawa M, Matsubara H (2010) miR-145, miR-133a and miR-133b: tumor suppressive miRNAs target FSCN1 in esophageal squamous cell carcinoma. Int J Cancer 127:2804–2814
84. Maru DM, Singh RR, Hannah C, Albarracin CT, Li YX, Abraham R, Romans AM, Yao H, Luthra MG, Anandasabapathy S, Swisher SG, Hofstetter WL, Rashid A, Luthra R (2009) MicroRNA-196a is a potential marker of progression during Barrett's metaplasia-dysplasia-invasive adenocarcinoma sequence in esophagus. Am J Pathol 174:1940–1948
85. Guo Y, Chen Z, Zhang L, Zhou F, Shi S, Feng X, Li B, Meng X, Ma X, Luo M, Shao K, Li N, Qiu B, Mitchelson K, Cheng J, He J (2008) Distinctive microRNA profiles relating to patient survival in esophageal squamous cell carcinoma. Cancer Res 68:26–33
86. Hiyoshi Y, Kamohara H, Karashima R, Sato N, Imamura Y, Nagai Y, Yoshida N, Toyama E, Hayashi N, Watanabe M, Baba H (2009) MicroRNA-21 regulates the proliferation and invasion in esophageal squamous cell carcinoma. Clin Cancer Res 15:1915–1922
87. Ogawa R, Ishiguro H, Kuwabara Y, Kimura M, Mitsui A, Katada T, Harata K, Tanaka T, Fujii Y (2009) Expression profiling of micro-RNAs in human esophageal squamous cell carcinoma using RT-PCR. Med Mol Morphol 42:102–109
88. Kan T, Sato F, Ito T, Matsumura N, David S, Cheng Y, Agarwal R, Paun BC, Jin Z, Olaru AV, Selaru FM, Hamilton JP, Yang J, Abraham JM, Mori Y, Meltzer SJ (2009) The miR-106b-25 polycistron, activated by genomic amplification, functions as an oncogene by suppressing p21 and Bim. Gastroenterology 136:1689–1700
89. Ivanovska I, Ball AS, Diaz RL, Magnus JF, Kibukawa M, Schelter JM, Kobayashi SV, Lim L, Burchard J, Jackson AL, Linsley PS, Cleary MA (2008) MicroRNAs in the miR-106b family regulate p21/CDKN1A and promote cell cycle progression. Mol Cell Biol 28:2167–2174
90. Petrocca F, Visone R, Onelli MR, Shah MH, Nicoloso MS, de Martino I, Iliopoulos D, Pilozzi E, Liu CG, Negrini M, Cavazzini L, Volinia S, Alder H, Ruco LP, Baldassarre G, Croce CM, Vecchione A (2008) E2F1-regulated microRNAs impair TGFbeta-dependent cell-cycle arrest and apoptosis in gastric cancer. Cancer Cell 13:272–286
91. Shackelford RE, Kaufmann WK, Paules RS (2000) Oxidative stress and cell cycle checkpoint function. Free Radic Biol Med 28:1387–1404
92. Kan T, Meltzer SJ (2009) MicroRNAs in Barrett's esophagus and esophageal adenocarcinoma. Curr Opin Pharmacol 9:727–732
93. Chen C, Ridzon DA, Broomer AJ, Zhou Z, Lee DH, Nguyen JT, Barbisin M, Xu NL, Mahuvakar VR, Andersen MR, Lao KQ, Livak KJ, Guegler KJ (2005) Real-time quantification of microRNAs by stem-loop RT-PCR. Nucleic Acids Res 33:e179
94. Zhou SL, Wang LD (2010) Circulating microRNAs: novel biomarkers for esophageal cancer. World J Gastroenterol 16:2348–2354
95. Seitz HK, Stickel F (2007) Molecular mechanisms of alcohol-mediated carcinogenesis. Nat Rev Cancer 7:599–612
96. Raghunathan L, Hsu LC, Klisak I, Sparkes RS, Yoshida A, Mohandas T (1988) Regional localization of the human genes for aldehyde dehydrogenase-1 and aldehyde dehydrogenase-2. Genomics 2:267–269
97. Hsu LC, Chang WC, Yoshida A (1989) Genomic structure of the human cytosolic aldehyde dehydrogenase gene. Genomics 5:857–865
98. Novoradovsky A, Tsai SJ, Goldfarb L, Peterson R, Long JC, Goldman D (1995) Mitochondrial aldehyde dehydrogenase polymorphism in Asian and American Indian populations: detection of new ALDH2 alleles. Alcohol Clin Exp Res 19:1105–1110
99. Yoshida A, Huang IY, Ikawa M (1984) Molecular abnormality of an inactive aldehyde dehydrogenase variant commonly found in Orientals. Proc Natl Acad Sci USA 81:258–261

100. Enomoto N, Takase S, Yasuhara M, Takada A (1991) Acetaldehyde metabolism in different aldehyde dehydrogenase-2 genotypes. Alcohol Clin Exp Res 15:141–144
101. Brooks PJ, Enoch MA, Goldman D, Li TK, Yokoyama A (2009) The alcohol flushing response: an unrecognized risk factor for esophageal cancer from alcohol consumption. PLoS Med 6:e50
102. Matsuda T, Yabushita H, Kanaly RA, Shibutani S, Yokoyama A (2006) Increased DNA damage in ALDH2-deficient alcoholics. Chem Res Toxicol 19:1374–1378
103. Lewis SJ, Smith GD (2005) Alcohol, ALDH2, and esophageal cancer: a meta-analysis which illustrates the potentials and limitations of a Mendelian randomization approach. Cancer Epidemiol Biomarkers Prev 14:1967–1971
104. Yokoyama A, Muramatsu T, Ohmori T, Higuchi S, Hayashida M, Ishii H (1996) Esophageal cancer and aldehyde dehydrogenase-2 genotypes in Japanese males. Cancer Epidemiol Biomarkers Prev 5:99–102
105. Yokoyama A, Muramatsu T, Omori T, Yokoyama T, Matsushita S, Higuchi S, Maruyama K, Ishii H (2001) Alcohol and aldehyde dehydrogenase gene polymorphisms and oropharyngolaryngeal, esophageal and stomach cancers in Japanese alcoholics. Carcinogenesis 22:433–439
106. Matsuo K, Hamajima N, Shinoda M, Hatooka S, Inoue M, Takezaki T, Tajima K (2001) Gene–environment interaction between an aldehyde dehydrogenase-2 (ALDH2) polymorphism and alcohol consumption for the risk of esophageal cancer. Carcinogenesis 22:913–916
107. Landi S, Gemignani F, Gioia-Patricola L, Chabrier A, Canzian F (2003) Evaluation of a microarray for genotyping polymorphisms related to xenobiotic metabolism and DNA repair. Biotechniques 35:816–820, 822, 824–7
108. Itoga S, Nanmoku T, Uchimoto T, Sunaga M, Nezu M, Tomonaga T, Harada S, Nomura F (2004) Comparative analyses of four different methods of genotyping ALDH2. Alcohol Clin Exp Res 28(8 Suppl Proceedings):117S–122S
109. Guillem PG (2005) How to make a Barrett esophagus: pathophysiology of columnar metaplasia of the esophagus. Dig Dis Sci 50:415–424
110. Silberg DG, Furth EE, Taylor JK, Schuck T, Chiou T, Traber PG (1997) CDX1 protein expression in normal, metaplastic, and neoplastic human alimentary tract epithelium. Gastroenterology 113:478–486
111. Mutoh H, Hakamata Y, Sato K, Eda A, Yanaka I, Honda S, Osawa H, Kaneko Y, Sugano K (2002) Conversion of gastric mucosa to intestinal metaplasia in Cdx2-expressing transgenic mice. Biochem Biophys Res Commun 294:470–479
112. Silberg DG, Sullivan J, Kang E, Swain GP, Moffett J, Sund NJ, Sackett SD, Kaestner KH (2002) Cdx2 ectopic expression induces gastric intestinal metaplasia in transgenic mice. Gastroenterology 122:689–696
113. Mutoh H, Sakurai S, Satoh K, Osawa H, Hakamata Y, Takeuchi T, Sugano K (2004) Cdx1 induced intestinal metaplasia in the transgenic mouse stomach: comparative study with Cdx2 transgenic mice. Gut 53:1416–1423
114. Mutoh H, Satoh K, Kita H, Sakamoto H, Hayakawa H, Yamamoto H, Isoda N, Tamada K, Ido K, Sugano K (2005) Cdx2 specifies the differentiation of morphological as well as functional absorptive enterocytes of the small intestine. Int J Dev Biol 49:867–871
115. Chawengsaksophak K, James R, Hammond VE, Kontgen F, Beck F (1997) Homeosis and intestinal tumours in Cdx2 mutant mice. Nature 386:84–87
116. Tamai Y, Nakajima R, Ishikawa T, Takaku K, Seldin MF, Taketo MM (1999) Colonic hamartoma development by anomalous duplication in Cdx2 knockout mice. Cancer Res 59:2965–2970
117. Gao N, White P, Kaestner KH (2009) Establishment of intestinal identity and epithelial mesenchymal signaling by Cdx2. Dev Cell 16:588–599
118. Vallböhmer D, DeMeester SR, Peters JH, Oh DS, Kuramochi H, Shimizu D, Hagen JA, Danenberg KD, Danenberg PV, DeMeester TR, Chandrasoma PT (2006) Cdx-2 expression in squamous and metaplastic columnar epithelia of the esophagus. Dis Esophagus 19:260–266
119. Phillips RW, Frierson HF Jr, Moskaluk CA (2003) Cdx2 as a marker of epithelial intestinal differentiation in the esophagus. Am J Surg Pathol 27:1442–1447

120. Groisman GM, Amar M, Meir A (2004) Expression of the intestinal marker Cdx2 in the columnar-lined esophagus with and without intestinal (Barrett's) metaplasia. Mod Pathol 17:1282–1288
121. Slack JM, Colleypriest BJ, Quinlan JM, Yu WY, Farrant MJ, Tosh D (2010) Barrett's metaplasia: molecular mechanisms and nutritional influences. Biochem Soc Trans 38:313–319
122. Stairs DB, Kong J, Lynch JP (2010) Cdx genes, inflammation, and the pathogenesis of intestinal metaplasia. Prog Mol Biol Transl Sci 96:231–270
123. Weimann A, Zimmermann M, Gross M, Slevogt H, Rieger A, Morawietz L (2010) CDX2 and LI-cadherin expression in esophageal mucosa: use of both markers can facilitate the histologic diagnosis of Barrett's esophagus and carcinoma. Int J Surg Pathol 18:330–337
124. Weimann A, Rieger A, Zimmermann M, Gross M, Hoffmann P, Slevogt H, Morawietz L (2010) Comparison of six immunohistochemical markers for the histologic diagnosis of neoplasia in Barrett's esophagus. Virchows Arch 457:537–545
125. Clarke CA, McConnell RB (1954) Six cases of carcinoma of the oesophagus occurring in one family. BMJ 2:1137–1138
126. Howel-Evans W, McConnell RB, Clarke CA, Sheppard PM (1958) Carcinoma of the oesophagus with keratosis palmaris et plantaris (tylosis). A study of two families. Q J Med 27:413–442
127. Lucker GPH, Van de Kerkhof PCM, Steijlen PM (1994) The hereditary palmoplantar keratoses: an updated review and classification. Br J Dermatol 131:1–14
128. Kelsell DP, Stevens HP (1999) The palmoplantar keratodermas: much more than palms and soles. Mol Med Today 36:107–113
129. Stevens HP, Kelsell DP, Bryant SP, Bishop DT, Spurr NK, Weissenbach J, Marger D, Marger RS, Leigh IM (1996) Linkage of an American pedigree with palmoplantar keratoderma and malignancy to 17q24: literature survey and proposed updated classification of the keratodermas. Arch Dermatol 132:640–651
130. Hennies HC, Hagedorn M, Reis A (1995) Palmoplantar keratoderma in association with carcinoma of the esophagus maps to chromosome 17q distal the keratin gene cluster. Genomics 29:537–540
131. Risk JM, Evans KE, Jones J, Langan JE, Rowbottom L, McRonald FE, Mills HS, Ellis A, Shaw JM, Leigh IM, Kelsell DP, Field JK (2002) Characterisation of a 500kb region on 17q25 and the exclusion of candidate genes as the familial tylosis oesophageal cancer (TOC) locus. Oncogene 21:6395–6402
132. Risk JM, Field EA, Field JK, Whittaker J, Fryer A, Ellis A, Shaw JM, Friedmann PS, Bishop DT, Bodmer J et al (1994) Tylosis oesophageal cancer mapped. Nat Genet 8:319–321
133. Kelsell DP, Risk JM, Leigh IM, Stevens HP, Ellis A, Hennies HC, Reis A, Weissenbach J, Bishop DT, Spurr NK, Field JK (1996) Close mapping of the focal non-epidermolytic palmoplantar keratoderma locus associated with oesophageal cancer. Hum Mol Genet 5:857–860
134. Langan JE, Cole CG, Huckle EJ, Byrne S, McRonald FE, Rowbottom L, Ellis A, Shaw JM, Leigh IM, Kelsell DP, Dunham I, Field JK, Risk JM (2004) Novel microsatellite markers and single nucleotide polymorphisms refine the tylosis with oesophageal cancer (TOC) minimal region on 17q25 to 42.5kb: sequencing does not identify causative gene. Hum Genet 114:534–540
135. Risk JM, Mills HS, Garde J, Dunn JR, Evans KE, Hollstein M, Field JK (1999) The tylosis oesophageal cancer (TOC) locus: more than just a familial cancer gene. Dis Esophagus 12:173–176
136. VonBrevern M, Hollstein MC, Risk JM, Garde J, Bennett WP, Harris CC, Muehlbauer KR, Field JK (1998) Loss of heterozygosity in sporadic oesophageal tumours in the tylosis oesophageal cancer (TOC) gene region of chromosome 17q. Oncogene 17:2101–2105
137. Iwaya T, Maesawa C, Kimura T, Ogasawara S, Ikeda K, Kimura Y, Noda Y, Ishida K, Sato N, Saito K, Masuda T (2005) Infrequent mutation of the human envoplakin gene is closely linked to the tylosis oesophageal cancer locus in sporadic oesophageal squamous cell carcinomas. Oncol Rep 13:703–707
138. Shahibi M, Noori Daloii MR, Langan JE et al (2004) An investigation of the tylosis with oesophageal cancer (TOC) locus in Iranian patients with oesophageal squamous cell carcinoma. Int J Oncol 25:389–395

139. Iwaya T, Maesawa C, Ogasawara S, Tamura G (1998) Tylosis esophageal cancer locus on chromosome 17q25.1 is commonly deleted in sporadic human esophageal cancer. Gastroenterology 114:1206–1210
140. McRonald FE, Liloglou T, Xinarianos G, Hill L, Rowbottom L, Langan JE, Ellis A, Shaw JM, Field JK, Risk JM (2006) Down-regulation of the cytoglobin gene, located on 17q25, in tylosis with oesophageal cancer (TOC): evidence for trans-allele repression. Hum Mol Genet 15:1271–1277
141. Bassett DR, Abel M, Moellering RC Jr, Rosenblatt G, Stokes J 3rd (1969) Dietary intake, smoking history, energy balance, and "stress" in relation to age, and to coronary heart disease risk in Hawaiian and Japanese men in Hawaii. Am J Clin Nutr 22:1504–1520
142. Coggon D, Osmond C, Barker DJ (1990) Stomach cancer and migration with England and Wales. Br J Cancer 61:573–574
143. International Agency for Research on Cancer (1994) IARC monograph on the evaluation of carcinogenic risks to humans. In: Schistosomes, liver flukes and *Helicobacter pylori*, vol 61. International Agency for Research on Cancer, Lyon
144. Danesh J (1999) *Helicobacter pylori* infection and gastric cancer: systematic review of the epidemiological studies. Aliment Pharmacol Ther 13:851–856
145. Eslick GD, Lim LL, Byles JE, Xia HH, Talley NJ (1999) Association of *Helicobacter pylori* infection with gastric carcinoma: a meta-analysis. Am J Gastroenterol 94:2373–2379
146. Fukase K, Kato M, Kikuchi S, Inoue K, Uemura N, Okamoto S, Terao S, Amagai K, Hayashi S, Asaka M (2008) Effect of eradication of *Helicobacter pylori* on incidence of metachronous gastric carcinoma after endoscopic resection of early gastric cancer: an open-label, randomised controlled trial. Lancet 372:392–397
147. Wong BC, Lam SK, Wong WM, Chen JS, Zheng TT, Feng RE, Lai KC, Hu WH, Yuen ST, Leung SY, Fong DY, Ho J, Ching CK, Chen JS, China Gastric Cancer Study Group (2004) *Helicobacter pylori* eradication to prevent gastric cancer in a high-risk region of China: a randomized controlled trial. JAMA 291:187–194
148. Kandulski A, Selgrad M, Malfertheiner P (2008) *Helicobacter pylori* infection: a clinical overview. Dig Liver Dis 40:619–626
149. Peek RM Jr, Blaser MJ (2002) *Helicobacter pylori* and gastrointestinal tract adenocarcinomas. Nat Rev Cancer 2:28–37
150. Hamajima N, Naito M, Kondo T, Goto Y (2006) Genetic factors involved in the development of *Helicobacter pylori*-related gastric cancer. Cancer Sci 97:1129–1138
151. Bagchi D, Bhattacharya G, Stohs SJ (1996) Production of reactive oxygen species by gastric cells in association with *Helicobacter pylori*. Free Radic Res 24:439–450
152. Papa A, Danese S, Sgambato A, Ardito R, Zannoni G, Rinelli A, Vecchio FM, Gentiloni-Silveri N, Cittadini A, Gasbarrini G, Gasbarrini A (2002) Role of *Helicobacter pylori* CagA+infection in determining oxidative DNA damage in gastric mucosa. Scand J Gastroenterol 37:409–413
153. Farinati F, Cardin R, Russo VM, Busatto G, Franco M, Rugge M (2003) *Helicobacter pylori* CagA status, mucosal oxidative damage and gastritis phenotype: a potential pathway to cancer? Helicobacter 8:227–234
154. Shirin H, Pinto JT, Liu LU, Merzianu M, Sordillo EM, Moss SF (2001) *Helicobacter pylori* decreases gastric mucosal glutathione. Cancer Lett 164:127–133
155. Machado AM, Figueiredo C, Touati E, Máximo V, Sousa S, Michel V, Carneiro F, Nielsen FC, Seruca R, Rasmussen LJ (2009) *Helicobacter pylori* infection induces genetic instability of nuclear and mitochondrial DNA in gastric cells. Clin Cancer Res 15:2995–3002
156. Crew KD, Neugut AI (2006) Epidemiology of gastric cancer. World J Gastroenterol 12:354–362
157. Tatematsu M, Takahashi M, Fukushima S, Hananouchi M, Shirai T (1975) Effects in rats of sodium chloride on experimental gastric cancers induced by N-methyl-N-nitro-N-nitrosoguanidine or 4-nitroquinoline-1-oxide. J Natl Cancer Inst 55:101–106
158. Hirayama T (1986) A large scale cohort study on cancer risk by diet with special reference to the risk reducing effects of greenyellow vegetable consumption. In: Hayashi Y, Nagao M, Sugimura T (ed) Diet, nutrition and cancer: proceedings of the 16th international symposium of the princess Takamatsu cancer research fund, VNU Science, Utrecht/Tokyo, pp 41–53

159. Hertog MG, Bueno-de-Mesquita HB, Fehily AM, Sweetnam PM, Elwood PC, Kromhout D (1996) Fruit and vegetable consumption and cancer mortality in the Caerphilly study. Cancer Epidemiol Biomarkers Prev 5:673–677
160. Kobayashi M, Tsubono Y, Sasazuki S, Sasaki S, Tsugane S (2002) Vegetables, fruit and risk of gastric cancer in Japan: a 10-year follow-up of the JPHC study cohort I. Int J Cancer 102:39–44
161. Wang ZY, Cheng SJ, Zhou ZC, Athar M, Khan WA, Bickers DR, Mukhtar H (1989) Antimutagenic activity of green tea polyphenols. Mutat Res 223:273–285
162. Wang ZY, Hong JY, Huang MT, Reuhl KR, Conney AH, Yang CS (1992) Inhibition of N-nitrosodiethylamine- and 4-(methylnitrosamino)-1-(3-pyridyl)-1-butanone-induced tumorigenesis in A/J mice by green tea and black tea. Cancer Res 52:1943–1947
163. Xu Y, Ho CT, Amin SG, Han C, Chung FL (1992) Inhibition of tobacco-specific nitrosamine-induced lung tumorigenesis in A/J mice by green tea and its major polyphenol as antioxidants. Cancer Res 52:3875–3879
164. Boehm K, Borrelli F, Ernst E, Habacher G, Hung SK, Milazzo S, Horneber M (2009) Green tea (*Camellia sinensis*) for the prevention of cancer. Cochrane Database Syst Rev 3:CD005004. doi:10.1002/14651858.RevCD005004.pub2
165. Sjödahl K, Lu Y, Nilsen TI, Ye W, Hveem K, Vatten L, Lagergren J (2007) Smoking and alcohol drinking in relation to risk of gastric cancer: a population-based, prospective cohort study. Int J Cancer 120:128–132
166. Chao A, Thun MJ, Henley SJ, Jacobs EJ, McCullough ML, Calle EE (2002) Cigarette smoking, use of other tobacco products and stomach cancer mortality in US adults: the cancer prevention study II. Int J Cancer 101:380–389
167. Lagergren J, Bergstrom R, Nyren O (1999) Association between body mass and adenocarcinoma of the esophagus and gastric cardia. Ann Intern Med 130:883–890
168. Ekstrom AM, Serafini M, Nyren O, Hansson LE, Ye W, Wolk A (2000) Dietary antioxidant intake and the risk of cardia cancer and noncardia cancer of the intestinal and diffuse types: a population-basedcase-control study in Sweden. Int J Cancer 87:133–140
169. Pharoah PD, Guilford P, Caldas C (2001) International gastric cancer linkage consortium. Incidence of gastric cancer and breast cancer in CDH1 E-cadherin. Mutation carriers from hereditary diffuse gastric cancer families. Gastroenterology 121:1348–1353
170. Matsukuma KE, Mullins FM, Dietz L, Zehnder JL, Ford JM, Chun NM, Schrijver I (2001) Hereditary diffuse gastric cancer due to a previously undescribed CDH1 splice site mutation. Hum Pathol 41:1200–1203
171. Jones EG (1964) Familial gastric cancer. N Z Med J 63:287–296
172. Guilford P, Hopkins J, Harraway J, McLeod M, McLeod N, Harawira P, Taite H, Scoular R, Miller A, Reeve AE (1998) E-cadherin germline mutations in familial gastric cancer. Nature 392:402–405
173. Gayther SA, Gorringe KL, Ramus SJ, Huntsman D, Roviello F, Grehan N, Machado JC, Pinto E, Seruca R, Halling K, MacLeod P, Powell SM, Jackson CE, Ponder BA, Caldas C (1998) Identification of germ-line E-cadherin mutations in gastric cancer families of European origin. Cancer Res 58:4086–4089
174. Richards FM, McKee SA, Rajpar MH, Cole TR, Evans DG, Jankowski JA, McKeown C, Sanders DS, Maher ER (1999) Germline E-cadherin gene (CDH1) mutations predispose to familial gastric cancer and colorectal cancer. Hum Mol Genet 8:607–610
175. Kaurah P, MacMillan A, Boyd N, Senz J, De Luca A, Chun N, Suriano G, Zaor S, Van Manen L, Gilpin C, Nikkel S, Connolly-Wilson M, Weissman S, Rubinstein WS, Sebold C, Greenstein R, Stroop J, Yim D, Panzini B, McKinnon W, Greenblatt M, Wirtzfeld D, Fontaine D, Coit D, Yoon S, Chung D, Lauwers G, Pizzuti A, Vaccaro C, Redal MA, Oliveira C, Tischkowitz M, Olschwang S, Gallinger S, Lynch H, Green J, Ford J, Pharoah P, Fernandez B, Huntsman D (2007) Founder and recurrent CDH1 mutations in families with hereditary diffuse gastric cancer. JAMA 297:2360–2372
176. Lugli A, Zlobec I, Singer G, Kopp Lugli A, Terracciano LM, Genta RM (2007) Napoleon Bonaparte's gastric cancer: a clinicopathologic approach to staging, pathogenesis, and etiology. Nat Clin Pract Gastroenterol Hepatol 4:52–57

177. Caldas C, Carneiro F, Lynch HT, Yokota J, Wiesner GL, Powell SM, Lewis FR, Huntsman DG, Pharoah PD, Jankowski JA, MacLeod P, Vogelsang H, Keller G, Park KG, Richards FM, Maher ER, Gayther SA, Oliveira C, Grehan N, Wight D, Seruca R, Roviello F, Ponder BA, Jackson CE (1999) Familial gastric cancer: overview and guidelines for management. J Med Genet 36:873–880
178. Suriano G, Yew S, Ferreira P, Senz J, Kaurah P, Ford JM, Longacre TA, Norton JA, Chun N, Young S, Oliveira MJ, Macgillivray B, Rao A, Sears D, Jackson CE, Boyd J, Yee C, Deters C, Pai GS, Hammond LS, McGivern BJ, Medgyesy D, Sartz D, Arun B, Oelschlager BK, Upton MP, Neufeld-Kaiser W, Silva OE, Donenberg TR, Kooby DA, Sharma S, Jonsson BA, Gronberg H, Gallinger S, Seruca R, Lynch H, Huntsman DG (2005) Characterization of a recurrent germ line mutation of the E-cadherin gene: implications for genetic testing and clinical management. Clin Cancer Res 11:5401–5409
179. Joensuu H (2006) Gastrointestinal stromal tumor (GIST). Ann Oncol 17:280–286
180. West RB, Corless CL, Chen X, Rubin BP, Subramanian S (2004) The novel marker, DOG1, is expressed ubiquitously in gastrointestinal stromal tumors irrespective of KIT or PDGFRA mutation status. Am J Pathol 165:107–113
181. Kim KM, Kang DW, Moon WS, Park JB, Park CK, Sohn JH, Jeong JS, Cho MY, Jin SY, Choi JS, Kang DY, Gastrointestinal Stromal Tumor Committee, The Korean Gastrointestinal Pathology Study Group (2005) Gastrointestinal stromal tumors in Koreans: incidence and the clinical, pathologic and immunohistochemical findings. J Korean Med Sci 20:977–984
182. Tryggvason G, Gislason HG, Magnusson MK, Jónasson JG (2005) Gastrointestinal stromal tumors in Iceland, 1990–2003: the Icelandic GIST study, a population-based incidence and pathologic risk stratification study. Int J Cancer 117:289–293
183. Goettsch WG, Bos SD, Breekveldt-Postma N, Casparie M, Herings RM, Hogendoorn PC (2005) Incidence of gastrointestinal stromal tumours is underestimated: results of a nation-wide study. Eur J Cancer 41:2868–2872
184. Agaram NP, Besmer P, Wong CC, Tianhua G, Socci ND, Maki RG, De Santis D, Brennan MF, Singer S, De Matteo RP, Antonescu CR (2007) Pathologic and molecular heterogeneity in imatinib-stable or imatinib-responsive gastrointestinal stromal tumors. Clin Cancer Res 13:170–181
185. Kim TW, Lee H, Kang YK, Choe MS, Ryu MH, Chang HM, Kim JS, Yook JH, Kim BS, Lee JS (2004) Prognostic significance of c-kit mutation in localized gastrointestinal stromal tumors. Clin Cancer Res 10:3076–3081
186. Heinrich MC, Maki RG, Corless CL, Antonescu CR, Harlow A, Griffith D, Town A, McKinley A, Ou WB, Fletcher JA, Fletcher CD, Huang X, Cohen DP, Baum CM, Demetri GD (2008) Primary and secondary kinase genotypes correlate with the biological and clinical activity of sunitinib in imatinib-resistant gastrointestinal stromal tumor. J Clin Oncol 26:5352–5359
187. Wordsworth S, Papanicolas I, Buchanan J, Frayling I, Taylor J, Tomlinson I (2008) Molecular testing for somatic cancer mutations: a survey of current and future testing in UK laboratories. J Clin Pathol 61:373–376
188. Kontogianni-Katsarou K, Dimitriadis E, Lariou C, Kairi-Vassilatou E, Pandis N, Kondi-Paphiti A (2008) KIT exon 11 codon 557/558 deletion/insertion mutations define a subset of gastrointestinal stromal tumors with malignant potential. World J Gastroenterol 14:1891–1897

Chapter 7
Molecular-Genetic Testing in Hepatocellular Carcinoma and Its Premalignant Conditions

Rodney E. Shackelford, Greg Mayhall, Shankar Japa, Aejaz Nasir, Mokenge Malafa, and Domenico Coppola

Contents

R.E. Shackelford, DO, Ph.D. • G. Mayhall, M.D. • S. Japa, Ph.D.
Department of Pathology and Laboratory Medicine, Tulane University School of Medicine, 1430 Tulane Avenue, SL-79, New Orleans, LA 70112, USA

A. Nasir
Diagnostic & Experimental Pathology & Tailored Therapeutics Program, Eli Lilly & Company, Indianapolis, IN, USA

M. Malafa
Department of Surgical Oncology, H. Lee Moffitt Cancer Center & Research Institute, 12902 Magnolia Drive, Tampa, FL 33612, USA

Department of Oncological Sciences, University of South Florida College of Medicine, Tampa, FL, USA

D. Coppola, M.D. (✉)
Department of Pathology, H. Lee Moffitt Cancer Center & Research Institute, 12902 Magnolia Drive, Tampa, FL 33612, USA

Department of Oncological Sciences, University of South Florida College of Medicine, Tampa, FL, USA
e-mail: Domenico.Coppola@moffitt.org

D. Coppola (ed.), *Molecular Pathology and Diagnostics of Cancer*, Cancer Growth and Progression 16, DOI 10.1007/978-94-007-7192-5_7,

Abstract Hepatocellular carcinoma (HCC) is the fifth most common malignancy worldwide and the third most common cause of malignancy-associated death. Presently there are relatively few molecular genetic testing directly performed on HCC. However, many molecular genetic tests are performed on conditions that increase the risk for HCC or modify drug treatments for conditions that increase HCC risk, including hepatitis B and C, hemochromatosis, and interleukin-28b testing. Here we review the common molecular diagnostic genetic tests associated with HCC diagnosis and treatment.

Keywords Hepatocellular carcinoma (HCC) • Hepatitis B (HBV) • Hepatitis C (HCV) • Hemochromatosis • Interleukin-28b • p53 • MicroRNA

7.1 Introduction

Hepatocellular carcinoma (HCC) is the fifth most common neoplasm worldwide and the third most common cause of malignancy-associated death. In 2008 more than 70,000 cases of HCC where diagnosed worldwide, with ~85 % occurring in the developing countries. The greatest incidence is seen in Eastern Asia and parts of sub-Saharan Africa. HCC has a high fatality rate, as only a minority of afflicted individuals are candidates for potentially curative treatments such as liver transplantation, resection, or complete ablation, making the overall mortality to incidence ratio an abysmal 0.93. The vast majority (70–90 %) of HHCs arise in a background of established chronic liver disease, especially cirrhosis and hepatic steatosis [1, 2].

7.2 Environmental Protective and HCC

The worldwide HCC incidence reflects regional differences in chronic liver disease risk factors, particularly to those causing cirrhosis. In Eastern Asian and sub-Saharan Africa where 80 % of HCCs occur, the main risk factor is chronic hepatitis B (HBV) infection, often combined with other risk factors, such as alcohol and aflatoxin B1 exposure. In Japan, Europe, and North America, the main risk factor is chronic hepatitis C (HCV) infection, often combined with alcohol abuse. Epidemiologically, the HCC incidence has developed in parallel with the spread of HCV in Japan, Europe, and North America. Once HCV induces cirrhosis, the HCC risk is high, with 3–5 % of affected individuals developing HCC/year [1–4]. Not surprisingly, the HCC risk increases with the increased hepatitis viral load and with the duration of infection, and it is likely decreased by anti-HBV vaccination programs and by the effective use of antiviral agents [5–7]. Co-infection with HIV and HBV or HCV causes a more rapid progression to liver disease and an increased risk for HCC once cirrhosis has developed [8].

Other risk factors for HCC include iron overload, either from dietary sources and the genetic disease hereditary hemochromatosis (HH) [9–11]. The mechanisms by which excess iron leads to hepatocarcinogenesis likely involves redox-active labile iron causing the formation of toxic reactive oxygen species via Fenton and Haber-Weiss chemistries, leading to chronic oxidative stress with concomitant lipid peroxide formation, DNA damage, mutagenesis, and eventual hepatocarcinogenesis [9, 10, 12]. A well-known example of dietary iron overload is seen in Southern and Central Africa where large volumes of traditional beer are consumed that has been fermented in cast iron containers. Under the acidic fermentation conditions ionized, highly bioavailable iron leaches from the fermentation vessel. High iron levels accumulate in the hepatocytes, causing portal fibrosis and eventual HCC. For individuals with the highest hepatic iron levels, the relative risk for HCC is 23.5 [9, 13]. Not surprisingly, hepatic iron overload, combined with either chronic HBV or aflatoxin B1 exposure increases an individual's HCC risk [9]. Smoking, heavy alcohol use, and diabetes are also risk factors for HCC, especially when they are combined with concurrent HBV or HCV infections [14, 15]. Interestingly, coffee consumption lowers HCC risk [16]. Less common environmental risk factors for liver cancer includes vinyl chloride exposure that can cause hepatic angiosarcoma and liver flukes, which can increase the risk for development of cholangiosarcoma [17].

7.3 Genetic Factors for HCC Risk

Multiple genetic factors can increase HCC risk, including HH, single nucleotide polymorphisms (SNPs) that modify HBV and HCV related HCC risk, family history, and epidermal growth factor polymorphisms. Many of these genetic factors interact with and modify environmental risk factors, especially those associated with viral hepatitis (see below).

Individuals with HH have an increased HCC risk, with early studies showing up to a 200-fold increased risk, prior to the use of repeated phlebotomy treatment to lower overall iron load [9, 10, 18–20]. HH is caused by multiple mutations in five different genes, with HFE mutation at 6p21.3 being the most common in Northern European populations [10]. Most HH results from decreased hepcidin synthesis, resulting in increased enteric iron import via ferroportin activity [10]. Given time, iron accumulates causing complications such as fatigue, diabetes mellitus, cardiac arrhythmias, heart failure, hypothyroidism, cirrhosis, and HCC [9–11, 18, 21]. Most data indicates that HCC arises in individuals with HH who have hepatic cirrhosis due to iron overload, as individuals with HH in whom cirrhosis is prevented by repeated phlebotomy have the same long-term survival as individuals without HH [10, 17, 21, 22].

Host genetic factors can also modify environmental risk factors for HCC. For example, genome-wide association studies have indicated that SNPs at 1p36.22 and 8p12 promote HBV-associated HCC [23, 24]. Similar studies have shown that six different SNPs effecting T-cell receptor activity, immune surveillance, and genes associated with antigen presentation and processing correlated strongly with the risk for HBV or HCV-induced HCC versus liver cirrhosis [25]. One SNP (an $A \rightarrow G$ transition) at 61 in the 5′ untranslated region of the epidermal growth factor gene causes a fourfold increased HCC risk, following adjustment for age, sex, race, etiology, and severity of cirrhosis [26]. Lastly, a family history of a first-degree relative with HCC confers a roughly fourfold greater risk for developing HCC, independently of having viral hepatitis [27]. Undoubtedly, the genetic risk for HCC is polygenetic and many more genetic variations will be found that modify individual HCC risk.

7.4 Hepatocarcinogenesis

Hepatocarcinogenesis is a complex, multistage event that usually progresses from chronic viral hepatitis/chronic liver disease, to cirrhosis, low- and high-grade dysplastic nodule formation, low-grade HCC, and advanced HCC (Fig. 7.1, [28]). While most of these stages are histologically well defined, several can be diagnostically difficult, such as the discrimination between a high-grade dysplastic nodule and low-grade HCC, although in some cases stromal invasion can help in differentiating the two conditions [29]. Recent molecular studies have identified gene expression patterns associated with HCC development, recurrence risk, and prognosis. For example, Hoshida et al. [30] employed genome- wide expression profiling to indentify 186 genes whose expression correlated with HCC recurrence risk and survival prognosis. Similarly, other studies employing serial analysis of gene expression (SAGE) and gene expression and methylation profiling have indentified

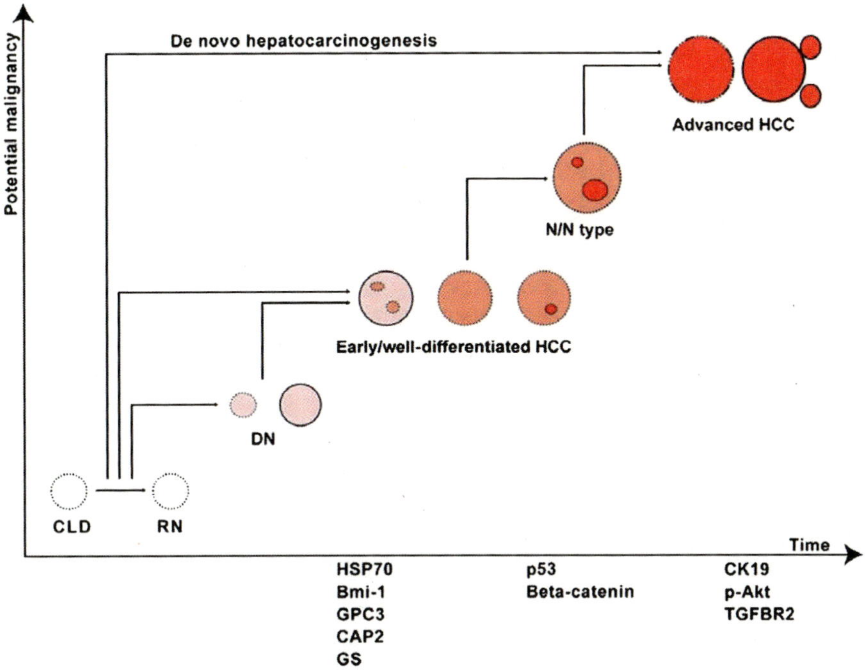

Fig. 7.1 HCC evolution and its related molecular and immunological markers. *CLD* chronic liver disease, *RN* regenerative nodule, *DN* dysplastic nodule, *N/N* nodule-in-nodule [28]

alterations in HCC gene expression and methylation patterns that correlate with hepatocarcinogenesis. Most of these genes are involved in cell proliferation and survival, biosynthesis, signal transduction, and cellular transport [31, 32]. Recently, several molecular signatures have been identified whose immunohistochemical expression correlates with early/well-differentiated HCC and advanced HCC (Fig. 7.1). Although most of these immunohistochemical markers are not completely specific for HCC, they can be useful adjunctive tools in histologically difficult cases. Here several are reviewed:

7.4.1 Heat Shock Protein 70 (HSP70)

HSP70 is a family of 70-kDa chaperone stress proteins that assists in a wide range of protein folding processes, including the folding and assembly of newly synthesized proteins, refolding of misfolded, denatured, or aggregated proteins, and the membranous translocation of proteins [33]. HSP70 is a potent antiapoptotic cellular survival factor, whose overexpression promotes cell cycle progression, and plays a role in tumorigenesis, with high expression levels associated with adverse outcomes in endometrial, colorectal, breast, prostate cancers and some leukemias [34–39]. Chuma et al. [40] analyzed the expression of ~12,600 genes in seven nodular HCCs and seven corresponding noncancerous hepatic tissue. HSP70 was overexpressed in early HCC compared to most high-grade dysplastic nodules, and was further increased in high-grade HCC. Interestingly, non-malignant/benign nodules, focal nodular hyperplasia, and hepatocellular adenomas showed low HSP70 expression [40, 41]. HSP70 expression is not entirely specific for HCC, as ~5 % of high-grade dysplastic nodules overexpress this protein [41].

7.4.2 Bmi-1

Bmi-1 is identified as a stem cell gene based on the observation that Bmi-1 deficiency compromises adult stem cell function [42]. Bmi-1 encodes a 37 kDa member of the Polycomb gene group which imparts stem cell features to malignant cells, including the induction of telomerase activity and the negative regulation of the p16 and p19 tumor suppressor genes [43, 44]. Bmi-1 overexpression correlates with therapy failure in many different human malignancies [45–47]. Interestingly, down regulation of BMi-1 results in apoptosis and senescence, and in increased cellular sensitivity to cytotoxic agents [48]. Bmi-1 expression is increased in early and well-differentiated HCC usually appearing as small dots within the nucleus. In one study 65 % of well differentiated, 45 % of moderately differentiated, and 50 % of poorly differentiated HCCs expressed Bmi-1 [49].

7.4.3 Glutamine Synthetase (GS)

GS is found predominantly in the brain, kidneys, and liver, where plays a central role in nitrogen metabolism by catalyzing the condensation of ammonia and glutamate to glutamine [50]. Interestingly, glutamine is known to act as an energy source for tumor cells [51]. In normal liver GS expression is found in the hepatocytes surrounding the terminal hepatic venules, while in HCC there is diffuse and extensive accumulation of GS in the malignant hepatocytes [52]. One study demonstrated increased GS expression in 14 % of high-grade dysplastic hepatic nodules as compared to 59 % of well-differentiated HCCs, and 86 % of moderately to poorly differentiated HCCs [41]. GC overexpression is associated with β-catenin mutations or activation of the β-catenin pathway [53, 54]. Interestingly, increasing GS expression appears to promote HCC progression and metastasis [55, 56]. GS is not entirely specific as increased expression is seen in 14 % of high-grade dysplastic hepatic nodules and in the β-catenin-activated hepatocellular adenoma subtype [41, 57].

7.4.4 α-Fetoprotein (AFP)

AFP is a well established serum marker for HCC, with ~50 % of individuals with HCC showing elevated AFP and plasma levels above 400–500 ng/ml AFP being virtually diagnostic of HCC [58]. Unfortunately APF levels are seldom elevated in early HCC and it has low sensitivity as a tissue marker, being expressed in only about 17–68 % of paraffin embedded HCC sections [58, 59]. In addition, AFP levels are usually not elevated in the fibrolamellar subtype of HCC.

7.4.5 Cyclase-Associated Protein 2 (CAP2)

CAP2 is a member of the cyclase-associated protein family and is involved in multicellular organism development, vesicle trafficking, and endocytosis, via regulating adenylyl cyclase [60, 61]. CAPS expression is increased with increasingly higher grades of HCC [62].

7.4.6 Glypican-3 (GPC3)

GPC3 is a cell-surface heperan sulfate proteoglycan normally expressed in fetal liver and placenta, but not in normal adult liver. Recently, GPC3 has been established as a serum and tissue maker for HCC. One recent study demonstrated GPC3 immunoreactivity in 69 % of well differentiated and 81 % of moderately to poorly differentiated HCCs. Only 9 % of high-grade dysplastic nodules and no low-grade nodules were positive [41]. GPC3 immunoreactivity shows 77 % sensitivity and 96 % specificity for small HHC, demonstrating that positivity for this immunostain can support the diagnosis of HCC. GPC3 typically shows a cytoplasmic staining pattern, although canicular or membranous patterns are also seen [41, 63, 64]. GPC3 immunopositivity needs to be interpreted in the correct clinical and histological context, as benign liver lesions with active inflammation and regeneration, and melanocytic lesions can also be GPC3 immunopositive [65, 66].

7.4.7 Immunostain Combinations for HCC

Like for immunohistochemical procedures, various immunostain combinations give better result in the diagnosis of HCC then a single stain. The combination of GPC3, HSP70, and GS allowed 72 % sensitivity and 100 % specificity in well differentiated HCC detection when two immunostains were positive. GPC3 and HSP70 alone gave a 59 % sensitivity and 100 % specificity for well-differentiated HCC. These results are significantly better than those achieved with any single immunostain [41].

7.5 Molecular-Genetic Testing for HCC

Currently, there are relatively few molecular-genetic tests routinely performed for HCC. Presently the Association for Molecular Pathology Solid Tumors Test Directory lists p53 mutational analysis for HCC, offered by two labs and no other tests [67]. However, there are several important molecular tests related to HCC risk and several areas of molecular pathology research that are likely to lead to new molecular diagnostic tests for HCC.

7.6 Hereditary Hemochromatosis

HH is one of the most common genetic diseases, affecting about one in 200–300, with Northern Europeans showing the highest known incidence. HH increased an affected individuals HCC risk, with different HH types often conferring a different risk. Presently there are five different known molecular causes of HH. Since untreated HH can result in cirrhosis and HCC, and can be inherited, molecular testing for HH followed by correct clinical care is necessary [10]. Presently, molecular diagnostic tests are available and routinely preformed in many labs, with HFE gene mutation being the most common.

7.6.1 Indications for HH Testing

The initial diagnosis of HH can be difficult due to the protean manifestations of HH. The symptoms of HH can include heart failure/cardiac arrhythmias, cirrhosis, diabetes, arthritis, joint pain, skin bronzing, fatigue, hypogonadism, hypothyroidism, and HCC [9–11]. It is important to identify individuals with HH as early as possible. While some manifestations of HH can be reversed by therapeutic phlebotomy, such as the liver and skin manifestations, other complications, such as hypogonadism, arthropathy, and diabetes, are irreversible once they have occurred [68]. Should an individual have a family history of HH, molecular testing is warranted to avoid missing HH in its earliest and most treatable form [10, 68]. Evaluation of iron overload should first consider non-genetic causes, many of which are more common than HH.

Iron overload can be measured by several tests, including total iron binding capacity, transferrin saturation, liver biopsy, and serum ferritin (SF). Initial testing is often performed by serum ferritin analysis, which is highly sensitive for iron overload, showing hyperferritinemia. Care must be taken in interpreting the test result, as SF is an acute phase reactant and hyperferritinemia also occurs in inflammatory processes, diabetes, chronic alcohol use, and liver damage [10]. Testing should be performed to exclude other disease processes. Santos et al. [69] proposed the following four-step strategy:

1. *Rule out other causes of hyperferritinemia.* Taking a personal and family history, performing a clinical exam, and performing tests such as iron parameters,

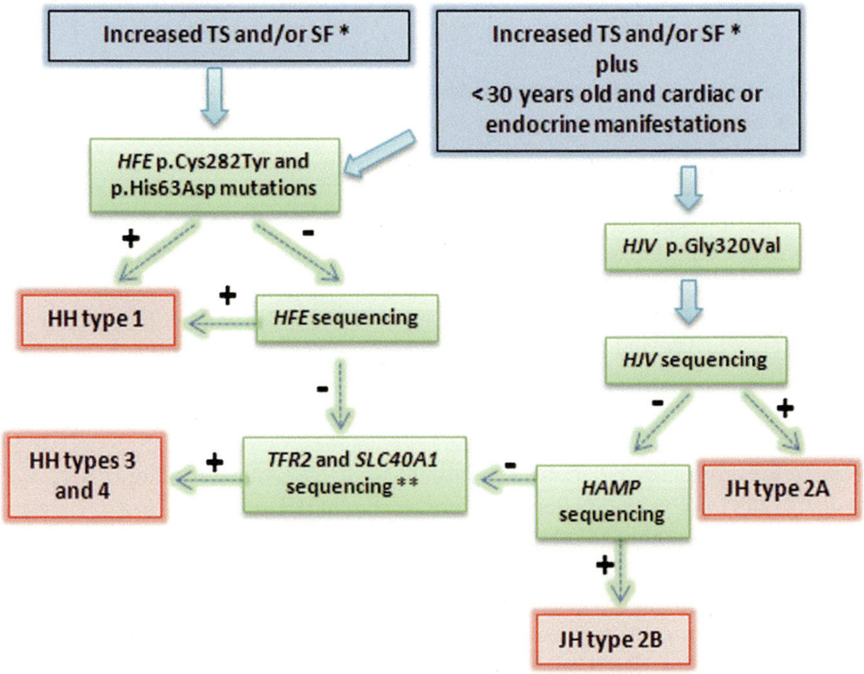

Fig. 7.2 Representation of diagnostic strategy for patients suspected HH. Recommendations report TS > 45 %, SF > 200 μg/L in females and >300 μg/L in males; or in advanced stages: TS > 50 % in females and TS > 60 % in males, in the absence of secondary causes. Some patients with primary iron overload may not present mutation during this genetic approach. Very rare mutations in other genes can be involved. *TS* transferrin saturation, *SF* serum ferritin, *JH* juveline hemochromatosis. + means positive result, and – means negative result; lane 7, heterozygous for C282Y, wild-type for H63D; lane 8, wild-type for both C282Y and H63D [10]

C-reactive protein, hemoglobin, and alanine aminotransferase and aspartate aminotransferase will usually give a diagnosis of acquired hyperferritinemia and avoid unnecessary molecular testing.

2. *Confirm iron overload.* Since SF levels can vary throughout the day, repeating SF can be useful. Along with other iron studies and diagnosis of iron overload can be rendered. Possible causes of iron overload include excessive iron supplementation (oral, parenteral, or transfusions), chronic liver disease (alcoholic, viral or metabolic), end stage liver disease, chronic anemia (thalassemia major, myelodysplastic syndrome, sideroblastic anemia, chronic hemolysis), and porphyria cutanea tarda.
3. *Assess hepatic iron stores.* This can be done via liver biopsy or magnetic resonance imaging. Hepatic iron store analysis may be necessary where other iron studies fail to give definitive results.
4. *Perform molecular genetic testing for HH.* While mutations of the HH gene are most common, other genetic causes of HH must also be considered. An algorithm for molecular genetic testing protocols is given in Fig. 7.2.

7.6.2 *HFE Testing*

The gene encoding *HFE* is located at 6p21.3 and encodes a seven exon, six protein domains, 47.5 kDa protein similar in structure to the major histocompatibility class I-like proteins. The exoms encode an initial signal sequence, three extracellular domains, a transmembrane region and a short cytoplasmic tail, forming a 4.2 kb long transcript. The seventh exon does not appear to be expressed [70]. HFE is mainly expressed in the liver, duodenum, small intestine, spleen, and heart. Several alternatively spliced variants are expressed at low levels in many human tissues [70–76]. Most cases of HH are caused by two single nucleotide polymorphisms (SNP), Cys282Tyr and His63Asp, making the inheritance autosomal recessive. Some 20 other less common HFE mutations are linked to HH, which contribute to the phenotypic heterogeneity of the disease. Most commonly, individuals with HH are homozygous for Cys282Tyr, or heterozygous for Cys282Tyr/His63Asp [10]. In Northern European populations, roughly 90 % of *HFE* mutations are Cys282Tyr, with Cys282Tyr/Cys282Tyr being the most common HH genotype. Homozygousity for His63Asp does not cause HH, but this SNP contributes to increased hepatic iron levels when the Cys282Tyr SNP is also present [76]. *HFE* mutation causes excess iron accumulation via reducing the amount of hepcidin levels, resulting in increase ferroportin activity and increased enteric iron import [77].

HFE testing for HH is performed employing a variety of different molecular tests. Usually the testing modalities include a combination of PCR amplification, restriction enzyme digest, allele- specific PCR, heteroduplex analysis, sequencing, and single-strand conformation polymorphism testing. Here a few of these techniques are reviewed.

7.6.2.1 Mutliplex PCR with Restriction Endonuclease Digestion

Stott et al. [78] employed a combination of mutliplex PCR with primer mismatches, followed by restriction endonuclease digestion to identify the Cys282Tyr and His63Asp mutations in peripheral blood samples. Five milliliter of blood was taken via venipuncture and the DNA was extracted. The DNA was then PCR amplified with the primers depicted in Fig. 7.3a. Note that the Cys282Tyr and His63Asp each had a different set of mismatched primers that introduced a *Bbr*PI restriction site into the wild type, but not in either mutant amplicon. The amplification was carried out under standard conditions with a 2 min denaturation at 96 °C, followed by an initial annealing step of 30 s at 55 °C, with 30 cycles each of 30 s at 72 °C, 30 s at 94 °C, and 15 s at 55 °C. A final extension period of 10 min at 72 °C completed the PCR.

The entire PCR reactions were then subjected to *Bbr*PI restriction digestion for 4 h using five Units of enzyme. The restriction fragments were separated by gel electrophoresis using 3 % Nusieve:Agarose (3:1) gels for 50–60 min at 100 V. Products were visualized by staining in 1 mg/L ethidium bromide followed by transillumination at 302 nm. Each possible combination of the two SNPs and wild type sequence are represented in Fig. 7.3b. Each combination gave a specific and reproducible pattern that allowed identification of the two common *HFE* SNPs.

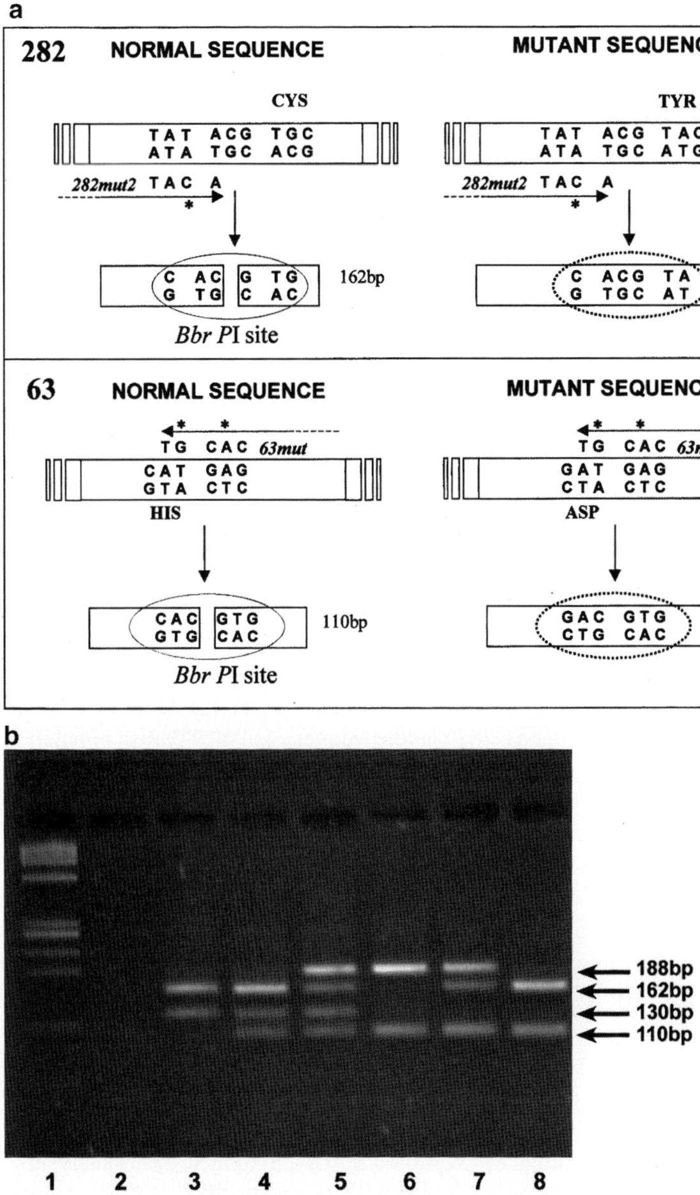

Fig. 7.3 (**a**) Schematic outline of PCR and restriction digestion used to determine the presence of HFE gene mutations and detection of both hemochromatosis mutations, C282Y and H63D, by PCR and restriction digestion (**b**). The site of mutation and primer mismatches are shown for the 282 locus (*top*) and for the 63 locus (*bottom*). (**b**) Restriction fragments were separated on 3 % Nusieve:Agarose. Results representative of all six possible genotypes are shown. Lane 1, PHI-X174-HaeIII molecular mass marker; lane 2, negative control; lane 3, wild-type for C282Y, homozygous for H63D; lane 4, wild-type for C282Y, heterozygous for H63D; lane 5, heterozygous for C282Y, heterozygous for H63D (compound heterozygote); lane 6, homozygous for C282Y, wild-type for H63D [79]

7.6.2.2 Allele-Specific PCR (ARMS)

ARMS takes advantage of the 10^{-3} to 10^{-6} lower amplification efficiency of the *Taq* DNA polymerase initiating from mismatched template-primer 3′-termini [79]. Through the use of primers specific for either a wild type or SNP sequence, it is possible to design primers that will preferentially amplify the sequence they share 100 % homology with [80]. In some systems ARMS technology can detect one mutant allele in a background of 104 wild-type alleles [81]. Sánchez et al. [81] used ARMS to analyze the blood of 5,370 Spanish blood donors for the Cys282Tyr and His63Asp *HFE* mutations. DNA was isolated via cell lysis, high-speed centrifugation, multiple washing steps, and protein removal by proteinase K digestion [82, 83]. The DNA was subjected to PCR amplification with the following probes:

Cys282Tyr	His63Asp
C282Y-R1: CCACTGATGACTCCAATGACTA	63Fw: AGCTGT TCGTGTTCTATGATC
C282Y-Rm: CCTGGGTGCTCCACCTGGT	HFE187Gas: CTCCACACGGCGACTCTCATC
C282Y-Fw: GGGAAGAGCAGAGATATACGTG	HFEEx2U: GCTCCCCTCCTACTACACAT
C282Y-F: TGGCAAGGGTAAACAGATCC	HFEEx2L: GGTCCCTATTTCCACCATCC

The allele-specific PCR was preformed under standard conditions for 35 cycles and the resulting amplicons were analyzed. Of the 5,370 blood samples analyzed, 8 C282Y homozygotes (0.15 %) and 74 compound C282Y/H63D heterozygotes (1.38 %) were identified, giving a C282Y allele frequency in the Spanish population of 3.16+/−0.46 %, or 1 homozygote in every 1,004 individuals. The H63D homozygote frequency was 20.8 %, or 1 in every 23 individuals. The allelic frequencies were not significantly different between men and women. To confirm that the above assay worked, the researchers employed the assay by Stott et al. [78] and found a 100 % results concordance. Four of the 8 C282Y homozygotes, all men, had high serum ferritin and transferring iron saturation, while only 1 of the 74 C282Y/H63D heterozygotes had the same serum results, demonstrating that the compound heterozygotes were less likely to develop HH.

7.6.2.3 DNA Sequencing

AHH is characterized by a number of common SNPs and in most cases analysis of these SNPs by techniques, such as ARMS, will locate specific *HFE* gene mutations. However, since HH can be caused by loss of *HFE* expression, resulting in increased ferroportin activity [10], other less common mutations that result in the loss of *HFE* protein expression can also cause HH. Sequencing is the ideal technique to locate these HFE gene variants, as it gives the specific nucleotide type at each point interrogated by the molecular assay. Cukjati et al. [83] analyzed a 47-year-old man, with no family history of HH, who had repeated high serum iron levels without any history of chronic anemia, infectious liver disease, alcohol abuse, or oral or parenteral iron administration. The patient's blood and the blood from 22 Slovenian patients with HH was collected and the DNA was extracted using a QIamp DNA Blood Mini Isolation Kit. RT-PCR analysis for the common HFE mutations (C282Y, H63D, and S65C) was performed on these blood samples. Of the 22 Slovenian patients with HH, four did not carry any of the common *HFE* gene SNPs tested for above. Additionally, the patient and his son were negative for all three common *HFE* gene SNPs.

To further analyze this set of patients, exons 1→6 with PCR amplified and subjected to Sanger sequencing using an ABI PRISM Big Dye Terminator Cycle Sequencing Ready Reaction Kit (Applied Biosystems) and analyzed on an ABI PRISM 310 Gene Analyzer. In three patients with HH, no mutations were identified by this analysis method, while the 47-year-old had a frameshift homozygous mutation of the A nucleotide in exon 3, at position 471 (c.471del, p.A158fs), which resulted in a prematurely truncated protein. The patient was also homozygous at both HLA-A and HLA-B, suggesting that loss of heterozygosity might have occurred during mitotic recombination. While rare, unusual *HFE* gene mutations require testing by sequencing or other molecular techniques capable of interrogating every nucleotide within the DNA sequence being analyzed. Although not performed often, HFE gene mutations have also been analyzed by DNA pyrosequencing with good results [84].

7.6.2.4 Genotyping HFE Gene Mutations by Melting Point Analysis

DNA melting point analysis typically involves PCR amplification followed by allele-specific fluorescent probe melting profile analysis. This technique is commonly employed to locate changes in nucleic acid sequences, although by itself it does identify specific nucleotide changes. It has the advantage of allowing melting analysis to be performed on the closed PCR reaction without the need of opening the reaction tube once amplicon amplification is complete. This significantly lowers the chances of sample contamination.

Bach et al. [85] used this technique to analyze genomic DNA from over 3,500 donor samples to look for the presence of the C282Y (845G>A), H63D (187C>G), and S65C (193A>T) *HFE* gene mutations. The mutations were amplified with the following primers:

C282Y	H63D and S65C
F5′-TGGCAAGGGTAAACAGATCC-3′	F5′-GCTCTGTCTCCAGGTTCACACTC-3′
R5′-CTCAGGCACTCCTCTCAACC-3′	R5′-CCCTCTCCACATACCCTTGC-3′

The amplification was performed as follows: denaturation 1 cycle 95 °C 10 min, followed by 45 cycles of 95 °C 10 s, 55 °C 10 s, and 72 °C 10 s, with a temperature transition rate of 20 °C/s. The melting curve was performed at 95 °C for 5 s and 45 °C for 15 s with a temperature transition rate of 20 °C/s ramping to 85 °C at 0.1 °C/s. The C282Y/845A>T transition was measured with a 3′-fluorescein-labeled sensor (5′-GAG ATA TAC GTG CCA GGT GGA GCA C-3′) and a

5′-LC-Red640-labeled anchor probe (5′-AGG CCT GGA TCA GCC CCT CAT TGT-3′). The H63D/187C>G was monitored with a 5′-LC-Red705-labeled anchor (5′-CTG GTA TCC ACG TAG CCC AAA GCT TCA A-3′) and a 3′-fluorescein-labeled sensor (5′-GG CGA CTC TCA TGA TCA TAG AAC ACG AAC A-3′) probe. This second probe- anchor combination was also used to monitor the S65C/193A>T mutation as the SNP was located only six nucleotides away from the H63D/187C>G mutation. Abnormal melting curves were analyzed by Sanger sequencing on an ABI PRISM 310 Gene Analyzer. By this method two new *HFE* gene substitutions were identified and one melting curve typical of the C282Y/845A>T transition was actually G>A transition located two nucleotides away from the C282Y/845A>T transition, giving the same melting curve. The authors concluded that this analysis method works well, but in some cases results should be further analyzed by DNA sequencing or restriction endonuclease digest.

7.6.3 Juvenile Hemochromatosis (JH)

JH or Type 2 HH is a rare autosomal recessive disorder that leads to significant iron overload before the age of 30 and is characterized by cardiomyopathy, liver damage, endocrine dysfunction, hypogonadotrophic hypogonadism. JH typically has a rapidly progressive clinical course, making the rapid initiation of therapy vital for patient care and also allowing the clinical differentiation from HFE mutation-induced HH (see Fig. 7.2). Molecular analyses have demonstrated that two genes are mutated in JH; *HJV* and *HAMP*, leading to JH types 2A and 2B, respectively. The *HJV* gene consists of four exons, encoding the hemojuvelin protein Individuals with *HJV* gene mutations and *HJV* knockout mice have low hepcidin, suggesting that hemojuvelin is involved in regulating hepcidin expression. The *HAMP* gene encodes three exons and encodes hepcidin, a peptide hormone produced in hepatocytes that plays a role in iron absorption and ferroportin degradation in intestinal enterocytes [10].

7.6.3.1 HJV Gene Analysis

The *HJV* gene has a large number of mutations that lead to JH 2A, with the most common one being a Gly320Val change [86–89]. Due to the rarity of *HVJ* gene mutations and the relatively large number of mutations that can cause type 2A JH, sequencing has often been chosen to analyze *JHV* gene mutations. Lee et al. [89] employed these primers to amplify the HJC gene exons in unrelated kinships in the Southeastern US in which HJ had been identified:

HJV	Primer sequence	Fragment size in BP
HJ Ex 1 F	GTACTCTGGCCAGCCATATACT	286
HJ Ex 1 R	CGAGAGACATCCAAGTAGGTGT	

(continued)

(continued)

HJV	Primer sequence	Fragment size in BP
HJ Ex 2 F	ATCTCCCCAAATTCCAGTCTG	359
HJ Ex 2 R	ACATAGCAGCCTACCCTCTAG	
HJ Ex 3 F	GCAAACTACACTCCGATAGAG	669
HJ Ex 3 R	GAATCTCATGAGGTGGATCGG	
HJ Ex 4A F	TAGTCCTGCATCTCTACTTGG	394
HJEx4AR	TGCAGGTCCTGTTCAGCTG	
HJ Ex 4B F	ATGGAGGTGACCGACCTGG	374
HJEx4BR	AGCTGCCACGGTAAAGTTGG	
HJ Ex 4C F	GCTCTCCTTCTCCATCAAGG	430
HJEx4CR	AAACTAGTAATGGGACTGATGG	
HJ Ex 4D F	TGTGGGCTCTTTGTTCTGTG	407
HJEx4DR	GTCTTCTGCTTTCAGCTCTTG	
HJ Ex 4E F	ATAAGTTTAGAGGTCATGAAGG	404
HJEx4ER	GCCCTCTTTCAGTGGAGTG	

The amplicons were purified using a Qiaquick PCR purification kit and the genotypes were determined by direct sequencing with an ABI 3100 DNA sequencer. By this method first group had two novel *HVJ* gene mutations, while to second group had two previously identified mutations.

7.6.3.2 HAMP Gene Analysis

HAMP gene mutations in HJ are very rare [10, 90]. *HAMP* gene mutations are usually identified by PCR amplification of the three gene exons, followed by DNA sequencing [90, 91].

7.6.4 Transferrin 2 Gene Mutation (TFR2) *and Hemochromatosis*

TFR2 gene mutations cause Type 3 HH, an HH type with similar clinical manifestations the HFE mutation-induced HH [10, 92]. The *TFR2* gene encodes an 18 exon, 801 amino acid protein that shares 45 % identity with TFRC. The protein mediates cellular iron import and has two predominant transcripts (alpha and beta), with the alpha form expressed mainly in the liver, spleen, lung, muscle, prostate, and peripheral blood mononuclear cells, and the beta form expressed in all tissue examined [92, 93]. Once identified, Type 3 HH is treated with periodic phlebotomies, like most other HH types [10].

TFR2 genes mutations leading to HH are relatively rare [10]. Roetto et al. [94] examined four different families with HH unrelated to *HFE* gene mutations. DNA was prepared from peripheral blood by standard phenol-chloroform extraction. The DNA was PCR amplified in a Thermal Cycler using 10 pmol of primers specific to all 18 *TFR2* exons. A total of 32 PCR cycles (denaturation, 94 °C for 30 s; annealing, 56 °C for 45 s; extension, 72 °C for 45 s) were performed. The amplicons were then transcribed into RNA with 10 units T7 RNA polymerase in an appropriate buffer with ^{35}S-UTP and subjected to gel etectrophoresis, drying, and autoradiography. Bands showing altered electrophoretic mobility were directly sequenced. Direct sequencing was performed on the purified PCR amplicons using a Thermo Squenase Cy5.5 dye terminator cycle sequencing kit. After removal of the unincorporated dye, the sequence was identified via electrophoresis on an automatic sequencer (model 373A; Applied Biosystem). The *Mae*I enzyme was used to detect the previously described Y250X mutant within the amplicon for exon 6.

Of the patients with altered *TFR2* gene exon electrophoretic mobility two patients had a previously described Y250X mutation in exon 6. In one large inbred family a frameshift mutation (84–88 insC; E60X) in exon 2 was identified which formed a premature stop codon. A single patient with nonfamilial HH carried a T→A transversion (T515A). All patients with a non-protein expressing phenotype showed severe clinical complications.

In another study, Biasiotto et al. [92] used denaturing high-performance liquid chromatography to analyze TFR2 gene mutations using blood samples from 657 individuals from Northern Italy who either had a diagnosis of HH or serum ferritin concentrations greater than 400 μg/L or a transferrin saturation above 50 %. The *HFE* gene C282Y and H63D mutations were identified by endonuclease digestion before this study was carried out. Genomic DNA was isolated from 0.2 ml of blood with a QIAamp DNA Blood Mini Kit and portions of the *hepcidin*, *HFE*, and *TFR2* genes were PCR amplified with appropriate primers. Specifically, exons 2, 4, and 6 of the *TFR2* gene were amplified. These exons were chosen for analysis as previous studies had shown mutations in these exons [92–94]. The resulting amplicons were heated to 94 °C for 10 min cooled at 56 °C for 60 min to obtain heteroduplexes. Mutations were analyzed by denaturing high-performance liquid chromatography on a Transgenomic WAVE® System with a preheated C_{18} reversed-phase column. Eight μL of the PCR mixture were loaded into column duplexes were eluted at a flow rate of 0.9 μL/min. DNA was detected by monitoring the absorbance at 260 nm and DNA fragment melting characteristics were predicted by Wavemaker™ software. The samples with altered elution profiles were subjected to DNA sequencing. As this technique does not detect homozygous mutations, the amplicons were also mixed with equal amounts of wild-type DNA, denatured, reannealed, and analyzed for heteroduplexes. All identified C282Y and H63D *HFE* gene mutations were confirmed by enzymatic digestion. No discrepancies between endonuclease assay- indentified C282Y and H63D *HFE* gene mutations and denaturing high-performance liquid chromatography *HFE* gene mutation results were detected, indicating that the chromatographic assay worked well and had 100 % sensitivity, at least for these two mutations.

Out of the 657 individuals tested, three new intronic variations, a previously identified IVS5-9T>A transition, and a new Val22→ILE *TFR2* gene mutation where found. Only one individual (72 years old and hepatitis B surface antigen positive) with *TFR2* gene mutations and no concomitant *HFE* gene mutations had a high serum ferritin value, possibly due to viral hepatitis. Based on these results, the authors concluded that *HFE* and *TFR1* gene mutations are often associated in HH and that HH due solely to the rare *TFR2* mutations is uncommon.

7.6.5 SLC40A1 *Gene Mutation and Type 4 HH*

The *SLC40A1* gene mutations cause a rare autosomal dominant HH, showing unusual clinical features including high serum ferritin levels with low or normal transferrin saturation until the end stage of the disease. Additionally, urinary hepcidin is usually reduced. Strangely, it may initially present as mild iron-deficient anemia with a reduced tolerance to therapeutic phlebotomy. *SLC40A1* consists of eight exons and encodes the ferroportin protein – a multipass transmembrane protein located on the basolateral membrane of enterocytes that regulates iron export into the circulation [10, 95]. Ferroportin also regulates the efflux of iron from macrophages of the spleen, liver, and bone marrow, and Type 4 HH is unique in that it often shows increased Kupffer cell iron ([10, 95, 96], Fig. 7.3a, b). *SLC40A1* gene mutations lead to increased iron loading, often due to ferroportin losing its responsiveness to hepcidin [97].

Like molecular testing for HH types 2 and 3, *SLC40A1* gene mutation analysis is not commonly performed, due to the rarity of the disease. Most molecular tests involve sequencing the entire coding region of the gene. Montosi et al. [98] examined genomic DNA isolated from peripheral blood from an Italian pedigree that included 15 individuals with iron overload, resulting in hepatic fibrosis, diabetes, impotence, and cardiac arrhythmias. None of these 15 individuals carried the C282Y *HFE* gene mutation [99]. The ferroportin exons were PCR amplified, sequenced, and compared to control sequences. Individuals with iron overload, but not those with normal iron levels, showed an exon 3 mutation that converted an alanine at residue 77 to an aspartic acid (GCC → GAC). The authors hypothesized that this mutations resulted in a gain of protein function that resulted in increased dietary iron accumulation. At least 26 other ferroptorin mutations have been identified by various molecular tests [10].

7.6.6 Genetic Testing for HH

While most cases of HH are due to *HFE* gene mutations in European populations, a subset of HH in this population and non-European populations can carry different gene mutations. Santos et al. [10] recommended the testing algorithm shown in Table 7.1.

Table 7.1 Common serological patterns associated with HBV infection (105–107)

HBsAg	Negative	
Anti-HBsAg	Negative	Susceptible to Infection
Anti-HBcAg	Negative	
HBsAg	Negative	Immune due to Natural Infection
Anti-HBsAg	Positive	
Anti-HBcAg	Positive	
HBsAg	Negative	Immune due to HVB Vaccination
Anti-HBsAg	Positive	
Anti-HBcAg	Negative	
HBsAg	Positive	
Anti-HBcAg	Positive	Acute infection
IgM anti-HBcAg	Positive	
Anti-HBsAg	Negative	
HBsAg	Positive	
Anti-HBcAg	Positive	Chronically Infected
IgM anti-HBcAg	Negative	
Anti-HBsAg	Negative	
HBsAg	Negative	Several Possibilities:
Anti-HBsAg	Negative	1. Resolved HVB Infection
Anti-HBcAg	Positive	2. False-Positive anti-HBcAg
		3. Low-Level Chronic Infection
		4. Resolving Acute Infection

7.7 Molecular Diagnostic Testing for Hepatitis B and C

Chronic HBV, HCV, and the satellite virus of HBV, hepatitis D (HDV), are major risk factors for HCC, with approximately 500 million people infected with viral hepatitis worldwide [1–4]. Proper medical management of chronic viral hepatitis requires timely and accurate diagnosis, staging, and disease monitoring. In general serological markers are commonly used for viral hepatitis diagnosis and staging, while molecular diagnostic tools are used for the identification of specific viral strains and for assessing drug responses. The end-point of such treatment is obtaining a sustained virological response, preferably with undetectable serum viral RNA, 6 months post-therapy completion [1–4, 99, 100]. Here we will review the serological and molecular testing for HBV, HCV, and HDV, with emphasis on molecular diagnostic techniques.

7.7.1 HBV

The WHO estimates that over two billion people have been infected with HBV and currently some 350 million people are chronically infected worldwide, with about 75 % living in the Asia Pacific region. Chronic HBV confers an increased risk for hepatic decompensation, cirrhosis, and HHC, and it is estimated that the worldwide mortality from this disease is 0.5–1.2 million deaths per year. In adults, most HBV infections are eventually cleared with only about 5 % resulting in chronic infections. In neonates, however, over 90 % fail to clear the virus and become chronically infected. HBV is spread parenterally by percutaneous or permucosal exposure to infected body fluids, especially blood. Risk factors for HBV infection include re-using syringes in between intravenous drug users, transfusions with untested blood, tattooing with unsterilized instruments, sexual promiscuity, working in a health-care setting, and living in a correctional facility [101, 102].

HBV is a double-stranded (ds), circular, enveloped 3,200 base pair DNA virus of the hepadenaviridae family. HBV has at least eight major genotypes (A through H), which shows a greater than 8 % divergence in viral nucleic acid sequence. Following entrance of the HBV into the hepatocyte, the viral genome enters the nucleus and integrates into the host genome, where the viral DNA functions as a transcriptional template making viral RNA. Unfortunately, because HBV integrates into the host genome and remains as an intercellular replicative intermediary (covalently closed circular DNA) complete elimination of HBV from an infected individual is not usually possible. Some of the viral RNA intermediates are reversed transcribed into DNA. The transcription products are used to make viral proteins, including the HBV surface and e antigens. Although HBV has a strong preference for the liver, viral DNA can be found in the kidneys, pancreas, and mononuclear cells of infected individuals. In acute infections the HBV infection becomes apparent roughly 45–180 days post initial infection, with the first 6 months of infections defined as acute phase of infection. Typically clearance of the HBV infection begins several weeks prior to the onset of clinical symptoms, and it is caused by antiviral cytokines produced by the adaptive and innate immune responses. Later, a cytologic immune response causes hepatocyte necrosis and apoptosis, responsible for the concomitant onset of clinical symptoms, and a rise in serum alanine aminotransferase (ALT). Individuals with a strong and specific CD4/CD8 immune response will usually clear the HBV, while a weaker response is associated with chronic HBV [101, 102].

7.7.1.1 HBV Serologic and Histopathologic Testing

Liver damage and function are typically analyzed serum ALT, bilirubin, and albumin levels, and the prothrombin time. Liver biopsy is used to quantify the grade of inflammation and the stage of fibrosis. Non-invasive methods such as ultrasound or rising alpha-fetoprotein levels can, on the other hand, often detect cirrhosis and HCC. Several serologic tests are employed in HBV infection and serum analysis based assays are presently the mainstay testing modality. Detectable HBV surface antigen (HBsAg) is a marker of chronic infection, while viral core antigen (HBcAg) indicates high hepatic viral replication. Loss of serum HBcAg with concomitant raise in anti-HBcAg antibodies (termed seroconversion) is associated with clinical improvement and reduced serum ALT, hepatitis, and reduced HBV DNA levels

[101–103]. Serum analysis of HBV-related antigens and antibodies identify the different phases of the infection and are summarized in Table 7.1 [101–103].

7.7.1.2 HBV Molecular Genetic Testing

Molecular HBV testing is usually employed in the diagnosis and management of HBV infection; quantification of viral load, genotyping, drug resistance, mutation analysis, and core promoter/precore mutation assays. Of these assays, the quantification of viral load is the most commonly used test [103].

7.7.1.2.1 HBV Viral Load Quantification

HBV viral load quantification is usually performed on plasma or serum. It is used to measure the viral load prior to the initiation of therapy, to monitor the effectiveness of anti-viral therapy, and to identify "occult" HBV viral infections, where the serologic tests can fail to detect HBV infections. It is also important in liver transplantation to avoid unnecessary HBV transmission [101–103]. In general, individuals with chronic HBV that are HBsAg positive, HBeAg negative, anti-HBeAg positive and serum HBV DNA levels below 10^5 copies/ml (>20,000 IU/ml) show histologically mild HVB-induced hepatic lesion as graded according to Ishak et al. [104, 105].

7.7.1.2.2 Nucleic Acid Hybridization Assays for HBV Quantification

The first molecular assay employed to quantify HBV viral loads were hybridization assays. Although these assays worked well, they were less sensitive and more cumbersome to perform that most PCR-based assays and are now seldom performed [104]. The degree of HBV probe hybridization does directly quantify the amount of serum HBV DNA present and correlates closely with infectivity [106]. Guo et al. [107] employed digoxigenin-labeled probes to detect HBV DNA in serum. Full-length HBV was inserted into a pBR322 plasmid at a *PstI* site, grown up in bacteria, subjected to restriction endonuclease digestion and isolated by gel electrophoresis. The probed DNA was purified by ion-exchange chromatography and either labeled with [α-^{32}P]dATP with a random labeling heximer or with a digoxigenin-11-dUTP labeling according to Boehringer Mannheim kit protocol. HBV DNA was isolated from human sera by two means: phenol-chloroform extraction followed by ethanol precipitation, or by alkaline denaturation in 1 M NaOH, followed by neutralization. Both samples were applied to nitrocellulose prewetted with appropriate buffers, baked to attach the HBV DNA to the nitrocellulose, pre-hybridized, hybridized with the HBV probes, washed, dried, and exposed to X-ray film. For the digoxigenin-labeled probes, the labeled DNA was detected immunologically using an antibody-enzyme conjugate, anti-digoxigenin-alkaline phosphatase with an enzyme-linked color reaction. Both assays included a standard curve within the same blot. Both assays yielded a lower detection limit of ~0.25 pg, corresponding to 7.0×10^4 genome copies. Since this number is close to the 10^5/ml copy number that defines viral loads that are not usually damaging to the liver. The sensitivity of this hybridization assay is adequate, but the sensitivity of the PCR assay is greater. Additionally, the digoxigenin-based assay had a longer shelf life and is safer to work with than the ^{32}P-based assay.

7.7.1.2.3 Branched DNA Technology in HBV Detection

Branched chain DNA (bDNA) is a sensitive, specific, and reliable tool for the diagnosis of viral infections and in monitoring drug response and/or disease progression. It has been successfully on multiple microorganisms, including T. *bricei,* cytomegalovirus, human papilloma virus, HIV, HCV, and HBV. bDNA does not depend on nucleic amplification, but instead uses a bDNA probe that hybridizes to the target sequence(s), resulting in a complex of probes and target sequences that can be quantified with great accuracy.

To perform this assay HBV is isolated from patient serum and treated to insure that the DNA can bind the assay "extender probe". The assay is usually performed on a multi-well plate, such as a 96 well plate. Attached to the walls and floor of the plate are many "capture probes". Extender probes are added under the correct buffer conditions to allow the capture and extender probes to hybridize. Part of the extender probe binds to the capture probe while the other, non-bound, single-stranded portions hybridizes to the target HBV DNA. A "label extender" is then added which binds to contiguous regions of the bound target HBV DNA. A "preamplifer oligonucleotide" is added which hybridizes to the label extender. This oligonucleotide partially hybridizes to the label extender and also usually has multiple branched oligonucleotides that hybridize to an amplifier oligonucleotide having alkaline phosphatase attached to it. After the required multiple washing steps, the amount of HBV target DNA present in the serum sample will be directly related to the signal created by the reporter molecule (alkaline phosphatase). A standard curve with positive and negative controls is used to estimate the number of HBV genomes in the serum sample. Essentially this assay depends on the HBV DNA linking the fixed capture probe to the amplifier/reporter, allowing the amount of HBV DNA to be quantified [108, 109]. The procedure may be summarized as follows:

Well → Capture Probe → Label Extender → HBV Target DNA → Label Extender → Preamplifier Oligonucleotide → Amplifier Oligonucleotide-Alkaline Phosphatase Conjugate

The advantages of bDNA technology include the fact that the technique lacks any amplification steps (therefore lowering the chances of cross contamination), that it is easy to automate, and is not labor intensive. Its sensitivity is usually less than that of PCR-based assays, but its reproducibility and specificity are excellent. Thus this assay would work well in patient populations that typically have higher HBV titers [109].

7.7.1.2.4 HVB Quantification by PCR

PCR has the advantages of high sensitivity and specificity and has largely replaced hybridization assays for serum HBV DNA quantification. While the sensitivity of hybridization assays is limited to about 70,000 viral genomes/ml, many PCR assays can reliably detect serum viral genomes over a 10^1 and 10^8/ml range [107, 110]. Abe et al. [110] developed an early RT-PCR assay for quantifying serum HBV. To begin this work, nucleotides 1–2,182 of the HBV genome were inserted into a BlueScript II SK(+) plasmid (Stratagen), grown in bacteria, and the recombinant plasmid was purified and then quantified by the optical density at 260 nm. Real-time detection PCR was performed on the HBV DNA with three sets of PCR primers and a probe; two primer sets would amplify the HBV surface (S) antigen gene and one the viral X gene. The amplified HBV viral gene segments were chosen based on being highly conserved between different viral strains, on having high sensitivity/specificity, and being placed relatively widely apart within the viral genome.

To quantify the HBV load, DNA was extracted from 100 μl of plasma and place into 20 μl of water. 10 μl of this DNA was amplified in a 50 μl volume with one of the primer-probe sets, *Taq* polymerase, appropriate buffer conditions, and nucleotide triphosphates. The mix was subjected to amplification cycles of 95 °C for 20 s and 60 °C for 1 min. The amount of target DNA was quantified by measuring the increase in probe fluorescence, following probe degradation with concomitant probe-quencher disassociation, normalized to an unchanging passive reference signal. The amount of target DNA amplified was thus the change in probe fluorescence minus the reference signal measured at the beginning of the PCR reaction. The threshold Ct value was calculated on the mean baseline of the first 15 amplification rounds and set at 10 standard deviations above this mean. The amount of HBV target DNA was measured against a standard HBV DNA curve ranging over 10^1 to 10^8 copies/reaction. A linear relationship was obtained between the Ct and the number of HBV viral copies. In parallel experiments employing HBV DNA quantification by bDNA technology, the detection limit was found to be 7×10^5 viral copies/ml. When applied to the sera of HBV infected and viral-free individuals, this PCR protocol was able to detect HBV viral DNA over a life range (10^1–10^8 copies/reaction) and have similar sensitivity of bDNA technology. This assay was also able to detect HBV DNA in patients who had undetectable HBV level by the bDNA testing method. The authors of this early study conclude that this assay was superior to other methods for HBV viral DNA quantification in its sensitivity, specificity, simplicity, and reproducibility.

Since this study, RT-PCR has become the gold standard for HBV DNA detection in patient sera and this technique is routinely employed in the automated detection of serum HBV [111–113]. However, RT-PCR still has limitations in detecting very low HBV loads. Wang et al. [114] used a locked nucleic acid PCR (LNA-PCR) probe to quantify serum HBV loads compared to standard TaqMan RT-PCR probe and achieved a significant increase in the viral detection limit. LNAs carry 2-methyele units between the O_2 and C_4 of ribose, locking the ribose in the 3′-endo (North) conformation, often found in A DNA. This locked conformation enhances base stacking and increases the melting temperature 2–8 °C compared to unmodified RNA or DNA oligonucleotides, increasing mismatch discrimination [115]. Wang et al. [114] used an LNA or an unmodified oligonucleotide probe designed to match the HBV X gene and produce a 114 base pair amplicon. The same oligonucleotide primers were used in both reactions:

Primer 1	GACCACCAAATGCCCCTAT
Primer 2	CCRAGAYYGAGATCTTCTGCGAC
LNA probe	FAM-TCGTCTAACAACAGT-BHQ1 (underlines denote methylene bridge)
TaqMan probe	FAM-TCGTCTAACAACAGT(TAMMRA)AGTTTCCGGAAGTGT-P

Serum samples were taken from 39 individuals, previously demonstrated by have chronic HBV by ELISA. These samples were divided into three groups: (1) 15 cases that were HBsAg positive only, (2) 10 cases that were HBsAg and HBeAg positive, and (3) 14 cases that were HBsAg, HBeAg, and HBc positive. Additionally, 19 cases of normal serum were taken from volunteers. The HBV DNA was isolated from 100 μl serum and 2 μl of purified DNA were used per reaction out of a final 25 μl volume. The amplification reaction consisted of 40 μl of 200 nM each primer, 75 nM LNA probe, dGTP, dATP, dCTP, and dUTP, 3.5 mM $MgCl_2$, 2 U HotSartTaq DNA polymerase, 0.5 U uracil DNA glycosylase and, 2 μl of purified DNA. The amplification was carried out in a iCycler iQ5 (Bio-Rad) consisting of an initial activation of UDG at 37 °C for 5 min, activation of HotStarTaq DNA polymerase and template denaturation at 95 °C for 3 min, and 40 cycles in two steps: 95 °C for 5 s, 60 °C for 30 s. Standard curves were created in the range of $40–4 \times 10^7$ IU/ml by 1:10 serial dilutions of an HBV standard. All samples were run in duplicate.

A linear relationship was obtained between the Ct values and the log10 concentrations of HBV DNA. Over a serial dilution of $40–4 \times 10^7$ IU/ml the maximum sensitivity of the standard oligonucleotide primers was 80 IU/ml, while the maximum sensitivity for the LNA probe was 40 IU/ml. Thus the LNS probe roughly doubled detection sensitivity compared to the standard oligonucleotide probe. When applied to patient samples, both probe types were able to detect HBV DNA in patient samples. Interestingly, in the 15 HBsAg positive only samples with low HBV DNA, the LNA probes were able to detect HBV DNA in four samples determined to be HBV DNA negative by standard probes. The authors concluded that LNA probe has higher precision, an improved signal to noise ration, and a better detection limit in clinical assays compared to standard probes.

7.7.1.2.5 HBV Molecular Genotyping Assays

HBV has at least eight different genotypes, A–H, which show greater than 8 % genomic variation between the viral types and numerous subtypes which show at least 4 % genomic variation. Most likely these variations have arisen due to the relatively high rate of nucleotide replication substitution ($1.4–4.57 \times 10^{-5}$ per base pair/year) seen in HBV. Phylogenetic evidence suggests that human HBV is a relatively recent viral pathogen, that first appeared about 3,000 years ago [116, 117]. Many of the HBV genotypes show significant differences in: (1) geographic distribution, (2) clinical course, (3) treatment responses, and (4) modes of transmission. For example, HBV genotype A is more common in Northwest Europe and the USA, while HBV genotype C is more common in Asia and the Pacific region. The HBV genotype C induces a more severe disease, characterized by higher fibrosis scores and a more frequent progression to cirrhosis than does HBV genotype B, while the D genotype appears to cause a higher incidence of HCC [118–122]. Additionally, while all HBV genotypes appear to respond equally well to nucleoside/nucleotide analogue treatment, genotypes A and B respond better to pegylated interferon-α than do genotypes C and D following 52 weeks of treatment [123, 124]. Last, different HBV genotypes are preferentially spread by different modes of transmission, although all genotypes can be spread by the common transmission modes. For example, HBV genotype A has been associated with sexual transmission while the D genotype is often transmitted by blood transfusions and IV drug abuse. Interestingly, genotype A appears to also be preferentially transmitted by homosexual or bisexual contact [125, 126].

Presently there are roughly ten different HBV genotyping techniques that entirely or partially use molecular technology (for review, [127]). Here these techniques will be briefly reviewed and the advantages and disadvantages of each technique discussed.

7.7.1.2.6 Direct HBV Sequencing

Sequencing remains the gold standard for HBV genotyping and presently commercial kits are available for this purpose, such as HBV sequencing test kit offered by Abbott Molecular (Illinois, USA). Sequencing has the advantage of directly interrogating every nucleotide within the viral genome or viral gene being sequenced, allowing the identification of new sequence variations, and it can be a relatively sensitive test. Since all nucleotides are interrogated, sequencing works equally well for genotyping, identifying drug resistant HBV clones, and other mutation testing. The drawback of this technique is that it can be expensive, time-consuming, and can easily miss less commonly represented HBV genotypes within a genotype mix [127].

Okamoto et al. [117] developed an early method for Sanger sequencing of the HBV genome. HBV DNA was isolated from 20 ml of serum taken from individuals demonstrated to have HBV by solid phase immunoassay for HBsAg and by dot blot hybridization for HBV DNA. The gapped region of the HBV genome was repaired with an endogenous DNA polymerase and the HBV DNA was cloned into a pSP65 plasmid *Bam*HI, grown in bacteria, and subcloned into different phage vectors. The HBV genomic fragments were removed with the appropriate restriction endonuclease and subjected to standard Sanger sequencing. A total of 18 HBV genomes were sequenced, five of which comprised newly identified viral subtypes. Although an early study, this work did demonstrate that Sanger sequencing is an excellent, although slow way to analyze HBV viral sequence variations.

Since the eight different HBV genotypes show significant sequence variation, efficient and accurate genotyping methods employing Sanger sequencing combined with genotype-specific PCR primers have been developed. The commercial TRUGENE HBV Genotyping commercial kit (Siemens Medical Solutions Diagnostics, NY, USA, [128]) uses these techniques. First, DNA is extracted from serum and the HBsAg gene is amplified via PCR. The resulting amplicons are then bidirectionally Sanger sequenced and compared to the known A through H HBV genotypes via a bioinformatics program. The bidirectional Sanger sequencing improves accuracy, as each sequence is effectively read twice. The detection limit of this assay is approximately 2.0×10^3 HBV genome copies/ml. Although less commonly used, pyrosequencing has worked well for some HBV sequencing applications, such as the analysis of specific nucleotide substitutions associated with dug resistance [129].

7.7.1.2.7 Multiplex Polymerase Chain Reaction

Multiplex PCR has been used to analyze HBV genotypes A through H in an accurate and cost-effective manner. Liu et al. [130] employed this technique to analyze the HBV genotypes in the sera of 441 HBV DNA-positive patients and compare it to restriction fragment length polymorphism analysis. The primers employed in this study were designed by analyzing 369 HBV full-length nucleotide sequences in GenBank which had been classified into eight different genotypes (A–H) using the Clustal X1.81, GenDoc2.6.002 and Mega2 software. From this database, genotype-specific primers were designed that were specific to at least 90 % of the viral isolates corresponding to the genotype.

Following patient DNA isolation, the HBV DNA was amplified by multiplex PCR performed with a GeneAmp PCY System 9600 in a 50 ml volume. The amplification protocol incubated the samples for 5 min at 94°, followed by 40 cycles consisting of 94° for 1 min, 59.5° for 1 min, and 72° for 2 min. The amplicons were visualized by electrophoresis in a 4 % agarose gel, stained with ethidium bromide, and evaluated under UV light. Each primer set gave an amplicon with a different molecular weight, allowing identification of the HBV genotype. HBV infections containing different genotypes gave multiple bands of different sizes. In order to be detected, a co-infecting HBV genotype had to represent at least 10 % of the total HBV infection load. When the results of the multiplex PCR were compared to genotyping results obtained by restriction fragment length polymorphism (RFLP) analysis a 93 % concordance was achieved, indicating that genotyping with multiplex PCR is relatively accurate. The authors concluded that this genotyping method could be applied only to areas where HBV genotypes A–G are prevalent. It could also provide an efficient alternative for clinical diagnosis and large-scale studies due to its low cost and fast turnaround time. PCR has also been combined with melting curve analysis to identify different HBV genotypes. This technique allowed as little as 100 HBV genome copies/ml sera and was more accurate than RFLP analysis [131].

7.7.1.2.8 Restriction Fragment Length Polymorphism (RFLP) Analysis

RFLP analysis interrogates the sequence difference between to homologous DNA sequences by using restriction endonucleases to cut the DNA into fragments of different lengths based on the sequences having sites cut by different restriction endonucleases. The resulting DNA fragments are often resolved by gel electrophoresis. Lindh et al. [132] used RFLP to genotype HBV. Seventy-three HBV sequences were obtained through the Entrez database of the National Center for Biotechnology Information (NCBI, Bethesda, MD) and analyzed with MacVector DNA analysis software (International Biotechnologies, New Haven, CT). A restriction endonuclease fingerprint pattern was predicted following treatment with the *Tsp509*I, *Hinf*I, and *Bsr*I endonucleases. To test the predicted fingerprint pattern, 187 HBeAg-positive chronic HBV carriers who resided in western Sweden were then analyzed by a commercial HBV genotyping serology kit (Abbott, Abbott Park, IL), or by RFLP. To perform the RFLP DNA was prepared from 30 μl of patient serum and the segment between nucleotides 256 and 796 were PCR amplified by 40 PCR cycles. Three minutes denaturation at 94 °C, 40 cycles of amplification, including denaturation for 45 s at 94 °C, annealing for 60 s at 53 °C, and extension for 90 s at 72 °C (prolonged by 3 s/cycle), were done and followed by a final 7 min extension at 72 °C.

The resulting amplicon was incubated for 3 h with either the *Tsp509*I or the *Hinf*I restriction endonucleases. The cut amplicons were then run into a composite gel containing 2 % NuSieve agarose and 1 % standard agarose, with uncut amplicon as a negative control. In some cases the cut amplicons were cut further with the *Bsr*I endonuclease. The DNA fragments were identified with ethidium bromide staining and the restriction fragment pattern read visually. One hundred and sixty-six of the samples fell into one of ten major patterns, each corresponding to specific HBV genotype. Seven additional patterns appeared to represent rare HBV genotypes. Thus roughly 92 % of the HBV genotypes were easily identified. Of the others, 14 samples were incubated with *Bsr*I, allowing seven additional cases to be genotyped. Comparison of this method to serological testing showed a 100 % genotyping correlation for those samples that could be RFLP analyzed.

Lee et al. [133] used RFLP combined with matrix-assisted laser desorption/ ionization-time- of-flight mass spectrometry to indentify the tyrosine-methionine-aspartate motif associated with lamivudine drug resistance. This detection technique, although expensive, had a lower detection limit of 100 copies/ml. than that of gel-based methods.

7.7.1.2.9 Oligonucleotide Microchip Arrays

Many different molecular assays employ specific gene sequences attached to a solid matrix, combined with washing steps and a hybridization detection reporter, to identify specific nucleic acid sequences within a complex mix. Often these methods show very high sensitivity and specificity [134–137]. Gauthier et al. [138] employed the Affymetrix in situ synthesis (Affymetrix) to design an HBV microarray consisting of 520,327 different 20-mer oligonucleotide probes allocated to detect HBV polymorphisms/mutations. The array was designed to detect 994 mutants located at 298 genomic positions in the HJBV genome, including positions in the S, C, P, and X viral genes. The fluorescence hybridization patterns were detected via DNAEM automated software (bioM erieux, Marcy-l'Etoile, France) and the fluorescence intensities were translated into sequence information by selecting the most probable nucleotide at each interrogated position.

A total of 253 patient sera that had been previously analyzed by Sanger sequencing were used in this study. DNA was extracted from the seras and amplified in a duplex PCR reaction as previously described [139]. Those amplifications that failed to give an expected 1.5 and 1.7 kb pair fragments were subjected to an alternative nested-PCR amplification procedure to produce an analyzable amplicon. The amplicons where cleaved and fluorescently labeled by successively adding 5 μl RNase-free water, 5 μl of PCR product, 5 μl of M bis-biotin-phenylmethyl-diazomethyl, and 5 μl of 20 mM HCl and incubating for 25 min at 95 °C. The labeled fragments were purified, hybridized on the microarray, and stained. The microarrays were immediately scanned at 570 nm. Analysis of the genotyping performance revealed that samples containing less than 400 HBV genome copies/ml could be successfully analyzed by this technique, demonstrating a high sensitivity. The results were 94 % concordant with Sanger sequencing. The technique also worked well for indentifying HBV sequences associated with adefovir and entecavir drug resistance, and with precore mutations. The authors concluded that this microarray technology could have clinical, epidemiological, and research applications for HBV analysis. Although relatively time-consuming and expensive, this technique is superior to the Sanger sequencing as it gives exhaustive information at multiple positions over the entire 3.2 kb HBV genome in a single reaction.

7.7.1.2.10 INNO-LiPA HBV Assay

The INNO-LiPA HBV assay is a commercially available reverse hybridization line probe assay (Innogenetics, Belgium) that is easy to performed and capable of identifying mixed HBV genotypic infections. In this assay HBV DNA is PCR amplified with biotinylated primers complementary to the conserved S/pre-S ORF. The amplicons are then hybridized to probes immobilized on a strip that has targets corresponding to HBV genotypes A though H. Following washing steps, alkaline phosphatase-labeled streptavidin added, followed by another washing step. The position of the hybridized biotin-labeled amplicon is visualized by the deposition of an insoluble purple/brown precipitate created by alkaline phosphatase catalysis acting on a soluble substrate. The INNO-LiPA HBV assay identifies mixed HBV infections.

Ali et al. [140] compared the INNO-LiPA HBV assay, direct sequencing, and subtractive PCR-RFLP for HBV genotyping. All three assays were performed on 80 consecutive HBV DNA positive serum samples obtained from individuals with

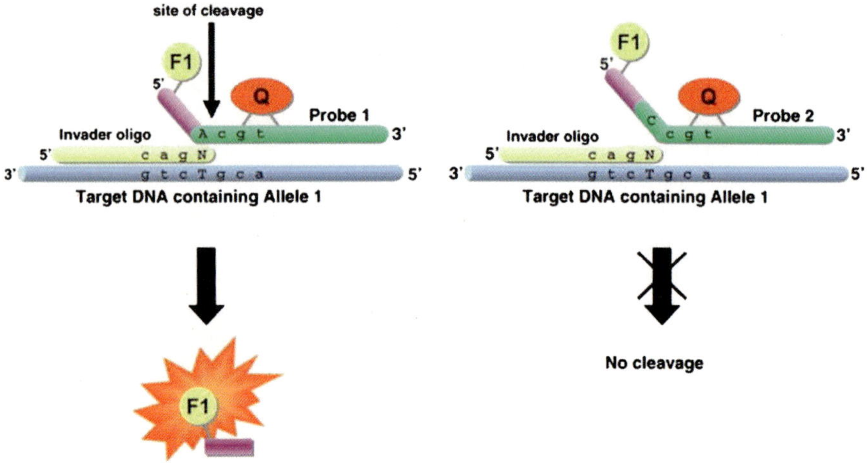

Fig. 7.4 The Invader assay from Ref. [146]

chromic HBV. The DNA was isolated with a High Pure Template Preparation Kit (Roche Applied Science, Germany). Ten μl out of a final 100 μl volume was used as a template for the HBV DNA amplification. The HBV DNA was amplified by nested PCR and the amplicons were hybridized to genotype-specific probes impregnated on membrane strips, and analyzed as described above. The INNO-LiPA HBV assay and direct sequencing both identified 63, 4, and 13 of the HBV strains as genotype D, genotype A, and mixed genotypes A and D, respectively. The PCR-RFLP-based method was less accurate, identifying all four A genotypes, but only 53 of the 63 D genotypes. In fact, seven HBV strains, previously categorized as genotype D, were identified as indeterminate. The authors concluded that the PCR-RFLP-based method failed to identify some genotype D HBV strains and it was therefore a less useful genotyping method as compared to the other assays. Additionally, since the INNO-LiPA HBV assay is available as a largely complete kit and does not require automated sequencing, it lends itself to use by less sophisticated laboratories.

7.7.1.2.11 PCR Invader Assay

HBV has been successfully genotyped by PCR invader assay. The advantage of this assay is that, when compared to the commonly used HBV genotyping methods (direct sequencing and PCR-RFLP analysis), it is less expensive and less difficult to perform for most routine clinical applications. In this assay the basic mechanism involves two specific oligonucleotide probes that bind to target DNA, forming a tripartite structure that can be recognized and cut by a thermostable structure-specific flap endonuclease or "DNA cleavase" (Fig. 7.4) [141]. The first probe, called the "Invader", is complementary to the 3′ end of the target DNA, but the last base is a mismatch with the target DNA. The second probe in this assay, the "allele-specific probe", contains the base complementary to the mismatched Invader probe and extends 5′ of this nucleotide with additional non-complementary nucleotides. Once the two probes anneal to the target DNA, they form a three-dimensional structure over the mismatched single nucleotide that can be cut by the DNA cleavase. Commonly the Invader probe is designed to permanently anneal to the target DNA at the assay temperature. The allele-specific probe is designed to have a melting temperature close to the assay temperature and therefore constantly anneal and detach. This allows the DNA cleavase to cut multiple allele-specific probes in succession and up to 3,000 allele-specific probe molecules can be cut/target over a 90-min period [141]. Additionally, a fluorophore is often added to the 5′ end of the allele-specific probe and a quencher placed at the 3′ end to the fluorophore such that DNA cleavase activity separates the two allowing the fluorophore signal to be measured. In tripartite structures where the allele-specific probe does not match the base mismatched by the Invader probe, the DNA cleavase does not cut the tripartite structure. Since the DNA cleavase is highly specific in its activity, doubly mismatched tripartite structures are cut at a very low rate and the Invader assay in highly specific for matched target DNA-allele-specific probe tripartite structures.

Tadokoro et al. [142] used the Invader assay to genotype HBV DNA taken from 505 HBsAg positive serum samples obtained from Toranoman Hospital, Japan. Initially the HBV genotypes were determined by two assays; (1) ELISA assay using an HBV genotyping EIA, and (2) a genotype- specific probe assay using seven oligonucleotides corresponding to sequences in the preS1 region. The viral strains were classified as genotypes A–F by ELISA and genotypes A–G by genotype-specific probe assay.

The genotype-specific Invader probes were designed by analyzing 491 individual complete HBV genomes from the National Center for Biotechnology Information (NCBI) database. The Invader Technology Creator (TWT, Madison WI) was used to design the specific probe/invasive oligonucleotides. The oligonucleotide probes were either labeled with FAM (carboxyfluorescein) or RED (REDmond RED). The HBV DNA for the Invader assay was extracted from 100 μl of serum and the HBV S and core gene sequences were amplified by PCR:

S gene	Sense: 5′-GGTCACYATATTCTTGGGAACAAGAKCTA-3′
	Anti-sense: 5′-CTGACTGCCGATTGGTRGAGGCAG-3′
Core gene	Sense: 5′-TATAAAGAATTTGGAGCTWCTGTGGAGTT-3′
	Anti-sense: 5′-GCGGCGATTGAGAYCTKCKT-3′

The Invader reactions were performed in 384-well plates with a Cleavage XI Invader core reagent kit containing 2 μl purified HBV amplicon. The plates were incubated at 65 °C for 15 min in a DNA thermocycler and the fluorescent intensities were measured from zero time to 15 min. Second fluorescent intensities were measured continuously on a Cytoflour 4000 fluorescence plate reader (Applied Biosystems) for FAM (carboxyfluorescein) (wave-length/bandwidth: excitation, 485/20 nm; emission, 530/25 nm) and RED (REDmond RED) (excitation, 560/20 nm;

emission, 620/40 nm) dyes. The genotype was identified by calculation of fold-over-zero (FOZ) values. Twenty-one sera without HBV-DNA were used to determine the cut-off value of FOZ. The mean plus 5 S.D. of the FOZ value of these sera in each well was calculated to be 1.21–1.51 (L1–12) of FAM-FOZ and 1.20–1.64 (L1–12) of RED-FOZ. Therefore, the cut-off level was set at 2.00. Four HBV genotypes and two subgenotypes (Ae, Ba, Bj, C, D) were also amplified, cloned, and sequenced for use in detection sensitivity assays for single and mixed genotype preparations.

The detection threshold for the PCR Invader assay was about ten HBV copies/reaction. Mixtures of two genotypes could be detected even where the ratio of the two genotypes was 1,000:10. All eight genotypes and four subgenotypes were identified by this assay. Thus the assay had a high sensitivity and specificity. In 168 serum samples with HBV, the ELISA and Invader assays gave identical results in 165 (98.2 %) of the samples, with three of the samples (1.8 %) not agreeing. When the three discordant samples were sequenced, the genotypes were found to be those determined by the Invader assay. Comparison of the genotyping results for the Invader and genotype-specific probe assays were in agreement, with 333 of 343 (97.1 %) samples having identical genotypes. Ten samples (2.9 %) were discrepant and could not be genotyped by the genotype-specific probe assay, but were genotyped by the Invader assay. The authors concluded that this assay is sensitive, accurate, relatively low in cost compared to other genotyping methods, and has a short, 7-hour turn-around time. Thus the Invader assay would be very useful in both the clinical and research settings.

7.7.1.2.12 Serological HBV Genotype Testing

HBV is commonly genotyped by serological methods. Typically antibodies directed towards genotype-specific HBsAg epitopes are employed, with antibodies to one constant determinant and two or more antibodies directed to mutually exclusive HBV HBsAg epitopes. Serological HBV genotyping is often used and it is cost-effective, has a high throughput, and it is easy to perform. Serological assays are also superior to molecular genotyping methods in typing HBV-PCR-negative carriers [127].

7.7.1.2.13 HBV Drug Resistance Assays and Promoter/Precore Mutation Testing

Molecular genetic testing is often performed on HBV to detect the development or presence of drug resistance and promoter/precore mutations. Most of the assays described above have been employed in this type of testing, especially sequencing, which interrogates all the nucleotides examined. In addition, other assays have been developed specifically for these purposes. For example, Innogenetics has developed a commercial INNO-LiPA assay that detects lamivudine, telbivudine, emtricitabine, adefovir, and entecavir resistance-associated HBV mutations [143]. Additionally,

Quest Diagnostics offers both HBV drug resistance and precore mutation testing performed by PCR amplification, followed by sequencing at specific codons [144].

7.7.2 *HCV*

The WHO estimates that three to four million people are newly infected with HCV every year and about 170 million people, or ~3 % of the world's population, are chronically infected and are therefore at risk for HCV-related cirrhosis and HCC. The highest HCV infections prevalence (>3.5 %) is found in Central and East Asia, North Africa, and the Middle East. Southern Asia, sub-Saharan Africa, and most of South and Central America have a moderate HCV infection prevalence (1.5–3.5 %), while the Asian Pacific and North America have a low prevalence (<1.5 %, [145]). Like HBV, HCV is a significant risk factor for cirrhosis and HCC and globally, it is the leading cause of liver transplantation. In the US HCV is the most common cause of liver disease related death (1–4, 145, 146). HCV is an enveloped, single-stranded positive-sense RNA virus of the *Flaviviridae* family consisting of approximately 9,600 nucleotides with two short untranslated regions at each end and a single open reading frame (ORF) of about 9,000 nucleotides. The HCV ORF, known as the polyprotein, encodes three structural proteins known as core, E1, and E2, and seven non-structural proteins; P7, NS2, NS3, NS4A, NS4B, NS5A, and NS5B. The ORF is initially translated into a large polyprotein that is later cut by cellular and viral proteases into smaller proteins. The virus replicates in hepatocytes and peripheral blood mononuclear cells, by the action of an RNA-dependent RNA polymerase and a negative RNA strand intermediate [147]. HCV has at least six major genotypes that show 30–35 % nucleotide divergence [147–150]. Not surprisingly, each HCV genotype exhibits a unique geographical distribution and response to different HCV directed therapies [150]. Thus optimal HCV treatment regimes requires knowledge of the HCV genotype, as well as of the serial viral titers. It also requires evaluation of livers biopsies and analysis of liver enzymes. In fact multiple patient parameters can effect the clinical course of HCV, including the viral genotype and load, hepatic iron load, gender, alcohol use, ethnicity, length of infection, patient adherence to medication regimens, obesity, and co-infection with HIV [151]. Numerous molecular genetic tests are performed on HCV, including the quantification of viral load and genotyping [152]. Additionally, IL-28B molecular testing is a powerful predictor of a patient's chance of achieving a sustained virologic response following interferon-based HCV therapy [153].

7.7.2.1 HCV Viral Load Quantification

Like HBV load quantification, there are many different molecular genetic tests employed in HCV load quantification. The main uses of HCV load quantification are to establish a prognosis, to evaluate treatment options, to guide possible changes in treatment, and to consider further treatment(s) [154, 155]. Here we will review the most commonly used molecular techniques. Most of them are similar to those used for HBV load tests, with the important difference that the nucleic acid analyzed in HCV testing is RNA, while for HBV the main nucleic acid tested is DNA [101, 102, 147].

7.7.2.1.1 Reverse Transcriptase PCR for HCV (RT-PCR)

RT-PCR is often used to quantify the HCV serum load and is currently the main HCV load quantification testing method [152]. Kleiber et al. [156] used RT-PCR to quantify serum HCV levels and were able to distinguish therapy responders from nonresponders and responder-relapsers. In their study three HCV RNA-positive samples with viral titers ranging from 4,000 to 1,600,000 IU/ml were used the analyze test precision. The specificity was determined by analyzing a set of 100 HCV negative plasma samples. The ability of the assay to monitor changes in viral load was analyzed by taking serial samples from three individuals being treated with five million units of interferon-α 3 times/week. Different HCV genotypes were generated by transcribing cloned HCV plasmid DNA genotypes 1a, 1b, 2a, 2b, 3a, 4, and 5 into RNA, isolating and quantifying the RNA, and diluting the samples to 100,000 copies/ml. These were serially diluted in HCV negative human plasma.

HCV RNA was isolated from 200 μl serum or plasma. A 250 base pair target sequence located in the highly conserved 5′ untranslated HCV genomic region was amplified. The reverse transcription and amplification steps were performed with a modified version of the *Thermus* species ZO5 DNA polymerase, which under appropriate buffer conditions has both reverse transcriptase and DNA polymerase activities occurring within the same reaction. The reaction was performed with HCV-specific oligonucleotides and fluorescently labeled probe oligonucleotides. The thermocycling parameters were 50 °C for 4 min, 30 min at 61 °C, two PCR cycles of 15 s at 95 °C and 50 s at 58 °C, and 48 PCR cycles of 15 s at 91 °C and 50 s at 58 °C. An ABI Prism 7700 Sequence Detector System measured fluorescent emissions, which increased in direct proportion to the increase of amplified product during the PCR amplification. The amount of HCV RNA was quantified by running a set of five external HCV RNA standards covering a four log concentration range, that were reverse transcribed and amplified in separate reaction run in parallel. The limit of detection for this assay proved to be 100 viral copies/ml. The different viral genotypes tested were all amplified with comparable efficiency with only small variations in amplification efficiency. The addition of significant amounts of nucleic acids from adenovirus types 2, 3, and 7, *Chlamydia trachomatis, coxsackievirus* B1, cytomegalovirus, echovirus 1, hepatitis A, hepatitis B, herpes simplex types 1 and 2, human herpesvirus, HIV-1, Group M subtypes A–E and G and Group O, *P. acnes*, *S. aureus*, *S. epidermis,* and varicella zoster did not result in the assay showing HCV positivity. Last, of the 100 negative plasma samples 96 were negative for HCV and four gave invalid results. Thus this assay showed high specificity. The linear range of the assay was determined to be over a braid 64 and 4,180,000 IU/ml range. Last, the assay was able to detect changes in HCV load during interferon therapy which paralleled changes in serum ALT, demonstrating that this assay could have value in monitoring patient response to therapy. Last, the test showed high precision as the assay highly repeatable results over a 10-day period where the assay was repeated 180 times. The authors concluded that this test has better sensitivity, a grater dynamic range, and a higher throughput than many other current HCV tests.

Currently many companies offer real-time PCR testing on serum from HCV infected individuals. For example, two real-time PCR tests offered by Roche and Abbott were analyzed by Halfon et al. [157] who concluded that both assays had high sensitivities and large dynamic ranges that were fully adequate for the clinical and therapeutic management of HCV. Other less often used methods of HCV load quantification included branched chain amplification and transcription mediated amplification assays [152].

7.7.2.2 HCV Genotyping Assays

Like HBV, different HCV genotypes typically have different clinical responses to treatment. For example, individuals with HCV genotypes 2 or 3 are three to six times more likely to achieve a sustained virological response to pegylated interferon than is genotype 1 [158, 159]. Unfortunately, data on how to treat HCV genotypes 4, 5, and 6 is scarce, but currently these genotypes are given the same treatment regime as HCV genotype 1 [158–162]. Thus HCV genotype testing plays an important role in predicting the clinical response to therapy. Similar to HBV infections, a sustained virological response for HCV is defined as a 6-month period negative HCV testing following the cessation of anti-viral therapy.

7.7.2.2.1 HCV Genotyping Strip Assays

As for other molecular applications, strip assays typically show high sensitivity and accuracy, and can be performed at a relatively low cost, usually from a commercial kit. Innogenetics provides a commercial kit for HCV genotyping (VERSANT® HCV Genotype 2.0 Products). The strip assay based technology can process up to 48 assays simultaneously and identify HCV genotypes 1–6. For most viral types, subtype information is also obtained. Verbeeck et al. [163] evaluated this assay by analyzing 326 HCV-positive clinical specimens consisting of either serum or EDTA plasma samples with viral loads about 2,000 IU/ml. RNA was collected from these samples using a QIAamp DSP virus kit in combination with a QIAvac 24 Plus vacuum system (Qiagen GmbH, Germany). Each extraction included positive and negative controls from the kit. The 5′ UTR region (NS5b) and the core region of the HCV genome were reverse transcribed and amplified using the kit. This was performed in two steps, with the first step involving reverse transcription and the second PCR activated by high heat with simultaneously denaturation of the reverse transcriptase and activation of the DNA polymerase. The primer sets were biotinylated, yielding two biotinylated amplicons of 240 and 270 base pairs, corresponding to the 5′ UTR and core HCV viral regions, respectively. The amplicons were hybridized to oligonucleotide probes immobilized on nitrocellulose. Following washing steps the strip are incubated with alkaline phosphatase labeled strepavidin and the hybridized bands are visualized with BCIP/NBT chromogen. The Versant HCV genotype (LiPA) 1.0 assay was used in this study as a reference assay.

Specific genotypes were identified by comparison to the patterns produced by known positive controls. Of the 326 samples analyzed, 93.3 % (304/326) gave interpretable genotyping results, with 2.1 % (7/326) failing to amplify and 4.6 % (15/326) amplifying with uninterpretable results. Of the 313 samples that did yield interpretable results, 99/4 % (311/313) agreed with the reference assay method. The method also showed very high reproducibility. The authors concluded that this genotyping method is accurate, rapid, and reliable, out performing the previous Versant HCV genotype (LiPA) 1.0 assay, and recommended it for large-scale genotyping.

7.7.2.2.2 HCV Sequencing Assays

HCV Genotyping by sequencing is commonly performed and considered the Gold Standard in genotyping assays. Both Sanger and pyrosequencing methods are commonly used [164, 165]. Most studies have demonstrated that sequencing works well and gives close or does give 100 % concordant results with assays such as the LiPA assay above [165]. The main difference between HBC and HCV genotyping by sequencing is that HCV has an RNA genome, usually requiring a reverse transcription step to convert the RNA genome into DNA prior to Sanger or pyrosequencing [164, 165].

7.7.2.2.3 Other HCV Genotyping Methods

HCV has been successfully genotyped with Invader technology, genotype-specific primers in reverse transcription PCR technology, and with the assays described above. Most of them are commercially available [158–166]. Since HCV genotyping methods are very similar to those employed for HBV genotyping, they will not be extensively reviewed here.

IL-28B Testing for HCV

As of 2011, it is estimated that 130–170 million people worldwide are chronically infected with HCV. HCV complications include increased risk of cirrhosis, HCC, and liver failure. PEG-INF-α plus Ribavirin therapy remains a mainstay HCV treatment, despite the fact that fewer than half of patients are able to achieve sustained viral response with this therapy. Moreover, treatment response and HCV clearing capability seem to differ among different ethnic groups infected with the same HCV genotype, suggesting a genetic predisposition, for some patients, to be more responsive to therapy than others [146–150]. Recent studies have shown that single nucleotide polymorphisms (SNPs) within the IL-28B gene locus are found in HCV infected patients. Patients with a common variant of the gene (rs12979860 CC) are significantly more likely to respond to PEG-IFN-α plus Ribavirin treatment [158–162]. These results have led to a more personalized approach to HCV management, with many medical centers now offering IL-28B testing to predict therapy response.

IL-28B is a member of the type III IFN-gamma cytokines and it is located on chromosome 19. Just like IFN-gamma, IL-28B and other INFs can be triggered by viral infection, inducing antiviral activity through both cellular and humoral immune pathways. IL-28B acts through pathways such as JAK-STAT and NF-kappaB to activate IFN stimulated genes (ISGs) in a viral infection. Successful induction of ISGs in response to IFN treatment is associated with favorable SNPs within the IL-28B gene. The independent effect of different SNPs in IL-28B suggests a major role in the regulation of antiviral activity against HCV [167, 168]. Ge et al. [169] first showed an association between SNPs and sustained virological response (SVR); a variable region of IL-28B (rs12979860) in a non-coding region 4 kb upstream the gene. In a multi-ethnic study of patients affected with HCV genotype 1, patient homozygous for the major allele of rs12979860 (CC) of IL-28B were twice as likely to achieve SVR as patients with even one copy of the minor allele (TT or CC) following combination therapy. Later McCarthy et al. [170] confirmed these findings in another multi-ethnic study involving patients infected with HCC genotypes 1, 2 and 3. Thus, the SNP status of this gene has remained the single strongest predictive factor for SVR.

SVR is affected in several ways by the favorable CC genotype. For instance, these patients show a higher likelihood of clearing the virus spontaneously even without treatment [170]. Differences in the antiviral cytokine response conveyed by IL-28B polymorphisms can also lead to different inflammatory states with the unfavorable genotype leading to higher frequencies of hepatic steatosis and fibrosis [146–150]. Due to its predictive value, IL-28B genotyping is now frequently used as a molecular test for HCV. Methods used to determine SNPs include RFLP, direct sequencing, high-resolution melting, sequencing, denaturing high-performance liquid chromatography, and allele- specific PCR. In most cases these assays have a near 100 % concordance [171–174].

The role of IL-28B in chronic HCV infection is an example of how personalized genotyping can be incorporated into the clinical arena affecting therapeutic decisions. Even with the recent introduction of new direct acting antiviral agents, the test is still useful in predicting treatment outcomes. It's useful in helping predict or control re-infection following liver transplantation [175]. In addition, extensive studies of IL-28B have yielded novel insights into the antiviral response to HCV. For example, the therapeutic role of INF-α is being studied as a less toxic alternative to INF-α therapy. Future studies may provide additional insights into ISG response that may even extend beyond the scope of HCV.

7.8 Direct HCC Molecular Tests

Presently there are relatively few molecular diagnostics tests that are performed directly on HCC and most molecular testing is directed towards conditions such as HH, hepatitis B and C, and IL-28B testing which modify an individual's risk for HCC and other liver diseases. The main importance of these tests, as related to HCC, is that the vast majority of HCC arises in the context of chronic liver disease and cirrhosis, which HH, and hepatitis B and C cause. While several direct HCC molecular tests show promise, a few are presently done and the main diagnostic tool for HCC remains a combination of imaging and histological analysis supplemented with immunohistochemistry [28, 175]. Here we will briefly review these tests.

7.8.1 Gene Expression Profiling in HCC

A major cause of morbidity and mortality for individuals with HCCs small enough to be enough to be surgically respected is eventual recurrence, which happens in most patients [176, 177]. Histological parameters are useful in predicting recurrence, including tumor multinodularity and vascular invasion [176]. Hoshida et al. [30] used gene-expression profiling to identify gene expression patterns associated with HCC recurrence. Initially, tissue samples from 106 patients with primary HCC were collected and the patients' clinical outcomes were followed over period of 7.8 years. Later a "validation set" of 234 HCCs from different patients were also obtained. The formalin-fixed, paraffin-embedded tumor samples were cut into 10 μM thick sections, after being macrodissected to isolate the HCC and adjacent benign liver, and were subjected to RNA extraction. The gene profiling was done by DNA-mediated annealing, extension, and ligation assay hybridized to a 6,100 transcriptionally informative gene array. Genes whose expression was associated with disease-specific survival and recurrence time were selected via Cox score analysis. One hundred and eighty six genes were identified that correlated with recurrence. Genes associated with a better prognosis were usually related to normal liver function and to drug metabolism, while those associated with a poor prognosis were involved in inflammation, interferon signaling, NF-κB, and TNF-α. The downstream targets of IL-6 were especially associated with a poor prognosis. These results were applied to 225 HCC tumor samples from the US and Europe and, despite a modest follow-up period (2.2 years), a significant difference in survival was seen that strongly correlated with the expression pattern of the 186 previously identified genes. Although this assay would be difficult to apply to a clinical setting, in the future simpler strip assays may be a useful prognostic test for HCC recurrence.

Similarly, several different studies have used gene expression profiling and similar techniques to demonstrate differences between hepatic dysplastic nodules and early HCC [40, 178–180]. Llovet et al. [180] identified 12 genes that were significantly differently expressed between hepatic dysplastic nodules and early HCC.

These genes included TETm GPC3, gankyrin, survivin, TOP2A, LYVE1, E-cadherin, IGFBP3, PDGFRA, TGFA, cyclin D1, and HGF. Analysis of these genes allowed a 94 % discriminative accuracy. Interestingly, GPC3 immunostaining was found to be 100 % expressed in HHC and not at all in dysplastic nodules.

7.8.2 *MicroRNA Testing in Hepatocellular Carcinoma*

miRNAs are major regulators of gene expression and are associated with HCC and other liver diseases. They are evolutionarily conserved, endogenously expressed non-coding ssRNA sequences usually 20–24 nucleotides long. They regulate the integrity and translational stability of up to 500 different mRNAs, enabling them to often control entire transcriptional programs that determine cellular properties and behavior. Interestingly, it has been estimated that 20–80 % of transcribed human genes are in part miRNA regulated. The dysregulated expression level of specific miRNAs has been shown to influence liver disease from fibrosis to HCC development, progression, and metastasis [181].

Recently, several studies have shown dysregulated miRNA expression in HCC compared to benign liver, with some of these miRNAs found to be aberrantly expressed in more than one study. Among the upregulated miRNAs are miR-18, miR-21, miR-221, miR-222, and miR-224. Among the downregulated miRNAs are miR-122, miR-125, miR-130a, miR-150, miR-199 and miR-200 [182]. For example, the liver-specific tumor suppressor miR-122 is significantly downregulated in HCC tissues. It functions by suppressing Cyclin G1 protein expression; a cyclin that promotes cell cycle progression. ADAM17 (a disintegrin and metalloprotease family 17) is involved in metastasis and is also suppressed by miR-122. There are also many mechanisms by which tumor-promoting miRNAs affect target genes. For example, miR-221 suppresses the cyclin-dependent kinase inhibitors CDKN1B/p27 and CDKN1C/p57, shifting hepatocytes from G_1 to S phase and facilitating cell cycle progression [181, 182]. The amount of data gathered on miRNAs and HCC is impressive and specific miRNAs have been associated with HCC differentiation, metastatic potential, recurrence, and patient survival. Interestingly miRNAs are also able to differentiate between HBV and HCV infections [183–188]. Quantitative real-time reverse transcriptase PCR is most commonly used to identify and quantify specific miRNAs in HCC [189, 190]. Other researchers have successfully used microarray analysis to analyze the expression patterns of several dozen miRNAs simultaneously, in HCC [191].

7.8.3 *Promoter Methylation in HCC*

Like most tumors examined, HCC shows epigenetic changes often involving specific CpG island promoter cytosine hypermethylation, often resulting in lowered expression of tumor suppressor genes [192–196]. Yang et al. [32] examined the tissue from 62 patients who had undergone resection for HCC with curative intent. Following surgery the patients were seen every 3–6 months and assessed for tumor recurrence by such parameters as serum α-fetoprotein and high-resolution, high-detection CT. Gene expression and methylation profiling were performed on the 62 HCCs and 139 adjacent benign liver samples by initial RNA isolation followed by amplification, labeling with strepavidin-Cy3, and hybridized to an Illumina Human-6 BeadChip (Illumina Inc., CA, USA). The arrays were scanned with an Illumina BeadArray Reader confocal scanner (BeadStation 500GXDW, Illumina, Inc). Gene expression profiles of 48,803 probes from the benign liver and HCC tissue were obtained. DNA was also extracted with the QIAamp DNA Mini Kit and checked for quality by gel electrophoresis. The EZ DNA methylation kit (Zymo Research, Orange, CA, USA) was used for the bisulfite conversion of 2 μg of genomic DNA. Following this treatment and further standard treatments, the DNA was analyzed with the Infinium HumanMethylation27 V1.o BeadChip array from Illumina to genotype bisulfite-converted and unconverted CpG sites of over 14,000 genes. The DNA was biotinylated and assay oligonucleotides were added and hybridized to resuspended DNA. Allele-specific extension and ligation of the hybridized oligonucleotides was performed; fluor-labeled strands were then hybridized to the Illumina HumanMethylation27 BeadChip. Arrays were scanned with an Illumina BeadArray Reader confocal scanner. The chip interrogates 27,578 CpG sites of over 14,000 genes. Within the HCC tissue samples, 12 genes were identified showing Cog site hypermethylation with concomitant lowered mRNA expression and a significant association with HCC recurrence. An additional 25 genes showed CpG site hypomethylation, increased concomitant mRNA expression, and a significant association with HCC recurrence. While encouraging, the author state that their results need further validation, but may eventually have prognostic and diagnostic value.

7.8.4 Specific Genes Dysregulated/Mutated in HCC

Several gene have been identified which are often mutated in HCCs. Some of these gene alterations can be tested in HCC, but only a few are routinely done presently.

p 53 Testing p53 is mutated in over 50 % of human malignancies [197]. p53 is the most commonly mutated tumor suppressor gene in HCC, with 27 % showing p53 mutations (range 0–67 %), and is correlated with tumor grade, progression, survival, and recurrence [198–203]. p53 is analyzed by many different methods, although immunohistochemistry and Sanger sequencing have been the most commonly used [203, 204].

β-catenin β-catenin (CTNNB1) is mutated in approximately 30 %, making it the commonly mutated oncogene in HCC [205]. HCCs with β-catenin mutations tend to show increased chromosomal instability, a well-differentiated histology, and cholestasis [206]. Molecular testing for β-catenin mutations is usually done via DNA isolation followed by PCR amplification of specific exons, followed by sequencing

[205]. β-catenin mutation testing in HCC is predominately performed for research purposes and has few clinical applications.

CK19 CK19 is not normally expressed by benign hepatocytes, although normal bile duct cells express it. CK19 expression is significantly higher in HCC lymph node metastases and its expression is a predictor of early postoperative recurrence due to increased invasiveness. CK19 testing is almost always performed by immunohistochemistry and molecular techniques are seldom used in its analysis [207].

H-Tert H-Tert is widely over expressed in many human malignancies [208]. Yang et al. [209] used real-time quantitative fluorescent PCR to quantify H-Tert in the Plasma samples were collected from 60 HCC patients, 21 patients with hepatitis B virus (HBV) and 29 healthy controls. H-Tert DNA was significantly higher in the plasma of individuals with HCC compared to those with HBV and normal controls. Thus plasma H-Tert DNA may have some value in screening for and detecting HCC.

Metastatic Liver Disease The majority of hepatic malignancies are metastatic to the liver with HCC far less common [210]. Molecular diagnostics performed on malignancies metastatic to the liver are those done for the primary tumor, such as KRAS testing performed on colorectal carcinoma metastatic to the liver [211].

References

1. Ferlay J, Shin HR, Bray F, Forman D, Mathers C, Parkin DM (2010) Estimates of worldwide burden of cancer in 2008: GLOBOCAN 2008. Int J Cancer 127:2893–2917
2. Forner A, Llovet JM, Bruix J (2012) Hepatocellular carcinoma. Lancet 379:1245–1255
3. Bosetti C, Levi F, Boffetta P, Lucchini F, Negri E, La Vecchia C (2008) Trends in mortality from hepatocellular carcinoma in Europe, 1980–2004. Hepatology 48:137–145
4. Qiu D, Katanoda K, Marugame T, Sobue T (2009) A Joinpoint regression analysis of long-term trends in cancer mortality in Japan (1958–2004). Int J Cancer 124:443–448
5. Chen CJ, Yang HI, Su J, Jen CL, You SL, Lu SN, Huang GT, Iloeje UH (2006) Risk of hepatocellular carcinoma across a biological gradient of serum hepatitis B virus DNA level. JAMA 295:65–73
6. Chang MH, Chen CJ, Lai MS, Hsu HM, Wu TC, Kong MS, Liang DC, Shau WY, Chen DS (1997) Universal hepatitis B vaccination in Taiwan and the incidence of hepatocellular carcinoma in children. Taiwan Childhood Hepatoma Study Group. N Engl J Med 336:1855–1859
7. Papatheodoridis GV, Lampertico P, Manolakopoulos S, Lok A (2010) Incidence of hepatocellular carcinoma in chronic hepatitis B patients receiving nucleos(t)ide therapy: a systematic review. J Hepatol 53:348–356
8. MacDonald DC, Nelson M, Bower M, Powles T (2008) Hepatocellular carcinoma, human immunodeficiency virus and viral hepatitis in the HAART era. World J Gastroenterol 14:1657–1663
9. Kew MC (2009) Hepatic iron overload and hepatocellular carcinoma. Cancer Lett 286:38–43
10. Santos PC, Krieger JE, Pereira AC (2012) Molecular diagnostic and pathogenesis of hereditary hemochromatosis. Int J Mol Sci 13:1497–1511
11. Strachan AS (1929) Hemosiderosis and hemochromatosis in South African natives with a comment on the aetiology of hemochromatosis. M.D. thesis, University of Glasgow, Glasgow

12. Shackelford RE, Kaufmann WK, Paules RS (2000) Oxidative stress and cell cycle checkpoint function. Free Radic Biol Med 28:1387–1404
13. Gordeuk VR, McLaren CE, MacPhail AP, Deichsel D, Bothwell TH (1996) Associations of iron overload in Africa and hepatocellular carcinoma and tuberculosis. Blood 87:3470–3476
14. Trichopoulos D, Bamia C, Lagiou P et al (2011) Hepatocellular carcinoma risk factors and disease burden in a European cohort: a nested case–control study. J Natl Cancer Inst 103:1686–1695
15. Bravi F, Bosetti C, Tavani A, Bagnardi V, Gallus S, Negri E, Franceschi S, La Vecchia C (2007) Coffee drinking and hepatocellular carcinoma risk: a meta-analysis. Hepatology 46:430–435
16. Yu MC, Yuan JM (2004) Environmental factors and risk for hepatocellular carcinoma. Gastroenterology 127:S72–S78
17. Chuang SC, La Vecchia C, Boffetta P (2009) Liver cancer: descriptive epidemiology and risk factors other than HBV and HCV infection. Cancer Lett 286:9–14
18. Pietrangelo A (2004) Hereditary hemochromatosis – a new look at an old disease. N Engl J Med 350:2383–2397
19. Bradbear RA, Bain C, Siskind V, Schofield FD, Webb S, Axelsen EM, Halliday JW, Bassett ML, Powell LW (1985) Cohort study of internal malignancy in genetic hemochromatosis and other chronic non- alcoholic liver diseases. J Natl Cancer Inst 75:81–84
20. Strohmeyer G, Niederau C, Stremmel W (1988) Survival and causes of death in hemochromatosis. Observations in 163 patients. Ann N Y Acad Sci 526:245–257
21. Bacon BR (2012) Hemochromatosis: discovery of the HFE gene. Mo Med 109:133–136
22. Adams PC, Speechley M, Kertesz AE (1991) Long-term survival analysis inhereditary hemochromatosis. Gastroenterology 101:368–372
23. Zhang H, Zhai Y, Hu Z, Wu C, Qian J et al (2010) Genome-wide association study identifies 1p36.22 as a new susceptibility locus for hepatocellular carcinoma in chronic hepatitis B virus carriers. Nat Genet 42:755–758
24. Chan KY, Wong CM, Kwan JS et al (2011) Genome-wide association study of hepatocellular carcinoma in Southern Chinese patients with chronic hepatitis B virus infection. PLoS One 6:e28798
25. Clifford RJ, Zhang J, Meerzaman DM, Lyu MS et al (2010) Genetic variations at loci involved in the immune response are risk factors for hepatocellular carcinoma. Hepatology 52:2034–2043
26. Tanabe KK, Lemoine A, Finkelstein DM, Kawasaki H et al (2008) Epidermal growth factor gene functional polymorphism and the risk of hepatocellular carcinoma in patients with cirrhosis. JAMA 299:53–60
27. Hassan MM, Spitz MR, Thomas MB et al (2009) The association of family history of liver cancer with hepatocellular carcinoma: a case–control study in the United States. J Hepatol 50:334–341
28. Sakamoto M, Effendi K, Masugi Y (2010) Molecular diagnosis of multistage hepatocarcinogenesis. Jpn J Clin Oncol 40:891–896
29. International Consensus Group for Hepatocellular Neoplasia (2009) Pathologic diagnosis of early hepatocellular carcinoma: a report of the international consensus group for hepatocellular neoplasia. Hepatology 49:658–664
30. Hoshida Y, Villanueva A, Kobayashi M et al (2008) Gene expression in fixed tissues and outcome in hepatocellular carcinoma. N Engl J Med 359:1995–2004
31. Dong H, Ge X, Shen Y, Chen L et al (2009) Gene expression profile analysis of human hepatocellular carcinoma using SAGE and LongSAGE. BMC Med Genomics 2:5
32. Yang J, Seol SY, Leem SH et al (2011) Genes associated with recurrence of hepatocellular carcinoma: integrated analysis by gene expression and methylation profiling. J Korean Med Sci 26:1428–1438
33. Evans CG, Chang L, Gestwicki JE (2010) Heat shock protein 70 (hsp70) as an emerging drug target. J Med Chem 53:4585–4602
34. Garrido C, Gurbuxani S, Ravagnan L, Kroemer G (2001) Heat shock proteins: endogenous modulators of apoptotic cell death. Biochem Biophys Res Commun 286:433–442

35. Helmbrecht K, Zeise E, Rensing L (2000) Chaperones in cell cycle regulation and mitogenic signal transduction: a review. Cell Prolif 33:341–365
36. Ciocca DR, Calderwood SK (2005) Heat shock proteins in cancer: diagnostic, prognostic, predictive, and treatment implications. Cell Stress Chaperones 10:86–103
37. Rohde M, Daugaard M, Jensen MH, Helin K, Nylandsted J, Jaattela M (2005) Members of the heat- shock protein 70 family promote cancer cell growth by distinct mechanisms. Genes Dev 19:570–582
38. Sliutz G, Karlseder J, Tempfer C, Orel L, Holzer G, Simon MM (1996) Drug resistance against gemcitabine and topotecan mediated by constitutive hsp70 overexpression in vitro: implication of quercetin as sensitiser in chemotherapy. Br J Cancer 74:172–177
39. Seo JS, Park YM, Kim JI, Shim EH, Kim CW, Jang JJ, Kim SH, Lee WH (1996) T cell lymphoma in transgenic mice expressing the human Hsp70 gene. Biochem Biophys Res Commun 218:582–587
40. Chuma M, Sakamoto M, Yamazaki K et al (2003) Expression profiling in multistage hepatocarcinogenesis: identification of HSP70 as a molecular marker of early hepatocellular carcinoma. Hepatology 37(1):198–207
41. Di Tommaso L, Franchi G, Park YN et al (2007) Diagnostic value of HSP70, glypican 3, and glutamine synthetase in hepatocellular nodules in cirrhosis. Hepatology 45:725–734
42. Park IK, Qian D, Kiel M, Becker MW, Pihalja M, Weissman IL, Morrison SJ, Clarke MF (2003) Bmi-1 is required for maintenance of adult self-renewing haematopoietic stem cells. Nature 23:302–305
43. Valk-Lingbeek ME, Bruggeman SW, van Lohuizen M (2004) Stem cells and cancer; the polycomb connection. Cell 118:409–418
44. Dimri GP, Martinez JL, Jacobs JJ, Keblusek P, Itahana K, Van Lohuizen M et al (2002) The Bmi-1 oncogene induces telomerase activity and immortalizes human mammary epithelial cells. Cancer Res 62:4736–4745
45. Glinsky GV (2007) Stem cell origin of death-from-cancer phenotypes of human prostate and breast cancers. Stem Cell Rev 3:79–93
46. Wang H, Pan K, Zhang HK, Weng DS, Zhou J, Li JJ, Huang W, Song HF, Chen MS, Xia JC (2008) Increased polycomb-group oncogene Bmi-1 expression correlates with poor prognosis in hepatocellular carcinoma. J Cancer Res Clin Oncol 134:535–541
47. Li DW, Tang HM, Fan JW, Yan DW, Zhou CZ, Li SX, Wang XL, Peng ZH (2010) Expression level of Bmi-1 oncoprotein is associated with progression and prognosis in colon cancer. J Cancer Res Clin Oncol 136:997–1006
48. Wu Z, Min L, Chen D, Hao D, Duan Y, Qiu G, Wang Y (2011) Overexpression of BMI-1 promotes cell growth and resistance to cisplatin treatment in osteosarcoma. PLoS One 6:e14648
49. Effendi K, Mori T, Komuta M, Masugi Y, Du W, Sakamoto M (2010) Bmi-1 gene is upregulated in early-stage hepatocellular carcinoma and correlates with ATP-binding cassette transporter B1 expression. Cancer Sci 101:666–672
50. Liaw SH, Kuo I, Eisenberg D (1995) Discovery of the ammonium substrate site on glutamine synthetase, a third cation binding site. Protein Sci 4:2358–2365
51. Reitzer LJ, Wice BM, Kennell D (1979) Evidence that glutamine, not sugar, is the major energy source for cultured HeLa cells. J Biol Chem 254:2669–2676
52. Moorman AF, de Boer PA, Geerts WJ et al (1988) Complementary distribution of carbamoylphosphate synthetase (ammonia) and glutamine synthetase in rat liver acinus is regulated at a pretranslational level. J Histochem Cytochem 36:751–755
53. Zucman-Rossi J, Benhamouche S, Godard C et al (2007) Differential effects of inactivated Axin1 and activated beta-catenin mutations in human hepatocellular carcinomas. Oncogene 26:774–780
54. Cadoret A, Ovejero C, Terris B et al (2002) New targets of beta-catenin signaling in the liver are involved in the glutamine metabolism. Oncogene 21:8293–8301
55. Christa L, Simon MT, Flinois JP et al (1994) Overexpression of glutamine synthetase in human primary liver cancer. Gastroenterology 106:1312–1320

56. Osada T, Sakamoto M, Nagawa H et al (1999) Acquisition of glutamine synthetase expression in human hepatocarcinogenesis: relation to disease recurrence and possible regulation by ubiquitin-dependent proteolysis. Cancer 85:819–831
57. Bioulac-Sage P, Rebouissou S, Thomas C et al (2007) Hepatocellular adenoma subtype classification using molecular markers and immunohistochemistry. Hepatology 46:740–748
58. Bialecki ES, Di Bisceglie AM (2005) Diagnosis of hepatocellular carcinoma. HPB (Oxford) 7:26–34
59. Varma V, Cohen C (2004) Immunohistochemical and molecular markers in the diagnosis of hepatocellular carcinoma. Adv Anat Pathol 11:239–249
60. Hubberstey AV, Mottillo EP (2002) Cyclase-associated proteins: CAPacity for linking signal transduction and actin polymerization. FASEB J 16:487–499
61. Yu G, Swiston J, Young D (1994) Comparison of human CAP and CAP2, homologs of the yeast adenylyl cyclase-associated proteins. J Cell Sci 107:1671–1678
62. Shibata R, Mori T, Du W, Chuma M, Gotoh M, Shimazu M et al (2006) Overexpression of cyclase-associated protein 2 in multistage hepatocarcinogenesis. Clin Cancer Res 12:5363–5368
63. Libbrecht L, Severi T, Cassiman D et al (2006) Glypican-3 expression distinguishes small hepatocellular carcinomas from cirrhosis, dysplastic nodules, and focal nodular hyperplasia-like nodules. Am J Surg Pathol 30:1405–1411
64. Wang XY, Degos F, Dubois S, Tessiore S et al (2006) Glypican-3 expression in hepatocellular tumors: diagnostic value for preneoplastic lesions and hepatocellular carcinomas. Hum Pathol 37:1435–1441
65. Abdul-Al HM, Makhlou HR, Wang G, Goodman ZD (2008) Glypican-3 expression in benign liver tissue with active hepatitis C: implications for the diagnosis of hepatocellular carcinoma. Hum Pathol 39:209–212
66. Nakatsuka T, Kageshita T, Ito S, Wakamatsu K, Monji M, Ikuta Y et al (2004) Identification of glypican-3 as a novel tumor marker for melanoma. Clin Cancer Res 10:6612–6621
67. http://www.amptestdirectory.org/index.cfm
68. Gan EK, Powell LW, Olynyk JK (2011) Natural history and management of HFE-hemochromatosis. Semin Liver Dis 31:293–301
69. Santos PC, Dinardo CL, Cançado RD et al (2012) Non-HFE hemochromatosis. Rev Bras Hematol Hemoter 34:311–316
70. Feder JN, Gnirke A, Thomas W, Tsuchihashi Z, Ruddy DA et al (1996) A novel MHC class-I gene is mutated in patients with hereditary haemochromatosis. Nat Genet 13:399–408
71. Sanchez M, Bruguera M, Rodes J, Oliva R (2001) Complete characterization of the 39 region of the human and mouse hereditary hemochromatosis HFE gene and detection of novel splicing forms. Blood Cells Mol Dis 27:35–43
72. Jeffrey GP, Basclain K, Hajek J, Chakrabarti S, Adams PC (1999) Alternate splicing produces a soluble form of the hereditary hemochromatosis protein HFE. Blood Cells Mol Dis 25:61–67
73. Rhodes DA, Trowsdale J (1999) Alternate splice variants of the hemochromatosis gene HFE. Immunogenetics 49:357–359
74. Thenie A, Orhant M, Gicquel I, Fergelot P, Le Gall JY et al (2000) The HFE gene undergoes alternate splicing processes. Blood Cells Mol Dis 26:155–162
75. Martins R, Silva B, Proenca D, Faustino P (2011) Differential HFE gene expression is regulated by alternative splicing in human tissues. PLoS One 6:e17542
76. Worwood M, Shearman JD, Wallace DF, Dooley LS, Merryweather- Clarke AT, Pointon LL et al (1997) A simple genetic test identifies 90 % of UK patients with haemochromatosis. Gut 41:841–844
77. Bridle KR, Frazer DM, Wilkins SJ, Dixon JL, Purdie DM, Crawford DH, Subramaniam VN, Powell LW, Anderson GJ, Ramm GA (2003) Disrupted hepcidin regulation in HFE-associated haemochromatosis and the liver as a regulator of body iron homoeostasis. Lancet 361:669–673
78. Stott MK, Fellowes AP, Upton JD, Burt MJ, George PM (1999) Simple multiplex PCR for the simultaneous detection of the C282Y and H63D hemochromatosis (HFE) gene mutations. Clin Chem 45:426–428

79. Huang MM, Arnheim N, Goodman MF (1992) Extension of base mispairs by Taq DNA polymerase: implications for single nucleotide discrimination in PCR. Nucleic Acids Res 20:4567–4573
80. Kimura H, Kasahara K, Kawaishi M, Kunitoh H, Tamura T, Holloway B, Nishio K (2006) Detection of epidermal growth factor receptor mutations in serum as a predictor of the response to gefitinib in patients with non-small-cell lung cancer. Clin Cancer Res 12:3915–3921
81. Sánchez M, Villa M, Ingelmo M et al (2003) Population screening for hemochromatosis: a study in 5370 Spanish blood donors. J Hepatol 38:745–750
82. Higuchi R (1989) DNA from whole blood for PCR. Amplifications 2:1–3
83. Cukjati M, Koren S, Curin Serbec V, Vidan-Jeras B, Rupreht R (2007) A novel homozygous frameshift deletion c.471del of HFE associated with hemochromatosis. Clin Genet 71:350–353
84. Gemmati D, Zeri G, Orioli E, De Gaetano FE et al (2012) Polymorphisms in the genes coding for iron binding and transporting proteins are associated with disability, severity, and early progression in multiple sclerosis. BMC Med Genet 13:70
85. Bach V, Barceló MJ, Altés A et al (2006) Genotyping the HFE gene by melting point analysis with the LightCycler system: pros and cons. Blood Cells Mol Dis 36:288–291
86. Aguilar-Martinez P, Lok CY, Cunat S, Cadet E, Robson K, Rochette J (2007) Juvenile hemochromatosis caused by a novel combination of hemojuvelin G320V/R176C mutations in a 5-year old girl. Haematologica 92:421–422
87. De Lima Santos PC, Pereira AC, Cancado RD, Schettert IT, Hirata RD, Hirata MH, Figueiredo MS, Chiattone CS, Krieger JE, Guerra-Shinohara EM (2010) Hemojuvelin and hepcidin genes sequencing in Brazilian patients with primary iron overload. Genet Test Mol Biomark 14:803–806
88. Lanzara C, Roetto A, Daraio F, Rivard S, Ficarella R, Simard H, Cox TM, Cazzola M, Piperno A, Gimenez-Roqueplo AP et al (2004) Spectrum of hemojuvelin gene mutations in 1q-linked juvenile hemochromatosis. Blood 103:4317–4321
89. Lee PL, Beutler E, Rao SV, Barton JC (2004) Genetic abnormalities and juvenile hemochromatosis: mutations of the HJV gene encoding hemojuvelin. Blood 103:4669–4671
90. Roetto A, Papanikolaou G, Politou M et al (2003) Mutant antimicrobial peptide hepcidin is associated with severe juvenile hemochromatosis. Nat Genet 33:21–22
91. Hattori A, Tomosugi N, Tatsumi Y et al (2012) Identification of a novel mutation in the HAMP gene that causes non-detectable hepcidin molecules in a Japanese male patient with juvenile hemochromatosis. Blood Cells Mol Dis 48:179–182
92. Biasiotto G, Belloli S, Ruggeri G et al (2003) Identification of new mutations of the HFE, hepcidin, and transferrin receptor 2 genes by denaturing HPLC analysis of individuals with biochemical indications of iron overload. Clin Chem 49:1981–1988
93. Kawabata H, Yang R, Hirama T, Vuong PT, Kawano S, Gombart AF, Koeffler HP (1999) Molecular cloning of transferrin receptor 2: a new member of the transferrin receptor-like family. J Biol Chem 274:20826–20832
94. Roetto A, Totaro A, Piperno A et al (2001) New mutations inactivating transferrin receptor 2 in hemochromatosis type 3. Blood 97:2555–2560
95. Anderson GJ, Vulpe CD (2009) Mammalian iron transport. Cell Mol Life Sci 66:3241–3261
96. Yang F, Liu X, Quinones M, Melby PC, Ghio A, Haile DJ (2002) Regulation of reticuloendothelial iron transporter MTP1 (Slc11a3) by inflammation. J Biol Chem 277:39786–39791
97. Pietrangelo A, Caleffi A, Corradini E (2011) Non-HFE hepatic iron overload. Semin Liver Dis 31:302–318
98. Montosi G, Donovan A, Totaro A et al (2001) Autosomal-dominant hemochromatosis is associated with a mutation in the ferroportin (SLC11A3) gene. J Clin Invest 108:619–623
99. Pietrangelo A, Montosi G, Totaro A et al (1999) Hereditary hemochromatosis in adults without pathogenic mutations in the hemochromatosis gene. N Engl J Med 341:725–732
100. Lavanchy D (2004) Hepatitis B, virus epidemiology, disease burden, treatment, and current and emerging prevention and control measures. J Viral Hepat 11:97–107

101. Liaw YF, Chu CM (2009) Hepatitis B virus infection. Lancet 373:582–592
102. Dienstag JL (2008) Hepatitis B, virus infection. N Engl J Med 359:1486–1500
103. Valsamakis A (2007) Molecular testing in the diagnosis and management of chronic hepatitis B. Clin Microbiol Rev 20:426–439
104. Martinot-Peignoux M, Boyer N, Colombat M et al (2002) Serum hepatitis B virus DNA levels and liver histology in inactive HBsAg carriers. J Hepatol 36:543–546
105. Ishak K, Baptista A, Bianchi L et al (1995) Histological grading and staging of chronic hepatitis. J Hepatol 22:696–699
106. Berninger M, Hammer M, Hoyer B, Gerin J (1982) An assay for the detection of the DNA genome of hepatitis B virus in serum. J Med Virol 9:57–68
107. Guo KJ, Bowden DS (1991) Digoxigenin-labeled probes for the detection of hepatitis B virus DNA in serum. J Clin Microbiol 29:506–509
108. Tsongalis GJ (2006) Branched DNA, technology in molecular diagnostics. Am J Clin Pathol 126:448–453
109. Chen CH, Wang JT, Lee CZ et al (1995) Quantitative detection of hepatitis B virus DNA in human sera by branched-DNA signal amplification. J Virol Methods 53:131–137
110. Abe A, Inoue K, Tanaka T et al (1999) Quantitation of hepatitis B virus genomic DNA by real-time detection PCR. J Clin Microbiol 37:2899–2903
111. Mackay IM, Arden KE, Nitsche A (2002) Real-time PCR in virology. Nucleic Acids Res 30:1292–1305
112. Nolan T, Hands RE, Bustin SA (2006) Quantification of mRNA using real-time RT-PCR. Nat Protoc 1:1559–1582
113. Germer JJ, Qutub MO, Mandrekar JN et al (2006) Quantification of hepatitis B virus (HBV) DNA with a TaqMan HBV analyte-specific reagent following sample processing with the MagNA pure LC instrument. J Clin Microbiol 44:1490–1494
114. Wang Q, Wang X, Zhang J, Song G (2012) LNA real-time PCR probe quantification of hepatitis B virus DNA. Exp Ther Med 3:503–508
115. Veedu RN, Wengel J (2010) Locked nucleic acids: promising nucleic acid analogs for therapeutic applications. Chem Biodivers 7:536–542
116. Orito E, Mizokami M, Ina Y, Moriyama EN et al (1989) Host-independent evolution and a genetic classification of the hepadnavirus family based on nucleotide sequences. Proc Natl Acad Sci U S A 86:7059–7062
117. Okamoto H, Tsuda F, Sakugawa H et al (1988) Typing hepatitis B virus by homology in nucleotide sequence: comparison of surface antigen subtypes. J Gen Virol 69:2575–2583
118. Stuyver L, De Gendt S, Van Geyt C et al (2000) A new genotype of hepatitis B virus: complete genome and phylogenetic relatedness. J Gen Virol 81:67–74
119. Miyakawa Y, Mizokami M (2003) Classifying hepatitis B virus genotypes. Intervirology 46:329–338
120. Kidd-Ljunggren K, Miyakawa Y, Kidd AH (2002) Genetic variability in hepatitis B viruses. J Gen Virol 83:1267–1280
121. Kao JH, Chen PJ, Lai MY, Chen DS (2000) Hepatitis B genotypes correlate with clinical outcomes in patients with chronic hepatitis B. Gastroenterology 118:554–559
122. Thakur V, Guptan RC, Kazim SN et al (2002) Profile, spectrum and significance of HBV genotypes in chronic liver disease patients in the Indian subcontinent. J Gastroenterol Hepatol 17:165–170
123. Wiegand J, Hasenclever D, Tillmann HL (2008) Should treatment of hepatitis B depend on hepatitis B virus genotypes? A hypothesis generated from an explorative analysis of published evidence. Antivir Ther 13:211–220
124. Janssen HL, van Zonneveld M, Senturk H et al (2005) Pegylated interferon alfa-2b alone or in combination with lamivudine for HBeAg-positive chronic hepatitis B: a randomised trial. Lancet 365:123–129
125. Koedijk FD, van Houdt R, Op de Coul EL et al (2008) Hepatitis B virus transmission patterns in the Netherlands, 2004. Ned Tijdschr Geneeskd 152:2673–2680
126. Alam MM, Zaidi SZ, Shaukat S et al (2007) Common genotypes of hepatitis B virus prevalent in injecting drug abusers (addicts) of North West Frontier Province of Pakistan. Virol J 4:63

127. Guirgis BS, Abbas RO, Azzazy HM (2010) Hepatitis B virus genotyping: current methods and clinical implications. Int J Infect Dis 14:e941–e953
128. http://www.medical-siemens.com.
129. Lindstom A, Odeberg J, Albert J (2004) Pyrosequencing for detection of lamivudine-resistant hepatitis B virus. J Clin Microbiol 42:4788–4795
130. Liu WC, Lindh M, Buti M et al (2008) Genotyping of hepatitis B virus – genotypes a to g by multiplex polymerase chain reaction. Intervirology 51:247–252
131. Yeh SH, Tsai CY, Kao JH et al (2004) Quantification and genotyping of hepatitis B virus in a single reaction by real-time PCR and melting curve analysis. J Hepatol 41:659–666
132. Lindh M, Andersson AS, Gusdal A (1997) Genotypes, nt 1858 variants, and geographic origin of hepatitis B virus – large-scale analysis using a new genotyping method. J Infect Dis 175:1285–1293
133. Lee JM, Ahn SH, Chang HY et al (2004) Reappraisal of HBV genotypes and clinical significance in Koreans using MALDI-TOF mass spectrometry. Korean J Hepatol 10:260–270
134. Kriegshäuser G, Auner V, Schuster E et al (2011) KRAS mutation analysis in genomic DNA isolated from formalin-fixed paraffin-embedded ovarian tissue: evaluation of a strip-based reverse-hybridisation assay. J Clin Pathol 64:252–256
135. Prix L, Uciechowski P, Böckmann B, Giesing M, Schuetz AJ (2002) Diagnostic biochip array for fast and sensitive detection of K-ras mutations in stool. Clin Chem 48:428–435
136. Ausch C, Buxhofer-Ausch V, Oberkanins C et al (2009) Sensitive detection of KRAS mutations in archived formalin-fixed paraffin-embedded tissue using mutant-enriched PCR and reverse-hybridization. J Mol Diagn 11:508–513
137. Fariña Sarasqueta A, Moerland E, de Bruyne H et al (2011) SNaPshot and StripAssay as valuable alternatives to direct sequencing for KRAS mutation detection in colon cancer routine diagnostics. J Mol Diagn 13:199–205
138. Gauthier M, Bonnaud B, Arsac M et al (2010) Microarray for hepatitis B virus genotyping and detection of 994 mutations along the genome. J Clin Microbiol 48:4207–4215
139. Tran N, Berne R, Chann R et al (2006) European multicenter evaluation of high-density DNA probe arrays for detection of hepatitis B virus resistance mutations and identification of genotypes. J Clin Microbiol 44:2792–2800
140. Ali MM, Hasan F, Ahmad S, Al-Nakib W (2010) Comparative evaluation of INNO-LiPA HBV assay, direct DNA sequencing and subtractive PCR-RFLP for genotyping of clinical HBV isolates. Virol J 7:111
141. Olivier M (2005) The Invader assay for SNP genotyping. Mutat Res 573:103–110
142. Tadokoro K, Kobayashi M, Yamaguchi T et al (2006) Classification of hepatitis B virus genotypes by the PCR-Invader method with genotype-specific probes. J Virol Methods 138:30–39
143. http://www.innogenetics.com/infectiousdiseases_detail.html?id=9
144. http://www.questdiagnostics.com/testcenter/testguide.action?dc=TS_HBV_Genotype_BCP_
145. Hanafiah KM, Groeger J, Flaxman AD, Wiersma ST (2012) Global epidemiology of hepatitis C virus infection: new estimates of age-specific antibody to hepatitis C virus seroprevalence. Hepatology. doi:10.1002/hep.26141
146. Kim WR (2002) The burden of hepatitis C in the United States. Hepatology 36:S30–S34
147. Robertson B, Myers G, Howard C et al (1998) Classification, nomenclature, and database development for hepatitis C virus (HCV) and related viruses: proposals for standardization. Arch Virol 143:2493–2503
148. NIH Consens State Sci Statements (2002) 19:1–46
149. Robertson B, Myers G, Howard C et al (1998) Classification, nomenclature, and database development for hepatitis C virus (HCV) and related viruses: proposals for standardization. International Committee on Virus Taxonomy. Arch Virol 143:2493–2503
150. Hnatyszyn HJ (2005) Chronic hepatitis C and genotyping: the clinical significance of determining HCV genotypes. Antivir Ther 10:1–11
151. http://www.hepatitis.va.gov/patient/treat/decisions-single-page.asp
152. Scott JD, Gretch DR (2007) Molecular diagnostics of hepatitis C virus infection: a systematic review. JAMA 297:724–732

153. Pearlman BL (2011) The IL-28 genotype: how it will affect the care of patients with hepatitis C virus infection. Curr Gastroenterol Rep 13:78–86
154. Bonetti P, Chemello L, Antona C et al (1997) Treatment of chronic hepatitis C with interferon-alpha by monitoring the response according to viraemia. J Viral Hepat 4:107–112
155. Tong MJ, Blatt LM, Tong LT et al (1998) Long-term retreatment in chronic hepatitis C patients who were non-responders to an initial course of interferon-alpha 2b. J Viral Hepat 5:323–331
156. Kleiber J, Walter T, Haberhausen G et al (2000) Performance characteristics of a quantitative, homogeneous TaqMan RT-PCR test for HCV RNA. J Mol Diagn 2:158–166
157. Halfon P, Bourlière M, Pénaranda G et al (2006) Real-time PCR assays for hepatitis C virus (HCV) RNA quantitation are adequate for clinical management of patients with chronic HCV infection. J Clin Microbiol 44:2507–2511
158. Fried MW, Shiffman ML, Reddy KR et al (2002) Peginterferon alfa-2a plus ribavirin for chronic hepatitis C virus infection. N Engl J Med 347:975–982
159. Manns MP, McHutchison JG, Gordon SC et al (2001) Peginterferon alfa-2b plus ribavirin compared with interferon alfa-2b plus ribavirin for initial treatment of chronic hepatitis C: a randomized trial. Lancet 358:958–965
160. Verbeeck J, Maes P, Lemey P, Pybus OG et al (2006) Investigating the origin and spread of hepatitis C virus genotype 5a. J Virol 80:4220–4226
161. Nguyen MH, Keeffe EB (2005) Prevalence and treatment of hepatitis C virus genotypes 4, 5 and 6. Clin Gastroenterol Hepatol 3:S97–S101
162. Legrand-Abravanel F, Sandres-Saune K, Barange L et al (2004) Hepatitis C virus genotype 5: epidemiological characteristics and sensitivity to combination therapy with interferon-alpha plus ribavirine. J Infect Dis 189:1397–1400
163. Verbeeck J, Stanley MJ, Shieh J et al (2008) Evaluation of Versant hepatitis C virus genotype assay (LiPA) 2.0. J Clin Microbiol 46:1901–1906
164. Elahi E, Pourmand N, Chaung R et al (2003) Determination of hepatitis C virus genotype by Pyrosequencing. J Virol Methods 109:171–176
165. Nakatani SM, Santos CA, Riediger IN et al (2011) Comparative performance evaluation of hepatitis C virus genotyping based on the 5′ untranslated region versus partial sequencing of the NS5B region of Brazilian patients with chronic hepatitis C. Virol J 8:459
166. Schutzbank TE, Sefers SE, Kahmann N et al (2006) Comparative evaluation of three commercially available methodologies for hepatitis C virus genotyping. J Clin Microbiol 44:3797–3798
167. Ank N, Paludan SR (2009) Type III interferons: new layers of complexity in innate antiviral immunity. Biofactors 35:82–87
168. Pagliaccetti NE, Eduardo R, Kleinstein SH et al (2008) Interleukin-29 (inteferon-lambda1) functions cooperatively with interferon to induce antiviral gene expression and inhibit hepatitis C replication. J Biol Chem 283:30079–30089
169. Ge D, Fellay J, Thompson AJ et al (2009) Genetic variation in IL28B predicts hepatitis C treatment-induced viral clearance. Nature 461:399–401
170. McCarthy JJ, Li JH, Thompson A, Suchindran S et al (2010) Replicated association between an IL28B gene variant and a sustained response to pegylated interferon and ribavirin. Gastroenterology 138:2307–2314
171. Fiorina L, Paolucci S, Papadimitriou S, Baldanti F (2012) Comparison of three different methods for the evaluation of IL28 and ITPA polymorphisms in patients infected with HCV. J Virol Methods 184:103–105
172. Cook L, Diem K, Kim W et al (2012) Allele-specific PCR for determination of IL28B genotype. J Clin Microbiol 50:4144–4146
173. Sharafi H, Pouryasin H, Alavian SM et al (2012) Development and validation of a simple, rapid and inexpensive PCR-RFLP method for genotyping of common IL28B polymorphisms: a useful pharmacogenetic tool for prediction of hepatitis C treatment response. Hepat Mon 12:190–195
174. Ito K, Higami K et al (2011) The rs8099917 polymorphism, when determined by a suitable genotyping method, is a better predictor for response to pegylated alpha interferon/ribavirin

therapy in Japanese patients than other single nucleotide polymorphisms associated with interleukin-28B. J Clin Microbiol 49:1853–1860
175. Eurich D, Boas-Knoop S, Ruehl M et al (2011) Relationship between the interleukin-28b gene polymorphism and the histological severity of hepatitis C virus-induced graft inflammation and the response to antiviral therapy after liver transplantation. Liver Transpl 17:289–298
176. Llovet JM, Burroughs A, Bruix J (2003) Hepatocellular carcinoma. Lancet 362:1907–1917
177. Llovet JM, Bruix J (2008) Novel advancements in the management of hepatocellular carcinoma in 2008. J Hepatol 48(Suppl 1):S20–S37
178. Paradis V, Bièche I, Dargère D et al (2003) Molecular profiling of hepatocellular carcinomas (HCC) using a large-scale real-time RT-PCR approach: determination of a molecular diagnostic index. Am J Pathol 163:733–741
179. Nam SW, Park JY, Ramasamy A et al (2005) Molecular changes from dysplastic nodule to hepatocellular carcinoma through gene expression profiling. Hepatology 42:809–818
180. Llovet JM, Chen Y, Wurmbach E et al (2006) A molecular signature to discriminate dysplastic nodules from early hepatocellular carcinoma in HCV cirrhosis. Gastroenterology 131:1758–1767
181. Haybaeck J et al (2011) The parallel universe: microRNAs and their role in chronic hepatitis, liver tissue damage and hepatocarcinogenesis. Swiss Med Wkly 141:w13287
182. Gramantieri L et al (2008) MicroRNA involvement in hepatocellular carcinoma. J Cell Mol Med 12:2189–2204
183. Coulouarn C, Factor VM, Andersen JB et al (2009) Loss of miR-122 expression in liver cancer correlates with suppression of the hepatic phenotype and gain of metastatic properties. Oncogene 28:3526–3536
184. Budhu A, Jia HL, Forgues M et al (2008) Identification of metastasis-related microRNAs in hepatocellular carcinoma. Hepatology 47:897–907
185. Zhang J, Yang Y, Yang T et al (2010) MicroRNA-22, downregulated in hepatocellular carcinoma and correlated with prognosis, suppresses cell proliferation and tumourigenicity. Br J Cancer 103:1215–1220
186. Ura S, Honda M, Yamashita T et al (2009) Differential microRNA expression between hepatitis B and hepatitis C leading disease progression to hepatocellular carcinoma. Hepatology 49:1098–1112
187. Chung GE, Yoon JH, Myung SJ et al (2010) High expression of microRNA-15b predicts a low risk of tumor recurrence following curative resection of hepatocellular carcinoma. Oncol Rep 23:113–119
188. Ji J, Shi J, Budhu A et al (2009) MicroRNA expression, survival, and response to interferon in liver cancer. N Engl J Med 361:1437–1447
189. Wang W, Zhao LJ, Tan YX et al (2012) MiR-138 induces cell cycle arrest by targeting cyclin D3 in hepatocellular carcinoma. Carcinogenesis 33:1113–1120
190. He XX, Chang Y, Meng FY et al (2012) MicroRNA-375 targets AEG-1 in hepatocellular carcinoma and suppresses liver cancer cell growth in vitro and in vivo. Oncogene 31:3357–3369
191. Huang YS, Dai Y, Yu XF et al (2008) Microarray analysis of microRNA expression in hepatocellular carcinoma and non-tumorous tissues without viral hepatitis. J Gastroenterol Hepatol 23:87–94
192. Antequera F, Bird A (1993) Number of CpG islands and genes in human and mouse. Proc Natl Acad Sci U S A 90:11995–11999
193. Antequera F, Boyes J, Bird A (1990) High levels of de novo methylation and altered chromatin structure at CpG islands in cell lines. Cell 62:503–514
194. Baylin SB, Hoppener JW, de Bustros A et al (1986) DNA methylation patterns of the calcitonin gene in human lung cancers and lymphomas. Cancer Res 46:2917–2922
195. Baylin SB, Fearon ER, Vogelstein B et al (1987) Hypermethylation of the 5′ region of the calcitonin gene is a property of human lymphoid and acute myeloid malignancies. Blood 70:412–417

196. de Bustros A, Nelkin BD, Silverman A et al (1985) The short arm of chromosome 11 is a "hot spot" for hypermethylation in human neoplasia. Proc Natl Acad Sci U S A 85:5693–5697
197. Jeng KS, Sheen IS, Chen BF, Wu JY (2000) Is the p53 gene mutation of prognostic value in hepatocellular carcinoma after resection? Arch Surg 135:1329–1333
198. Katiyar S, Dash BC, Thakur V, Guptan RC, Sarin SK, Das BC (2000) p53 tumor suppressor gene mutations in hepatocellular carcinoma patients in India. Cancer 88:1565–1573
199. Honda K, Sbisa E, Tullo A, Papeo PA et al (1998) p53 mutation is a poor prognostic indicator for survival in patients with hepatocellular carcinoma undergoing surgical tumour ablation. Br J Cancer 77:776–782
200. Heinze T, Jonas S, Karsten A, Neuhaus P (1999) Determination of the oncogenes p53 and C-erb B2 in the tumour cytosols of advanced hepatocellular carcinoma (HCC) and correlation to survival time. Anticancer Res 19:2501–2503
201. Malkin D (2001) The role of p53 in human cancer. J Neurooncol 51:231–243
202. Ryan KM, Phillips AC, Vousden KH (2001) Regulation and function of the p53 tumor suppressor protein. Curr Opin Cell Biol 13:332–337
203. Chen GG, Merchant JL, Lai PB et al (2003) Mutation of p53 in recurrent hepatocellular carcinoma and its association with the expression of ZBP-89. Am J Pathol 162:1823–1829
204. Hsia CC, Nakashima Y, Thorgeirsson SS et al (2000) Correlation of immunohistochemical staining and mutations of p53 in human hepatocellular carcinoma. Oncol Rep 7:353–356
205. Laurent-Puig P, Legoix P, Bluteau O et al (2001) Genetic alterations associated with hepatocellular carcinomas define distinct pathways of hepatocarcinogenesis. Gastroenterology 120:1763–1773
206. Audard V, Grimber G, Elie C et al (2007) Cholestasis is a marker for hepatocellular carcinomas displaying β-catenin mutations. J Pathol 212:345–352
207. Uenishi T, Kubo S, Yamamoto T et al (2003) Cytokeratin 19 expression in hepatocellular carcinoma predicts early postoperative recurrence. Cancer Sci 94:851–857
208. Kirkpatrick KL, Mokbel K (2001) The significance of human telomerase reverse transcriptase (hTERT) in cancer. Eur J Surg Oncol 27:754–760
209. Yang YJ, Chen H, Huang P, Li CH et al (2011) Quantification of plasma hTERT DNA in hepatocellular carcinoma patients by quantitative fluorescent polymerase chain reaction. Clin Invest Med 34:E238
210. Bosch FX, Ribes J, Diaz M, Cleries R (2004) Primary liver cancer: worldwide incidence and trends. Gastroenterology 127:S5–S16
211. Shackelford RE, Whitling NA, McNab P et al (2012) KRAS testing: a tool for the implementation of personalized medicine. Genes Cancer 3:459–466

Chapter 8
Molecular Diagnostics of Pancreatic Cancer

Edward J. Richards, William Kong, Mokenge Malafa, Jin Q. Cheng, and Domenico Coppola

Contents

E.J. Richards • W. Kong • J.Q. Cheng
Department of Molecular Oncology, H. Lee Moffitt Cancer Center and Research Institute, 12902 Magnolia Drive, Tampa, FL 33612, USA

M. Malafa, M.D.
Department of Surgical Oncology, H. Lee Moffitt Cancer Center and Research Institute, 12902 Magnolia Drive, Tampa, FL 33612, USA

Department of Oncological Sciences, University of South Florida College of Medicine, Tampa, USA

D. Coppola, M.D. (✉)
Department of Anatomic Pathology, H. Lee Moffitt Cancer Center and Research Institute, 12902 Magnolia Drive, Tampa, FL 33612, USA

Department of Oncological Sciences, University of South Florida College of Medicine, Tampa, USA

Department of Pathology and Cell Biology, H. Lee Moffitt Cancer Center, 12902 Magnolia Drive, Tampa, FL 33612, USA
e-mail: Domenico.coppola@moffitt.org

D. Coppola (ed.), *Molecular Pathology and Diagnostics of Cancer*, Cancer Growth and Progression 16, DOI 10.1007/978-94-007-7192-5_8,

Abstract Pancreatic cancer is a malignant disease relating to uncontrollable cell growth in the tissues of the pancreas. The vast majority of pancreatic cancers are ductal adenocarcinomas, originating in the epithelial layer of the exocrine pancreas, however some pancreatic cancers do originate in the endocrine compartment. Ductal adenocarcinomas are very aggressive cancers, associating with poor prognosis and late staging upon discovery. One reason for this is that many patients do not present symptoms until late onset of disease. Numerous research efforts have been put forth to earlier diagnose pancreatic cancer. Understanding of pancreatic cancer etiology and identification of associated tumor markers has progressed, however there is a clear need for more specific and sensitive technologies. This chapter aims to address current status of molecular diagnostics in pancreatic cancer.

Keywords Pancreatic cancer • Molecular diagnostics • Tumor markers • KRAS • Micro RNA

Abbreviations

CA-19-19	Carbohydrate antigen 19 9
CA-242	Carbohydrate antigen 242
CEA	Carcinoembryonic antigen
CK7/17/20	Cytokeratin 7/17/20
CTCs	Circulating tumor cells
GWAS	Genome wide association study
IPMNs	Intraductal papillary mucinous neoplasms

MCNs	Mucinous cystic neoplasms
MIC-1	Macrophage inhibitory cytokine 1
miRNA	MicroRNA
MSLN	Mesothelin
mtDNA	mitochondrial DNA
MUC4	Mucin 4
OPN	Osteopontin
PanINs	Pancreatic intraepithelial neoplasias
PDAC	Pancreatic ductal adenocarcinoma
SELDI	Surface enhanced laser desorption and ionization
SNP	Single nucleotide polymorphism
TPS	Tissue polypeptide specific antigen

8.1 Introduction

Pancreatic cancer ranks fourth among cancer related death in the United States. It is estimated that in 2012 there will be 43,920 new pancreatic cancer cases and that 37,390 patients will die of this disease [1]. Pancreatic cancer has a very poor prognosis with a 5-years survival of 6 % when considering tumors of all stages [2]. The majority of pancreatic cancers are ductal adenocarcinomas originating in the epithelial tissue of the exocrine pancreas, responsible for almost 95 % of cases. Though, a small percentage of pancreatic cancers can initiate in the endocrine component of the pancreas. Exocrine pancreatic cancers have a poorer prognosis compared to that of endocrine pancreatic cancers, and 5-year survival is 1 % and 15 % respectively in stage 4 presentation of disease [2]. There are three well characterized precursor lesions believed to progress to pancreatic cancer, and it is well established that such progression occurs through the accumulation of genetic mutations [3].

Pancreatic ductal adenocarcinoma is commonly diagnosed as a high stage tumor and absolute removal by surgery is not always a therapeutic option. In these cases, chemo- or radiation therapy has shown limited benefit [4]. Timely detection and diagnosis is critical to increase survival rate of this disease.

This chapter aims to address pancreatic cancer development and the current state of molecular diagnostics. The understanding in both is vital for appropriately diagnosing a patient at the earliest stage of disease. Numerous serum, pancreatic juice, and tissue markers have been evaluated for their diagnostic utility. Of greatest importance, discussed will be the recent advances in technology that have provided more specific and sensitive assays in molecular diagnosis of pancreatic cancer.

8.2 Precursor Lesions of the Pancreas

Ideally, detection of pancreatic cancer would occur prior to malignant presentation of the disease. Three well defined precursor lesions have been associated with pre-invasive disease with the potential to progress to pancreatic cancer.

8.2.1 Mucinous Cystic Neoplasms (MCNs)

MCNs occur almost exclusively in women and arise in the mucin-producing epithelial layer of cells. MCNs typically occur in the head or tail region of the pancreas and do not directly communicate with the pancreatic ductal system [5, 6]. Their defining diagnostic and histological feature is that the mucinous cystic neoplasm is supported by “ovarian-type” stroma [7]. Patients presenting with these lesions typically are on average 40–50 years of age and 5–10 years younger than those presenting invasive disease [8]. MCNs are graded as low, moderate, or high grade based upon the degree of dysplasia and architectural atypia present. One third of these lesions progress into invasive carcinoma [5, 6].

8.2.2 Intraductal Papillary Mucinous Neoplasms (IPMNs)

IPMNs arise within the epithelium of the main pancreatic duct or corresponding branch. They are mucin producing, and papillary in structure [9]. IPMNs are the most common pancreatic cystic lesion and likely to occur in the head of the pancreas in males between 60 and 70 years of age [10, 11]. It is possible to identify IPMNs using the current imaging technology available because of their large size [12]. Upon diagnosis, IMPNs are subcategorized according to the same metrics used for MCNs, and about 40 % of them progress to invasive neoplasms [13]. Both MCNs and IPMNs, if non-invasive, can be completely cured by surgical resection [14, 15].

8.2.3 Pancreatic Intraepithelial Neoplasias (PanINs)

PanINs are microscopic (<5 mm) lesions that arise in the epithelium of the pancreatic ducts, with prevalence commonly increasing with age [16]. PanINs are columnar to cuboidal cells containing mucin and displaying different degrees of architectural atypia [17]. Classified into grades based on histological analysis, these lesions are pathologically characterized as PanIN-1, PanIN-2, and PanIN-3 [16]. At the molecular level, many of the same genetic alterations seen in invasive carcinoma are also found in PanINs. For this reason, PanINs are closely associated with the genetic progression model towards low-grade neoplasia, high-grade PanIN, and eventually invasive carcinoma [18].

8.3 Molecular Pathogenesis of Pancreatic Cancer

In recent years, the molecular pathways associated with pancreatic cancer tumorigenesis have become more evident through exhaustive research efforts. Four central genetic alterations are commonly associated with malignant disease, yet these alterations can be present at the premalignant stage. Precursor lesions presenting any of these alterations should be considered to have a high risk of progression to cancer.

8.3.1 KRAS2

A member of the GTPase superfamily of proteins responsible for a range of biological functions, KRAS2 is locates at chromosome 12p12.1 and if is frequently mutated in pancreatic cancer. It is estimated that more than 90 % of pancreatic ductal adenocarcinomas harbor an activating point mutation in KRAS2, with the majority of these mutations causing an amino acid substitution at codon 12 or 13 [19, 20]. Constitutive activation derives from this mutation and results in the locking of KRAS2 in a GTP-bound active conformation. In this state KRAS2 generates aberrant signaling to downstream members of the phosphoinositide-3-kinase (PI3K) and RAF-mitogen-activated protein kinase (MAPK) pathways [21]. A small subset of pancreatic cancer without a point mutation in the KRAS2 oncogene can alternatively present with a gain-of-function point mutation in BRAF, a serine/threonine kinase downstream of KRAS2 [22].

8.3.2 p16/CDKN2A

Loss of function of the 16/CDKN2A gene (INK4A) is the most frequently observed tumor suppressor deficiency occurring in almost all pancreatic cancers [23]. Interestingly, selective inactivation of INK4A occurs through a variety of mechanisms: homozygous deletion (40 %), intragenic loss-of-function mutation of one allele and loss of second allele (40 %), and hypermethylation of the gene promoter (20 %) [23, 24]. This gene critically functions as a cyclin-dependent-kinase (CDK) inhibitor at the G1/S checkpoint of cell cycle and division therefore preventing Rb phosphorylation by CDKs and cyclin-CDK complexes [25, 26].

8.3.3 TP53

Loss of TP53 activity is the most common abnormality in human cancer and occurs in more than 50 % of pancreatic cancers. Inactivation of the TP53 tumor suppressor predominantly arises through intragenic loss-of-function mutation of one allele and loss of second allele [27]. TP53 plays a critical role in cell cycle arrest and the DNA damage response. Importantly, the p53 transcriptional targets 14-3-3 and p21 can no longer be induced for expression by a mutated p53 and fail to function in mediating these biological processes [28, 29].

8.3.4 DPC4/SMAD4

The tumor suppressor deleted-in-pancreatic-carcinoma-4 gene (DPC4 or SMAD4) loses function through homozygous deletion (30 %) or intragenic loss-of-function mutation of one allele and loss of second allele (25 %). This alteration is present in 55 % of pancreatic cancers [30]. SMAD4 signaling occurs through the transforming growth factor-beta (TGF-B) pathway with activation resulting in phosphorylation and nuclear trafficking of SMAD transcription factors and subsequent growth inhibitory effects [31, 32]. Loss of SMAD4 can be found in PanIN-3 lesions, but not in IPMNs and MCNs, and it is almost exclusive to pancreatic ductal adenocarcinoma [33, 34].

8.4 Pancreatic Tumor Markers

Numerous markers are under evaluation for their diagnostic utility in pancreatic cancer. A pancreatic tumor marker is defined as any molecule elevated to a significant degree in the diseased state that can be present in the bodily fluids and tissue. Serum carbohydrate antigen 19 9 (CA-19-9) is currently the only marker accepted for clinical use, and there is a clear need for further candidates.

8.4.1 Serum Markers

8.4.1.1 Carbohydrate Antigen 19–9 (CA-19-9)

CA-19-9 is the sialylated Lewis-a blood group oligosaccharide tumor associated antigen first identified through hybridoma antibodies generated from colorectal carcinoma [35]. It is still accepted as a clinically useful diagnostic marker for pancreatic cancer with some reservations. In 2006 the American Society of Clinical Oncology (ASCO) claimed that CA-19-9 is inadequate for reliable diagnosis when used alone, yet monitoring its levels can be of use in combination with other markers [36]. The National Academy of Clinical Biochemistry (NACB) guidelines reflect similar conclusions for its use in diagnostics, asserting that CA-19-9 can be useful in conjunction with imaging tests, such as computed tomography (CT) or endoscopic ultrasound (EUS) [37].

Nevertheless, CA-19-9 remains the standard to which performance of other candidate serum markers are compared. Two major reviews compiling 46 different studies evaluating CA-19-9 (cutoff 37 U/mL in the majority of studies) in comparison to controls groups have found the overall mean sensitivity to be 81 % and specificity to be 68 %, and the overall median sensitivity to be 79 % and specificity to be 82 % [38, 39].

There are several limitations in using CA-19-9 as a single diagnostic tool in pancreatic cancer. Namely, CA-19-9 has been shown to be elevated in other cancer types and numerous benign conditions such as acute and chronic pancreatitis, cholangitis, hepatic cirrhosis, obstructive jaundice, and choleocystitis [38–41]. Also, it is estimated that 5–10 % of Caucasian population lack the Lewis antigen, a condition in which CA19-9 cannot be detected [40, 42, 43].

8.4.1.2 Carbohydrate Antigen 242 (CA-242)

CA-242 marker was first isolated through immunization of mice with COLO 205, a human colon adenocarcinoma cell line [44]. The suggested antigenic determinant of CA-242 is sialylated carbohydrate structure related to type I chain, a similar but distinct epitope from CA-19-9 [45].

Numerous studies have been performed comparing CA-242 to other pancreatic cancer diagnostic markers including CA-19-9, carbohydrate antigen 50 (CA-50), and carcinoembryonic antigen (CEA) [46–50].

The general consensus remains that CA-242 is comparable in diagnostic performance to CA-19-9, and yet it has not proven to be superior [37]. The diagnostic utility and clinical usefulness of CA-242 is the fact that, in contrast to CA19.9, its expression is independent of Lewis-a secretor status [41].

8.4.1.3 CAM17.1

CAM17.1 antibody is a mucin based marker that detects an epitope of a sialylated blood group antigen, likely type I antigen related [51]. CAM17.1 was first assessed in pancreatic cancer through the development of an enzyme-linked antibody sandwich assay (CAM17.1/WGA) in combination with CA-19-9 assay with satisfactory results. CAM17.1 and CA-19-9 tested independently had comparable sensitivities, 78–77 %, yet CA-19-9 achieved greater specificity (88 % vs. 76 %). Combining the two assays increased sensitivity to 85 %, yet did not increase the specificity originally achieved with CAM17.1 alone [52].

Interestingly, in one study CAM17.1 significantly outscored CA-19-9 in specificity when comparing pancreatic cancer to chronic pancreatitis (90 % vs. 78 %) [53]. Equally remarkable is a large patient cohort comparing 250 patients with (n=89) and without (n=165) jaundice where CAM17.1 served to be a better marker in patients without jaundice. In this cohort both sensitivity and specificity increased (85–89 % and 81–94 % respectively) [54].

8.4.1.4 Tissue Polypeptide Specific Antigen (TPS)

TPS is an epitope derived from multiple fragments of soluble cytokeratin 18 and has shown to reflect active tumor growth rather than simple tumor burden providing diagnostic utility [55, 56]. The potential effectiveness of TPS as a useful marker in pancreatic cancer has been debatable and while outperforming CA-19-9 in monitoring palliative treatment response [57], it has not yet reached levels comparable to other diagnostic serum markers [58–60]. However, it is possible that these differences may likely be due to differential cutoffs and non-uniform study design.

More recently it has been shown that increasing the cutoff value of TPS could prove useful in discriminating pancreatic cancer versus chronic pancreatitis. When TPS (>100 U/L) and CA-19-9 (>37 U/mL) were assessed in the preoperative serum of pancreatic carcinoma patients, 100 % (46/46) patients had elevated levels of TPS compared to 70 % CA-19-9. In the same study, TPS and CA-19-9 were elevated in 22 % and 19 % of patients with chronic pancreatitis respectively. Further increasing the cutoff to 200 U/L significantly raised both sensitivity and specificity, facilitating almost complete discrimination between patient groups [53, 61].

8.4.1.5 Tissue Inhibitor of Matrix Metalloproteinase 1 (TIMP-1)

TIMP-1 gene is located at chromosome Xp11.3–p11.23 and encodes a protein capable of inhibiting the matrix metalloproteinase (MMP) family of enzymes that degrade the extracellular matrix. TIMP-1 RNA expression levels are elevated in both pancreatic tumor tissue and serum of pancreatic cancer patients [62].

In one study, TIMP-1 was significantly higher in pancreatic cancer patient sera compared to normal controls, with no correlation established between resectable versus unresectable groups. This may suggest elevated serum TIMP-1 as an early event in pancreatic tumor progression, and thus may carry diagnostic potential. When used as a single diagnostic marker, TIMP-1 did not meet the same standard as CA-19-9 in specificity, yet by combining measurements of TIMP-1, CEA, and CA-19-9, 100 % specificity was achieved [62].

8.4.1.6 Osteopontin (OPN)

OPN locates at chromosome 4q22.1 and encodes for an adhesive glycoprotein of ~44 kDa identified as a sialoprotein in bone [63]. OPN is secreted into most of the bodily fluids and is produced in osteoblasts, macrophages, smooth muscle, and other epithelia [64]. It has become clear that OPN aids in tumor progression and increases metastatic potential specifically through facilitating anchorage independent growth in transformed cells, increasing migration and invasion potential, and activating matrix metalloproteinases [65–67].

Numerous malignancies have demonstrated serum levels of OPN to be elevated, including colon, prostate, breast, and ovarian cancer, implicating its potential use as a biomarker in cancer [68, 69]. Global gene expression profiling technology first identified elevated levels of OPN in pancreatic cancer in 2002 [70]. Through the development of an ELISA based assay in initial studies, OPN demonstrated better performance in sensitivity (80 %) and specificity (97 %) as compared to CA-19-9 (sensitivity 62 % and specificity 79 %) [71].

8.4.1.7 Macrophage Inhibitory Cytokine 1 (MIC-1)

MIC-1 locates at 19p13.11 and is a divergent member of the transforming growth factor-beta (TGF-B) superfamily identified for its role inhibiting macrophage activation [72]. MIC-1 goes by several other names including growth differentiation factor 15 (GDF15), placental bone morphogenic protein (PLAB), placental transforming growth factor (PTGF-B), prostate derived factor (PDF), and non-steroidal anti-inflammatory drug-activated protein 1 (NAG-1). The MIC-1 gene product encodes a precursor peptide that is cleaved into a ~12 kDa mature form containing 7 conserved cysteine residues at the carboxyl-terminal and is secreted as a 25 kDa homodimer [72].

It has been shown that MIC-1 can perform adequately in comparison to CA-19-9 when used as a single marker in distinguishing pancreatic and periampullary adenocarcinomas from precursor lesions of the periampullary region. When combined, even greater diagnostic accuracy was achieved [73]. This same study demonstrated through a variety of molecular techniques that MIC-1 is significantly overexpressed in the cytoplasm of pancreatic tumor cells. MIC-1 levels in the serum were much lower for IPMNs and noncancerous neoplastic pancreatic cysts compared to invasive adenocarcinomas. This findings suggest that MIC-1 could be a useful marker to discriminate between these entities [73]. However, MIC-1 had limitations in differentiating between chronic pancreatitis and pancreatic adenocarcinoma and CA-19-9 still serves as a more specific marker in this regard [74]. Also, MIC-1 has been shown to be elevated in several other diseased states [75–77].

8.4.2 Tissue Markers

8.4.2.1 Cytokeratins (CK7, CK17, and CK20)

Cytokeratins, as the name implies, are cytoplasmic keratin polypeptides of intermediate size that function to provide scaffolding and structural support in epithelial cells [78]. Previously, epithelial carcinomas of unknown origin have been differentially diagnosed through the use of differential expression patterns of CK7 and CK20 [79, 80].

Two independent reports have shown similar differential CK7/CK20 expression profiles in assessing pancreatic adenocarcinomas. The results indicate that pancreatic adenocarcinomas are positive for both (CK7+/CK20+) in 65–62 % of cases.

Positivity for only CK7 (CK7+/CK20-)was seen between 26 % and 30 % of cases. The other cytokeratin profiles (CK7-/CK20+ and CK7-/CK20-), in both studies, were seen in less than 10 % of all cases [81, 82].

A later study comparing pancreatic carcinomas with nearby ampulla of Vater carcinomas demonstrated that through the use of another marker, CK17, adenocarcinomas of pancreatic origin can more readily be distinguished [83].

8.4.2.2 Mucins (MUC4)

Mucins are densely glycosylated proteins of the epithelia. These high molecular weight molecules are secreted in a gel-like form, which among other functions, facilitates their function as a protective barrier in the mucosal system. Two initial investigations of mucin expression, one using in situ hybridization and the another using immunohistochemistry, were consistent in reporting that mucin-1 (MUC1) was the predominant apomucin expressed in the normal pancreas [84, 85].

In comparing normal pancreas to pancreatic cancer using more sensitive techniques, like Northern blotting and RT-PCR, it was found that MUC4 was expressed in 75 % of pancreatic tumor tissue and 73 % of tumor cell lines, yet it was undetectable in normal pancreas and chronic pancreatitis [86]. Immunohistochemical analysis demonstrated up-regulation of MUC4 throughout pancreatic intraepithelial neoplasia progression (PanIN-1 [17 %], PanIN-2 [36 %], PanIN-3 [85 %]) that continued to elevate into invasive adenocarcinoma (89 %) [87]. This report recapitulates a progressive model for pancreatic cancer development.

8.4.2.3 Carcinoembryonic Antigen (CEA)

CEA is an anchored cell surface glycoprotein produced and utilized for cell adhesion in the developing fetus. Its expression is halted prior to birth. The fact of not being normally present in tissue and blood of healthy adults gives CEA diagnostic potential. Immunohistochemical analysis of tissue sections using dual antibody interrogation in one study demonstrated that pancreatic adenocarcinoma stained positive for CEA in 70–77 % of cases. Within this group, moderately and well differentiated tumors had a significantly greater proportion of positive cells. Normal pancreas was negative for detection using either antibody [88].

A later study using an indirect immunoperoxidase technique detected CEA in 20 of 22 pancreatic ductal adenocarcinomas. In this case, CEA detection was specific for the luminal membrane or cytoplasm of the malignant ducts, yet the surrounding normal pancreas was negative [89].

The clinical usefulness of CEA as a serum marker in pancreatic cancer diagnosis has been debatable. Studies have shown that CEA in combination with other serum markers gives limited benefit, and has proved inferior to CA-19-9 when used alone [59, 90].

8.4.2.4 Mesothelin (MSLN)

MSLN, located on chromosome 16p13.3, encodes a 69 kDa precursor that is proteolytically processed into two distinct protein products, megakaryocyte potentiating factor (MPF) and MSLN [91, 92]. MSLN results from the 40 kDa c-terminal fragment that potentially functions as a cell adhesion molecule via glycosylphosphotidylinositol (GPI) anchoring. Constitutive expression of MSLN has been confined to mesothelial cells in normal tissue of the pleura, peritoneum, and pericardium, with the potential to be overexpressed in solid tumor malignancy [91, 93].

Serial analysis of gene expression (SAGE) identified the MSLN transcript to be over-expressed in pancreatic adenocarcinoma in comparison to normal pancreas [94]. More in depth analysis combining RTqPCR, in situ hybridization, and immunohistochemistry techniques supported that MSLN is over-expressed in the vast majority of pancreatic adenocarcinomas at both RNA and protein levels [95]. Further analysis has revealed MSLN as a reliable discriminatory marker to differentiate pancreatic adenocarcinomas from both normal pancreas and chronic pancreatitis [96].

8.4.3 Pancreatic Juice Markers

8.4.3.1 DNA Methylation Alterations

It is common observation in human cancer to detect hypermethylation of CpG islands within particular gene promoters through methylation specific PCR analysis (MSP) [97]. In one study, pancreatic juice from 155 patients suspected to have pancreatic disease was collected surgically or endoscopically and analyzed using conventional MSP. Methylation in promoter regions was detected in 71.3 % of the 13-gene panel in patients confirmed to have pancreatic cancer, in comparison to chronic pancreatitis (26.7 %) and normal controls (10.9 %). Using the six most promising markers within this panel (Cyclin D2, FOXE1, NPTX2, ppENK, p16, and TFP12), quantitative MSP was able to detect pancreatic cancer with 82 % sensitivity and 100 % specificity [98].

In another study, global gene expression analysis was performed following treatment with a DNA demethylating agent to determine candidate genes that became preferentially upregulated. Three candidate genes (NPTX2, SARP2, and CLDN5) were selected and assessed for methylation status in pancreatic cancer and pancreatic juice in comparison to normal epithelia. Of these three genes, aberrant methylation of at least one was detected in 100 % of primary pancreatic carcinoma and in 75 % of pancreatic juice in known cases of cancer [99]. The results suggest DNA methylation signatures can help discriminate in the molecular diagnosis of pancreatic cancer.

8.4.3.2 KRAS Mutations in DNA

It has been well documented that KRAS point mutations occur as an early event in pancreatic tumorigenesis including precursory benign states, and therefore its identification could be of significant value in prevention and diagnostics [100–102]. A study including three groups, no pancreatic disease, benign pancreatic disease, and pancreatic cancer, assessed the presence of KRAS mutations in the pancreatic juice. Analysis using PCR mediated restriction length polymorphism (PCR/RFLP) demonstrated 0 % KRAS mutations in the groups with no pancreatic disease and benign pancreatic conditions. Yet, KRAS mutations were detected in 77 % of patients known to have malignant pancreatic cancer [103].

Another similar study found KRAS mutant alleles in the pancreatic juice via PCR/RFLP at a rate of 87.8 % of pancreatic cancer patients in comparison to 23.9 % of benign pancreatic disease. This study also compared diagnostic usefulness of detecting mutant KRAS to mutant p53 in the pancreatic juice, with KRAS significantly outperforming the latter [104].

Recently, newer technology has been developed to detect and quantify single nucleotide differences in a more sensitive manner. The LigAmp Assay, which utilizes a two-oligonucleotide interrogation system and qPCR step, has been applied to identify KRAS2 mutations in the pancreatic juice. Follow-up studies are needed, however the assay has shown to accurately quantify levels of KRAS2 mutant DNA which may prove effective in aiding early diagnosis given the fact that progressive mutation events are associated with disease progression [105].

8.5 Advances in Molecular Diagnostics of Pancreatic Cancer

In the past decade many resources and efforts have been put forth to developing better molecular based assays to detect cancer at earlier stages through more sensitive means. Despite the fact that no kits are currently commercially available for the molecular diagnosis of pancreatic cancer, the rate at which this research progresses gives a clear hint that this trend will end soon. Below is a summary of the current assays being developed likely to be soon available for use in the clinical arena in the near future.

8.5.1 MicroRNA (miRNA) Expression Profiling

MicroRNAs (miRNAs) are evolutionarily conserved short (~22 nt) non-coding RNA molecules that directly affect biological function through inhibition of target messenger RNA (mRNA) [106]. Cleavage of a precursor and trafficking of miRNA from the nucleus to the cytoplasm has previously been described in detail [107–109].

After processing, a mature form, capable of perfect or imperfect base pairing at the seed sites on mRNA, results in degradation of the transcript via the RNA induced silencing complex (RISC) or inhibition of translation through interaction with the 3′ untranslated region (3′ UTR) [110, 111]. A major attraction to miRNAs is that they are stable and can be quantified by means of real-time PCR using limited starting material required.

Initial investigations of miRNA expression profiles (miRNome) compared normal pancreas (n = 5), chronic pancreatitis (n = 6), pancreatic ductal adenocarinoma (n = 8), and pancreatic cancer cell lines (n = 6), to a reference set of 33 human tissues. Pancreatic tissue was characterized by miR-216 and miR-217 expression, and lacking miR133a expression. Twenty-six miRNAs were identified as being dysregulated in pancreatic cancer, with miR-217 and miR-196a levels sufficient to discriminate between normal pancreas, chronic pancreatitis, and other cancer tissues [112].

A similar study comparing ductal adenocarcinoma (n = 65) and adjacent normal pancreas (n = 65) identified 21 miRNAs up-regulated and 4 miRNAs down-regulated in pancreatic cancer. When comparing the same adenocarcinoma samples to chronic pancreatitis (n = 42), 15 miRNAs were found to be overexpressed while 8 miRNAs were down regulated. Notably, miR-21 and miR-155 were preferentially elevated and able to distinguish pancreatic ductal adenocarcinoma from normal pancreas and chronic pancreatitis [113]. However, further studies in pancreatic cancer miR expression profiling are needed, before specific miRNAs can be used as potential diagnostic markers in the clinic.

8.5.2 Cancer Genome Sequencing

Cancer can be classified as disease that manifests itself at the genetic level. Inherently, whole genome analysis and sequencing is a critical step in understanding the pathogenesis and progression of disease. Recent advances in massively parallel sequencing have made it possible to not only sequence the cancer genome for novel mutations [114], but also consider somatically acquired rearrangements in the context of cancer genomic instability [115]. The challenge that now faces researchers is making sense of this large amount of data, and will require efforts across multiple disciplines.

The pancreatic cancer genome was sequenced in 2008 and was analyzed for novel somatic mutations and deletions. In this study, a pattern emerged in which 12 major signaling pathways were consistently altered (ranging from 67 % to 100 % in frequency) in a given pancreatic tumor. The pathway playing the major role in driving tumorigenesis and tumor progression varied from case to case. This study has provided tremendous insight into our understanding of driver and passenger mutations in pancreatic tumorigenesis and cancer progression, and has contributed to a new perspective of personalized medicine and cancer prevention [116].

8.5.3 Mitochondrial Genome Analysis (mtDNA)

The human mitochondrial genome (mtDNA) is ~16.5 kb that encode the proteins and RNA elements essential for the organelle's processes and function. Due to its limited size, identifying mutations and copy number variation in mtDNA could prove valuable diagnostically because of the quick turn around in mitochondrial genome sequencing.

In one study, 15 pancreatic cancer cell lines (10) and xenografts (5) were analyzed for somatic mutation and copy number variation. Among the cell lines, 49 homoplasmic variations were identified that had not seen previously reported. Southern blot analysis demonstrated that mtDNA was amplified 6–7.7-fold in comparison to normal duodenal tissue in two patients [117].

It has been shown that mtDNA can be mutated and contain amplified gene copy number in response to damage through oxidative stress caused by smoking [118]. A recent study has linked higher mtDNA copy gene number and a significantly increased risk of developing pancreatic cancer in a cohort of male smokers [119]. These results suggest that mtDNA has potential for diagnostic utility for pancreatic cancer in certain populations.

8.5.4 Genome-Wide Association Study (GWAS) and Single Nucleotide Polymorphisms (SNPs)

In addition to the familial and heritable risk factors described above, newer techniques and analyses are critical for identifying a high risk population to target for the prevention and early detection of pancreatic cancer. GWASs and the identification of particular SNPs have demonstrated to be useful in regards to pancreatic cancer susceptibility.

In a two-stage GWAS initially comparing individuals with pancreatic cancer (n = 1,896) to healthy controls (n = 1,939) adjusted for age, sex, ancestry, and five principle components of population stratification, 558,542 SNPs were genotyped and analyzed. SNPs from three distinct genomic regions were fast tracked for replication, resulting in a strong association for locus rs505922 on chromosome 9q34 and pancreatic cancer [120]. This SNP, residing in intron 1 of the ABO blood group gene, is consistent with previous findings that A and B blood types are at higher risk for developing gastric and pancreatic cancer than blood type O [121, 122].

A complementary GWAS study was performed adding approximately 2,000 cases per affected and control cohorts above in order to identify additional susceptibility SNPs. Eight novel SNPs were identified within three genomic loci (13q22.1, 1q32.1, and 5p15.33) to be associated with common susceptibility in the development of pancreatic cancer [123].

8.5.5 *Microsatellite Marker Loss of Heterozygosity and K-Ras Mutation*

Current diagnostic modalities for pancreaticobiliary cancer (cholangiocarcinoma), or cancer located in the bile duct, requires endoscopic retrograde cholangiography to obtain brushings of cells for pathological evaluation. The process yields a very low diagnostic sensitivity (<60 %) due to the fact that determining malignancy is objective and based on cellularity and morphology [124–127].

As in most pancreatic cancers, numerous tumor suppressor genes are frequently deleted in pancreaticobiliary cancer. In one study, loss of heterozygosity (LOH) of a panel of 12 microsatellite markers linked to six common tumor suppressor genes (RIZ, VHL, APC, p16/CDKN2A, PTEN, TP53) was assessed via PCR in combination with KRAS point mutation at codon 12 for diagnostic utility in brush cytology specimens. Through traditional cytomorphological analysis in 17 patients comparing diseased tissue to a normal adjacent control, 8 were deemed malignant, 10 were indeterminate, and 8 were benign. Tissue categorized as malignant harbored numerous LOH with varying heterogeneity, likely due to intratumoral clonal expansion. All of these samples also contained KRAS mutation, with adjacent normal tissue and benign samples having no LOH. This study, although limited in sample size, proved his technique to have 100 % sensitivity, specificity, and accuracy [128].

A similar methodology was also applied for more accurate diagnosis when using routine endoscopic ultrasound guided fine needle aspiration (EUS-FNA). This procedure sometimes results in unnecessary surgery for patients with benign pancreatic conditions due to inconclusive cytology assessment. In comparing six known cases of benign disease to 15 cases of malignancy, a panel of 16 LOH microsatellite markers (located at 1p, 3p, 5q, 9p, 9q, 10q, 17p, 17q, 21q, and 22q) combined with presence of KRAS point mutation was able to reliably discriminate between masses using EUS-FNA samples [129].

RedPath Integrated Pathology, Inc., a leader in molecular diagnostics, presented results of a multi-institutional prospective study from 492 patient outcomes on integrated molecular pathology (IMP) at the recently held 2013 ACG Annual Meeting in San Diego, CA. Final data results validate the company's *PathFinderTG®* pancreas platform's high negative predictive value (NPV=97 %) for correctly identifying patients at very low risk of developing pancreatic cancer. Patients with low risk *PathFinderTG* diagnoses had a 97 % probability of follow up without malignancy. These low risk patients could be statistically differentiated from those with much higher risk of malignancy. Patients in the 'statistically higher risk' category have a 31-fold increased risk of cancer and those in the 'aggressive' category have a 76-fold increased risk of cancer, added Dr. Smith Redpath also offers similar tests for predicting esophageal cancer in background of Barrett's. Both tests are medicare approved [130].

8.5.6 Surface Enhanced Laser Desorption and Ionization (SELDI)

SELDI ProteinChip Arrays (Ciphergen Biosystems Inc., Fremont, CA) is a novel approach for more sensitive detection and differential profiling of serum proteins. The technique utilizes an energy absorbing matrix in combination with laser to ionize proteins of a given biological sample enabling molecular weight quantification via time-of-flight mass spectrometry [131]. SELDI offers a more high-throughput diagnostic assay for proteomic analysis and offers potential in developing predictive models in cancer. Initial studies have already demonstrated the potential success of SELDI in differentiating ovarian cancer [132, 133], prostate cancer [134–137], breast cancer [138], renal cell carcinoma [139], hepatocellular carcinoma [140] and bladder cancer [141].

Initial reports have identified two discriminatory peaks that could differentiate pancreatic cancer from healthy controls with a sensitivity of 78 % and a specificity of 97 %, proven to be significantly superior to using the CA-19-9 serum marker alone. Combining these two markers with CA-19-9 further improved diagnostic accuracy. SELDI profiling was again superior to CA-19-9 when differentiating pancreatic cancer from pancreatitis [142].

Another study combined SELDI with an artificial intelligence classification algorithm for serum screening. By using a panel of six peaks, this classification and algorithm was able to discriminate pancreatic cancer from controls with 88.9 % sensitivity and 74.1 % specificity. This methodology was challenged in a double blind test, results showed a sensitivity of 80 % and specificity of 84.6 % in differentiating pancreatic cancer from controls. Impressively, in 39 of the 47 of these cases, this technique was successful in determining patients with surgically resectable disease [143].

8.5.7 Circulating Tumor Cells (CTCs)

CTCs are malignant cells found in the peripheral blood that have detached from primary tumor site and have metastatic potential. Detecting CTCs in the context of prognosis has already proven useful, yet little is known about its potential in diagnostics [144]. Initial studies in pancreatic cancer patients found 11 of 26 (42 %) patients to be positive for CTC (1–105 cells/7.5 ml). None of the patients with chronic pancreatitis and healthy volunteers (100 %) had CTCs using CellSearch (Veridex, LLC, Raritan, NJ, USA). The presence of CTCs was significantly linked to poorer prognosis [145].

Efforts have been put forth to apply CTC detection for use in diagnostics as potential biomarkers. Two platforms, CellSearch (mentioned above) and isolation by size of epithelial tumor cells (ISET) (RareCell Diagnostics, Paris, FR), were used to compare blood samples from 54 patients. A major difference between the assays is that CellSearch captures cells expressing epithelial markers like EpCAM, and ISET is marker-independent and based on cell size and morphology. Similarly to the report above, CellSearch was able to detect CTCs in 40 % of patients, but was outperformed by ISET which detected CTCs in 93 % of cases. It is possible to account for this dramatic difference by the level of heterogeneity in epithelial markers expressed, as well as not detecting cells which may have undergone the epithelial to mesenchymal transition (EMT) [146].

It is evident that additional evaluation is needed before considering CTCs as a diagnostic tool, yet clear potential exists.

8.5.8 DNA Methylation Profiling

Epigenetic alterations and aberrant methylation of cytosine at CpG motifs are partly responsible for differential gene expression in cancer, and can be exploited in tumor profiling [147–149]. These modifications are critical events in tumorigenesis in the context of proto-oncogene and tumor suppressor gene promoters [150].

Global profiling of normal pancreas, pancreatic carcinoma, and pancreatic cancer cell lines was assessed for 807 gene promoters. The status of 289 markers were shown to be altered, and novel candidate genes for hypo- (23) and hypermethylation (35) were identified as potent oncogenes and tumor suppressors [151]. Notably, previously published markers specific to pancreatic cancer such as CCND2 and 14-3-3 also displayed an irregular methylation status in this study [152, 99].

8.6 Conclusions

Pancreatic cancer has a very poor survival due to diagnosis corresponding with later onset of disease. Clearly defined precursor lesions and the progressive molecular pathogenesis associated with pancreatic disease has provided a window of opportunity to detect pancreatic cancer prior to its development or at the earliest stage of malignancy. Over the past decade, there have been significant advancements in tumor marker identification and evaluation, yet it is clear that the majority of these markers have limitations. Recent advancements in technology and molecular diagnostics have put forth some promising alternatives with higher sensitivities and specificities. Despite the fact that commercial availability of specific diagnostic assays has yet to be approved for use in the clinic, it is evident that they will be available soon.

References

1. Siegel R, Naishadham D, Jemal A (2012) Cancer statistics, 2012. CA Cancer J Clin 62:10–29
2. American Cancer Society (2012) Pancreatic cancer, pancreatic cancer survival by stage. American Cancer Society, Atlanta
3. Vogelstein B, Kinzler KW (2004) Cancer genes and the pathways they control. Nat Med 10(8):789–799

4. Stathis A, Moore MJ (2010) Advanced pancreatic carcinoma: current treatment and future challenges. Nat Rev Clin Oncol 7(3):163–172
5. Wilentz RE, Albores-Saavedra J, Hruban RH (2000) Mucinous cystic neoplasms of the pancreas. Semin Diagn Pathol 17(1):31–42
6. Hruban RH, Klimstra DS, Pitman MB (2006) Tumors of the pancreas. Armed Forces Institute of Pathology, Washington, DC
7. Goh BK et al (2006) A review of mucinous cystic neoplasms of the pancreas defined by ovarian-type stroma: clinicopathological features of 344 patients. World J Surg 30(12):2236–2245
8. Hruban RH et al (2007) Precursors to pancreatic cancer. Gastroenterol Clin North Am 36(4):831–849, vi
9. Brat DJ et al (1998) Progression of pancreatic intraductal neoplasias to infiltrating adenocarcinoma of the pancreas. Am J Surg Pathol 22(2):163–169
10. Kosmahl M et al (2004) Cystic neoplasms of the pancreas and tumor-like lesions with cystic features: a review of 418 cases and a classification proposal. Virchows Archiv Int J Pathol 445(2):168–178
11. Kloppel G, Kosmahl M, Luttges J (2005) Intraductal neoplasms of the pancreas: cystic and common. Pathologe 26(1):31–36
12. Canto MI et al (2004) Screening for pancreatic neoplasia in high-risk individuals: an EUS-based approach. Clin Gastroenterol Hepatol Off Clin Pract J Am Gastroenterol Assoc 2(7):606–621
13. Sohn TA et al (2004) Intraductal papillary mucinous neoplasms of the pancreas: an updated experience. Ann Surg 239(6):788–797, discussion 797–9
14. D'Angelica M et al (2004) Intraductal papillary mucinous neoplasms of the pancreas: an analysis of clinicopathologic features and outcome. Ann Surg 239(3):400–408
15. Kimura W, Makuuchi M, Kuroda A (1998) Characteristics and treatment of mucin-producing tumor of the pancreas. Hepatogastroenterology 45(24):2001–2008
16. Hruban RH et al (2001) Pancreatic intraepithelial neoplasia: a new nomenclature and classification system for pancreatic duct lesions. Am J Surg Pathol 25(5):579–586
17. Hruban RH et al (2004) An illustrated consensus on the classification of pancreatic intraepithelial neoplasia and intraductal papillary mucinous neoplasms. Am J Surg Pathol 28(8):977–987
18. Maitra A, Kern SE, Hruban RH (2006) Molecular pathogenesis of pancreatic cancer. Best Pract Res Clin Gastroenterol 20(2):211–226
19. Almoguera C et al (1988) Most human carcinomas of the exocrine pancreas contain mutant c-K-ras genes. Cell 53(4):549–554
20. Hruban RH et al (1993) K-ras oncogene activation in adenocarcinoma of the human pancreas. A study of 82 carcinomas using a combination of mutant-enriched polymerase chain reaction analysis and allele-specific oligonucleotide hybridization. Am J Pathol 143(2):545–554
21. Hingorani SR, Tuveson DA (2003) Ras redux: rethinking how and where Ras acts. Curr Opin Genet Dev 13(1):6–13
22. Calhoun ES et al (2003) BRAF and FBXW7 (CDC4, FBW7, AGO, SEL10) mutations in distinct subsets of pancreatic cancer: potential therapeutic targets. Am J Pathol 163(4):1255–1260
23. Schutte M et al (1997) Abrogation of the Rb/p16 tumor-suppressive pathway in virtually all pancreatic carcinomas. Cancer Res 57(15):3126–3130
24. Caldas C et al (1994) Frequent somatic mutations and homozygous deletions of the p16 (MTS1) gene in pancreatic adenocarcinoma. Nat Genet 8(1):27–32
25. Russo AA et al (1998) Structural basis for inhibition of the cyclin-dependent kinase Cdk6 by the tumour suppressor p16INK4a. Nature 395(6699):237–243
26. Liggett WH Jr, Sidransky D (1998) Role of the p16 tumor suppressor gene in cancer. J Clin Oncol Off J Am Soc Clin Oncol 16(3):1197–1206
27. Redston MS et al (1994) p53 mutations in pancreatic carcinoma and evidence of common involvement of homocopolymer tracts in DNA microdeletions. Cancer Res 54(11):3025–3033

28. Hermeking H et al (1997) 14-3-3 sigma is a p53-regulated inhibitor of G2/M progression. Mol Cell 1(1):3–11
29. Chan TA et al (1999) 14-3-3Sigma is required to prevent mitotic catastrophe after DNA damage. Nature 401(6753):616–620
30. Hahn SA et al (1996) DPC4, a candidate tumor suppressor gene at human chromosome 18q21.1. Science 271(5247):350–353
31. Massague J, Blain SW, Lo RS (2000) TGFbeta signaling in growth control, cancer, and heritable disorders. Cell 103(2):295–309
32. Siegel PM, Massague J (2003) Cytostatic and apoptotic actions of TGF-beta in homeostasis and cancer. Nat Rev Cancer 3(11):807–821
33. Iacobuzio-Donahue CA et al (2000) Dpc4 protein in mucinous cystic neoplasms of the pancreas: frequent loss of expression in invasive carcinomas suggests a role in genetic progression. Am J Surg Pathol 24(11):1544–1548
34. Wilentz RE et al (2000) Loss of expression of Dpc4 in pancreatic intraepithelial neoplasia: evidence that DPC4 inactivation occurs late in neoplastic progression. Cancer Res 60(7): 2002–2006
35. Koprowski H et al (1979) Colorectal carcinoma antigens detected by hybridoma antibodies. Somatic Cell Genet 5(6):957–971
36. Locker GY, Hamilton S, Harris J, Jessup JM, Kemeny N, Macdonald JS, Somerfield MR, Hayes DF, Bast RC Jr, ASCO (2006) ASCO 2006 update of recommendations for the use of tumor markers in gastrointestinal cancer. Clin Oncol 24(33):5313–5327, Nov 20, Epub 2006 Oct 23
37. Diamandis P, Hoffman BR, Sturgeon CM (2208) National academy of clinical biochemistry laboratory medicine practice guidelines for the use of tumor markers. Clin Chem 54(11):1935–1939
38. Steinberg W (1990) The clinical utility of the CA 19–9 tumor-associated antigen. Am J Gastroenterol 85(4):350–355
39. Goonetilleke KS, Siriwardena AK (2007) Systematic review of carbohydrate antigen (CA 19–9) as a biochemical marker in the diagnosis of pancreatic cancer. Eur J Surg Oncol J Eur Soc Surg Oncol Br Assoc Surg Oncol 33(3):266–270
40. Duffy MJ (1998) CA 19–9 as a marker for gastrointestinal cancers: a review. Ann Clin Biochem 35(Pt 3):364–370
41. Lamerz R (1999) Role of tumour markers, cytogenetics. Ann Oncol 10(Suppl 4):145–149
42. Albert MB, Steinberg WM, Henry JP (1988) Elevated serum levels of tumor marker CA19-9 in acute cholangitis. Dig Dis Sci 33(10):1223–1225
43. Takasaki H et al (1988) Correlative study on expression of CA 19–9 and DU-PAN-2 in tumor tissue and in serum of pancreatic cancer patients. Cancer Res 48(6):1435–1438
44. Lindholm L, Johansson C, Jansson E-L, Hallberg C, Nilsson O (1985) An immunoradiometric assay (IRMA) for the CA-50 antigen. In: Holgren J (ed) Tumor marker antigen. Studentlitteratur, Lund, p 123
45. Nilsson O et al (1992) Sensitivity and specificity of CA242 in gastro-intestinal cancer. A comparison with CEA, CA50 and CA 19–9. Br J Cancer 65(2):215–221
46. Rothlin MA, Joller H, Largiader F (1993) CA 242 is a new tumor marker for pancreatic cancer. Cancer 71(3):701–707
47. Kawa S et al (1994) Comparative study of CA242 and CA19-9 for the diagnosis of pancreatic cancer. Br J Cancer 70(3):481–486
48. Haglund C et al (1994) CA 242, a new tumour marker for pancreatic cancer: a comparison with CA 19–9, CA 50 and CEA. Br J Cancer 70(3):487–492
49. Ventrucci M et al (1998) Serum CA 242: the search for a valid marker of pancreatic cancer. Clin Chem Lab Med CCLM/FESCC 36(3):179–184
50. Ozkan H, Kaya M, Cengiz A (2003) Comparison of tumor marker CA 242 with CA 19–9 and carcinoembryonic antigen (CEA) in pancreatic cancer. Hepatogastroenterology 50(53):1669–1674
51. Eccleston DW et al (1998) Pancreatic tumour marker anti-mucin antibody CAM 17.1 reacts with a sialyl blood group antigen, probably I, which is expressed throughout the human gastrointestinal tract. Digestion 59(6):665–670

52. Parker N et al (1992) A new enzyme-linked lectin/mucin antibody sandwich assay (CAM 17.1/WGA) assessed in combination with CA 19–9 and peanut lectin binding assay for the diagnosis of pancreatic cancer. Cancer 70(5):1062–1068
53. Gansauge F et al (1996) CAM 17.1–a new diagnostic marker in pancreatic cancer. Br J Cancer 74(12):1997–2002
54. Yiannakou JY et al (1997) Prospective study of CAM 17.1/WGA mucin assay for serological diagnosis of pancreatic cancer. Lancet 349(9049):389–392
55. Rydlander L et al (1996) Molecular characterization of a tissue-polypeptide-specific-antigen epitope and its relationship to human cytokeratin 18. Eur J Biochem/FEBS 241(2):309–314
56. Bjorklund B, Bjorklund V (1983) Specificity and basis of the tissue polypeptide antigen. Cancer Detect Prev 6(1–2):41–50
57. Kornek G et al (1995) Tissue polypeptide-specific antigen (TPS) in monitoring palliative treatment response of patients with gastrointestinal tumours. Br J Cancer 71(1):182–185
58. Banfi G et al (1993) Behavior of tumor markers CA19.9, CA195, CAM43, CA242, and TPS in the diagnosis and follow-up of pancreatic cancer. Clin Chem 39(3):420–423
59. Pasanen PA, Eskelinen M, Partanen K, Pikkarainen P, Penttilä I, Alhava E (1994) A prospective study of serum tumour markers carcinoembryonic antigen, carbohydrate antigens 50 and 242, tissue polypeptide antigen and tissue polypeptide specific antigen in the diagnosis of pancreatic cancer with special reference to multivariate diagnostic score. Br J Cancer 69(3):562–565
60. Plebani M et al (1993) Clinical utility of TPS, TPA and CA 19–9 measurement in pancreatic cancer. Oncology 50(6):436–440
61. Slesak B et al (2000) Tissue polypeptide specific antigen (TPS), a marker for differentiation between pancreatic carcinoma and chronic pancreatitis. A comparative study with CA 19–9. Cancer 89(1):83–88
62. Zhou W et al (1998) Identifying markers for pancreatic cancer by gene expression analysis. Cancer Epidemiol Biomarkers Prev Publ Am Assoc Cancer Res Cosponsored Am Soc Prev Oncol 7(2):109–112
63. Prince CW et al (1987) Isolation, characterization, and biosynthesis of a phosphorylated glycoprotein from rat bone. J Biol Chem 262(6):2900–2907
64. O'Brien ER et al (1994) Osteopontin is synthesized by macrophage, smooth muscle, and endothelial cells in primary and restenotic human coronary atherosclerotic plaques. Arterioscler Thromb J Vasc Biol/Am Heart Assoc 14(10):1648–1656
65. Rittling SR, Chambers AF (2004) Role of osteopontin in tumour progression. Br J Cancer 90(10):1877–1881
66. Wu Y, Denhardt DT, Rittling SR (2000) Osteopontin is required for full expression of the transformed phenotype by the ras oncogene. Br J Cancer 83(2):156–163
67. Philip S, Bulbule A, Kundu GC (2001) Osteopontin stimulates tumor growth and activation of promatrix metalloproteinase-2 through nuclear factor-kappa B-mediated induction of membrane type 1 matrix metalloproteinase in murine melanoma cells. J Biol Chem 276(48): 44926–44935
68. Fedarko NS et al (2001) Elevated serum bone sialoprotein and osteopontin in colon, breast, prostate, and lung cancer. Clin Cancer Res Off J Am Assoc Cancer Res 7(12):4060–4066
69. Kim JH et al (2002) Osteopontin as a potential diagnostic biomarker for ovarian cancer. JAMA 287(13):1671–1679
70. Iacobuzio-Donahue CA et al (2002) Discovery of novel tumor markers of pancreatic cancer using global gene expression technology. Am J Pathol 160(4):1239–1249
71. Koopmann J et al (2004) Evaluation of osteopontin as biomarker for pancreatic adenocarcinoma. Cancer Epidemiol Biomarkers Prev Publ Am Assoc Cancer Res Cosponsored Am Soc Prev Oncol 13(3):487–491
72. Bootcov MR et al (1997) MIC-1, a novel macrophage inhibitory cytokine, is a divergent member of the TGF-beta superfamily. Proc Natl Acad Sci U S A 94(21):11514–11519
73. Koopmann J et al (2004) Serum macrophage inhibitory cytokine 1 as a marker of pancreatic and other periampullary cancers. Clin Cancer Res Off J Am Assoc Cancer Res 10(7):2386–2392

74. Koopmann J et al (2006) Serum markers in patients with resectable pancreatic adenocarcinoma: macrophage inhibitory cytokine 1 versus CA19-9. Clin Cancer Res Off J Am Assoc Cancer Res 12(2):442–446
75. Buckhaults P et al (2001) Secreted and cell surface genes expressed in benign and malignant colorectal tumors. Cancer Res 61(19):6996–7001
76. Welsh JB et al (2003) Large-scale delineation of secreted protein biomarkers overexpressed in cancer tissue and serum. Proc Natl Acad Sci U S A 100(6):3410–3415
77. Welsh JB et al (2001) Analysis of gene expression identifies candidate markers and pharmacological targets in prostate cancer. Cancer Res 61(16):5974–5978
78. Franke WW, Schmid E, Osborn M, Weber K (1979) Intermediate-sized filaments of human endothelial cells. J Cell Biol 81(3):570–580
79. Miettinen M (1995) Keratin 20: immunohistochemical marker for gastrointestinal, urothelial, and Merkel cell carcinomas. Mod Pathol Off J US Can Acad Pathol 8(4):384–388
80. Ramaekers F et al (1990) Use of monoclonal antibodies to keratin 7 in the differential diagnosis of adenocarcinomas. Am J Pathol 136(3):641–655
81. Wang N, Zee S, Zarbo R et al (1995) Coordinate expression of cytokeratin 7 and 20 defines unique subsets of carcinomas. Appl Immunohistochem 3(2):99–107
82. Chu P, Wu E, Weiss LM (2000) Cytokeratin 7 and cytokeratin 20 expression in epithelial neoplasms: a survey of 435 cases. Mod Pathol Off J US Can Acad Pathol 13(9):962–972
83. Goldstein NS, Bassi D (2001) Cytokeratins 7, 17, and 20 reactivity in pancreatic and ampulla of vater adenocarcinomas. Percentage of positivity and distribution is affected by the cut-point threshold. Am J Clin Pathol 115(5):695–702
84. Balague C et al (1994) Altered expression of MUC2, MUC4, and MUC5 mucin genes in pancreas tissues and cancer cell lines. Gastroenterology 106(4):1054–1061
85. Terada T et al (1996) Expression of MUC apomucins in normal pancreas and pancreatic tumours. J Pathol 180(2):160–165
86. Andrianifahanana M et al (2001) Mucin (MUC) gene expression in human pancreatic adenocarcinoma and chronic pancreatitis: a potential role of MUC4 as a tumor marker of diagnostic significance. Clin Cancer Res Off J Am Assoc Cancer Res 7(12):4033–4040
87. Swartz MJ et al (2002) MUC4 expression increases progressively in pancreatic intraepithelial neoplasia. Am J Clin Pathol 117(5):791–796
88. Allum WH et al (1986) Demonstration of carcinoembryonic antigen (CEA) expression in normal, chronically inflamed, and malignant pancreatic tissue by immunohistochemistry. J Clin Pathol 39(6):610–614
89. Heyderman E et al (1990) Epithelial markers in pancreatic carcinoma: immunoperoxidase localisation of DD9, CEA, EMA and CAM 5.2. J Clin Pathol 43(6):448–452
90. Ni XG et al (2005) The clinical value of serum CEA, CA19-9, and CA242 in the diagnosis and prognosis of pancreatic cancer. Eur J Surg Oncol J Eur Soc Surg Oncol Br Assoc Surg Oncol 31(2):164–169
91. Chang K, Pastan I (1996) Molecular cloning of mesothelin, a differentiation antigen present on mesothelium, mesotheliomas, and ovarian cancers. Proc Natl Acad Sci U S A 93(1):136–140
92. Kojima T et al (1995) Molecular cloning and expression of megakaryocyte potentiating factor cDNA. J Biol Chem 270(37):21984–21990
93. Scholler N et al (1999) Soluble member(s) of the mesothelin/megakaryocyte potentiating factor family are detectable in sera from patients with ovarian carcinoma. Proc Natl Acad Sci U S A 96(20):11531–11536
94. Chang K, Pastan I, Willingham MC (1992) Isolation and characterization of a monoclonal antibody, K1, reactive with ovarian cancers and normal mesothelium. Int J Cancer 50(3):373–381
95. Argani P et al (2001) Mesothelin is overexpressed in the vast majority of ductal adenocarcinomas of the pancreas: identification of a new pancreatic cancer marker by serial analysis of gene expression (SAGE). Clin Cancer Res Off J Am Assoc Cancer Res 7(12):3862–3868

96. Hassan R et al (2005) Mesothelin is overexpressed in pancreaticobiliary adenocarcinomas but not in normal pancreas and chronic pancreatitis. Am J Clin Pathol 124(6):838–845
97. Feinberg AP, Tycko B (2004) The history of cancer epigenetics. Nat Rev Cancer 4(2):143–153
98. Matsubayashi H et al (2006) DNA methylation alterations in the pancreatic juice of patients with suspected pancreatic disease. Cancer Res 66(2):1208–1217
99. Sato N et al (2003) Discovery of novel targets for aberrant methylation in pancreatic carcinoma using high-throughput microarrays. Cancer Res 63(13):3735–3742
100. Bos JL et al (1987) Prevalence of ras gene mutations in human colorectal cancers. Nature 327(6120):293–297
101. Cerny WL, Mangold KA, Scarpelli DG (1992) K-ras mutation is an early event in pancreatic duct carcinogenesis in the Syrian golden hamster. Cancer Res 52(16):4507–4513
102. Luttges J et al (1999) The K-ras mutation pattern in pancreatic ductal adenocarcinoma usually is identical to that in associated normal, hyperplastic, and metaplastic ductal epithelium. Cancer 85(8):1703–1710
103. Berthelemy P et al (1995) Identification of K-ras mutations in pancreatic juice in the early diagnosis of pancreatic cancer. Ann Intern Med 123(3):188–191
104. Lu X et al (2002) Detecting K-ras and p53 gene mutation from stool and pancreatic juice for diagnosis of early pancreatic cancer. Chin Med J 115(11):1632–1636
105. Shi C et al (2004) LigAmp for sensitive detection of single-nucleotide differences. Nat Methods 1(2):141–147
106. Farh KK et al (2005) The widespread impact of mammalian MicroRNAs on mRNA repression and evolution. Science 310(5755):1817–1821
107. Lee Y et al (2003) The nuclear RNase III Drosha initiates microRNA processing. Nature 425(6956):415–419
108. Han J et al (2004) The Drosha-DGCR8 complex in primary microRNA processing. Genes Dev 18(24):3016–3027
109. Yi R et al (2003) Exportin-5 mediates the nuclear export of pre-microRNAs and short hairpin RNAs. Genes Dev 17(24):3011–3016
110. Tang G (2005) siRNA and miRNA: an insight into RISCs. Trends Biochem Sci 30(2):106–114
111. Gregory RI et al (2005) Human RISC couples microRNA biogenesis and posttranscriptional gene silencing. Cell 123(4):631–640
112. Szafranska AE et al (2007) MicroRNA expression alterations are linked to tumorigenesis and non-neoplastic processes in pancreatic ductal adenocarcinoma. Oncogene 26(30):4442–4452
113. Bloomston M et al (2007) MicroRNA expression patterns to differentiate pancreatic adenocarcinoma from normal pancreas and chronic pancreatitis. JAMA 297(17):1901–1908
114. Ley TJ et al (2008) DNA sequencing of a cytogenetically normal acute myeloid leukaemia genome. Nature 456(7218):66–72
115. Campbell PJ et al (2008) Identification of somatically acquired rearrangements in cancer using genome-wide massively parallel paired-end sequencing. Nat Genet 40(6):722–729
116. Jones S et al (2008) Core signaling pathways in human pancreatic cancers revealed by global genomic analyses. Science 321(5897):1801–1806
117. Jones JB et al (2001) Detection of mitochondrial DNA mutations in pancreatic cancer offers a "mass"-ive advantage over detection of nuclear DNA mutations. Cancer Res 61(4):1299–1304
118. Lee HC et al (1998) Aging- and smoking-associated alteration in the relative content of mitochondrial DNA in human lung. FEBS Lett 441(2):292–296
119. Lynch SM et al (2011) Mitochondrial DNA copy number and pancreatic cancer in the alpha-tocopherol beta-carotene cancer prevention study. Cancer Prev Res 4(11):1912–1919
120. Amundadottir L et al (2009) Genome-wide association study identifies variants in the ABO locus associated with susceptibility to pancreatic cancer. Nat Genet 41(9):986–990
121. Aird I, Bentall HH, Roberts JA (1953) A relationship between cancer of stomach and the ABO blood groups. Br Med J 1(4814):799–801
122. Marcus DM (1969) The ABO and Lewis blood-group system. Immunochemistry, genetics and relation to human disease. N Eng J Med 280(18):994–1006

123. Petersen GM et al (2010) A genome-wide association study identifies pancreatic cancer susceptibility loci on chromosomes 13q22.1, 1q32.1 and 5p15.33. Nat Genet 42(3):224–228
124. Stewart CJ et al (2001) Brush cytology in the assessment of pancreatico-biliary strictures: a review of 406 cases. J Clin Pathol 54(6):449–455
125. Pugliese V et al (2001) Pancreatic intraductal sampling during ERCP in patients with chronic pancreatitis and pancreatic cancer: cytologic studies and k-ras-2 codon 12 molecular analysis in 47 cases. Gastrointest Endosc 54(5):595–599
126. Farrell RJ et al (2001) The combination of stricture dilation, endoscopic needle aspiration, and biliary brushings significantly improves diagnostic yield from malignant bile duct strictures. Gastrointest Endosc 54(5):587–594
127. Glasbrenner B et al (1999) Prospective evaluation of brush cytology of biliary strictures during endoscopic retrograde cholangiopancreatography. Endoscopy 31(9):712–717
128. Khalid A et al (2004) Use of microsatellite marker loss of heterozygosity in accurate diagnosis of pancreaticobiliary malignancy from brush cytology samples. Gut 53(12):1860–1865
129. Khalid A et al (2006) Endoscopic ultrasound fine needle aspirate DNA analysis to differentiate malignant and benign pancreatic masses. Am J Gastroenterol 101(11):2493–2500
130. Khalid A et al (2009) Pancreatic cyst fluid DNA analysis in evaluating pancreatic cysts: a report of the PANDA study. Gastrointest Endosc 69(6):1095–1102
131. Merchant M, Weinberger SR (2000) Recent advancements in surface-enhanced laser desorption/ionization-time of flight-mass spectrometry. Electrophoresis 21(6):1164–1177
132. Petricoin EF et al (2002) Use of proteomic patterns in serum to identify ovarian cancer. Lancet 359(9306):572–577
133. Kozak KR et al (2003) Identification of biomarkers for ovarian cancer using strong anion-exchange ProteinChips: potential use in diagnosis and prognosis. Proc Natl Acad Sci U S A 100(21):12343–12348
134. Petricoin EF 3rd et al (2002) Serum proteomic patterns for detection of prostate cancer. J Natl Cancer Inst 94(20):1576–1578
135. Banez LL et al (2003) Diagnostic potential of serum proteomic patterns in prostate cancer. J Urol 170(2 Pt 1):442–446
136. Qu Y et al (2002) Boosted decision tree analysis of surface-enhanced laser desorption/ionization mass spectral serum profiles discriminates prostate cancer from noncancer patients. Clin Chem 48(10):1835–1843
137. Adam BL et al (2002) Serum protein fingerprinting coupled with a pattern-matching algorithm distinguishes prostate cancer from benign prostate hyperplasia and healthy men. Cancer Res 62(13):3609–3614
138. Li J et al (2002) Proteomics and bioinformatics approaches for identification of serum biomarkers to detect breast cancer. Clin Chem 48(8):1296–1304
139. Won Y et al (2003) Pattern analysis of serum proteome distinguishes renal cell carcinoma from other urologic diseases and healthy persons. Proteomics 3(12):2310–2316
140. Poon TC et al (2003) Comprehensive proteomic profiling identifies serum proteomic signatures for detection of hepatocellular carcinoma and its subtypes. Clin Chem 49(5):752–760
141. Vlahou A et al (2001) Development of a novel proteomic approach for the detection of transitional cell carcinoma of the bladder in urine. Am J Pathol 158(4):1491–1502
142. Koopmann J et al (2004) Serum diagnosis of pancreatic adenocarcinoma using surface-enhanced laser desorption and ionization mass spectrometry. Clin Cancer Res Off J Am Assoc Cancer Res 10(3):860–868
143. Yu Y et al (2005) Prediction of pancreatic cancer by serum biomarkers using surface-enhanced laser desorption/ionization-based decision tree classification. Oncology 68(1):79–86
144. Cristofanilli M et al (2004) Circulating tumor cells, disease progression, and survival in metastatic breast cancer. N Eng J Med 351(8):781–791
145. Kurihara T et al (2008) Detection of circulating tumor cells in patients with pancreatic cancer: a preliminary result. J Hepatobiliary Pancreat Surg 15(2):189–195
146. Khoja L et al (2012) A pilot study to explore circulating tumour cells in pancreatic cancer as a novel biomarker. Br J Cancer 106(3):508–516

147. Jones PA, Takai D (2001) The role of DNA methylation in mammalian epigenetics. Science 293(5532):1068–1070
148. Laird PW (2003) The power and the promise of DNA methylation markers. Nat Rev Cancer 3(4):253–266
149. Esteller M et al (2001) A gene hypermethylation profile of human cancer. Cancer Res 61(8):3225–3229
150. Yegnasubramanian S et al (2004) Hypermethylation of CpG islands in primary and metastatic human prostate cancer. Cancer Res 64(6):1975–1986
151. Tan AC et al (2009) Characterizing DNA methylation patterns in pancreatic cancer genome. Mol Oncol 3(5–6):425–438
152. Esteller M (2007) Cancer epigenomics: DNA methylomes and histone-modification maps. Nat Rev Genet 8(4):286–298

Chapter 9
Molecular Pathology and Diagnostics of Prostate Cancer

Rodney E. Shackelford, Janese Trimaldi, Philippe E. Spiess, Wade J. Sexton, Maisoun Qassim Abdelbaqi, and Shang-Tian Chuang

Contents

R.E. Shackelford
Department of Pathology and Laboratory Medicine, Tulane University School of Medicine, 1430 Tulane Avenue, SL-79, New Orleans, LA 70112, USA

J. Trimaldi
Department of Pathology, H. Lee Moffitt Cancer Center & Research Institute, 12902 Magnolia Drive, Tampa, FL 33612, USA

P.E. Spiess • W.J. Sexton
Department of Genitourinary Oncology, H. Lee Moffitt Cancer Center & Research Institute, 12902 Magnolia Drive, Tampa, FL 33612, USA

M.Q. Abdelbaqi
Department of Pathology, LSU Health Sciences Center Shreveport, 1501 Kings Highway, Shreveport, LA 71130, USA

S.-T. Chuang (✉)
Pathology, East Los Angeles Doctors Hospital, 4060 Whittier Blvd, Los Angeles, CA 90023, USA

4060 Whittier Blvd., Los Angeles, CA 90023-2523, USA
e-mail: tiansmail@yahoo.com

D. Coppola (ed.), *Molecular Pathology and Diagnostics of Cancer*, Cancer Growth and Progression 16, DOI 10.1007/978-94-007-7192-5_9,

Abstract Prostate cancer (PCa) is the most common malignancy among men and is the second leading cause of cancer-related deaths in the United States and Europe. The molecular alterations underlying PCa have recently been shown to be quite complex, involving many different genes, microRNA species, epigenetic and mitochondrial changes, and multiple gene translocations. Because of the highly complex molecular changes underlying this malignancy, PCa molecular diagnostics are exceptionally complex and have only recently led to useful molecular tests. Here, we will review several promising areas in the molecular diagnostics of PCa and try to indicate which ones may have clinical utility in the near future.

Keywords Prostate cancer • Translocation • PSA • Molecular diagnostics • Mitochondria • Prostatic intraepithelial neoplasia • Benign prostatic hypertrophy • Environmental risk factors • Genetic risk factors

Abbreviations

AMACR	Alpha-methylacyl-CoA racemase
BPH	Benign prostatic hypertrophy
BPSA	Benign prostate-specific antigen

COPA	Cancer outlier profile analysis
CTC	Circulating tumor cells
ECM	Extracellular matrix
ELISA	Enzyme-linked immunosorbent assay
EpCAM	Epithelial cell adhesion molecule
ETS	Erythroblast transformation-specific
FISH	Fluorescent in situ hybridization
fPSA	Free PSA
GOLPH2	Golgi Phosphoprotein 2
GST	Glutathione-S-transferase
GSTP1	Glutathione-S-transferase P1
hK2	Human glandular kallikrein 2
miRNA	MicroRNA
MMP	Matrix metalloproteinase
MSMB	Microdeminoprotein-ß
PBS	Phosphate-buffered saline
PCa	Prostate cancer
PCA3	Prostate cancer gene 3
PIN	Prostatic intraepithelial neoplasia
PSA	Prostate-specific antigen
RT-PCR	Reverse transcription-polymerase chain reaction
SNP	Single nucleotide polymorphism
uPA	Urokinase plasminogen activator
uPAR	Urokinase plasminogen activator receptor

9.1 Introduction

Prostate cancer (PCa) is the most common cancer in men within the United States (US) and is the second leading cause of cancer deaths in the US and Europe. One in six US men develops PCa at some point in their lives. Each year, 186,320 US men and 345,900 European men are diagnosed with PCa; of these men, 28,660 US and 87,400 European men will die of the disease. Since the incidence of PCa increases with age, the number of men with newly diagnosed PCa will probably continue to rise as life expectancy of the general population increases [1, 2]. The incidence of PCa is much lower in other parts of the world, with Eastern Europe, Asia, and Africa having a significantly lower incidence [3]. Within the US, the age-adjusted incidence of PCa-related mortality peaked in the early 1990s and declined by 4.17 % per year from 1994 to 2004, possibly due to early prostate-specific antigen (PSA) testing and more aggressive treatment of asymptomatic disease [4].

9.2 Environmental Versus Genetic Factors for Prostate Cancer Risk

Multiple environmental and genetic risk factors have been identified that play a role in determining PCa risk. Several studies have implicated diet, chronic inflammation, and obesity in the risk of developing PCa. Obesity confers an increased risk for aggressive PCa. Although poorly understood, the underlying causes may in part relate to the lower testosterone levels and higher levels of estrogens seen in obese men, which might facilitate tumor growth. Additionally, there may be bias against screening obese men for PCa, potentially leading to a delay in diagnosing early-stage disease [5]. A diet high in meat, particularly well-done red meat and highly processed meat, is associated with an increased risk of PCa. Interestingly, the increased risk is likely due to the mutagenic effects of heterocyclic amines, particularly rich in well-done/overcooked red meat, and not due to the effects of high levels of saturated fats found in red meat [6]. Additionally, a diet consisting of less than 35 g of protein/day, eating fish three or more times/week, and high dietary levels of genistein, curcumin, folate, and retinoic acid lowers the risk for PCa [7, 8]. Interestingly, agents such as genistein and curcumin may lower the risk for PCa by altering microRNA expression patterns [8]. Lastly, chronic inflammation plays a role in PCa development, as many factors that increase chronic inflammation/oxidative stress, such as mitochondrial dysfunction, loss of antioxidant defenses, and chronic prostatitis, stimulate cell proliferation in a background of increased genomic instability [9].

Studies of twins and families with strong histories of PCa, genetic studies of single nucleotide polymorphisms (SNPs), and genome-wide linkage studies have demonstrated a genetic component in approximately 42 % of all PCas [10, 11]. Several gene mutations have been implicated in either hereditary or sporadic PCa, including BRCA1 and 2, AR, PALB2, ELAC2, CHEK2, CYP17, CYP1B1, CYP3A4, GSTM1, GSTP1, GSTT1, PON1, SRD5A2, VDR ANXA7, KLF5, NKX3-1, and CDKN1B [12–15]. The relative contribution of each of these genes to PCa varies enormously. For example, BRCA mutations that play an important role in hereditary breast and ovarian cancers only account for 1–2 % of PCas [12, 15]. Similarly, a large number of SNPs have been implicated in PCa risk/susceptibility [14]. Presently, however, there is little molecular diagnostic testing for PCa directed at SNPs or gene mutations associated with increased cancer risk.

9.2.1 PCa Risk and Race

African American men present with PCa at a younger age, have a higher PCa incidence, often present with a more advanced stage, and have a worse clinical course than men of other races. In fact, African American ancestry is a well-recognized PCa risk factor, with African American men often having higher serum PSA and Gleason scores at diagnosis than Caucasian men [13]. Although some of these differences are due to socioeconomic and lifestyle factors, a significant component of the PCa racial disparity appears to be molecular-genetic factors found in African American men. Many of these factors have been indentified and include higher mean serum testosterone levels (a PCa risk factor), increased androgen receptors in benign prostatic tissue and PCa, variants of 5α-reductase that may convert testosterone to the more active dihydrotestosterone, less active cytochrome P450c17 (an enzyme that inactivates testosterone), increased epidermal growth factor expression, increased *Bcl-2* expression (which exerts anti-apoptosis effects), increased *MDM2* (which suppresses p53 expression promoting genomic instability), and patterns of microRNAs (which may promote PCa) (for review, see [14]).

9.3 PSA Testing

The US Food and Drug Administration approved the serum PSA test in 1986 for monitoring men with PCa. In 1994 the test was approved in conjunction with the digital rectal examination for the detection of PCa [2, 11]. PSA is a member of the Kallikrein gene family, which consists of at least 15 different proteins, all of which are found at 19q13.41. PSA has five exons, is regulated by steroid hormones, and functions as a serine protease [16–18]. PSA testing has been very successful and has led to a dramatic reduction in the incidence of advanced-stage disease, that is, those typically difficult to treat and carrying a poor prognosis [4, 19].

Serum PSA is elevated in benign conditions such as benign prostatic hypertrophy (BPH) and prostatitis, giving the test low specificity, especially in the "gray zone" of a total serum PSA between 4 and 10 ng/mL. In this PSA range, only 25 % of men will have detectable PCa upon biopsy [20]. Additionally, men with a total serum PSA below 4 ng/mL have a PCa risk similar to men with total serum PSA levels between 4 and 10 ng/mL, making clinical decision-making based on PSA values alone often difficult. Attempts to improve the positive predictive value of PSA for PCa detection have included lowering the PSA level threshold for recommending biopsies. The lowering of the PSA threshold has resulted in an increased number of positive PSA screening tests and an increased number of men undergoing prostate biopsies with no definite improvement in the detection of clinically significant PCas [21]. Thus, the sensitivity and specificity of PSA levels in PCa detection are not satisfactory, and others factors, including family history, body mass, race, and age, are usually included in the clinical decision making [20, 21]. Lastly, negative biopsies do not completely rule out the presence of PCa; conversely, many biopsies are performed on patients without PCa or on patients with clinically insignificant indolent tumors that would be better treated with active surveillance and less frequent biopsies. Thus, a major challenge in PCa testing, not met by the PSA test, is the stratification of men into those who need biopsy, those who do not, and those with indolent, clinically insignificant PCa who do not require aggressive local therapy (i.e., radical prostatectomy or radiotherapy) [20–22]. Several variations on serum PSA testing have been developed, which have led to greater clinical utility for PSA testing. Some of these include those listed below.

9.3.1 PSA Density

PSA Density compares the serum PSA value to the size of the prostate. A higher PSA value with a greatly enlarged prostate is far less concerning than an increased PSA with a normal to small sized prostate. One drawback with this test is that a man may have an enlarged prostate that harbors PCa [22].

9.3.2 PSA Velocity

PSA Velocity measures the changes in serum PSA over time. A relatively sudden increase in serum PSA levels may indicate the presence of PCa or a previously indolent PCa becoming more aggressive [22]. For example, Carter et al. [23] demonstrated that a serum PSA increase of over 0.35 ng/mL/year increased the relative risk of death from PCa compared to men with a velocity below 0.35 ng/mL/year. PSA velocity has been demonstrated to be a more accurate way to detect adverse clinical/pathological features rather than measuring the PSA doubling time [24].

9.3.3 Free Versus Bound PSA

This test measures two separate serum PSA forms, one free within the serum and the other attached to a carrier protein, such as serine protease inhibitor 1-antichymotrypsin. The free PSA (fPSA) assay is best utilized in men with serum PSA between 4 and 10 ng/mL. In PCa, a higher percentage of serum PSA is protein-bound compared to that shown with benign prostatic conditions. For instance, men without PCa have a higher likelihood of having a fPSA above 25 %. fPSA values between 10 % and 25 % are not predictive of PCa risk. Finally, men with fPSA values below 10 % have the highest possibility of having a PCa when their serum PSA is within the 4–10 ng/mL range [22, 25, 26].

9.3.4 Benign Prostate-Specific Antigen

Another form of PSA, called benign prostate-specific antigen (BPSA), is derived from the cleavage of fPSA between Lys182 and Ser183. The resulting peptide has a unique, measurable epitope that is found in the prostatic tissue, blood, and seminal fluid. BPSA is localized to the prostatic transitional zone of men with BPH, almost undetectable in healthy men, and increased in men with BPH. Serum BPSA levels correlate strongly with nodular hyperplasia of the prostate, especially with increased transition zone volume. BPSA is a better predictor of prostatic enlargement than serum PSA or free serum PSA and may have use in differentiating BPH from PCa [27–29].

9.4 Molecular-Genetic Testing for Prostate Cancer

Since the introduction of PSA testing in 1986, several other potential biomarkers of PCa have been examined in hopes of increasing PCa detection sensitivity and specificity. Among these markers, only a few have demonstrated clinical value, while others show some promise following further analysis. These include PSA derivatives, microdeminoprotein-β (MSMB), PCa gene 3 (PCA3), *TMPRSS2:ETS* fusions, *SPINK1* overexpression, the t(4;6)(q22;q15) chromosomal translocation, somatic mitochondrial DNA mutation, *C-MYC* amplification, *Bcl-2* overexpression, Kallikrein serum levels, Urokinase Plasminogen Activator activity, *GSTP-1* hypermethylation, alpha-methylacyl-CoA racemase (AMACR) levels, PCa microRNA expression patterns, and SNPs. Here, we will review several of them.

9.4.1 Microdeminoprotein-ß Urine Testing

PSA, prostate acid phosphatase, and microdeminoprotein-ß (MSMB) are the three most abundant proteins found in human semen [25]. MSMB, also known as PSP94 or β-inhibin, is found at 10q11.2 and encodes a cysteine-rich 16-kDa, 94 amino acid protein [30, 31]. MSMB is a strong inhibitor of follicle stimulating hormone. MSMB peptide fragments exert pro-apoptotic effects, inhibit matrix metalloproteinase-9 (MMP-9) secretion, antagonize tumor neovascularization, and inhibit tyrosine kinase pathways downstream of VEGF and PDGF, thus preventing intracellular signaling through the MAPK cascade [32–35]. MSMB is expressed in multiple tissues, including tracheobronchial tract and the cervix, although at levels much lower than are found in the prostate [36, 37].

MSMB expression is low to absent in PCa, but highly expressed in benign prostatic tissue and BPH [38–42]. MSMB loss may be an early event in the PCa development as its expression is lost in prostatic intraepithelial neoplasia (PIN), although some studies refute this finding [40, 42]. Additionally, in pubertal and adult normal prostates MSMB expression is most intense in the review of the peripheral zone, less intense in the transitional zone, and shows variable staining in the central zone. Thus, higher MSMB expression is found at prostatic anatomic sites most likely to develop PCa. Interestingly, no zonal differential expression was identified for PAP or PSA [40–42]. Lastly, MSMB is bound to proteins that in part regulate its bioavailability. One of these proteins, cysteine-rich secretory protein-3, is relatively low in benign prostatic tissue and elevated in PCa, and its expression is an independent predictor of disease recurrence following radical prostatectomy [42]. Taken together, the above data indicate that MSMB exerts tumor suppressor effects on PCa and its loss may have potential as a biomarker for this malignancy.

Two genome-wide association studies have identified a small nucleotide polymorphism, rs10993994 at 10q11.2, that is strongly associated with increased PCa risk ($p = 8.8 \times 10^{-18}$) [43–45]. rs10993994 is 57-bp centromeric of the first MSMB gene exon and has several 2-bp variants. The CT or CC variants express high levels of MSMB/reporter gene mRNA, while the TT variant expresses only about 13 % of the CT/CC variants, probably due to low CREB transcription factor binding to TT variant promoters [45, 46]. The TT variant occurs in about 30–40 % of European men and 70–80 % of men with African ancestry [47]. The low MSMB expression in the TT variant could lead to less suppression of prostatic epithelial cell growth and increased risk for malignant transformation [45].

9.4.2 Immunohistochemical Analysis of Urinary MSMB for PCa Molecular Diagnostic Testing

Until recently, MSMB has rarely been used in clinical testing, although low to absent levels in PCa have been detected by a variety of techniques, including immunohistochemistry, reverse transcription-polymerase chain reaction (RT-PCR), and enzyme-linked immunosorbent assay (ELISA) assays [38–42]. Recently, several studies have demonstrated that MSMB testing may have value in analyzing PCa risk, diagnosis, and disease monitoring. For example, Whitaker et al. [48] employed immunohistochemical (sandwich ELISA) analysis of urinary MSMB to detect PCa. The urine of 215 men with no history of PCa and 89 men with PCa was examined. Urine was collected prior to a digital rectal exam, aliquoted, and immediately frozen at −80 °C until needed. Plates for urine MSMB quantification were prepared by incubating 96-well plates overnight at 4 °C with mouse anti-PSP94 antibody at a 1:1,000 dilution in phosphate-buffered saline (PBS). The wells were washed three times between all steps with 0.05 % PBS-Tween. The wells were blocked with 1 % bovine serum albumen for 1 h and 50 μL of sample or standard was added to each well in duplicate and incubated at room temperature for 2 h. Serial dilutions of recombinant MSMB were used as a control and standard curve for MSMB quantification. Goat anti-MSMB was added to each well for 1 h and further incubated with anti-goat horseradish peroxidase-conjugated antibody for an additional 1 h. The amount of bound MSMB was quantified by the addition of 100 μL TMB for 15 min. The reaction was then stopped by acidification, and the absorbance was measured at 450 nm using a Lucy II spectrophotometer. Urinary and serum PSAs were quantified with a commercial kit.

Men with PCa showed a consistent and significant decrease in urinary MSMB compared to men without cancer, which correlated strongly with the rs10993994 TT variant. Urinary MSMB significantly improved upon urinary PSA for PCa diagnosis specificity and sensitivity in this cohort, particularly when the PCa was stratified into low (six and seven) and high (eight and nine) Gleason scores. It did not improve upon serum PSA for specificity and sensitivity. No correlation between urinary MSMB levels and BRCA1 and BRCA2 status was identified. As previously found, MSMB staining was lost in PIN and PCa and was significantly lower in men with the rs10993994 TT variant versus those with the CC variant. MSMB urine protein testing has the following advantages: (1) MSMB urine protein testing does not require digital rectal massage, (2) MSMB expression is not affected by hormonal status or BPH, and (3) urine MSMB has improved specificity and sensitivity over urine PSA. The authors conclude that urine MSMB may be a useful biomarker for screening for both PCa development and risk, although further studies are required to validate the assay.

9.4.3 Prostate Cancer Gene 3 (PCA3)

Prostate cancer gene 3 (PCA3), also known as "differential display 3," is found at 9q21-22 within intron 6 of the *BMCC1* gene, has four exons, and is transcribed into multiple RNA splice and polyadenylation variants. The PCA3 RNA carries many stop codons and hence appears to produce no detectable protein(s), and thus functions as a non-coding RNA. Interestingly, however, a recent detailed analysis revealed a novel PCA3 isoform with four putative open reading frames from a single ATG initiation site. Although no protein(s) has been found to be coded for by PCA3, some may exist [49–51]. PCA3 was discovered by differential display analysis of normal versus PCa, where it was highly overexpressed in 53 of 56 PCas compared to the same prostate samples taken from non-neoplastic areas. PCA3 expression is prostate-specific and was not detected in normal human artery, brain breast, bladder, colon, heart, duodenum, liver, lung, ovary, pancreas, placenta, seminal vesicles, skeletal muscle, spinal cord, or testis [49]. Although originally thought to be expressed only in PCa, PCA3 is expressed in benign prostate and is on average 66-fold up-regulated in 95 % of PCas (median 158.4×10^5 copies/μg tissue RNA in PCa compared to 2.5×10^5 copies/μg tissue RNA) [52].

9.4.3.1 PCa Molecular Diagnostics and PCA3

Many different molecular diagnostic protocols have been developed for PCA3 analysis. Most employ variations on RT-PCR with simultaneous amplification of control gene(s) products to normalized PCA3 transcript levels and confirm a yield of prostate-specific RNA. PSA is often employed as a normalization control as it is relatively prostate-specific and unlike PCA3 its mRNA levels are not increased in malignant prostatic tissue [51, 52]. Detection of PCA3 in urine is attractive as urine collection is noninvasive and since PCA3 RNA is prostate-specific [49–54], cells and urinary sediments from non-prostatic sources do not interfere with test specificity.

9.4.3.2 PCA3 Quantification in Urine

Hessels et al. [52] employed quantitative RT-PCR to analyze PCA3 in the urine of 108 men with serum PSA above 3 ng/mL. The urine was collected following a thorough rectal examination, cooled on ice to 4 °C, centrifuged at 700 g for 10 min, washed twice with ice-cold PBS, snap frozen in liquid nitrogen, and stored at –70 °C.

Total RNA was later extracted using TRIzol® reagent (Invitrogen). A cDNA was made by heating the purified RNA for 10 min at 68 °C and reverse transcribing the RNA at 37 °C for 1 h with an olido-d(T)$_{18}$ primer. The resulting PCA3 cDNA was PCR amplified with these PCA3-specific primers: forward 5′-TGGGAAGGA CCTGATGATACA-3′ and reverse 5′-CCCAGGGATCTCTGTGCTT-3′. After 35 amplification rounds, the products were quantified by time-resolved fluorescence-based hybridization assay on strepavidin-coated microtitration wells. Target-specific detection was achieved with a PCA3-detection probe labeled with Eu^{3+}. PSA RNA was amplified in a similar manner and detected with a Tb^{3+} labeled detection probe. The amount of PCA3 RNA in the sample was calculated by comparing detected PCA3 to a standard curve, to the PCA3 RNA found in normal prostate, and to the urine PSA RNA levels. Of the 108 men analyzed, 24 had PCa by prostate biopsy, with 84 being negative. Of the men with PCa, 16 were positive by PCA3 testing, giving a sensitivity of 67 % and a negative predictor value of 90 %. The authors concluded that PCA3 testing could have value in urine analysis for PCa and could reduce the number of unnecessary biopsies. However, a larger multi-center study should be performed to further analyze the usefulness of urine PCA3 in detecting PCa.

9.4.3.3 Transcription-Mediated Amplification Platform for Urine PCA3 Analysis

One major drawback of urine based RT-PCR for PCA3 analysis is that this method is too time-consuming and insensitive to lend itself to routine clinical molecular diagnostic testing. Up to ~20 % of all clinical specimens contained insufficient prostate cells for testing, thus giving an unacceptably low informative rate of ~80 % [52]. Groskope et al. [55] employed a transcription-mediated amplification (TMA) system combined with mRNA capture to achieve an informative rate of 98.2 %. Two hundred μL of urine and urine transport medium were initially used to facilitate RNA capture and increase RNA stability. The specimens were vortexed and incubated at 62 °C with magnetic particles with attached PSA or PCA3 RNA target-specific oligonucleotides. After 30 min, the magnetic particles with attached RNAs were placed on a Gen-Probe Target Capture System for 10 min to allow the magnetic particles to migrate to the sides of the tubes. The fluid was removed, the tubes were washed with 1 mL buffer, and the process was repeated once more for complete sample purification. Seventy-five μL of buffer and primers were added to the beads, and the samples were heated to 62 °C for 10 min. Twenty-five μL of enzyme reagents were added to each tube, and the TMA reaction was allowed to proceed for 1 h at 42 °C.

TMA amplifies nucleic acids isothermally and employs two primers and two enzymes: RNA polymerase and reverse transcriptase. One of the primers contains a promoter for RNA polymerase. Amplification is initiated when this primer hybridizes to the purified RNA at a defined site and the reverse transcriptase creates an dsRNA:DNA hybrid, which is rapidly degraded to ssDNA by the RNase activity of the reverse transcriptase. The second primer then binds the ssDNA, and the reverse transcriptase polymerizes a dsDNA. The RNA polymerase attaches to the DNA promoter sequence and initiates many rounds of transcription. The resulting RNA amplicons reenter the TMA cycle for new replication rounds. Up to one billion copies of the original RNA can be produced within 1 h. The amplicons were detected with specific gene probes in a hybridization protection assay employing a chemiluminescence detection format. All samples were run in triplicate.

To examine the clinical utility of this test, three groups were tested: (1) 70 men with serum PSAs ≥2.5 ng/mL and/or abnormal digital rectal exams, (2) 52 men under 45 years who had no PCa risk factors, and (3) 21 men who had undergone previous prostatectomies at least 3 months before their urine was analyzed. Additionally, the urine of six women was used as a negative control. Of the 70 men with elevated serum PSA, 68 yielded informative specimens. Of these, 16 were PCa positive by biopsy; of the remaining 52, 40 had BPH and/or inflammation. PCA3 analysis of this group gave a specificity of 67 % and a sensitivity of 79 %, while serum PSA yielded a specificity of 28 % and sensitivity of 81 %. The calculated media ratios (PCA3/PSA $\times 10^{-3}$) for healthy, biopsy negative, and biopsy positive groups were 4.5, 27.0, and 81.8, respectively, with the mean PCA3/PCA ratios of the three groups significantly different ($p<0.01$). The advantages of this system are as follows: (1) urine testing is noninvasive, (2) it has a high informative rate, (3) it has a higher specificity than serum PSA (69 % vs. 28 %), (4) it uses whole urine and not urine sediments, which simplifies specimen-processing, and (5) the assay can be completed in 6 h, giving a relatively short turn-around time.

9.4.3.4 PCA3 Detection by Analysis of Circulating Tumor Cells

Circulating tumor cells (CTCs) are found in 50–70 % of individuals with metastatic breast, colon, and PCas, and their appearance in advanced PCa correlates with a poor prognosis and treatment failure [56–59]. There are many different approaches for isolating and analyzing CTCs, each having different efficiencies and value for molecular analyses [60]. Jost et al. [61] developed an efficient immunomagnetic system for the capture and molecular analysis of circulating PCa cells. Magnetic particles were employed, which either had attached anti-epithelial cell adhesion molecule (EpCAM) or anti-EpCam combined with anti-prostate specific membrane antigen antibodies attached. To initially test this system, 10 mL of normal donor blood harvested by venipuncture into EDTA-containing Vacutainer tubes and 5 mL of the blood was spiked with five C4-2 prostate cell line cancer cells; 100 μL of antibody-coated magnetic particles were added, and the mix was incubated at room temperature for 30 min. The magnetic-bound fraction was subjected to three PBS washings and subsequently treated with Gen-Probe lysis buffer. The immunomagnetically-enriched fractions were analyzed for PSA mRNA expression via a TMA-based system similar to that employed by Groskope et al. [55]. Five C4-2 cells yielded slightly over 1,000 PSA mRNA copies/reaction. Similar reactions carried out without magnetic beads and/or attached anti-EpCAM antibodies failed to yield any PSA mRNA amplicons, demonstrating system component specificity. The system was also tested with LNCaP prostatic cell lines expressing green fluorescent protein, as measured by phase-contrast and fluorescent microscopy. The immunomagnetic particles bound only the transformed prostatic cells.

To analyze this system with patient samples, 5 mL of EDTA-containing blood from the following groups were examined: (1) 35 men diagnosed with advanced-stage PCa diagnosed by bone scan, (2) 29 men diagnosed with early-stage PCa diagnosed by biopsy, digital rectal exam, and serum PSA measurements, (3) five men diagnosed with BPH, and (4) five healthy men without prostate disease as controls. The CTCs were isolated as above, and PSA, PCA3, and the *TMPRSS2:ERG* gene fusion RNA levels were analyzed by TMA. The *TMPRSS2:ERG* gene fusion occurs in 15–50 % of PCas and confers a more aggressive PCa course in a transgenic murine model, is preferentially detected in metastatic PCa, and is linked with a more aggressive PCa phenotype in humans [62–67] (see below). mRNA for PSA was not detectable in any of the samples from men with BPH or men with early-stage (i.e., confined to the prostrate) PCa. Of the men with advanced-stage PCa, none with androgen-dependent PCa were PCA3 positive, while 31 % of those with androgen-independent PCa were PCA3 positive. Additionally, more of the patients with androgen-independent PCa were *TMPRSS2:ERG* gene fusion positive, compared to that shown in androgen-dependent PCa patients. The addition of anti-prostate specific membrane antigen to the magnetic beads coated with anti-EpCAM did not improve the yield of the TMA-amplified RNAs. The authors opined that this could be due to stochastic differences between the splitting of a sample containing very dilute number of CTCs. Lastly, the immunomagnetic bead-antibody method yielded a higher amplicon copy number than did analysis of cell-free plasma samples from the same patients, demonstrating that the higher complexity of this assay results in greater sensitivity. The authors concluded that, since this system lends itself well to automation and improves upon detecting RNA in plasma, it might have value in the molecular diagnostics of PCa. Additionally, they concluded that further studies are needed with larger patient samples to validify this technique.

9.4.3.5 PCA3 Utility in PCA Molecular Testing

Presently, the TMA-based PCA3 system is now commercially available in the US and Europe [68]. There are many studies demonstrating the value of PCA3 in the molecular diagnostic testing of PCa. In addition, many other studies have shown interesting biological correlates with PCA3 status. For example, Whitman et al. [69] found that a high PCA3:PSA amplicon ratio correlated with an increased incidence of extracapsular extension and greater tumor volume, with the PCA3 score having a 94 % specificity and 80 % positive predictive value for these events. Interestingly, this represents the first molecular marker to predict PCa extracapsular extension. Many of the studies dealing with new molecular diagnostic techniques will require extensive validation studies if they are to be implemented for routine PCa molecular diagnostics. Other techniques are presently too complex, time-consuming, poorly informative, and/or expensive to have clinical use.

Meta-analyses of PCA3 have demonstrated that PCA3 detection techniques have accepted diagnostics accuracy rates and can be used in the diagnosis of PCa. For example, Ruiz-Aragón et al. [70] performed a meta-analysis of 14 PCA3 studies done between 2000 and 2009 reported in MedLine, Embase, Cochrane Library, CRD, EGRI, Hayes, and cancer and urology databases and journals. The quality of the studies was evaluated by QUADAS criteria to determine the quality of the studies selected. Fourteen studies were selected that met the criteria for moderate to high quality. Of these, the study sensitivities were between 46.9 % and 82.3 %, and the specificities were between 56.3 % and 89 %. Combined with other parameters, the authors concluded PCA3 molecular testing would be a useful method for early PCA3 detection and would significantly reduce the number of repeat biopsies in patients with a PSA >3.0 ng/mL, who could be monitored by PCA3 testing. It should be remembered, however, that a low percentage of patients could have PCa with low to undetectable PCA3 levels.

9.4.4 Gene Fusions in PCa

Tomlins et al. [71] developed a bioinformatics approach to the discovery of candidate oncogenic chromosomal aberrations based on outlier gene expression, termed Cancer Outlier Profile Analysis (COPA). This analysis applies a simple numerical transformation based on the median and median absolute deviation of a gene expression profile. A compendium of 132 gene expression data sets representing 10,486 microarray experiments was analyzed via COPA analysis. COPA correctly identified several outlier profiles for genes in specific malignancies previously found to have recurrent gene rearrangements or high-level gene amplifications. When applied to PCa, COPA identified two erythroblast transformation-specific (*ETS)* family members, *ERG* (21q22.3) and *ETV1* (7p21.2), as strong outlier profiles. The authors reasoned that, because gene fusions involving the highly conserved DNA binding domains of the ETS family, such as *ERG* and *ETV1*, as found in Ewing sarcoma, are functionally redundant, they are therefore seldomly found together within a specific tumor. The same may be true for *ERG* and *ETV1* expressions in PCa. COPA analysis demonstrated that *ERG* and *ETV1* expression across several PCa data sets had invariably mutually exclusive outlier profiles, consistent with the hypothesis that *ERG* and *ETV1* expressions likely play functionally redundant roles in PCa carcinogenesis.

Further analysis of *ERG* and *ETV1* expression in cell lines and human metastatic PCa tumors revealed over- and underexpression of specific *ERG* and *ETV1* exons. For example, cells derived from metastatic PCa showed >90 % reduced *ETV1* exon 2 expression compared to exons 3–7. This selective exon expression suggested that gene rearrangements might be involved in the altered *ERG* and *ETV1* expression patterns. 5′-RNA ligase mediated rapid amplification of cDNA ends was employed to identify the complete 5′ transcripts of the overexpressed *ERG* and *ETV1* exons.

In this process, an RNA is collected that contains the target of interest. The sample is first treated with calf intestinal phosphatase to remove all 5′-phosphates of the RNA species that lack a cap structure, such as rRNA, tRNA, and all fragmented RNA species. The RNA polyermase II transcripts that have cap structures retain their 5′-phosphates. The calf intestinal phosphatase is removed, and the RNA is treated with tobacco acid pryrophosphatase to remove the RNA cap structure and leave an intact 5′-phosphate. A synthetic RNA oligonucleotide (adaptor sequence) is added to the reaction and ligated to the calf intestinal phosphatase/tobacco acid pryrophosphatase treated RNA. The ligation reaction can only happen on RNA with an intact 5′-phosphate, so only RNA polymerase II transcripts are ligated. The resulting RNA is then converted into cDNA with random primers and reverse transcriptase. The cDNAs were amplified with adaptor sequence primers and *ERG*/*ETV1* primers. The products were cloned and sequenced, revealing that the *ERG* and *ETV1* exons were fused with the prostate-specific and androgen-regulated transmembrane-serine protease gene (*TMPRSS2*, 21q22.2). Specifically, several different fusions were identified, including the following: (1) exon 1 of *TMPRSS2* was fused to exon 4 of *ERG,* (2) exon 1 of *TMPRSS2* with the beginning of *ETV1* exon 4, and (3) exons 1 and 2 of *TMPRSS2* with the beginning of *ETV1* exon 4.

Primers specific for these transcripts were then designed to exon 1 of *TMPRSS2* and exons 4 of *ERG* and *ETV1*, as well as exon 6 of *ERG* and exon 7 of *ETV1.* Amplicons were quantified with SYBR Green. Forty-two cases of clinically localized and metastatic PCas were chosen for *ERG* and *ETV1* overexpression as measured by previous microarray analyses. *ERG* and *ETV1* fusions were readily identified, with transcript size variations seen. Similarly, interphase fluorescent in situ hybridization was performed with red or green-labeled probes for *TMPRSS2, ERG* and *ETV1.* While peripheral lymphocytes showed two separate signals, some prostate cell lines and PCa cases showed *TMPRSS2:ETV1* or *TMPRSS2:ERG* rearrangements, confirming the RNA ligase mediated rapid amplification/PCR-derived data. Lastly, the *TMPRSS2:ERG* fusion was examined for androgen responsiveness. Quantitative PCR analysis of the *TMPRSS2:ERG* fusion was performed on the VCaP and LNCaP cell lines, with only the former expressing the fusion transcript. Although both cell lines responded to androgen exposure with increased PSA expression, the VCaP expressed 2,000-fold more *ERG* than the LNCaP cells and expressed increased *ERG* upon androgen exposure. Similar results were obtained with other *TMPRSS2:ERG* fusion positive cell lines, saved for those that express low androgen receptor levels. Thus, the *TMPRSS2:ERG* fusion is under androgen control and the aberrant *ERG* or *ETV1* expression seen in subsets of PCa may in part be explained by fusion with the androgen-responsive *TMPRSS2* gene.

Presently, the molecular effects exerted by the PCa gene fusions are incompletely understood. Transfection of different *TMPRSS2:ERG* fusion splice forms into primary prostatic epithelial cells or a PCa cell line promotes cell proliferation and increases cell motility and invasiveness. The relative activity of the fusions depended upon the 5′ structure and the presence or absence of *ERG* exon 8. Knockdown of the fusion inhibited cell proliferation and slowed tumor progression in an in vivo orthotopic murine model [72]. Other studies have examined altered gene expression patterns secondary to the presence of the *TMPRSS2:ERG* fusion. Barwick et al. [73] compared *TMPRSS2:ERG* fusion positive vs. fusion negative PCas with a 502 cancer-related gene microarray system using cDNA-mediated, annealing, selection, extension, and ligation to identify fusion-associated gene expression patterns. Sixty-nine patients with the fusion positive PCas were compared to 70 patients with fusion negative PCas. Fifty-one genes were identified as differentially regulated due to the presence of the fusion. Of these genes, 16 were associated with recurrence following radical prostatectomy and 11 were associated with non-recurrence. Recurrence associated genes included those involved in deoxyribosylthymine monophosphate biosynthesis, negative leukocyte regulation, and inhibition of cell matrix adhesion. Genes associated with non-recurrence generally increased cell-matrix adhesion and collagen binding.

Lastly, like other PCa markers [14], *TMPRSS2:ERG* gene fusions patterns show different expression patterns in different ethnicities. For example, Magi-Galluzzi et al. [74], found *TMPRSS2:ERG* gene fusions in 50 %, 31.3 %, and 15.9 % of African American, Caucasian, and Japanese men with PCa, respectively. Interestingly, the patterns by which the gene fusion arose was different in each group, with fusions arising from translocation, deletion, or both events seen in 61.9 %, 38.1 %, and 0 % of Caucasian men, 20 %, 60 %, and 20 % of African American men, and 71.4 %, 28.6 %, and 0 % of Japanese men.

9.4.5 Diversity of PCa Translocations

The ETS transcription factor family consists of 25 genes that share a conserved winged helix-turn-helix DNA binding domain which binds GGAA/T promoter/regulatory elements of over 200 different target genes. The ETS transcription factors function as positive or negative regulators of genes involved in cellular proliferation, differentiation, hematopoietic, apoptosis, tissue remodeling, angiogenesis, and malignant transformation [75]. Since the ETS transcription factors exert many shared and often-redundant effects, different ETS family genes have been found fused to the same 5′-transcript. For example, in Ewing sarcoma, *EWS* is found fused to the ETS family genes *FLI1, ERG, ETV1, ETV4,* and *FEV* [76]. Clark et al. [77] first demonstrated a high diversity within the *TMPRSS2:ERG* fusion transcripts by analyzing 26 PCas, 17 morphologically normal prostate, 31 BPH, and 20 samples of normal, non-prostate tissue for fusions with PCR primers to *5′-TMPRSS2* exon 1, *3′-ERG* exon 6, as previously employed by Tomlins et al. [71]. Of these samples, 14 distinct *TMPRSS2:ERG* fusion transcripts were detected. Included within these 14 samples were fusions of exons 1, 2, and 3 of *TMPRSS2* to exons 2, 3, 4, 5, or 6 of *ERG*. Five of these fusions contained in-frame stops and were unlikely to encode proteins. The most commonly detected fusions were *TMPRSS2* exon 1 fused to *ERG* exons 4 and 5 (designated T1/E4 and T1/E5, respectively), previously identified by Tomlins et al. [71]. Unlike most fusions, T1/E4 and T1/E5 occurred together within individual samples, indicating that they were probably alternative splices from the same fusion. Interestingly of the BPH samples examined, 6 % were fusion positive and shown to harbor PCa upon repeat histologic examination. Also of interest, Clark et al. [77] found that different separate regions of the same prostate with PCa can harbor different gene fusions, suggesting multifocal origins for PCa.

More recently over 20 different gene fusions have been identified in PCa, many of which have unique characteristics and biological behaviors. The 3′ *ETS* fusion genes identified in the fusions are *ERG, ETV1, RTV4,* and *ETV5*. All of these promote cellular self-renewal and proliferation [75]. The 5′ fusion partners are *TMPRSS2, SLC45A3, ACSL3, HERV-K, FOXP1, EST14, Chromosome 14(q13.3-21.1), C15orf21, HNRPA2B1, KLK2, CANT1,* and *DDX5*. *ERG* is nearly always paired with *TMPRSS2,* while *ETV1, RTV4,* and *ETV5* have multiple fusion partners. The 3′ portion of the fusion usually retains its *ETS* DNA binding capacity and is responsible for the transforming effects of the fusion. Most 5′ fusion partners are androgen regulated, placing the transforming effects under the control of androgen stimulation [78].

9.4.6 PCa Translocations in PCa Diagnosis and Prognosis

TMPRSS2:ETS fusions occur in about 50 % of PCas, making them the most prevalent gene fusions identified in any solid tumor [62, 71, 74, 78, 79]. Since some gene fusions are associated with specific clinical outcomes in other malignancies, there is considerable interest in the possible value of the PCa gene fusions as prognostic biomarkers. Multiple studies have addressed the importance of *TMPRSS2:ETS* fusions in PCa aggressiveness and clinical outcome; however, no consistent results have so far been obtained. For example, *TMPRSS2:ETS* fusions have been associated with a favorable [80–83], unfavorable [64, 84–93], and no effect on the clinical course and prognosis of PCa [94–98]. The reason for these divergent findings probably comes from several factors, such as different patient populations, different parameters and endpoints employed between different studies, and the molecular heterogeneity found in the *TMPRSS2:ETS* fusions [14, 62, 71, 77–98]. However, several specific gene fusion patterns have been found to correlate with a poor PCa clinical course and prognosis;

9.4.7 Concurrent TMPRSS2-ERG and PTEN Loss in PCa

King et al. [99] examined 121 *ERG* rearrangement positive and negative human PCas for *PTEN* copy number loss and *MYC* amplification. Gene loss or amplification was measured by high-resolution array-based comparative genome hybridization. *PTEN* loss and *ERG* rearrangements were significantly associated in PCa ($p < 0.002$), while *MYC* (commonly amplified in PCa) was not associated with *ERG* rearrangements ($p < 0.56$). Interestingly, transgenic mice that expressed high levels of the *TMPRSS2:ERG* fusion (~20-fold increased *ERG* expression) did not show higher rates of PCa than control mice. To further analyze this, transgenic mice bearing a *TMPRSS2:ERG* fusion were crossed with *Pten*$^{+/-}$ mice. At 6 months of age all 8 of 8 *TMPRSS2:ERG/Pten*$^{+/-}$ mice had clear histologic evidence of high-grade PIN while only one focus of low grade PIN was identified in one of the eight *Pten*$^{+/-}$ littermate controls. Similar crosses of *TMPRSS2:ERG* fusion mice with mice expressing high *MYC* transcripts did not show cooperativity in PCa development. Cooperativity was identified when *TMPRSS2:ERG* fusion mice were crossed with prostate-specific AKT overexpressing transgenic mice, where 8 of 8 bigenic mice developed florid PCa lesions by 10–12 months, while all of the AKT overexpressing mice developed low-grade PIN and did not progress to PCa. Other investigators found similar results [100], finding that *ERG* overexpression promoted cell migration, without affecting proliferation, and that *PTEN* loss was needed for increased cell proliferation, mediated by increased AKT activity. Interestingly, microarray expression analysis demonstrated that *ERG* overexpression increased *CXCR4* and *ADAMTS1* expression, two genes whose products promote cell migration, invasion, and angiogenesis.

Yoshimoto et al. [93] performed a retrospective study on 125 PCa cases with known clinical outcomes and examined *TMPRSS2:ERG* fusions and *PTEN* genomic deletions by fluorescent in situ hybridization (FISH). Forty-eight percent of the PCas had *TMPRSS2:ERG* fusions. Gleason grade ($p=0.0002$)/score ($p=0.001$), median tumor volume ($p=0.15$), preoperative PSA ($p=0.001$), and perineural invasion ($p=0.0304$) were associated with biochemical reoccurrence, while *TMPRSS2:ERG* fusion almost reached significance ($p=0.0523$). Interestingly, multivariate analysis revealed *PTEN* homozygous deletion ($p=0.013$) and concurrent *TMPRSS2:ERG* fusion with *PTEN* homozygous deletion ($p=0.036$). Kaplan-Meier and multivariate analysis both indicated that concurrent *TMPRSS2:ERG* fusion and *PTEN* loss predict earlier PCa biochemical recurrence.

9.4.8 Loss of the TMPRSS2 3′ Genomic Region of PCa with Concurrent Fusion Duplication

TMPRSS2 and ERG are located ~3 Mb apart on chromosome 21, allowing the *TMPRSS2:ERG* fusion to form via a translocation between chromosomes 21, or by interstitial deletions [86, 101]. Several studies have demonstrated that *TMPRSS2:ERG* fusions resulting from interstitial deletions have a worse prognosis than those arising from translocations. For example, Attard et al. [89] analyzed 445 PCas from conservatively managed patients. Individuals lacking *ERG* alterations exhibited a favorable clinical course, with a 90 % survival at 8 years. Conversely, individuals with duplications of the *TMPRSS2:ERG* fusions (2+Edel) resulting from interstitial 3′ deletions had an extremely poor clinical course, with 25 % survival at 8 years. Multivariant analysis revealed 2+Edel provided significant prognostic information ($p=0.003$), in addition to that provided by Gleason score and PSA levels.

In another study, Gopalan et al. [87] analyzed 521 patients who underwent radical prostatectomies using FISH probes to 3′ *ERG*, 5′*TMPRSS2*, and 3′ *TMPRSS2* clones. Since FISH measures genomic structural alterations and is therefore an indirect test for gene fusions, 67 PCas previously analyzed for fusions by oligonucleotide arrays were analyzed by FISH. FISH was less sensitive than oligonucleotide arrays and preferentially detected PCas with higher *ERG* expression. Of the 521 PCas analyzed, 217 (42 %) had *TMPRSS2:ERG* alterations; of these, 128 (59 %) were 3′ *TMPRSS2* deletions, or a total of 12 % of the 521 PCas. *ERG* expression alone was not significantly different between patients with and without biochemical recurrence, but did correlate with overall survival and metastases, and was associated with a lower Gleason score. Interestingly, increased *ERG* or *TMPRSS2* copy number without fusion was significantly associated with high (≥7) Gleason scores, while increased copy number of the *TMPRSS2:ERG* deletion fusion was significantly ($p < 0.01$) associated with increased metastases and poorer outcomes. Lastly, *ETV1* rearrangements failed to show an association with poorer survival [102].

Wang et al. [88] found that different *TMPRSS2:ERG* isoforms are associated with aggressive PCa. Specifically, *TMPRSS2:ERG* fusion isoforms in which the native ATG of *TMPRSS2* is in frame with exon 4 of *ERG* was associated with early biochemical recurrence following radical prostatectomy, aggressive disease, and death from PCa. Similarly, fusions with the native *ERG* ATG in exon 3 were associated with seminal vesicle invasion and poor outcome following radical prostatectomy. Interestingly, PCas not having these fusions isoforms tended to have higher overall fusion mRNA expression. Wang et al. [88] concluded that both the level of fusion mRNA expression and the specific isoform likely effect PCa progression.

9.5 Specific TMPRSS2:ETS Gene Fusion Detection Techniques

Several different molecular techniques have proven useful in the detection of *TMPRSS2:ETS* gene fusions. Among them are many variations of PCR, FISH, microarray, DNA sequencing techniques, and immunohistochemistry. Here we will review a few of these techniques.

9.5.1 PCR

Many *TMPRSS2:ETS* fusion detection methods utilize PCR, with amplicon detection achieved via various detection methods. Wang et al. [88] extracted RNA from 19 normal (peripheral zone), 18 early recurrence (less than 1 year), 16 late recurrence (recurrence after 1–5 years), and 20 non-recurrent radical prostatectomy samples. Five micrograms of RNA were reverse transcribed in cDNA in a total volume of 100 μL in an iScript cDNA synthesis kit, according to the manufacturer's protocol.

Five μL of cDNA template were amplified with *TMPRSS2* RT forward 5′-CAGGAGGCGGAGGCGGA-3′ and *TMPRSS2:ERG* RT reverse 5′-GGCGTT GTAGCTGGGGGTGAG-3′ in a volume of 25 μL, using a standard three-step protocol with an annealing temperature of 65 °C. The resulting amplicons were detected on a 1.2 % agarose gel stained ethidium bromide. The different sized amplicons were cloned into a PCR 2.1-Topo vector cloning kit. Plasmids were prepared using a Qiagen Spin Mini-Prep kit and sequenced by M13R and M13F primers. The sequences were analyzed by National Center for Biotechnology Information BLAST software. Additionally, quantitative real-time PCR was performed using β-actin as an amplification control and SYBR green fluorescence as the detection method. Fifty-nine percent of the prostatectomies showed *TMPRSS2:ERG* fusions. As mentioned above, those fusions carrying native *TMPRSS2* or *ERG* translation initiation codons had a significantly worse prognosis.

9.5.2 FISH

FISH has commonly been used to detect *TMPRSS2:ERG* fusions and has the advantage of giving information concerning chromosomal structure that PCR does not give. Attard et al. [89] used overlapping bacterial artificial chromosome probes to the centromeric 3′-end (red) and probes to the telomeric 5′-end (green) to analyze different *TMPRSS2:ETS* fusion isoforms. By this assay, unrearranged *ERG* loci appeared as immediately adjacent green and red signals in interphase nuclei. When the *TMPRSS2:ERG* fusion isoform was *TMPRSS2* exons 1 or 2 fused to *ERG* exons 2, 3, or 4 (common isoforms) [71, 77], *ERG* occurred as separated red and green signals. As previously mentioned, duplication of these deletion isoforms (2+Edel) resulted in an extremely poor clinical course.

9.5.3 Gene Fusion Detected in PCa by Immunohistochemistry

Park et al. [103] employed tissue microarrays to analyze 131 men who underwent radical prostatectomies. The tissue microassays were constructed from benign and malignant formalin-fixed paraffin-embedded tissue blocks from the prostatectomies. The selection of tissue samples and review of each case's pathological findings were conducted and performed by the study pathologists. The primary rabbit antibody was obtained from Epitomics (San Diego, CA) and was carefully characterized for use in tissue microarray studies compared to two color interphase FISH. Immunohistochemical tissue microarray reactivity was highly concordant with two color interphase FISH. The tissue microarray was carried out using an automated DiscoveryXT staining platform from Ventana Medical Systems. Antigen recovery was conducted using heat retrieval with the slides incubated with 1:100 primary *ERG* antibody for 1 h at room temperature. The primary antibody was detected using a ChromoMapDAB anti-rabbit horseradish peroxidase conjugated antibody that was applied for 16 min followed by washing and detection. ERG protein expression was subjectively evaluated using a negative (0), weakly positive (+1), moderately positive (+2), and strongly positive (+3) scale.

ERG expression was confined to the PCa cells and high-grade PIN that was associated with *ERG*-positive PCa. It was also identified in blood vessels and lymphocytes where it has a known biologic role. Analysis of the 131 cases compared to FISH revealed 95.7 % sensitivity and 96.5 % specificity. Since immunohistochemical studies are technically easier and less expensive than FISH analyses, molecular PCa subtyping by immunohistochemistry may have clinical utility, especially for prostate needle core biopsies.

9.5.4 *SPINK1* Overexpression in PCa

Tomlins et al. [104] employed COPA analysis on seven PCa profiling studies in the Oncomine database to identify candidate outlier genes in *ETS* negative PCas. Twenty-nine genes were identified as possible outliers in three of the seven databases, with 11 genes identified in at least four of the databases. The first outlier out of all of the databases was *ERG*, with the COPA analysis performed as previously described [71]. One gene, *SPINK1* (serine peptidase inhibitor, Kazal type 1) was ranked as the second outlier, exhibiting overexpression in PCa compared to benign tissue and additionally having overexpression mutually exclusive of *ERG* and *ETV1*.

To confirm that *SPINK1* expression did not occur in *ETS* positive PCas, *SPINK1*, *ERG*, and *ETV1* expression was analyzed in 10 benign and 61 malignant prostate samples using quantitative PCR. Total RNA was isolated from the samples with Trizol, quantified, and 3–5 μg of total RNA was reversed transcribed into DNA using Superscript III in the presence of random primers. The cDNA was amplified with Power SYBR Green Master Mix in the presence of 25 ng SPINK1 f-CAAAAATCTG GGCCTTGCTGAGAAC and SPINK1 r- AGGCCTCGCGGTGACCTGAT and forward and reverse primers for *ERG*, *ETV1*, and *GAPDH* and *HMBS* as housekeeping gene controls. The primers for these last four genes were the same as those employed by Tomlins et al. [71]. Serial dilutions of the primers on pooled PCA cDNA demonstrated approximately equal primers efficiencies. All reactions were subjected to melt curve analyses. *ERG*, *ETV1*, and *SPINK1* were expressed in 41 %, 6.5 %, and 6.5 % of the 61 PCas and none of the 10 benign samples and exhibited mutually exclusive expression patterns. Additionally, FISH analysis for *SPINK1* and *TMPRSS2:ERG* fusion was performed on two tissue microarrays representing 392 PCa cases. *SPINK1* overexpression was identified in 13.3 % of cases, while *TMPRSS2:ERG* fusion overexpression was identified in 48 % of cases; again, no concurrent *SPINK1-TMPRSS2:ERG* fusion was seen.

Examination of three independent cohorts consisting of 79, 75, and 817 PCa cases that underwent radical prostatectomies revealed that *SPINK1* overexpressing cases had a significantly higher risk for PCa recurrence than those cases without overexpression.

Multivariate Cox proportional-hazards regression analysis confirmed that *SPINK1* outlier status was a significant predictor of PCa recurrence and was independent of Gleason score, lymph node status, surgical margin status, seminal vesicle invasion, extraprostatic extension, and preoperative PSA levels. Tomlins et al. [104] hypothesized that in *ETS* negativity may predispose PCas to *SPINK1* overexpression. Although not commonly used in the molecular diagnostic of PCa, *SPINK1* overexpression shows promise as a predictor of a more aggressive PCa clinical course and an increased recurrence rate following radical prostatectomy.

9.5.5 *t(4;6)(q22;q15) in PCa*

A t(4;6)(q22;q15) chromosomal translocation has been indentified in PCa lines and human PCas using multiplex FISH and FISH for this translocation on tissue microarrays [105, 106]. Of 667 PCas analyzed by tissue microarray, 11.7 % were positive for the t(4;6)(q22;q15) translocation [105]. The presence of this translocation did not affect cause-specific or overall survival. Its presence did, however, correlate with a higher Gleason score, clinical stage, baseline PSA, and tumor volume upon biopsy. Adding the t(4;6)(q22;q15) translocation to a Multivariate Cox model, which included the Gleason score, baseline PSA, extent of disease, and age at diagnosis, did not significantly improve the model. Interestingly, t(4;6)(q22;q15) did occur more frequently in 2+Edel positive samples than negative samples, although the correlation did not reach significance ($p = 0.0628$) [105]. The authors concluded that, while this translocation does not independently affect patient outcome, it may define specific cohort of PCas, thus warranting further investigation.

Since the work by Tomlins et al. [71], PCa has been found to harbor over 20 different translocations, some of which are known to alter the clinical course of PCa, while others either have little effect, or require further study [62, 64, 71–106]. While extremely complex, some of these translocations appear to have value in the molecular diagnostics of PCa and are likely be incorporated into clinical testing within the next few years.

9.6 Somatic Mitochondrial DNA Mutations in PCa

Mitochondrial mutations have been identified in many different malignancies, including, breast, ovarian, colorectal, gastric, hepatic, brain, thyroid, esophageal, pancreatic, renal, and PCas [107]. In a recent study, Parr et al. [108] examined somatic DNA mitochondrial mutations in PCa via full mitochondrial genome sequencing. Thirty-six patients were selected for the study. Twenty-four patients had undergone radical prostatectomy for advanced PCa, and 12 patients were symptomatic (i.e., had elevated PSA) but free of detectable PCa by biopsy. DNA was recovered from histologically malignant and benign paraffin-embedded prostate glands by laser capture microdissection. DNA was also isolated from whole blood draws taken from the 36 patients and a subset of the patients' maternal relatives recruited for the study. The complete mitochondrial genome was PCR amplified with 34 primer sets, sequenced, and analyzed by Sequencher Software (Gene Codes Corp.). Sequence polymorphic variations were identified by comparing the blood samples to the revised Cambridge reference sequence. Additionally, nuclear-embedded mitochondrial pseudogenes sequences that co-amplified were prepared from an osteosarcoma cell line. The resulting amplicons were extensively analyzed and compared to hetero- and homoplasmic sites in the sequence data to preclude any inclusions of paralogue nuclear mutations in the mitochondrial final data set.

Sixteen of the 24 PCa samples (66.7 %) had mitochondrial mutations in all three examined prostatic compartments. 91.7 % had mutations in the histologically malignant prostatic glands, 79.2 % had mutations in histologically benign prostatic glands near the PCA, and 91.7 % had mutations in distant, histologically benign prostatic glands. The average mitochondrial genome sequence coverage was 78 % which leaved 3.6 kb unexamined. A total of 273 somatic mitochondrial mutations were identified. The maternal relative blood samples showed few differences between genomes, indicating that the mutations were not merely age-associated events.

Since mutations were found in histologically benign glands, the disease specificity of the mutations was examined. The symptomatic benign group had far fewer mutations, most of which occurred in known polymorphic loci on non-coding genomic regions. The histologically malignant glands did not differ in the non-coding genomic region mutations, but had significantly increased coding region mutations compared to all the histologically benign glands. The authors concluded that genomic mutations precede malignant histology and accumulate with malignancy progression. Additionally, with tumor progression, very specific mutations became increasingly common, with six linked mutations seen in 44 % of the PCas and one (mutation 15,527) identified in 74 % of PCas. Since cells typically carry a high mitochondrial genome copy number and mitochondrial DNA can be easily isolated and analyzed for specific mutations, the use of high-frequency mitochondrial genome mutations associated with PCa may have eventual utility in PCa molecular diagnostics. Methods such as microarray and allele-specific PCR would allow for high-throughput analysis of mutations. Presently, further work is required to analyze and validify PCa mitochondrial mutation frequencies and association with PCa.

9.6.1 C-MYC Amplification in PCa

C-*MYC* is found at 8q24.12 to 8q24.13 and belongs to the Myc family that also includes *Myc/MAD/MAX* basic helix-loop-helix leucine zipper domain transcription factors. *C-MYC* is a multifunctional nuclear phosphoprotein that plays a role in regulating cell cycle entry and progression, transcription, differentiation, apoptosis, and cellular motility. *C-MYC* is dysregulated in several malignancies, including breast, colon, gynecological, and hepatocellular malignancies, and those of hematopoietic lineage. *C-MYC* appears to bind DNA nonspecifically, although it also recognizes the core sequence 5′-CAC[GA]TG-3′ where it activates the expression of growth-related genes [109, 110]. Fleming et al. [111] first demonstrated *C-MYC* overexpression in PCa vs. BPH with Northern blotting. Since then, data derived from FISH analyses have shown that *C-MYC* is expressed in PIN, PCa, and metastatic PCa, with the *C-MYC* levels increasing with tumor progression [112–114]. Additionally, Sato et al. [114] used dual-probe FISH with a centromere-specific probe for chromosome 8 and one region-specific probe for *C-MYC* to examine changes in 50 Japanese PCa patients who had undergone retropubic prostatectomies. *C-MYC* expression correlated strongly with higher histopathologic grade, Gleason score, earlier disease progression, and earlier PCa-related death. Lastly, *C-MYC* overexpression was a predictor of biochemical recurrence, and higher *C-MYC* mRNA levels significantly correlated with positive surgical margins upon prostatectomy, higher Gleason score, and pathologic stage [115]. Interestingly, *C-MYC* expression varies in different neoplastic lesions within the same prostate, similar to many of the other molecular alterations identified in PCa carcinogenesis and progression [62, 64, 71–106, 115].

C-MYC levels in PCa have been quantified via FISH, RT-PCR, and microarray [112–116]. While all these methods have worked well and reliably, RT-PCR is comparatively low-cost, has a short turn-around time, and high sensitivity. Hawksworth et al. [115] employed RT-PCR quantify C-MYC expression in 182 specimens taken from 91 retropubic prostatectomies, using laser capture microdissection to isolate benign and neoplastic prostatic epithelial cells. Quantitative gene expression was performed by extracting total RNA with a MicroRNA kit, quantifying the RNA yield with RiboGreen dye and a VersaLour fluorimeter, converting to cDNA by Sensiscript (Qiagen oligonucleotide primers with reverse transcriptase), and finally PCR amplifying with a forward primer, 5′-ACCACCAGCAGCGACTCTGA-3′, reverse primer, 5′-TCC AGCAGAAGGTGATCCAGA CT-3′, and a probe 5′-ACCTTTTGCCAGGAGCCTGCCTCT-3′. The reactions were carried out with a TaqMan-based QRT-PRC on an ABI 7700 with 50 cycles; 95 °C for 15 s and 60 °C for 1 min. *GAPDH* was amplified as a control gene. Gene-expression results were obtained as average threshold values (C_t value) of duplicate samples. As mentioned above, higher *C-MYC* expression significantly correlated with biochemical recurrence, positive surgical margins, and higher Gleason score and pathologic stage [115]. Interestingly, the common *TMPRSS2:ERG* fusion activates *C-MYC* expression and not surprisingly, *C-MYC* overexpression and the *TMPRSS2:ERG* fusion commonly occur together [117].

9.6.2 Bcl-2

Bcl-2, or B-cell lymphoma 2, is found at 18q21.3 and plays a central role in regulating apoptosis and is induced by a wide variety of divergent stimuli. *Bcl-2* is part of a larger protein family that is involved in regulating cell death by promoting or inhibiting apoptosis. The ratio of the pro-apoptotic to anti-apoptotic determines cell survival and vulnerability to toxic stimuli by inhibiting the activation of the pro-apoptotic proteins *Bax* and *Bak* on the outer mitochondrial membrane. Thus, *Bcl-2* overexpression confers a survival advantage [118–120]. In normal prostate, *Bcl-2* expression is limited to the basilar glandular epithelium, where its expression is androgen independent. In PCa, *Bcl-2* expression is significantly increased in androgen-independent PCa, but to a far lesser degree in androgen-dependent PCa. Based on this, it is thought that *Bcl-2* overexpression is one factor in allowing the survival and spread of androgen-independent PCa [121].

Although not commonly employed in the molecular diagnostics of PCa, *Bcl-2* overexpression confers are worse PCa prognosis. For example, Concato et al. [122] analyzed 1,007 PCa cases for Bcl-2 expression, with an average patient age of 72 years at PCa diagnosis. The patients were followed for over 15 years. At the end of this period, 71.8 % had died of any cause, with 21.5 % due to PCa. The median overall survival was 7.7 years. Multivariate analysis of this cohort revealed that increasing age, higher PSA levels (over 20 μg/mL), and moderately to poorly differentiated PCa were strongly associated with shorter survival. *Bcl-2* overexpression was associated with an increased long-term death risk from PCa, with an adjusted hazard ratio of 1.61. Interestingly, the same study revealed that p53 overexpression and the upper three quartiles of microvessel density were also associated with a long-term death risk from PCa, having adjusted hazard ratios of 1.48 and 3.20, respectively. *Bcl-2* expression has mainly been examined by immunohistochemical staining [121–124].

9.6.3 Kallikrein

In addition to PSA, another member of the kallikrein family, human glandular kallikrein 2 (hK2), may also be useful in detecting early PCa. In the bloodstream, hK2 is present at 1–2 % of the total PSA serum concentration with up to 20 % of which can be complexed with α_1-antichymotrypsin [125]. Of detectable hK2 in blood, 80–90 % occurs as free, non-complexed 30-kDa form. Both hK2 and PSA are produced mainly in the prostate under the control of androgen stimulation [126, 127]. hK2 shows an age dependency, but less than is seen with PSA. Men in their 40s and 50s seem to have similar hK2 concentrations, while men in the 60s show an increase in hK2, but once again less than that seen for PSA. hK2 functions as a trypsin-like protease and among the kallikrein variants it has the highest homology to PSA, having about 80 % sequence identity. Because of this high level of homology, previous assays utilizing monoclonal antibodies that were raised against PSA could also detect hK2 [128]. The physiological link between these two proteins may be the ability of hK2 to cleave the propeptide of inactive pro-PSA, converting it into its mature active form [129, 130].

hK2 and PSA expression differ in that PSA is more intensely expressed in BPH than in PCa. Additionally, PSA expression is higher in low-grade than in high-grade PCas.

In contrast, hK2 shows higher staining intensity in high-grade PCa and lymph node metastasis than it does in low-grade PCa or BPH [131, 132]. Similar to PSA, hK2 exists in different molecular forms. In vitro, it complexes with several protease inhibitors, including α2-antiplasmin, AT, antithrombin III, α2-macroglobulin, C1-inactivator, and plasminogen activator inhibitor-1 [133–135]. Both free and complexed forms have been found in biological fluids. In seminal fluid, the protein is mainly complexed to protein C inhibitor [136]. However, in the bloodstream, 80–95 % is uncomplexed [127, 137] while in PCa patients with high hK2 levels, up to 20 % is complexed to ACT [125]. As previously mentioned, an inactive zymogen form (pro-hK2) is found in blood [138].

Because of its low circulating levels, immunoassays for hK2 must have low detection limits with excellent reproducibility. The first assay developed to measure hK2 employed an immunoflurometric technique using two separate incubations, one to inhibit subsequent reactions of both free and complexed PSA using MAb2H11 (which does not cross react with hK2) and a second using biotinylated MabH50 (which cross reacts with hK2 by epitope overlapping with Mab2H11, binding only hK2 on streptavidin microtitration wells). A third step utilized eu-labeled MAb117, which cross reacted with hK2 and detected the immobilized hK2. The assay was calibrated with a recombinant hK2, giving a detection limit of 0.1 μg/L, and cross reactivity with PSA of <0.7 %. However, up to 57 % of samples had hK2 concentrations below the detection limit [126].

Since then, more sensitive and specific assays have been developed using hK2 specific monoclonal antibodies. These, with the addition of ultrasensitive immunoassays for measuring free and total hK2 in serum, yield detection limits of 0.0008 μg/mL for total hK2 and 0.001 μg/mL for the free hK2. This technique was developed to achieve the required sensitivity to measure blood hK2. The limit of quantification (intraassay CV <15 %) in serum matrix for total hK2 was 0.003 and 0.010 μg/L for free hK2. The results revealed hK2 concentrations of 1–5 % of the total PSA (range, 0.1–58 %; median, 3.6 %), with a median total hK2 concentration of 0.022 μg/L [139]. Previous studies revealed hK2 concentrations to be 1–4 % of PSA concentrations [126, 140, 141]. The median hK2 concentration was lower than the reported value of 0.026 μg/L [142] but higher than the value of 0.016 μg/L reported by other authors [141]. In addition, the correlation coefficient was low between the two proteins, particularly in the "gray diagnostic area" for PSA (4–10 ng/mL), suggesting PSA and hK2 may have different elimination patterns and that hK2 may therefore be able to provide clinical information independent from PSA [139].

Interestingly, while hK2 concentrations did not significantly differ between PCa and BPH patients, the ratio of hK2 to fPSA (percent hK2) did allow the discrimination of PCa from BPH within the 4–10-ng/mL PSA range over percent fPSA alone [143]. Similar findings of a nonsignificant relationship of hK2 concentrations and PCa have been reported [144–146]; however, later studies found significantly higher levels of hK2 in PCa versus BPH or non-PCa samples [147–154]. The percent hK2 enhanced the discrimination between PCa and non-PCa patients in multiple studies [144–146, 148, 150–152]. Within the 2.5–10-ng/mL PSA range, the predictive value of percent hK2 was greater than percent fPSA in most studies [144, 145, 151, 152], although a different large study found a higher predictive value for percent fPSA [145]. In addition, other studies found that for PSA levels <4 ng/mL, the predictive value of percent hK2 performed worse than percent fPSA [145, 152].

Several studies examined the relationship between PCa stage and grade, revealing that hK2 can differentiate high- from low-grade tumors and organ versus non-organ confined disease [155–159]. Several studies also revealed that hK2 levels were significantly higher in organ confined versus non-organ confined disease, although after Gleason grade and clinical stage were added to a multivariate logistic regression model, the improvements were only marginal [182–184]. A current study has confirmed these findings [153]. In contrast, others showed that hK2 was of no to little value in predicting tumor stage and grade [160, 161]. In summary, most studies show significantly elevated levels of hK2 in men with PCa than in men without PCa, although several other studies did not. An increased predictive value for percent hK2 over percent fPSA alone is supported by most studies. Most studies show a limited increase in predicting stage and tumor grade after addition of hK2 or hK2 incorporated ratios with fPSA or total PSA.

9.6.4 Urokinase Plasminogen Activator

Most patients that experience relapsed or advanced disease respond initially to androgen ablation therapy because early PCa is often androgen dependent. However, many PCas eventually progress to hormone refractory PCa, which is refractory to androgen ablation, thus limiting treatment options thus far for metastatic PCa.

Metastatic PCa often follows lymphatic and hematogenous routes to regional lymph nodes and bone, especially the spine. Although the mechanism(s) of tumor progression is incompletely understood, several proteolytic enzymes are involved in degrading the basement membrane and extracellular matrix (ECM), thereby increasing PCa metastatic potential. One proteolytic enzyme and receptor involved in this process are the urokinase plasminogen activator (uPA) and its receptor (uPAR). uPA is a serine protease family member linked to many different malignancies. It is synthesized as a pro-enzyme, a single chain known as pro-uPA, which binds to uPAR with high affinity. Binding converts inactive plasminogen into plasmin, which then can cleave various ECM components including fibrin, collagen, laminin, fibronectin, and vitronectin. Plasmin can also activate matrix metalloproteinases (MMPs) and elastase, causing further ECM degradation. It is thought that these processes lead to increased tumor invasiveness and metastatic potential. Binding of uPA to uPAR also increases the affinity of uPAR for the ECM protein vitronectin and for integrin adhesion receptors [162].

Activity of uPA is regulated by two serine protease inhibitors (PAI1 and PAI2) and by uPAR. PAI1 and PAI2 form SDS-stable 1:1 complexes with uPA. PAI1 is a 43-kDa single chain glycoprotein and is likely the primary inhibitor of the uPA. PAI2 has 2 forms, one 47-kDa form that is intracellular and non-glycosolated and one 60-kDa form that is extracellular and glycosolated. The interaction of PAI1/uPA/uPAR leads to internalization of the ternary complex, which causes cell proliferation. In PCa cells, this complex enters the cell via receptor-mediated endocytosis mediated by the low-density lipoprotein receptor-related protein. The discovery of this mechanism may facilitate the transfer of cytotoxic therapies to uPA-positive cancer cells, as inhibiting uPA by plasminogen activator inhibitor-2 results in accelerated clearance of uPA from the cell membrane [163].

uPAR is not only responsible for lateral protein-protein interactions that contribute to cell adhesion and migration via the integrin family but also contributes to signal transduction cascades within uPAR expressing cells, including the JAK-STAT, mitogen-activated, and Ras/extracellular signal regulated kinase pathway proteins, which regulate genes responsible for proliferation, survival, and apoptosis [164–166]. Interestingly, in a murine model, anti-sense oligonucleotides down-regulated uPAR expression, decreasing FAK/JNK/Jun phosphorylation, inhibiting cyclins A, B, D1 and D3 synthesis, and causing a G_2 phase cell cycle checkpoint, resulting in unaffected adhesion, but impaired proliferation and invasion, and a subsequent decrease in PCa bone metastasis [167].

The uPAR protein consists of three homologous three-finger domains, in which the amino terminal domain I is required in order for uPA binding. Domain 1 contains the N-terminal. Removal of this domain from the cell surface drastically reduces the capacity of cells to bind to uPA. When bound, uPA cleaves uPAR between domains I and II freeing domain I (uPAR1), leaving domains II and III (uPARII-III) attached to the cell surface. Additionally, uPAR can be cleaved from the cell's surface at its lipid anchor by either phospholipases or proteases, generating a full-length uPAR(I-III) and/or uPAR(II-III) [168, 169]. Immunoassays capable of detecting intact and cleaved forms of the receptor have been developed, and certain forms of the cleaved receptor, such as uPAR1 and uPARII-III, are found at higher levels in PCa than in benign disease. In men with a serum PSA of 2–10 μg/L, the combination of percent fPSA with the uPAR1/uPARI-III ratio, had a greater area under the ROC curve (0.73), compared to percent fPSA alone (0.68) [170, 171].

A number of studies have demonstrated increased levels of uPA and uPAR in prostate PCa [172, 173]. Others have shown an association of uPA overexpression with extracapsular extension [174]. Elevated levels of both have also been demonstrated in high-grade tumors (Gleason > 7), using immunohistochemistry and tissue microarrays. Elevated levels have also been seen to be associated with metastasis [175–177]. Stromal expression of uPA and its receptor have also been found to have significance. TMAs have demonstrated expression not only in PCa cells, but also in stromal cells in high Gleason score cancers [177]. By releasing chemotactic factors, the PCa epithelia can induce stromal cells to contribute to an environment conducive to metastasis through their release of cytokines, growth factors, and proteolytic enzymes. MMPs are synthesized by both cancer and stromal cells [178], and elevations in uPA and uPAR have been associated with an increase in these enzymes [179–181]. These findings suggest that increased uPA/uPAR in PCa may stimulate stromal paracine MMP synthesis, increasing PCa metastatic potential.

uPA/uPAR are the targets of several new potential treatments. The tyrosine kinase inhibitors, genistein and tyrphostin AG-1478, profoundly reduce uPA/uPAR production and mRNA levels in PCa cells and inhibit invasive potential [182–185]. Because PAI2 is stable in vitro and is unlikely to be subject to inactivation in oxidizing environments such as inflammation and laboratory testing, it is a potential vector for targeted therapy. By forming radioimmunoconjugates through the labeling of PAI2 with α-emitting radionucleotide ^{213}Bi-uPA positive cancer cells were induced to apoptosis in vitro. This could be done on monolayer PCa cells alone or in conjunction with other radioimmunoconjugates as multi-targeted alpha therapy. In vivo studies using nude mice showed that this strategy leads to a dose-dependent complete regression or delay of tumor growth, along with a decreased incidence of lymph node metastasis [186–188]. RNA interference is a sequence specific, post-transcriptional gene-silencing mechanism that utilizes double stranded RNA homologous to the target gene sequence. Silencing of the uPA/uPAR genes was performed using single plasmid constructs expressing small hairpin RNAs for both uPA and uPAR. This leads to reduced cell viability, apoptosis, and interference of downstream signaling of the ERK1/2 pathway (responsible for cancer cell invasion, proliferation, and survival) and Stat 3. This substantiates the theory that complex signaling networks downstream of uPA/uPAR are responsible for tumor cell invasion, proliferation, and survival of PCa cells [189].

9.6.5 GSTP-1 Promoter Hypermethylation

The detoxifying glutathione-S-transferases (GSTs) comprise a large supergene family that includes members of eight classes based on sequence similarity: Alpha, Mu, Theta, Kappa, Zeta, Omega, and Sigma. GSTs detoxify a wide variety of exogenous and endogenous compounds, such as reactive oxygen species produced by normal cellular functions, and exogenous toxins, such as polycyclic aromatic hydrocarbons. GSTs function by catalyzing the nucleophilic attack of glutathione on electrophilic substrates, reducing their reactivity with cellular constituents [190, 191]. Interestingly, some data indicate that GSTs may have non-detoxifying activities, such as selective inhibition of oncogenic ras-p21-induced mitogenic signaling via Jun kinase inhibition [192].

Because GSTs play an important role in the detoxification and hence inhibition of endogenous and exogenous toxins, loss of these proteins is pro-mutagenic [193]. In fact, the GSTs are lost in a large number of different malignancies, including squamous cell carcinoma, nasopharyngeal carcinoma, non-small cell lung cancers, and PCa [193–196]. Within PCa, hypermethylation of glutathione-S-transferase P1 (GSTP1) promoter CpG islands are the most consistent DNA alterations identified in PCas, having been identified in ~70 % of high-grade PIN and over 90 % of PCas [196]. GSTP1 CpG island promoter methylation has been detected by a variety of different methods, such as digestion of normal and PCa DNA with endonucleases that cut at non-methylated, but not methylated cytosine residues, followed by PRC amplification, or methylation-specific PCR techniques [196, 197].

9.6.6 Methylation-Specific PCR

Methylation-specific PCR (MSP) is commonly employed in the analysis of CpG promoter hypermethylation. In this technique, genomic DNA (~1 μg) is isolated and denatured in NaOH for 10 min at 37 °C. Samples with low (nanogram) quantities of DNA often have carrier DNA, such as salmon sperm DNA, added to the subsequent reactions. Next, fresh hydroquinone and sodium bisulfite are added to the reaction at pH 5, and the samples are mixed and incubated for ~16 h at 50 °C. The bisulfite treatment changes cytosine to uracil while not altering methyl-cytosine. Thus, following bisulfite treatment, methylated and unmethylated cytosines can be distinguished by binding to either guanine (methyl-cytosine) or adenine (uracil). The modified DNA is then purified, and different sets of oliogonucleotide primers are employed to analyze the DNA for the presence or absence of methyl-cytosine(s) [198]. Esteller et al. [199] employed bisulfite-modified DNA from more than 300 primary tumors for GSTP1 aberrant promoter methylation and included tumor DNA from endometrial, ovarian, bladder, pancreatic, lung, head and neck, leukemias, melanomas, meningiomas, and PCas. Primers for the unmethylated reactions were *5′-GATGTTTGGGOTGTA*GTGGTTGTT-3′and5′-CCACCCCAATACTAAATCAC AACA-3′ while primers for the methylated reactions were 5′-TTCGGGGTGTAG CGCTCGTC-3′ and 5′-GCCCCAATA CTAAATCAGACG-3′. The annealing PCR temperature was 59 °C, and the resulting amplicons were analyzed on nondenaturing polyacrylamide gels stained with ethidium bromide and visualized under UV-illumination. Normal lymphocytes, breast, kidney, and liver had completely unmethylated GSTP1 promoters, while PCas showed a very high level of methylation. Much lower methylation levels were identified in lung and colon cancers and non-Hodgkin lymphomas. The endometrial, ovarian, bladder, pancreatic, head and neck cancers, melanomas, and meningiomas showed no GSTP1 promoter methylation. GSTP1 methylation has been analyzed in urinary sediments following prostatic massage and found to have an overall sensitivity of 73 % and a specificity of 98 % in a relatively small patient cohort [200].

Although there is utility for promoter methylation analysis, including GSTP1 PCa promoter methylation, it is relatively cumbersome, time-consuming, complex to perform, and often difficult to get to work reliably, as ~90 % of the DNA is often lost in the bisulfite treatment step. The loss of so much DNA with the bisulfite treatment step makes this assay difficult to apply to human testing, as often very little DNA is obtained from sources such as blood or urine sediments. Lastly, methylation-specific promoter design can be very complex. For these reasons, MSP is not often used routinely in molecular diagnostics.

9.6.7 Alpha-Methylacyl-CoA Racemase (AMACR)

Alpha-methylacyl-CoA racemase (AMACR) is encoded in the p504S gene found at 5p13. It is localized to the peroxisomes and mitochondria, where it interconverts a large variety of *(R)*- and *(S)*-2-methyl-branched-chain-fatty acyl-CoAs, an activity necessary for the degradation of these substrates by peroxisomal β-oxidation [201–203]. AMACR levels are increased in PCa compared to benign prostatic epithelium, as measured by immunohistochemistry, Western blotting, microarray, and RT-PCR [204–206]. With immunohistochemical staining, AMACR shows 97 % sensitivity and 100 % specificity for PCa detection [206]. The major drawback of employing AMACR in PCa testing is that AMACR levels are increased in other malignancies and normal tissues. Increased AMACR can be seen in lesions such as metanephric adenomas and papillary renal cell carcinoma [207, 208]. Presently, AMACR immunohistochemical staining, often combined with p63 immunohistochemical staining, is mainly employed in the interpretation of diagnostically difficult prostate needle core biopsies, where p63 staining identifies basal myoepithelial cells and AMACR identifies PCa [205].

9.6.8 MicroRNA Expression in PCa

MicroRNAs (miRNAs) are small noncoding RNAs that regulate the translational efficiency of target mRNAs. They typically bind to 3′ or 5′ untranslated regions of the target mRNAs, leading to lowered stability or decreased translation efficiency [209]. It is estimated that ~30 % of gene expression is regulated by miRNAs, and they have been demonstrated to be dysregulated in a variety of human malignancies. Interestingly, some miRNAs function as tumor suppressors and others act as oncogenes, with the former suppressed and the latter overexpressed in human malignancies [209–212]. Multiple studies have shown that PCa shows an altered miRNA expression pattern, with more than 50 miRNA species dysregulated in this disease [213]. Interestingly, some of the dysregulated miRNAs give biochemical information about the specific PCa. For example, miR-21 expression is significantly higher in androgen-independent than in androgen-dependent PCa cells while expression of miR-203 correlates with PCa progression and metastases [214, 215]. Although presently mainly a research tool, miRNA expression profiling in PCa may eventually have value in the diagnosis and treatment of PCa. miRNA expression appears to lend itself more easily to profiling analysis, as miRNA typically regulates about 200 different mRNAs [209–212]. Thus, a relatively low number of miRNA species studied may be superior to profiling the expression of hundreds of different mRNAs in PCa. One study supports this contention, where miRNA was highly informative in analyzing human tumors, whereas mRNA profiling was highly inaccurate when applied to the same system [216].

9.6.9 Single Nucleotide Polymorphisms

A large number of single nucleotide polymorphisms (SNPs) have been implicated in the risk of developing PCa, including SNPs in the ATM, AR, E-cadherin, ICAM-1s, -4, and -5, APE1, VDR, p53, CDKN1A, CCND1, MDM2, hOGG1,

VEGF, EGF, and HIF-1α genes [14, 229–238]. Presently, SNP analysis is largely confined to basic research and not used in the clinical molecular diagnostics of PCa. It is likely within the next few years that SNP analysis will be employed as part of an algorithm to establish an individual's relative risk for the development of PCa and other pathologies. Such an analysis would be facilitated by accurate and low-cost whole genome sequencing technologies [217].

9.6.10 Golgi Phosphoprotein 2 (GOLPH2)

Golgi phosphoprotein 2 (GOLPH2) is a type II Golgi membrane phosphoprotein that plays a role in liver disease and may be a potential serum marker for hepatocellular carcinoma [218–221]. Laxman et al. [222] obtained urine samples from 276 men prior to prostrate needle biopsy ($n = 216$) or radical prostatectomy ($n = 60$). The urine was collected following mild digital pressure to the prostate, and RNA was isolated and analyzed via quantitative PCR. *GOLPH2* mRNA expression analysis outperformed serum PSA as a predictor of PCa. Similarly, other investigators found *GOLPH2* overexpression in PCa by immunohistochemistry, microarray, and RT-PCR [223, 224]. Although not presently used in the molecular diagnostic of PCa, *GOLPH2* expression analysis may be used in PCa diagnosis in the future, particularly as part of a panel [222, 225] (see below).

9.6.11 Biomarker Panels in PCa Molecular Diagnostics

The above data indicate that molecular pathology underlying PCa is exceptionally complex, with many different genetic events playing a role in the development and progression of PCa. Many of the molecular alterations seen in PCa are present only in a subset of PCas or carry altered prognostic significance only when accompanied by other concomitant molecular alterations; the poorer prognosis seen with concomitant *TMPRSS2:ERG* fusion and *PTEN* loss are examples [93]. Several studies have addressed this issue. For example, Laxman et al. [222] found by univariant analysis that increased *GOLPH2, SPINK1, PCA3*, and *TMPRSS2-ERG* fusion all were significant predictors of PCa. However, multivariate regression analysis demonstrated that a multiplexed model incorporating all of the biomarkers outperformed both serum PSA and PCA3 by itself in detecting PCa. Similarly, Vener et al. [225] developed a multiplexed, methylation-specific PCR array consisting of three methylation markers for *GSTP1, RARB,* and *APC,* along with one endogenous control *ACTB*, in a closed-tube, homogeneous assay format. A total of 234 urine samples were examined following digital rectal examinations in two independent cohorts of men with PSA ≥2.5 μg/L. Combined with factors such as race, patient age, and serum PSA, the addition of these markers improved PCa detection. It is likely that future PCa molecular diagnostic testing will often involve gene expression/mutation panels to increase assay sensitivity and specificity.

9.7 Conclusion

The spectrum of PCa ranges from relatively indolent tumors, where an active surveillance approach offers maximum benefit to the patient, to PCa cases with metastatic progression and death occurring within a matter of months. Obviously, many cases require aggressive clinical intervention [226–228]. Presently, our ability to differentiate between these distinct entities is poor, thus leaving some patients overtreated and others tragically undertreated. Although current PCa molecular diagnostics are extremely limited, our understanding of this disease has vastly increased in a relatively short period of time. Within the next few years, molecular diagnostics will very likely be applied to PCa on a routine basis and prove a useful tool for patient risk stratification and a personalized therapeutic approach to each individual patient.

References

1. Jemal A, Siegel R, Ward E, Hao Y, Xu J, Murray T, Thun MJ (2008) Cancer statistics. CA Cancer J Clin 58:71–96
2. Ferlay J, Autier P, Boniol M, Heanue M, Colombet M, Boyle P (2007) Estimates of the cancer incidence and mortality in Europe in 2006. Ann Oncol 18:581–592
3. http://www.wcrf.org/cancer_facts/prostate-cancer-worldwide.php
4. Osório-Costa F, Rocha GZ, Dias MM, Carvalheira JB (2009) Epidemiological and molecular mechanisms aspects linking obesity and cancer. Arq Bras Endocrinol Metabol 53:213–226
5. Freedland SJ, Platz EA (2007) Obesity and prostate cancer: making sense out of apparently conflicting data. Epidemiol Rev 29:88–97
6. Zheng W, Lee SA (2009) Well-done meat intake, heterocyclic amine exposure, and cancer risk. Nutr Cancer 61:437–446
7. Khan N, Afaq F, Mukhtar H (2010) Lifestyle as risk factor for cancer: evidence from human studies. Cancer Lett 293:133–143
8. Saini S, Majid S, Dahiya R (2010) Diet, microRNAs and prostate cancer. Pharm Res 27:1014–1026
9. Khandrika L, Kumar B, Koul S, Maroni P, Koul HK (2009) Oxidative stress in prostate cancer. Cancer Lett 282:125–136
10. Lichtenstein P, Holm NV, Verkasalo PK, Iliadou A, Kaprio J, Koskenvuo M, Pukkala E, Skytthe A, Hemminki K (2000) Environmental and heritable factors in the causation of cancer-analyses of cohorts of twins from Sweden, Denmark, and Finland. N Engl J Med 343:78–85
11. Dianat SS, Margreiter M, Eckersberger E, Finkelstein J, Kuehas F, Herwig R, Ayati M, Lepor H, Djavan B (2009) Gene polymorphisms and prostate cancer: the evidence. BJU Int 104:1560–1572
12. Ostrander EA, Udler MS (2008) The role of the BRCA2 gene in susceptibility to prostate cancer revisited. Cancer Epidemiol Biomarkers Prev 17:1843–1848
13. Berger AD, Satagopan J, Lee P, Taneja SS, Osman I (2006) Differences in clinicopathologic features of prostate cancer between black and white patients treated in the 1990s and 2000s. Urology 67:120–124
14. Hatcher D, Daniels G, Osman I, Lee P (2009) Molecular mechanisms involving prostate cancer racial disparity. Am J Transl Res 1:235–248

15. Tischkowitz M, Sabbaghian N, Ray AM, Lange EM, Foulkes WD, Cooney KA (2008) Analysis of the gene coding for the BRCA2-interacting protein PALB2 in hereditary prostate cancer. Prostate 68:675–678
16. Lundwall A (1989) Characterization of the gene for prostate-specific antigen, a human glandular kallikrein. Biochem Biophys Res Commun 161:1151–1159
17. Stephenson SA, Verity K, Ashworth LK, Clements JA (1999) Localization of a new prostate-specific antigen-related serine protease gene, KLK4, is evidence for an expanded human kallikrein gene family cluster on chromosome 19q13.3-13.4. J Biol Chem 274:23210–23214
18. Yousef GM, Diamandis EP (2001) The new human tissue kallikrein gene family: structure, function, and association to disease. Endocr Rev 22:184–204
19. Ung JO, Richie JP, Chen MH, Renshaw AA, D'Amico AV (2002) Evolution of the presentation and pathologic and biochemical outcomes after radical prostatectomy for patients with clinically localized prostate cancer diagnosed during the PSA era. Urology 60:458–463
20. Scattoni V, Zlotta A, Montironi R, Schulman C, Rigatti P, Montorsi F (2007) Extended and saturation prostatic biopsy in the diagnosis and characterisation of prostate cancer: a critical analysis of the literature. Eur Urol 52:1309–1322
21. Thompson IM, Goodman PJ, Tangen CM, Lucia MS, Miller GJ, Ford LG, Lieber MM, Cespedes RD, Atkins JN, Lippman SM, Carlin SM, Ryan A, Szczepanek CM, Crowley JJ, Coltman CA Jr (2003) The influence of finasteride on the development of prostate cancer. N Engl J Med 349:215–224
22. http://www.ncbi.nlm.nih.gov/bookshelf/br.fcgi?book=es63
23. Carter HB, Ferrucci L, Kettermann A, Landis P, Wright EJ, Epstein JI, Trock BJ, Metter EJ (2006) Detection of life-threatening prostate cancer with prostate-specific antigen velocity during a window of curability. J Natl Cancer Inst 98:1521–1527
24. Ng MK, Van As N, Thomas K, Woode-Amissah R, Horwich A, Huddart R, Khoo V, Thompson A, Dearnaley D, Parker C (2009) Prostate-specific antigen (PSA) kinetics in untreated, localized prostate cancer: PSA velocity vs PSA doubling time. BJU Int 103:872–876
25. Uemura H, Nakamura M, Hasumi H, Sugiura S, Fujinami K, Miyoshi Y, Yao M, Kubota Y (2004) Effectiveness of percent free prostate specific antigen as a predictor of prostate cancer detection on repeat biopsy. Int J Urol 11:494–500
26. Walz J, Haese A, Scattoni V, Steuber T, Chun FK, Briganti A, Montorsi F, Graefen M, Huland H, Karakiewicz PI (2008) Percent free prostate-specific antigen (PSA) is an accurate predictor of prostate cancer risk in men with serum PSA 2.5 ng/mL and lower. Cancer 113:2695–2703
27. Mikolajczyk SD, Millar LS, Wang TJ, Rittenhouse HG, Wolfert RL, Marks LS, Song W, Wheeler TM, Slawin KM (2000) "BPSA," a specific molecular form of free prostate-specific antigen, is found predominantly in the transition zone of patients with nodular benign prostatic hyperplasia. Urology 55:41–45
28. Slawin KM, Shariat S, Canto E (2005) BPSA: a novel serum marker for benign prostatic hyperplasia. Rev Urol 7(Suppl 8):S52–S56
29. Canto EI, Singh H, Shariat SF, Lamb DJ, Mikolajczyk SD, Linton HJ, Rittenhouse HG, Kadmon D, Miles BJ, Slawin KM (2004) Serum BPSA outperforms both total PSA and free PSA as a predictor of prostatic enlargement in men without prostate cancer. Urology 63:905–910
30. Lilja H, Abrahamsson PA (1988) Three predominant proteins secreted by the human prostate gland. Prostate 12:29–38
31. Dubé JY, Frenette G, Paquin R, Chapdelaine P, Tremblay J, Tremblay RR, Lazure C, Seidah N, Chrétien M (1987) Isolation from human seminal plasma of an abundant 16-kDa protein originating from the prostate, its identification with a 94-residue peptide originally described as beta-inhibin. J Androl 8:182–189
32. Garde SV, Basrur VS, Li L, Finkelman MA, Krishan A, Wellham L, Ben-Josef E, Haddad M, Taylor JD, Porter AT, Tang DG (1999) Prostate secretory protein (PSP94) suppresses the growth of androgen-independent prostate cancer cell line (PC3) and xenografts by inducing apoptosis. Prostate 38:118–125

33. Porter AT, F A C R O, Ben-Josef E (2001) Humoral mechanisms in prostate cancer: a role for FSH. Urol Oncol 6:131–138
34. Lamy S, Ruiz MT, Wisniewski J, Garde S, Rabbani SA, Panchal C, Wu JJ, Annabi B (2006) A prostate secretory protein94-derived synthetic peptide PCK3145 inhibits VEGF signaling in endothelial cells: implication in tumor angiogenesis. Int J Cancer 118:2350–2358
35. Ulvsbäck M, Lindström C, Weiber H, Abrahamsson PA, Lilja H, Lundwall A (1989) Molecular cloning of a small prostate protein, known as beta-microsemenoprotein, PSP94 or beta-inhibin, and demonstration of transcripts in non-genital tissues. Biochem Biophys Res Commun 164:1310–1315
36. Baijal-Gupta M, Clarke MW, Finkelman MA, McLachlin CM, Han VK (2000) Prostatic secretory protein (PSP94) expression in human female reproductive tissues, breast and in endometrial cancer cell lines. J Endocrinol 165:425–433
37. Weiber H, Andersson C, Murne A, Rannevik G, Lindström C, Lilja H, Fernlund P (1990) Beta microseminoprotein is not a prostate-specific protein. Its identification in mucous glands and secretions. Am J Pathol 137:593–603
38. Doctor VM, Sheth AR, Simha MM, Arbatti NJ, Aaveri JP, Sheth NA (1986) Studies on immunocytochemical localization of inhibin-like material in human prostatic tissue: comparison of its distribution in normal, benign and malignant prostates. Br J Cancer 53:547–554
39. Imasato Y, Xuan JW, Sakai H, Izawa JI, Saito Y, Chin JL, Moussa M (2000) PSP94 expression after androgen deprivation therapy: a comparative study with prostate specific antigen in benign prostate and prostate cancer. J Urol 164:1819–1824
40. Bjartell AS, Al-Ahmadie H, Serio AM, Eastham JA, Eggener SE, Fine SW, Udby L, Gerald WL, Vickers AJ, Lilja H, Reuter VE, Scardino PT (2007) Association of cysteine-rich secretory protein 3 and beta-microseminoprotein with outcome after radical prostatectomy. Clin Cancer Res 13:4130–4138
41. Sakai H, Tsurusaki T, Kanda S, Koji T, Xuan JW, Saito Y (1999) Prognostic significance of beta-microseminoprotein mRNA expression in prostate cancer. Prostate 38:278–284
42. Chan PS, Chan LW, Xuan JW, Chin JL, Choi HL, Chan FL (1999) In situ hybridization study of PSP94 (prostatic secretory protein of 94 amino acids) expression in human prostates. Prostate 41:99–109
43. Hamdy FC, Dearnaley DP, Muir KR, Smith C, Bagnato M, Ardern-Jones AT, Hall AL, O'Brien LT, Gehr-Swain BN, Wilkinson RA, Cox A, Lewis S, Brown PM, Jhavar SG, Tymrakiewicz M, Lophatananon A, Bryant SL, Horwich A, Huddart RA, Khoo VS, Parker CC, Woodhouse CJ, Thompson A, Christmas T, Ogden C, Fisher C, Jamieson C, Cooper CS, English DR, Hopper JL, Neal DE, Easton DF, UK Genetic Prostate Cancer Study Collaborators; British Association of Urological Surgeons' Section of Oncology, UK ProtecT Study Collaborators (2008) Multiple newly identified loci associated with prostate cancer susceptibility. Nat Genet 40:316–321
44. Thomas G, Jacobs KB, Yeager M, Kraft P, Wacholder S, Orr N, Yu K, Chatterjee N, Welch R, Hutchinson A, Crenshaw A, Cancel-Tassin G, Staats BJ, Wang Z, Gonzalez-Bosquet J, Fang J, Deng X, Berndt SI, Calle EE, Feigelson HS, Thun MJ, Rodriguez C, Albanes D, Virtamo J, Weinstein S, Schumacher FR, Giovannucci E, Willett WC, Cussenot O, Valeri A, Andriole GL, Crawford ED, Tucker M, Gerhard DS, Fraumeni JF Jr, Hoover R, Hayes RB, Hunter DJ, Chanock SJ (2008) Multiple loci identified in a genome-wide association study of prostate cancer. Nat Genet 40:310–315
45. Lou H, Yeager M, Li H, Bosquet JG, Hayes RB, Orr N, Yu K, Hutchinson A, Jacobs KB, Kraft P, Wacholder S, Chatterjee N, Feigelson HS, Thun MJ, Diver WR, Albanes D, Virtamo J, Weinstein S, Ma J, Gaziano JM, Stampfer M, Schumacher FR, Giovannucci E, Cancel-Tassin G, Cussenot O, Valeri A, Andriole GL, Crawford ED, Anderson SK, Tucker M, Hoover RN, Fraumeni JF Jr, Thomas G, Hunter DJ, Dean M, Chanock SJ (2009) Fine mapping and functional analysis of a common variant in MSMB on chromosome 10q11.2 associated with prostate cancer susceptibility. Proc Natl Acad Sci U S A 106:7933–7938

46. Chang BL, Cramer SD, Wiklund F, Isaacs SD, Stevens VL, Sun J, Smith S, Pruett K, Romero LM, Wiley KE, Kim ST, Zhu Y, Zhang Z, Hsu FC, Turner AR, Adolfsson J, Liu W, Kim JW, Duggan D, Carpten J, Zheng SL, Rodriguez C, Isaacs WB, Grönberg H, Xu J (2009) Fine mapping association study and functional analysis implicate a SNP in MSMB at 10q11 as a causal variant for prostate cancer risk. Hum Mol Genet 18:1368–1375
47. Kader AK, Sun J, Isaacs SD, Wiley KE, Yan G, Kim ST, Fedor H, DeMarzo AM, Epstein JI, Walsh PC, Partin AW, Trock B, Zheng SL, Xu J, Isaacs W (2009) Individual and cumulative effect of prostate cancer risk-associated variants on clinicopathologic variables in 5,895 prostate cancer patients. Prostate 69:1195–1205
48. Whitaker HC, Kote-Jarai Z, Ross-Adams H, Warren AY, Burge J, George A, Bancroft E, Jhavar S, Leongamornlert D, Tymrakiewicz M, Saunders E, Page E, Mitra A, Mitchell G, Lindeman GJ, Evans DG, Blanco I, Mercer C, Rubinstein WS, Clowes V, Douglas F, Hodgson S, Walker L, Donaldson A, Izatt L, Dorkins H, Male A, Tucker K, Stapleton A, Lam J, Kirk J, Lilja H, Easton D; IMPACT Study Steering Committee; IMPACT Study Collaborators; UK GPCS Collaborators, Cooper C, Eeles R, Neal DE (2010) The rs10993994 risk allele for prostate cancer results in clinically relevant changes in microseminoprotein-beta expression in tissue and urine. PLoS One 5:e13363
49. Bussemakers MJ, van Bokhoven A, Verhaegh GW, Smit FP, Karthaus HF, Schalken JA, Debruyne FM, Ru N, Isaacs WB (1999) DD3: a new prostate-specific gene, highly overexpressed in prostate cancer. Cancer Res 59:5975–5979
50. Schalken JA, Hessels D, Verhaegh G (2003) New targets for therapy in prostate cancer: differential display code 3 (DD3(PCA3)), a highly prostate cancer-specific gene. Urology 62:34–43
51. Clarke RA, Zhao Z, Guo AY, Roper K, Teng L, Fang ZM, Samaratunga H, Lavin MF, Gardiner RA (2009) New genomic structure for prostate cancer specific gene PCA3 within BMCC1: implications for prostate cancer detection and progression. PLoS One 4:e4995
52. Hessels D, Klein Gunnewiek JM, van Oort I, Karthaus HF, van Leenders GJ, van Balken B, Kiemeney LA, Witjes JA, Schalken JA (2003) DD3(PCA3)-based molecular urine analysis for the diagnosis of prostate cancer. Eur Urol 44:8–15
53. Meng FJ, Shan A, Jin L, Young CY (2002) The expression of a variant prostate-specific antigen in human prostate. Cancer Epidemiol Biomarkers Prev 11:305–309
54. Magklara A, Scorilas A, Stephan C, Kristiansen GO, Hauptmann S, Jung K, Diamandis EP (2000) Decreased concentrations of prostate-specific antigen and human glandular kallikrein 2 in malignant versus nonmalignant prostatic tissue. Urology 56:527–532
55. Groskopf J, Aubin SM, Deras IL, Blase A, Bodrug S, Clark C, Brentano S, Mathis J, Pham J, Meyer T, Cass M, Hodge P, Macairan ML, Marks LS, Rittenhouse H (2006) APTIMA PCA3 molecular urine test: development of a method to aid in the diagnosis of prostate cancer. Clin Chem 52:1089–1095
56. Hayes DF, Smerage JB (2010) Circulating tumor cells. Prog Mol Biol Transl Sci 95:95–112
57. Moreno JG, Miller MC, Gross S, Allard WJ, Gomella LG, Terstappen LW (2005) Circulating tumor cells predict survival in patients with metastatic prostate cancer. Urology 65:713–718
58. Danila DC, Heller G, Gignac GA, Gonzalez-Espinoza R, Anand A, Tanaka E, Lilja H, Schwartz L, Larson S, Fleisher M, Scher HI (2007) Circulating tumor cell number and prognosis in progressive castration-resistant prostate cancer. Clin Cancer Res 13:7053–7058
59. Garcia JA, Rosenberg JE, Weinberg V, Scott J, Frohlich M, Park JW, Small EJ (2007) Evaluation and significance of circulating epithelial cells in patients with hormone-refractory prostate cancer. BJU Int 99:519–524
60. Morgan TM, Lange PH, Vessella RL (2007) Detection and characterization of circulating and disseminated prostate cancer cells. Front Biosci 12:3000–3009
61. Jost M, Day JR, Slaughter R, Koreckij TD, Gonzales D, Kinnunen M, Groskopf J, Rittenhouse HG, Vessella RL, Reynolds MA (2010) Molecular assays for the detection of prostate tumor derived nucleic acids in peripheral blood. Mol Cancer 9:174

62. Kumar-Sinha C, Tomlins SA, Chinnaiyan AM (2008) Recurrent gene fusions in prostate cancer. Nat Rev Cancer 8:497–511
63. Tomlins SA, Bjartell A, Chinnaiyan AM, Jenster G, Nam RK, Rubin MA, Schalken JA (2009) ETS gene fusions in prostate cancer: from discovery to daily clinical practice. Eur Urol 56:275–286
64. Tomlins SA, Laxman B, Varambally S, Cao X, Yu J, Helgeson BE, Cao Q, Prensner JR, Rubin MA, Shah RB, Mehra R, Chinnaiyan AM (2008) Role of the TMPRSS2-ERG gene fusion in prostate cancer. Neoplasia 10:177–188
65. Mehra R, Tomlins SA, Yu J, Cao X, Wang L, Menon A, Rubin MA, Pienta KJ, Shah RB, Chinnaiyan AM (2008) Characterization of TMPRSS2-ETS gene aberrations in androgen-independent metastatic prostate cancer. Cancer Res 68:3584–3590
66. Cai C, Hsieh CL, Omwancha J, Zheng Z, Chen SY, Baert JL, Shemshedini L (2007) ETV1 is a novel androgen receptor-regulated gene that mediates prostate cancer cell invasion. Mol Endocrinol 21:1835–1846
67. Perner S, Mosquera JM, Demichelis F, Hofer MD, Paris PL, Simko J, Collins C, Bismar TA, Chinnaiyan AM, De Marzo AM, Rubin MA (2007) TMPRSS2-ERG fusion prostate cancer: an early molecular event associated with invasion. Am J Surg Pathol 31:882–888
68. Hessels D, Schalken JA (2009) The use of PCA3 in the diagnosis of prostate cancer. Nat Rev Urol 6:255–261
69. Whitman EJ, Groskopf J, Ali A, Chen Y, Blase A, Furusato B, Petrovics G, Ibrahim M, Elsamanoudi S, Cullen J, Sesterhenn IA, Brassell S, Rittenhouse H, Srivastava S, McLeod DG (2008) PCA3 score before radical prostatectomy predicts extracapsular extension and tumor volume. J Urol 180:1975–1978
70. Ruiz-Aragón J, Márquez-Peláez S (2010) Assessment of the PCA3 test for prostate cancer diagnosis: a systematic review and meta-analysis. Actas Urol Esp 34:346–355
71. Tomlins SA, Rhodes DR, Perner S, Dhanasekaran SM, Mehra R, Sun XW, Varambally S, Cao X, Tchinda J, Kuefer R, Lee C, Montie JE, Shah RB, Pienta KJ, Rubin MA, Chinnaiyan AM (2005) Recurrent fusion of TMPRSS2 and ETS transcription factor genes in prostate cancer. Science 310:644–648
72. Wang J, Cai Y, Yu W, Ren C, Spencer DM, Ittmann M (2008) Pleiotropic biological activities of alternatively spliced TMPRSS2/ERG fusion gene transcripts. Cancer Res 68:8516–8524
73. Barwick BG, Abramovitz M, Kodani M, Moreno CS, Nam R, Tang W, Bouzyk M, Seth A, Leyland-Jones B (2010) Prostate cancer genes associated with TMPRSS2-ERG gene fusion and prognostic of biochemical recurrence in multiple cohorts. Br J Cancer 102:570–576
74. Magi-Galluzzi C, Tsusuki T, Elson P, Simmerman K, Lafargue C, Esgueva R, Klein E, Rubin MA, Zhou M (2011) TMPRSS2-ERG gene fusion prevalence and class are significantly different in prostate cancer of Caucasian, African-American and Japanese patients. Prostate 71(5):489–497
75. Hsu T, Trojanowska M, Watson DK (2004) Ets proteins in biological control and cancer. J Cell Biochem 91:896–903
76. Delattre O, Sevenet N (2002) Chromosome translocations in the Ewing family of tumors. Landes Bioscience, Austin
77. Clark J, Merson S, Jhavar S, Flohr P, Edwards S, Foster CS, Eeles R, Martin FL, Phillips DH, Crundwell M, Christmas T, Thompson A, Fisher C, Kovacs G, Cooper CS (2007) Diversity of TMPRSS2-ERG fusion transcripts in the human prostate. Oncogene 26:2667–2673
78. Clark JP, Cooper CS (2009) ETS gene fusions in prostate cancer. Nat Rev Urol 6:429–439
79. Soller MJ, Isaksson M, Elfving P, Soller W, Lundgren R, Panagopoulos I (2006) Confirmation of the high frequency of the TMPRSS2/ERG fusion gene in prostate cancer. Genes Chromosomes Cancer 45:717–719
80. Petrovics G, Liu A, Shaheduzzaman S, Furusato B, Sun C, Chen Y, Nau M, Ravindranath L, Chen Y, Dobi A, Srikantan V, Sesterhenn IA, McLeod DG, Vahey M, Moul JW, Srivastava S (2005) Frequent overexpression of ETS-related gene-1 (ERG1) in prostate cancer transcriptome. Oncogene 24:3847–3852

81. Winnes M, Lissbrant E, Damber JE, Stenman G (2007) Molecular genetic analyses of the TMPRSS2-ERG and TMPRSS2-ETV1 gene fusions in 50 cases of prostate cancer. Oncol Rep 17:1033–1036
82. Saramäki OR, Harjula AE, Martikainen PM, Vessella RL, Tammela TL, Visakorpi T (2008) TMPRSS2:ERG fusion identifies a subgroup of prostate cancers with a favorable prognosis. Clin Cancer Res 14:3395–3400
83. Hermans KG, Boormans JL, Gasi D, van Leenders GJ, Jenster G, Verhagen PC, Trapman J (2009) Overexpression of prostate-specific TMPRSS2(exon 0)-ERG fusion transcripts corresponds with favorable prognosis of prostate cancer. Clin Cancer Res 15:6398–6403
84. Rostad K, Hellwinkel OJ, Haukaas SA, Halvorsen OJ, Øyan AM, Haese A, Budäus L, Albrecht H, Akslen LA, Schlomm T, Kalland KH (2009) TMPRSS2:ERG fusion transcripts in urine from prostate cancer patients correlate with a less favorable prognosis. APMIS 117:575–582
85. Demichelis F, Fall K, Perner S, Andrén O, Schmidt F, Setlur SR, Hoshida Y, Mosquera JM, Pawitan Y, Lee C, Adami HO, Mucci LA, Kantoff PW, Andersson SO, Chinnaiyan AM, Johansson JE, Rubin MA (2007) TMPRSS2:ERG gene fusion associated with lethal prostate cancer in a watchful waiting cohort. Oncogene 26:4596–4599
86. Perner S, Demichelis F, Beroukhim R, Schmidt FH, Mosquera JM, Setlur S, Tchinda J, Tomlins SA, Hofer MD, Pienta KG, Kuefer R, Vessella R, Sun XW, Meyerson M, Lee C, Sellers WR, Chinnaiyan AM, Rubin MA (2006) TMPRSS2:ERG fusion-associated deletions provide insight into the heterogeneity of prostate cancer. Cancer Res 66:8337–8341
87. Gopalan A, Leversha MA, Satagopan JM, Zhou Q, Al-Ahmadie HA, Fine SW, Eastham JA, Scardino PT, Scher HI, Tickoo SK, Reuter VE, Gerald WL (2009) TMPRSS2-ERG gene fusion is not associated with outcome in patients treated by prostatectomy. Cancer Res 69:1400–1406
88. Wang J, Cai Y, Ren C, Ittmann M (2006) Expression of variant TMPRSS2/ERG fusion messenger RNAs is associated with aggressive prostate cancer. Cancer Res 66:8347–8351
89. Attard G, Clark J, Ambroisine L, Fisher G, Kovacs G, Flohr P, Berney D, Foster CS, Fletcher A, Gerald WL, Moller H, Reuter V, De Bono JS, Scardino P, Cuzick J, Cooper CS, Transatlantic Prostate Group (2008) Duplication of the fusion of TMPRSS2 to ERG sequences identifies fatal human prostate cancer. Oncogene 27:253–263
90. Rajput AB, Miller MA, De Luca A, Boyd N, Leung S, Hurtado-Coll A, Fazli L, Jones EC, Palmer JB, Gleave ME, Cox ME, Huntsman DG (2007) Frequency of the TMPRSS2:ERG gene fusion is increased in moderate to poorly differentiated prostate cancers. J Clin Pathol 60:1238–1243
91. Nam RK, Sugar L, Yang W, Srivastava S, Klotz LH, Yang LY, Stanimirovic A, Encioiu E, Neill M, Loblaw DA, Trachtenberg J, Narod SA, Seth A (2007) Expression of the TMPRSS2:ERG fusion gene predicts cancer recurrence after surgery for localised prostate cancer. Br J Cancer 97:1690–1695
92. Fine SW, Gopalan A, Leversha MA, Al-Ahmadie HA, Tickoo SK, Zhou Q, Satagopan JM, Scardino PT, Gerald WL, Reuter VE (2010) TMPRSS2-ERG gene fusion is associated with low Gleason scores and not with high-grade morphological features. Mod Pathol 23:1325–1333
93. Yoshimoto M, Joshua AM, Cunha IW, Coudry RA, Fonseca FP, Ludkovski O, Zielenska M, Soares FA, Squire JA (2008) Absence of TMPRSS2:ERG fusions and PTEN losses in prostate cancer is associated with a favorable outcome. Mod Pathol 21:1451–1460
94. Bonaccorsi L, Nesi G, Nuti F, Paglierani M, Krausz C, Masieri L, Serni S, Proietti-Pannunzi L, Fang Y, Jhanwar SC, Orlando C, Carini M, Forti G, Baldi E, Luzzatto L (2009) Persistence of expression of the TMPRSS2:ERG fusion gene after pre-surgery androgen ablation may be associated with early prostate specific antigen relapse of prostate cancer: preliminary results. J Endocrinol Invest 32:590–596
95. Lapointe J, Li C, Giacomini CP, Salari K, Huang S, Wang P, Ferrari M, Hernandez-Boussard T, Brooks JD, Pollack JR (2007) Genomic profiling reveals alternative genetic pathways of prostate tumorigenesis. Cancer Res 67:8504–8510

96. Tu JJ, Rohan S, Kao J, Kitabayashi N, Mathew S, Chen YT (2007) Gene fusions between TMPRSS2 and ETS family genes in prostate cancer: frequency and transcript variant analysis by RT-PCR and FISH on paraffin-embedded tissues. Mod Pathol 20:921–928
97. Furusato B, Gao CL, Ravindranath L, Chen Y, Cullen J, McLeod DG, Dobi A, Srivastava S, Petrovics G, Sesterhenn IA (2008) Mapping of TMPRSS2-ERG fusions in the context of multi-focal prostate cancer. Mod Pathol 21:67–75
98. Yoshimoto M, Joshua AM, Chilton-Macneill S, Bayani J, Selvarajah S, Evans AJ, Zielenska M, Squire JA (2006) Three-color FISH analysis of TMPRSS2/ERG fusions in prostate cancer indicates that genomic microdeletion of chromosome 21 is associated with rearrangement. Neoplasia 8:465–469
99. King JC, Xu J, Wongvipat J, Hieronymus H, Carver BS, Leung DH, Taylor BS, Sander C, Cardiff RD, Couto SS, Gerald WL, Sawyers CL (2009) Cooperativity of TMPRSS2-ERG with PI3-kinase pathway activation in prostate oncogenesis. Nat Genet 41:524–526
100. Carver BS, Tran J, Gopalan A, Chen Z, Shaikh S, Carracedo A, Alimonti A, Nardella C, Varmeh S, Scardino PT, Cordon-Cardo C, Gerald W, Pandolfi PP (2009) Aberrant ERG expression cooperates with loss of PTEN to promote cancer progression in the prostate. Nat Genet 41:619–624
101. Iljin K, Wolf M, Edgren H, Gupta S, Kilpinen S, Skotheim RI, Peltola M, Smit F, Verhaegh G, Schalken J, Nees M, Kallioniemi O (2006) TMPRSS2 fusions with oncogenic ETS factors in prostate cancer involve unbalanced genomic rearrangements and are associated with HDAC1 and epigenetic reprogramming. Cancer Res 66:10242–10246
102. Attard G, Clark J, Ambroisine L, Mills IG, Fisher G, Flohr P, Reid A, Edwards S, Kovacs G, Berney D, Foster C, Massie CE, Fletcher A, De Bono JS, Scardino P, Cuzick J, Cooper CS (2008) Heterogeneity and clinical significance of ETV1 translocations in human prostate cancer. Br J Cancer 99:314–320
103. Park K, Tomlins SA, Mudaliar KM, Chiu YL, Esgueva R, Mehra R, Suleman K, Varambally S, Brenner JC, MacDonald T, Srivastava A, Tewari AK, Sathyanarayana U, Nagy D, Pestano G, Kunju LP, Demichelis F, Chinnaiyan AM, Rubin MA (2010) Antibody-based detection of ERG rearrangement-positive prostate cancer. Neoplasia 12:590–598
104. Tomlins SA, Rhodes DR, Yu J, Varambally S, Mehra R, Perner S, Demichelis F, Helgeson BE, Laxman B, Morris DS, Cao Q, Cao X, Andrén O, Fall K, Johnson L, Wei JT, Shah RB, Al-Ahmadie H, Eastham JA, Eggener SE, Fine SW, Hotakainen K, Stenman UH, Tsodikov A, Gerald WL, Lilja H, Reuter VE, Kantoff PW, Scardino PT, Rubin MA, Bjartell AS, Chinnaiyan AM (2008) The role of SPINK1 in ETS rearrangement-negative prostate cancers. Cancer Cell 13:519–528
105. Shan L, Ambroisine L, Clark J, Yáñez-Muñoz RJ, Fisher G, Kudahetti SC, Yang J, Kia S, Mao X, Fletcher A, Flohr P, Edwards S, Attard G, De-Bono J, Young BD, Foster CS, Reuter V, Moller H, Oliver TD, Berney DM, Scardino P, Cuzick J, Cooper CS, Lu YJ, Transatlantic Prostate Group (2010) The identification of chromosomal translocation, t(4;6)(q22;q15), in prostate cancer. Prostate Cancer Prostatic Dis 13:117–125
106. Lane TM, Strefford JC, Yáñez-Muñoz RJ, Purkis P, Forsythe E, Nia T, Hines J, Lu YJ, Oliver RT (2007) Identification of a recurrent t(4;6) chromosomal translocation in prostate cancer. J Urol 177:1907–1912
107. Carew JS, Huang P (2002) Mitochondrial defects in cancer. Mol Cancer 1:9
108. Parr RL, Dakubo GD, Crandall KA, Maki J, Reguly B, Aguirre A, Wittock R, Robinson K, Alexander JS, Birch-Machin MA, Abdel-Malak M, Froberg MK, Diamandis EP, Thayer RE (2006) Somatic mitochondrial DNA mutations in prostate cancer and normal appearing adjacent glands in comparison to age-matched prostate samples without malignant histology. J Mol Diagn 8:312–319
109. Takahashi E, Hori T, O'Connell P, Leppert M, White R (1991) Mapping of the MYC gene to band 8q24.12–q24.13 by R-banding and distal to fra(8)(q24.11), FRA8E, by fluorescence in situ hybridization. Cytogenet Cell Genet 57:109–111
110. Vita M, Henriksson M (2006) The Myc oncoprotein as a therapeutic target for human cancer. Semin Cancer Biol 16:318–330

111. Fleming WH, Hamel A, MacDonald R, Ramsey E, Pettigrew NM, Johnston B, Dodd JG, Matusik RJ (1986) Expression of the c-myc protooncogene in human prostatic carcinoma and benign prostatic hyperplasia. Cancer Res 46:1535–1538
112. Jenkins RB, Qian J, Lieber MM, Bostwick DG (1997) Detection of c-myc oncogene amplification and chromosomal anomalies in metastatic prostatic carcinoma by fluorescence in situ hybridization. Cancer Res 57:524–531
113. Bubendorf L, Kononen J, Koivisto P, Schraml P, Moch H, Gasser TC, Willi N, Mihatsch MJ, Sauter G, Kallioniemi OP (1999) Survey of gene amplifications during prostate cancer progression by high-throughout fluorescence in situ hybridization on tissue microarrays. Cancer Res 59:803–806
114. Sato H, Minei S, Hachiya T, Yoshida T, Takimoto Y (2006) Fluorescence in situ hybridization analysis of c-myc amplification in stage TNM prostate cancer in Japanese patients. Int J Urol 13:761–766
115. Hawksworth D, Ravindranath L, Chen Y, Furusato B, Sesterhenn IA, McLeod DG, Srivastava S, Petrovics G (2010) Overexpression of C-MYC oncogene in prostate cancer predicts biochemical recurrence. Prostate Cancer Prostatic Dis 13:311–315
116. Chaib H, Cockrell EK, Rubin MA, Macoska JA (2001) Profiling and verification of gene expression patterns in normal and malignant human prostate tissues by cDNA microarray analysis. Neoplasia 3:43–52
117. Sun C, Dobi A, Mohamed A, Li H, Thangapazham RL, Furusato B, Shaheduzzaman S, Tan SH, Vaidyanathan G, Whitman E, Hawksworth DJ, Chen Y, Nau M, Patel V, Vahey M, Gutkind JS, Sreenath T, Petrovics G, Sesterhenn IA, McLeod DG, Srivastava S (2008) TMPRSS2-ERG fusion, a common genomic alteration in prostate cancer activates C-MYC and abrogates prostate epithelial differentiation. Oncogene 27:5348–5353
118. Reed JC (1997) Double identity for proteins of the Bcl-2 family. Nature 387:773–776
119. Lindsay J, Esposti MD, Gilmore AP (2011) Bcl-2 proteins and mitochondria-specificity in membrane targeting for death. Biochim Biophys Acta 1813(4):532–539
120. Reed JC (1994) Bcl-2 and the regulation of programmed cell death. J Cell Biol 124:1–6
121. McDonnell TJ, Troncoso P, Brisbay SM, Logothetis C, Chung LW, Hsieh JT, Tu SM, Campbell ML (1992) Expression of the protooncogene Bcl-2 in the prostate and its association with emergence of androgen-independent prostate cancer. Cancer Res 52:6940–6944
122. Concato J, Jain D, Uchio E, Risch H, Li WW, Wells CK (2009) Molecular markers and death from prostate cancer. Ann Intern Med 150:595–603
123. Bubendorf L, Sauter G, Moch H, Jordan P, Blöchlinger A, Gasser TC, Mihatsch MJ (1996) Prognostic significance of Bcl-2 in clinically localized prostate cancer. Am J Pathol 148:1557–1565
124. Colombel M, Symmans F, Gil S, O'Toole KM, Chopin D, Benson M, Olsson CA, Korsmeyer S, Buttyan R (1993) Detection of the apoptosis-suppressing oncoprotein Bc1-2 in hormone-refractory human prostate cancers. Am J Pathol 143:390–400
125. Grauer LS, Finlay JA, Mikolajczyk SD, Pusateri KD, Wolfert RL (1998) Detection of human glandular kallikrein, hK2, as its precursor form and in complex with protease inhibitors in prostate carcinomaserum. J Androl 19:407–411
126. Piironen T, Lovgren J, Karp M, Eerola R, Lundwall A, Dowell B, Lövgren T, Lilja H, Pettersson K (1996) Immunofluorometric assay for sensitive and specific measurement of human prostatic glandular kallikrein (hK2) in serum. Clin Chem 42:1034–1041
127. Becker C, Piironen T, Kiviniemi J, Lilja H, Pettersson K (2000) Sensitive and specific immunodetection of human glandular kallikrein 2 in serum. Clin Chem 46:198–206
128. Schedlich LJ, Bennetts BH, Morris BJ (1987) Primary structure of a human glandular kallikrein gene. DNA 6:429–437
129. Lovgren J, Airas K, Lilja H (1999) Enzymatic action of human glandular kallikrein 2 (hK2). Substrate specificity and regulation by Zn2_ and extracellular protease inhibitors. Eur J Biochem 262:781–789
130. Lovgren J, Rajakoski K, Karp M, Lundwall A, Lilja H (1997) Activation of the zymogen form of prostate-specific antigen by human glandular kallikrein 2. Biochem Biophys Res Commun 238:549–555

131. Darson MF, Pacelli A, Roche P, Rittenhouse HG, Wolfert RL, Young CY, Klee GG, Tindall DJ, Bostwick DG (1997) Human glandular kallikrein 2 (hK2) expression in prostatic intraepithelial neoplasia and adenocarcinoma: a novel prostate cancer marker. Urology 49:857–862
132. Darson MF, Pacelli A, Roche P, Rittenhouse HG, Wolfert RL, Saeid MS, Klee GG, Tindall DJ, Bostwick DG (1999) Human glandular kallikrein 2 expression in prostate adenocarcinoma and lymph node metastases. Urology 53:939–944
133. Frenette G, Deperthes D, Tremblay RR, Lazure C, Dube JY (1997) Purification of enzymatically active kallikrein hK2 from human seminal plasma. Biochim Biophys Acta 1334:109–115
134. Heeb MJ, Espana F (1998) β2-Macroglobulin and C1-inactivator are plasma inhibitors of human glandular kallikrein. Blood Cells Mol Dis 24:412–419
135. Mikolajczyk SD, Millar LS, Kumar A, Saedi MS (1999) Prostatic human kallikrein 2 inactivates and complexes with plasminogen activator inhibitor-1. Int J Cancer 81:438–442
136. Deperthes D, Chapdelaine P, Tremblay RR, Brunet C, Berton J, Hebert J, Lazure C, Dubé JY (1995) Isolation of prostatic kallikrein hK2, also known as hGK-1, in human seminal plasma. Biochem Biophys Acta 1245:311–316
137. Black MH, Magklara A, Obiezu CV, Melegos DN, Diamandis EP (1999) Development of an ultrasensitive immunoassay for human glandular kallikrein with no cross-reactivity from prostate-specific antigen. Clin Chem 45:790–799
138. Saedi MS, Hill TM, Kuus-Reichel K, Kumar A, Payne J, Mikolajczyk SD, Wolfert RL, Rittenhouse HG (1998) The precursor form of the human kallikrein 2, a kallikrein homologous to prostate-specific antigen, is present in human sera and is increased in prostate cancer and benign prostatic hyperplasia. Clin Chem 44:2115–2119
139. Vaisanen V, Eriksson S, Ivaska KK, Lilja H, Nurmi M, Pettersson K (2004) Development of sensitive immunoassays for free and total human glandular kallikrein 2. Clin Chem 50:91607–91617
140. Finlay JA, Evans CL, Day JR, Payne JK, Mikolajczyk SD, Millar LS, Kuus-Reichel K, Wolfert RL, Rittenhouse HG (1998) Development of monoclonal antibodies specific for human glandular kallikrein (hK2): development of a dual antibody immunoassay for hK2 with negligible prostate-specific antigen crossreactivity. Urology 51:804–809
141. Finlay JA, Day JR, Evans CL, Carlson R, Kuus-Reichel K, Millar LS, Mikolajczyk SD, Goodmanson M, Klee GG, Rittenhouse HG (2001) Development of a dual monoclonal antibody immunoassay for total human kallikrein 2. Clin Chem 47:1218–1224
142. Klee GG, Goodmanson MK, Jacobsen SJ, Young CY, Finlay JA, Rittenhouse HG, Wolfert RL, Tindall DJ (1999) Highly sensitive automated chemiluminometric assay for measuring free human glandular kallikrein-2. Clin Chem 45:800–806
143. Kwiatkowski MK, Recker F, Piironen T, Pettersson K, Otto T, Wernli M, Tscholl R (1998) In prostatism patients the ratio of human glandular kallikrein to free PSA improves the discrimination between prostate cancer and benign hyperplasia within the diagnostic "gray zone" of total PSA 4 to 10 ng/mL. Urology 52:360–365
144. Magklara A, Scorilas A, Catalona WJ, Diamandis EP (1999) The combination of human glandular kallikrein and free prostate-specific antigen (PSA) enhances discrimination between prostate cancer and benign prostatic hyperplasia in patients with moderately increased total PSA. Clin Chem 45:1956–1960
145. Partin AW, Catalona WJ, Finlay JA, Darte C, Tindall DJ, Young CY, Klee GG, Chan DW, Rittenhouse HG, Wolfert RL, Woodrum D (1999) Use of human glandular kallikrein 2 for the detection of prostate cancer: preliminary analysis. Urology 54:839–845
146. Stephan C, Jung K, Soosaipillai A, Yousef GM, Cammann H, Meyer H, Xu C, Diamandis EP (2005) Clinical utility of human glandular kallikrein 2 within a neural network for prostate cancer detection. BJU Int 96:521–527
147. Bangma CH, Wildhagen MF, Yurdakul G, Schroder FH, Blijenberg BG (2004) The value of (7, 5) pro-prostate-specific antigen and human kallikrein-2 as serum markers for grading prostate cancer. BJU Int 93:720–724
148. Becker C, Piironen T, Pettersson K, Björk T, Wojno KJ, Oesterling JE, Lilja H (2000) Discrimination of men with prostate cancer from those with benign disease by measurements of human glandular kallikrein 2 (HK2) in serum. J Urol 163:311–316

149. Becker C, Piironen T, Pettersson K, Hugosson J, Lilja H (2000) Clinical value of human glandular kallikrein 2 and free and total prostate-specific antigen in serum from a population of men with prostate-specific antigen levels 3.0 ng/mL or greater. Urology 55:694–699
150. Nam RK, Diamandis EP, Toi A, Trachtenberg J, Magklara A, Scorilas A, Papnastasiou PA, Jewett MA, Narod SA (2000) Serum human glandular kallikrein-2 protease levels predict the presence of prostate cancer among men with elevated prostate-specific antigen. J Clin Oncol 18:1036–1042
151. Recker F, Kwiatkowski MK, Piironen T, Pettersson K, Lümmen G, Wernli M, Wiefelspütz J, Graber SF, Goepel M, Huber A, Tscholl R (1998) The importance of human glandular kallikrein and its correlation with different prostate specific antigen serum forms in the detection of prostate carcinoma. Cancer 83:2540–2547
152. Scorilas A, Plebani M, Mazza S, Basso D, Soosaipillai AR, Katsaros N, Pagano F, Diamandis EP (2003) Serum human glandular kallikrein (hK2) and insulin-like growth factor 1 (IGF-1) improve the discrimination between prostate cancer and benign prostatic hyperplasia in combination with total and %free PSA. Prostate 54:220–229
153. Steuber T, Vickers A, Haese A, Kattan MW, Eastham JA, Scardino PT, Huland H, Lilja H (2007) Free PSA isoforms and intact and cleaved forms of urokinase plasminogen activator receptor in serum improve selection of patients for prostate cancer biopsy. Int J Cancer 120:1499–1504
154. Vickers AJ, Ulmert D, Serio AM, Björk T, Scardino PT, Eastham JA, Berglund G, Lilja H (2007) The predictive value of prostate cancer biomarkers depends on age and time to diagnosis: towards a biologically-based screening strategy. Int J Cancer 121:2212–2217
155. Haese A, Becker C, Noldus J, Graefen M, Huland E, Huland H, Lilja H (2000) Human glandular kallikrein 2: a potential serum marker for predicting the organ confined versus non-organ confined growth of prostate cancer. J Urol 163:1491–1497
156. Haese A, Graefen M, Becker C, Noldus J, Katz J, Cagiannos I, Kattan M, Scardino PT, Huland E, Huland H, Lilja H (2003) The role of human glandular kallikrein 2 for prediction of pathologically organ confined prostate cancer. Prostate 54:181–186
157. Haese A, Graefen M, Steuber T, Becker C, Pettersson K, Piironen T, Noldus J, Huland H, Lilja H (2001) Human glandular kallikrein 2 levels in serum for discrimination of pathologically organ-confined from locally-advanced prostate cancer in total PSA-levels below 10 ng/ml. Prostate 49:101–109
158. Recker F, Kwiatkowski MK, Piironen T, Pettersson K, Huber A, Lümmen G, Tscholl R (2000) Human glandular kallikrein as a tool to improve discrimination of poorly differentiated and non-organ-confined prostate cancer compared with prostate-specific antigen. Urology 55:481–485
159. Steuber T, Vickers AJ, Serio AM, Vaisanen V, Haese A, Pettersson K, Eastham JA, Scardino PT, Huland H, Lilja H (2007) Comparison of free and total forms of serum human kallikrein 2 and prostate specific antigen for prediction of locally advanced and recurrent prostate cancer. Clin Chem 53:233–240
160. Stephan C, Jung K, Nakamura T, Yousef GM, Kristiansen G, Diamandis EP (2006) Serum human glandular kallikrein 2 (hK2) for distinguishing stage and grade of prostate cancer. Int J Urol 13:238–243
161. Vaisanen V, Pettersson K, Alanen K, Viitanen T, Nurmi M (2006) Free and total human glandular kallikrein 2 in patients with prostate cancer. Urology 68:219–225
162. Chapman HA, Wei Y (2001) Protease crosstalk with integrins: the urokinase receptor paradigm. Thromb Haemost 86:124–129
163. Croucher D, Saunders DN, Ranson M (2006) The urokinase/PAI-2 complex: a new high affinity ligand for the endocytosis receptor low-density lipoprotein receptor-related protein. J Biol Chem 281:10206–10213
164. Rao JS (2003) Molecular mechanisms of glioma invasiveness: the role of proteases. Nat Rev Cancer 3:489–501
165. Ma Z, Webb DJ, Fo M, Gonias SL (2001) Endogenously produced urokinase-type plasminogen activator is a major determinant of the basal level of activated ERK/MAK kinase and prevents apoptosis in MDA-MB-231 breast cancer cells. J Cell Sci 114:3387–3396

166. Aguirre-Ghiso JA, Estrada Y, Liu D, Ossowski L (2003) ERK (MAPK) activity as a determinant of tumor growth and dormancy; regulation by p38 (SAPK). Cancer Res 63:1684–1695
167. Margheri F, D'Alessio S, Serrati S, Pucci M, Annunziato F, Cosmi L, Liotta F, Angeli R, Angelucci A, Gravina GL, Rucci N, Bologna M, Teti A, Monia B, Fibbi G, Del Rosso M (2005) Effects of blocking urokinase receptor signaling by antisense oligonucleotides in a mouse model of experimental prostate cancer bone metastases. Gene Ther 12(8):702–714
168. Wilhelm OG, Wilhelm S, Escott GM, Lutz V, Magdolen V, Schmitt M, Rifkin DB, Wilson EL, Graeff H, Brunner G (1999) Cellular glycosylphosphatidylinositol-specific phospholipase D regulates urokinase receptor shedding and cell surface expression. J Cell Physiol 180:225–235
169. Beaufort N, Leduc D, Rousselle JC, Magdolen V, Luther T, Namane A, Magdolen V, Luther T, Namane A, Chignard M, Pidard D (2004) Proteolytic regulation of the urokinase receptor/CD87 on monocytic cells by neutrophil elastase and cathepsin G. J Immunol 172:540–549
170. Piironen T, Laursen B, Pass J, List K, Gardsvoll H, Ploug M, Danø K, Høyer-Hansen G (2004) Specific immunoassays for detection of intact and cleaved forms of the urokinase receptor. Clin Chem 50:2059–2068
171. Piironen T, Haese A, Huland H, Steuber T, Christensen IJ, Brunner N, Danø K, Høyer-Hansen G, Lilja H (2006) Enhanced discrimination of benign from malignant prostatic disease by selective measurements of cleaved forms of urokinase receptor in serum. Clin Chem 52:838–844
172. Miyake H, Hara I, Yamanaka K, Arakawa S, Kamidono S (1999) Elevation of urokinase-type plasminogen activator and its receptor densities as new predictors of disease progression and prognosis in men with prostate cancer. Int J Oncol 14:535–541
173. Pulukuri SM, Estes N, Patel J, Rao JS (2007) Demethylation-linked activation of urokinase plasminogen activator is involved in progression of prostate cancer. Cancer Res 67:930–939
174. Van Veldhuizen PJ, Sadasivan R, Cherian R, Wyatt A (1996) Urokinasetype plasminogen activator expression in human prostate carcinomas. Am J Med Sci 312:8–11
175. Gavrilov D, Kenzior O, Evans M, Calaluce R, Folk WR (2001) Expression of urokinase plasminogen activator and receptor in conjunction with the ETS family and AP-1 complex transcription factors in high grade prostate cancers. Eur J Cancer 37:1033–1040
176. Linja MJ, Savinainen KJ, Saramaki OR, Tammela TLJ, Vessella T, Visakorpi T (2001) Amplification and overexpression of androgen receptor gene in hormone-refractory prostate cancer. Cancer Res 61:3550–3555
177. Cozzi PJ, Wang J, Delprado W, Madigan MC, Fairy S, Russell PJ, Li Y (2006) Evaluation of urokinase plasminogen activator and its receptor in different grades of human prostate cancer. Hum Pathol 37(11):1442–1451
178. Egeblad M, Werb Z (2002) New functions for the matrix metalloproteinases in cancer progression. Nat Rev 2(3):161–174
179. Quax PH, de Bart AC, Schalken JA, Verheijen JH (1997) Plasminogen activator and matrix metalloproteinase production and extracellular matrix degradation by rat prostate cancer cells in vitro: correlation with metastatic behavior in vivo. Prostate 32(3):196–204
180. Rabbani SA (1998) Metalloproteases and urokinase in angiogenesis and tumor progression. In Vivo 12:135–142
181. Festuccia C, Giunciuglio D, Guerra F, Villanova I, Angelucci A, Manduca P, Teti A, Albini A, Bologna M (1999) Osteoblasts modulate secretion of urokinasetype plasminogen activator (uPA) and matrix metalloproteinase-9 (MMP-9) in human prostate cancer cells promoting migration and matrigel invasion. Oncol Res 11:17–31
182. Skogseth H, Larsson E, Halgunset J (2005) Inhibitors of tyrosine kinase inhibit the production of urokinase plasminogen activator in human prostatic cancer cells. APMIS 113:332–339
183. Skogseth H, Larsson E, Halgunset J (2006) The invasive behaviour of prostatic cancer cells is suppressed by inhibitors of tyrosinekinase. APMIS 114:61–66
184. Skogseth H, Larsson E, Halgunset J (2006) Urokinase plasminogen activator receptor (uPAR) expression is reduced by tyrosinekinase inhibitors. APMIS 114:307–313
185. Skogseth H, Larsson E, Halgunset J (2006) Transcription levels of invasion-related genes in prostate cancer cells are modified by inhibitors of tyrosine kinase. APMIS 114:364–371

186. Li Y, Rizvi SM, Ranson M, Allen BJ (2002) ^{213}Bi-PAI2 conjugate selectively induces apoptosis in PC3 metastatic prostate cancer cell line and shows anti-cancer activity in a xenograft animal model. Br J Cancer 86:1197–1203
187. Li Y, Abbas Rizvi SM, Blair nee Brown JM, Cozzi PJ, Qu CF, Ow KT, Tam PN, Perkins AC, Russell PJ, Allen BJ (2004) Antigenic expression of human metastatic prostate cancer cell lines for in vitro multiple-targeted alpha-therapy with ^{213}Bi-conjugates. Int J Radiat Oncol Biol Phys 60:896–908
188. Wang J, Abbas Rizvi SM, Madigan MC, Cozzi PJ, Power CA, Qu CF, Morgenstern A, Apostolidis C, Russell PJ, Allen BJ, Li Y (2006) Control of prostate cancer spheroid growth using ^{213}Bi-labeled multiple targeted alpha radioimmunoconjugates. Prostate 66:1753–1767
189. Pulukuri SM, Gondi CS, Lakka SS, Jutla A, Estes N, Gujrati M, Rao J (2005) RNA interference-directed knockdown of urokinase plasminogen activator and urokinase plasminogen activator receptor inhibits prostate cancer cell invasion, survival, and tumorigenicity in vivo. J Biol Chem 280:36529–36540
190. Josephy PD (2010) Genetic variations in human glutathione transferase enzymes: significance for pharmacology and toxicology. Hum Genomics Proteomics 2010:876940
191. Armstrong RN (1997) Structure, catalytic mechanism, and evolution of the glutathione transferases. Chem Res Toxicol 10:2–18
192. Villafania A, Anwar K, Amar S, Chie L, Way D, Chung DL, Adler V, Ronai Z, Brandt-Rauf PW, Yamaizumii Z, Kung HF, Pincus MR (2000) Glutathione-S-Transferase as a selective inhibitor of oncogenic ras-p21-induced mitogenic signaling through blockade of activation of jun by jun-N-terminal kinase. Ann Clin Lab Sci 30:57–64
193. Zöchbauer-Müller S, Fong KM, Virmani AK, Geradts J, Gazdar AF, Minna JD (2001) Aberrant promoter methylation of multiple genes in non-small cell lung cancers. Cancer Res 61:249–255
194. He Y, Zhou GQ, Li X, Dong XJ, Chai XQ, Yao KT (2009) Correlation of polymorphism of the coding region of glutathione S-transferase M1 to susceptibility of nasopharyngeal carcinoma in South China population. Ai Zheng 28:5–7
195. Stephen JK, Chen KM, Raitanen M, Grénman S, Worsham MJ (2009) DNA hypermethylation profiles in squamous cell carcinoma of the vulva. Int J Gynecol Pathol 28:63–75
196. Lee WH, Isaacs WB, Bova GS, Nelson WG (1997) CG island methylation changes near the GSTP1 gene in prostatic carcinoma cells detected using the polymerase chain reaction: a new prostate cancer biomarker. Cancer Epidemiol Biomarkers Prev 6:443–450
197. Goessl C, Müller M, Miller K (2000) Methylation-specific PCR (MSP) for detection of tumour DNA in the blood plasma and serum of patients with prostate cancer. Prostate Cancer Prostatic Dis 3:S17
198. Herman JG, Graff JR, Myöhänen S, Nelkin BD, Baylin SB (1996) Methylation-specific PCR: a novel PCR assay for methylation status of CpG islands. Proc Natl Acad Sci U S A 93:9821–9826
199. Esteller M, Corn PG, Urena JM, Gabrielson E, Baylin SB, Herman JG (1998) Inactivation of glutathione S-transferase P1 gene by promoter hypermethylation in human neoplasia. Cancer Res 58:4515–4518
200. Cairns P, Esteller M, Herman JG, Schoenberg M, Jeronimo C, Sanchez-Cespedes M, Chow NH, Grasso M, Wu L, Westra WB, Sidransky D (2001) Molecular detection of prostate cancer in urine by GSTP1 hypermethylation. Clin Cancer Res 7:2727–2730
201. Schmitz W, Fingerhut R, Conzelmann E (1994) Purification and properties of an alpha-methylacyl-CoA racemase from rat liver. Eur J Biochem 222:313–323
202. Schmitz W, Albers C, Fingerhut R, Conzelmann E (1995) Purification and characterization of an alpha-methylacyl-CoA racemase from human liver. Eur J Biochem 231:815–822
203. Ferdinandusse S, Denis S, IJ Ist L, Dacremont G, Waterham HR, Wanders RJ (2000) Subcellular localization and physiological role of alpha-methylacyl-CoA racemase. J Lipid Res 41:1890–1896
204. Jiang Z, Woda BA, Rock KL, Xu Y, Savas L, Khan A, Pihan G, Cai F, Babcook JS, Rathanaswami P, Reed SG, Xu J, Fanger GR (2001) P504S: a new molecular marker for the detection of prostate carcinoma. Am J Surg Pathol 25:1397–1404

205. Luo J, Zha S, Gage WR, Dunn TA, Hicks JL, Bennett CJ, Ewing CM, Platz EA, Ferdinandusse S, Wanders RJ, Trent JM, Isaacs WB, De Marzo AM (2002) α-methylacyl-CoA racemase: a new molecular marker for prostate cancer. Cancer Res 62:2220–2226
206. Rubin MA, Zhou M, Dhanasekaran SM, Varambally S, Barrette TR, Sanda MG, Pienta KJ, Ghosh D, Chinnaiyan AM (2002) Alpha-Methylacyl coenzyme A racemase as a tissue biomarker for prostate cancer. JAMA 287:1662–1670
207. Olgac S, Hutchinson B, Tickoo SK, Reuter VE (2006) Alpha-methylacyl-CoA racemase as a marker in the differential diagnosis of metanephric adenoma. Mod Pathol 19:218–224
208. Higgins JP, Shinghal R, Gill H, Reese JH, Terris M, Cohen RJ, Fero M, Pollack JR, van de Rijn M, Brooks JD (2003) Gene expression patterns in renal cell carcinoma assessed by complementary DNA microarray. Am J Pathol 162:925–932
209. Bartel DP (2004) MicroRNAs: genomics, biogenesis, mechanism, and function. Cell 116:281–297
210. Xie X, Lu J, Kulbokas EJ, Golub TR, Mootha V, Lindblad-Toh K, Lander ES, Kellis M (2005) Systematic discovery of regulatory motifs in human promoters and 3′ UTRs by comparison of several mammals. Nature 434:338–345
211. Shyu AB, Wilkinson MF, van Hoof A (2008) Messenger RNA regulation: to translate or to degrade. EMBO J 27:471–481
212. Vrba L, Jensen TJ, Garbe JC, Heimark RL, Cress AE, Dickinson S, Stampfer MR, Futscher BW (2010) Role for DNA methylation in the regulation of miR-200c and miR-141 expression in normal and cancer cells. PLoS One 5:e8697
213. Li T, Li D, Sha J, Sun P, Huang Y (2009) MicroRNA-21 directly targets MARCKS and promotes apoptosis resistance and invasion in prostate cancer cells. Biochem Biophys Res Commun 383:280–285
214. Sun R, Fu X, Li Y, Xie Y, Mao Y (2009) Global gene expression analysis reveals reduced abundance of putative microRNA targets in human prostate tumours. BMC Genomics 10:93
215. Saini S, Majid S, Yamamura S, Tabatabai ZL, Suh SO, Shahryari V, Chen Y, Deng G, Tanaka Y, Dahiya R (2011) Regulatory role of miR-203 in prostate cancer progression and metastasis. Clin Cancer Res 17:5287–5298
216. Lu J, Getz G, Miska EA, Alvarez-Saavedra E, Lamb J, Peck D, Sweet-Cordero A, Ebert BL, Mak RH, Ferrando AA, Downing JR, Jacks T, Horvitz HR, Golub TR (2005) MicroRNA expression profiles classify human cancers. Nature 435:834–838
217. Synder M, Du J, Gerstein M (2010) Personal genome sequencing: current approaches and challenges. Genes Dev 24:423–431
218. Bachert C, Fimmel C, Linstedt A (2007) Endosomal trafficking and proprotein convertase cleavage of cis Golgi protein GP73 produces marker for hepatocellular carcinoma. Traffic 8:1415–1423
219. Kladney RD, Cui X, Bulla GA, Brunt EM, Fimmel CJ (2002) Expression of GP73, a resident Golgi membrane protein, in viral and nonviral liver disease. Hepatology 35:1431–1440
220. Iftikhar R, Kladney RD, Havlioglu N, Schmitt-Graff A, Gusmirovic I, Solomon H, Luxon BA, Bacon BR, Fimmel CJ (2004) Disease- and cell-specific expression of GP73 in human liver disease. Am J Gastroenterol 99:1087–1095
221. Marrero JA, Romano PR, Nikolaeva O, Steel L, Mehta A, Fimmel CJ, Comunale MA, D'Amelio A, Lok AS, Block TM (2005) GP73, a resident Golgi glycoprotein, is a novel serum marker for hepatocellular carcinoma. J Hepatol 43:1007–1012
222. Laxman B, Morris DS, Yu J, Siddiqui J, Cao J, Mehra R, Lonigro RJ, Tsodikov A, Wei JT, Tomlins SA, Chinnaiyan AM (2008) A first-generation multiplex biomarker analysis of urine for the early detection of prostate cancer. Cancer Res 68:645–649
223. Kristiansen G, Fritzsche FR, Wassermann K, Jäger C, Tölls A, Lein M, Stephan C, Jung K, Pilarsky C, Dietel M, Moch H (2008) GOLPH2 protein expression as a novel tissue biomarker for prostate cancer: implications for tissue-based diagnostics. Br J Cancer 99:939–948
224. Wei S, Dunn TA, Isaacs WB, De Marzo AM, Luo J (2008) GOLPH2 and MYO6: putative prostate cancer markers localized to the Golgi apparatus. Prostate 68:1387–1395

225. Vener T, Derecho C, Baden J, Wang H, Rajpurohit Y, Skelton J, Mehrotra J, Varde S, Chowdary D, Stallings W, Leibovich B, Robin H, Pelzer A, Schäfer G, Auprich M, Mannweiler S, Amersdorfer P, Mazumder A (2008) Development of a multiplexed urine assay for prostate cancer diagnosis. Clin Chem 54:874–882
226. Albertsen PC, Hanley JA, Fine J (2005) 20-year outcomes following conservative management of clinically localized prostate cancer. JAMA 293:2095–2101
227. Johansson JE, Holmberg L, Johansson S, Bergström R, Adami HO (1997) 15-year survival in prostate cancer. A prospective, population-based study in Sweden. JAMA 277:467–471
228. Halabi S, Small EJ, Kantoff PW, Kattan MW, Kaplan EB, Dawson NA, Levine EG, Blumenstein BA, Vogelzang NJ (2003) Prognostic model for predicting survival in men with hormone-refractory metastatic prostate cancer. J Clin Oncol 21:1232–1237
229. Amundadottir LT et al (2006) A common variant associated with prostate cancer in European and African populations. Nat Genet 38(6):652–658
230. Freedman ML et al (2006) Admixture mapping identifies 8q24 as a prostate cancer risk locus in African-American men. Proc Natl Acad Sci U S A 103(38):14068–14073
231. Severi G et al (2007) The common variant rs1447295 on chromosome 8q24 and prostate cancer risk: results from an Australian population-based case-control study. Cancer Epidemiol Biomarkers Prev 16(3):610–612
232. Yeager M et al (2007) Genome-wide association study of prostate cancer identifies a second risk locus at 8q24. Nat Genet 39(5):645–649
233. Gudmundsson J (2007) Genome-wide association study identifies a second prostate cancer susceptibility variant at 8q24. Nat Genet 39(5):631–637
234. Wang L et al (2007) Two common chromosome 8q24 variants are associated with increased risk for prostate cancer. Cancer Res 67(7):2944–2950
235. Schumacher FR et al (2007) A common 8q24 variant in prostate and breast cancer from a large nested case-control study. Cancer Res 67(7):2951–2956
236. Suuriniemi M et al (2007) Confirmation of a positive association between prostate cancer risk and a locus at chromosome 8q24. Cancer Epidemiol Biomarkers Prev 16(4):809–814
237. Cheng I et al (2008) 8q24 and prostate cancer: association with advanced disease and meta-analysis. Eur J Hum Genet 16(4):496–505
238. Zheng SL et al (2008) Cumulative association of five genetic variants with prostate cancer. New Engl J Med 358(9):910–919

Chapter 10
Molecular Diagnosis of Bladder and Kidney Cancer

Marino E. Leon, Dahui Qin, and Debra L. Zynger

Contents

Abstract This chapter will review the molecular diagnosis of bladder and kidney cancer. In current clinical practice, early detection and diagnosis of urothelial carcinoma is based on urinary cytology. UroVysion™ bladder cancer fluorescence in situ hybridization (FISH) has become a useful ancillary test in the detection of urothelial carcinoma for initial diagnosis and recurrence; this test is applicable to routine cytologic urine specimens. Multiple studies have shown that UroVysion™ FISH in voided urine and washing specimens can help in patient management due to its superior sensitivity over cytology in certain situations. Within the renal cortex,

---

M.E. Leon, M.D. (✉)
Department of Anatomic Pathology, H. Lee Moffitt Cancer Center and Research Institute, University of South Florida College of Medicine, 12902 Magnolia Drive, Tampa, FL 33612, USA
e-mail: marino.leon@moffitt.org

D. Qin, M.D., Ph.D.
Department of Hematopathology and Laboratory Medicine and Anatomic Pathology, H. Lee Moffitt Cancer Center and Research Institute, University of South Florida College of Medicine, 12902 Magnolia Drive, Tampa, FL 33612, USA

D.L. Zynger, M.D.
Department of Pathology, The Ohio State University, Wexner Medical Center, Columbus, OH, USA

D. Coppola (ed.), *Molecular Pathology and Diagnostics of Cancer*, Cancer Growth and Progression 16, DOI 10.1007/978-94-007-7192-5_10,

molecular studies have not achieved routine use; the most widely available tests are used to identify Xp11.2 translocations/TFE fusions for the subclassification of renal cell carcinoma.

Keywords Carcinoma • Bladder • Diagnosis • Molecular • Urothelial

Abbreviations

BCG	Bacillus Calmette-Guerin
BTA	Bladder Tumor Antigen
CEP	Chromosome Enumeration Probes
FDP	Fibrinogen Degradation Products
FDP	Fibrinogen Degradation
FGFR3	Fibroblast Growth Factor Receptor 3
FISH	Fluorescent in Situ Hybridization
hCFHrp	Human Complement Factor H Related Protein
LSI	Locus Specific Identifier
TPS	Tissue Polypeptide Specific

10.1 Introduction

This chapter will focus on the current clinical molecular diagnosis of neoplasms arising in the urothelium, the specialized form of transitional epithelium that lines the renal pelvis, ureters, bladder, and urethra. The urothelium is composed of a surface layer of large cells, the umbrella cells, and several layers of cells with smaller oval nuclei resting on a well developed basement membrane.

Urothelial carcinoma is more common in males than females [1]. This latter predominance may be explained by a higher prevalence of cigarette smoking in men. Tobacco use, especially cigarette smoking, is one of the leading causes of urothelial carcinoma in the Western hemisphere [1–3]. Additionally, other implicated toxins have been identified including 4-aminobiphenyl, benzidine, 2-naphthylamine and phenacetin-containing analgesics, and cancer chemotherapeutic agents, such as phosphoramide mustards [3]. In the Middle East and parts of Africa, Schistosoma bladder infection is the main cause of squamous cell carcinoma of the bladder [1, 3].

About 70 % of urothelial carcinomas are superficial including non-invasive low-grade papillary (Ta), carcinoma in situ (Tis) [4] and urothelial carcinomas with invasion of subepithelial connective tissue (T1) [5–7]. The remaining 30 % present as muscularis propria invasive disease (≥T2) and are associated with a poor prognosis [6]. Of the superficial urothelial carcinomas, most patients with non-invasive low-grade papillary urothelial neoplasms have a good prognosis [5, 8, 9] yet approximately 70 % of these patients have recurrences [8, 10], and less than 5 % of cases progress to invasive carcinoma [8, 10]. Patients with low-grade and lower

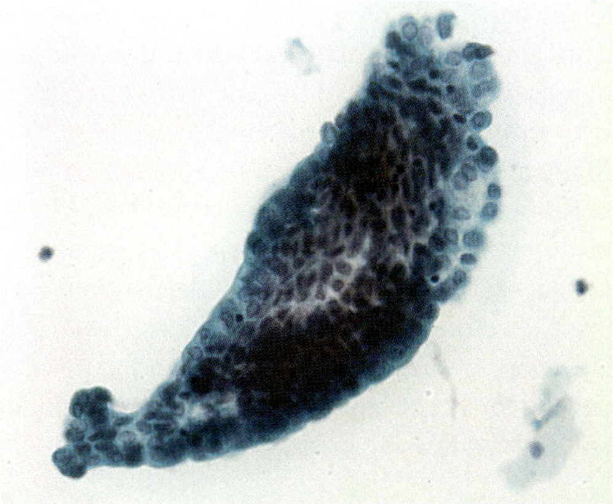

Fig. 10.1 Low-grade urothelial neoplasm with papillary architecture. Urine cytology specimen stained with Papanicolaou staining (original magnification 400×)

pathologic T stage tumors tend to have lower rates of recurrence, progression, and mortality than high-grade and/or higher pathologic stage, suggesting a different biology in tumors that are prone to recurrence [9].

Two main pathways are believed to be involved in urothelial carcinogenesis [11, 12]. One pathway involves the mutation of the *Fibroblast Growth Factor receptor 3* gene (*FGFR3*); this appears to be a favorable pathway giving rise to low-grade non-invasive papillary tumors that may recur but rarely invade [11–13]. The second pathway involves mutation and deletions in the *TP53* gene; tumors that harbor *TP53* gene mutations are high-grade, including high-grade papillary urothelial carcinoma and urothelial carcinoma in situ [11–13]. Supporting this genetic profile, expression array (cDNA) analysis shows specific mRNA signatures associated with either one of these two pathways [14]. Additionally, several other chromosomal abnormalities are observed in high-grade urothelial carcinoma. Alterations that involve chromosome 9 are frequent, including monosomy, and deletions of 9p and 9q [4, 15–19]. Loss of chromosomes 4 and 8, deletions of 2q, 8p, 11p, 13q, 14q, and 17p, and gains of chromosomes, 3, 7, and 17 are also reported [15, 16, 18–20]. Furthermore, papillary tumors and intraepithelial urothelial neoplasia show deletions of chromosome 9 [16, 18, 21]. Specifically, 9p21 deletion that affects the tumor suppressor gene p16 *(INK4a)* is seen [22]. A detailed discussion of the molecular mechanisms of urothelial carcinoma formation is beyond the scope of this review; recent publications are suggested for this purpose [12, 13, 23].

Urinary tract carcinoma presents with painless hematuria making early identification sometimes difficult [6, 24]. Patients with carcinoma in situ present with dysuria, nocturia, urinary frequency and urgency with microscopic hematuria [25]. In the current clinical practice, early detection and diagnosis is based on urinary cytology [6, 26, 27]. Urine cytology is the initial test of choice for screening and follow-up of urothelial carcinoma [27–32]. Cytology is a highly reliable, sensitive, and specific test in the diagnosis of high-grade urothelial carcinoma [27]. However, given the cytomorphologic features of a low-grade urothelial neoplasm, the findings may be equivocal or negative in a large proportion of patients yielding a low sensitivity for low-grade urothelial tumors (Fig. 10.1) [27]. Due to the low sensitivity of a single urine cytology study, several specimens may be needed to detect a tumor, justifying the use of three consecutive urine specimens [27]. Additionally, the diagnosis is difficult in patients with upper urinary tract neoplasms and in patients with urothelial carcinoma treated with bacillus Calmette-Guerin (BCG) [33–35]. Many ancillary studies used in conjunction with urine cytology have been explored to further characterize equivocal cytology [30, 32]. Unfortunately, an ideal ancillary test for screening and monitoring has yet to be created [30, 32, 36, 37].

Once the initial evaluation and detection with cytology is performed using voided urine specimens, the patients undergo cystoscopy with a confirmatory biopsy [32]. However, cystoscopy is invasive and expensive. Therefore, there is a need to the develop markers capable of identifying urothelial carcinoma by a more economical and/or less invasive methodology [8, 28, 31, 32].

10.2 UroVysion™ Fluorescent In Situ Hybridization (FISH) Test for Urothelial Carcinoma

The FISH technique allows for the visualization of a specific nucleic acid sequence area within a cell by the precise annealing of a fluorescent labeled single strand of DNA fragment, called a probe, to its complementary DNA target sequence on the chromosomes. The hybridization of the probes is visible in a fluorescent microscope as fluorescent dots. Each dot represents a copy of the targeted sequence.

Currently, FISH analysis of urothelial cells from urine has emerged as powerful ancillary technique addressing the limitations of cytopathology [33]. The commercially available UroVysion™ FISH multiprobe (Abbot, DesPlaines, IL) is a molecular test with proven clinical value [22, 33, 34, 38, 39] and it has become a well known and established test to further characterize urine cytology specimens [20, 22, 34, 38–41]. UroVysion™ is Food and Drug Administration (FDA)-approved for the detection of urothelial carcinoma in voided urine specimens from patients with gross or microscopic hematuria and no previous history of urothelial carcinoma and for the detection of recurrent urothelial carcinoma in voided urine specimens from patients with a prior history of urothelial carcinoma [39, 42].

UroVysion™ bladder cancer FISH kit is applicable to routine cytologic urine specimens fixed on slides. This kit consists of a four color, four probe mixture of DNA sequences to determined regions on chromosomes 3, 7, 9, and 17 [22, 39] including three Chromosome Enumeration Probes (CEP), CEP 3 SpectrumRed, CEP 7 SpectrumGreen, and CEP 17 SpectrumAqua, and a Locus Specific Identifier (LSI) 9p21 SpectrumGold (Fig. 10.2) [43]. Therefore, this test is capable of detecting increased copy numbers (polysomy) of the chromosomes 3, 7 and 17 and deletion of 9p21 (Figs. 10.3 and 10.4) [33, 39].

The criteria for a FISH positive result as suggested by the manufacturer of UroVysion™ are as follows: abnormal cells show a gain of multiple chromosomes (three or more signals of CEP 3, CEP 7, or CEP 17) or a homozygous loss of 9p21. This assay requires that a minimum of 25 morphologically abnormal cells are to be

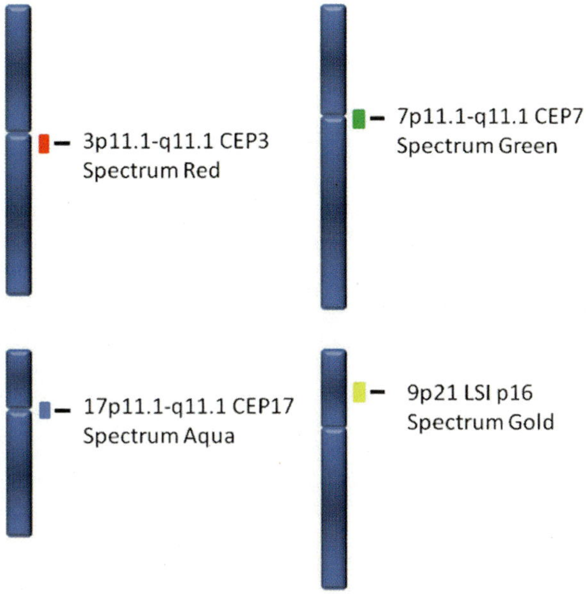

Fig. 10.2 The specific markers used on the UroVysion™ kit are shown in this graph. Note that chromosome enumeration probes (CEP) are used for chromosomes 3 (*Spectrum Red*), 7 (*Spectrum Green*) and 17 (*Spectrum Aqua*); a locus specific identifier is used in chromosome 9p21 (*Spectrum Gold*)

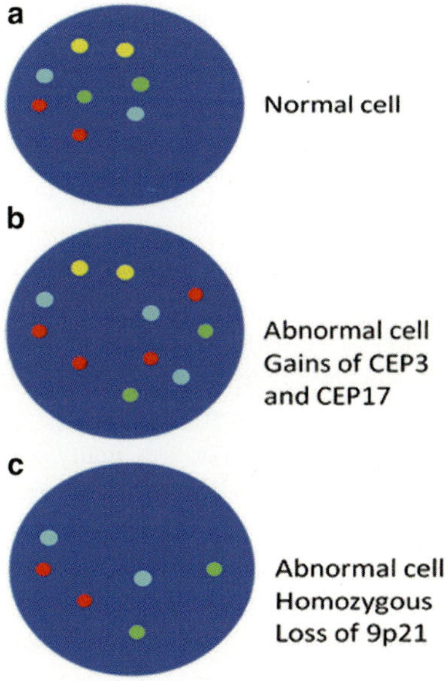

Fig. 10.3 (**a**) Diagram of a chromosomally normal cell nucleus with presence of all the tested probes; two of each CEP 3 *red*, CEP 7 *green*, CEP 17 *aqua*, and LIS 9p21 *gold* respectively. (**b**) Diagram of a chromosomally abnormal cell with additional signals for CEP 3, four signals, and CEP17, three signals. (**c**) Diagram of a chromosomally abnormal cell with homozygous loss of LSI 9p21 *gold* signals

analyzed [44]. Specifically, "analysis should continue until either ≥4 cells with gains of multiple chromosomes or ≥12 cells with homozygous loss of 9p21 are detected or the entire sample is analyzed. The total number of chromosomally abnormal cells, i.e. cells with gain of multiple chromosomes or homozygous loss of

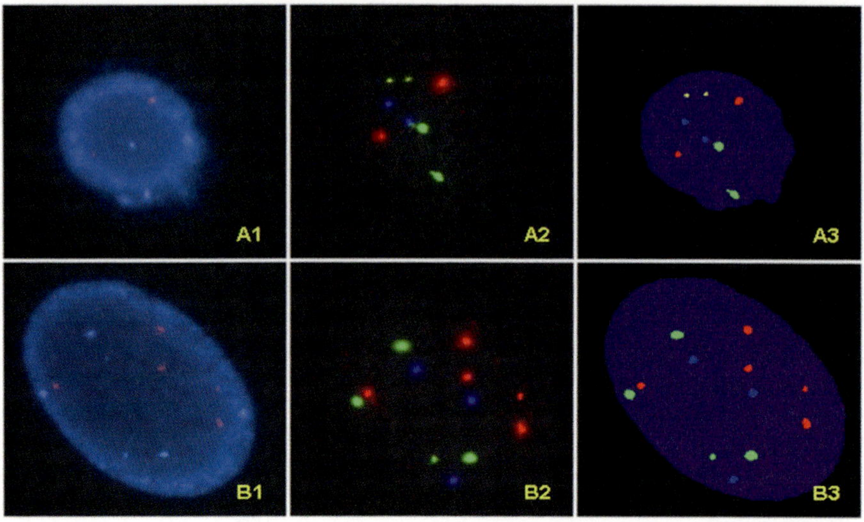

Fig. 10.4 *A1*. An UroVysion negative ("normal") cell observed with DAPI filter. *A2*. The same UroVysion negative cell observed with filters for *gold*, *green*, *red*, and *aqua* respectively; the actual photographs from different filters are overlapped using software. The results show normal 9p21 locus (two *gold signals*) and normal number of chromosomes 3 (two *red signals*), 7 (two *green signals*) and 17 (two *aqua signals*). *A3*. The overlapping images of the same UroVysion negative cell with computer generated pseudo-color. *B1*. An UroVysion abnormal cell observed with DAPI filter. *B2*. The same UroVysion abnormal cell observed with filters for *gold*, *red*, *green*, and *aqua* respectively; the actual photographs from different filters are overlapped using software; gains in chromosome 3 (five *red signals*), 7 (four *green signals*) and 17 (three *aqua signals*) are noted. Note that the signal for 9p21 (*gold*) is not present due to homozygous loss of 9p21. *B3*. The overlapping images of the same UroVysion abnormal cell with computer generated pseudo-color

9p21, are determined; results are reported as positive or negative" [44]. As such, a positive result is reported when either four or more cells with multiple chromosomal gains or 12 or more cells with loss of both signals for 9p21 are observed. When there is less than four cells with chromosome gain or less than 12 cells with 9q21 loss, a negative result is reported with a comment, indicating how many cells with chromosome gain or how many cells with 9q21 loss. The study may be aided using either FDA cleared systems BioView Duet™ System for Automated FISH scanning of UroVysion™ (Rehovot, Israel) or the *onco*FISH® bladder for automated UroVysion™ by Ikoniscope® Digital Microscopy System (Ikonisys, New Haven, Connecticut) [45–47]. When an automated system is used, the assay requires the screening of more cells before a negative result can be issued [48, 49]. In the case of BioView Duet™ System, at least 100 cells are needed to be screened for a negative case [48, 49]. These systems enhance the practice; however, they do not replace the microscopic evaluation by cytology professionals.

UroVysion™ may detect more abnormalities than cytology [20, 50]. Multiple studies have shown that UroVysion™ FISH in voided urine and washing specimens can help in patient management due to its superior sensitivity over cytology in different situations [50]. It can be particularly useful to clarify equivocal cytological findings [33]. UroVysion™ can aid in the clinical follow-up after BCG treatment to identify patients with therapy failure. In this clinical circumstance, UroVysion™ is also better than cytology [20, 41]. UroVysion™ FISH is more sensitive than cytology in diagnosing high-grade tumors than low-grade tumors and flat intraepithelial lesions [51], yet as with any test, clinical correlation is always recommended. Additionally, UroVysion™ may clarify cases with reactive epithelial atypia [35]. In these specimens, the overall sensitivity of cytology improves when coupled with UroVysion™ [52]. In patients followed with UroVysion™ for urothelial carcinoma, 27 % of patients without clinical evidence of tumor will demonstrate a positive UroVysion™ FISH result [53]. Interestingly, about 63 % of these patients will develop a clinically and pathologically recognizable recurrent tumor within 2 years [20, 53]. Although UroVysion™ FISH has a higher sensitivity than cytology, the specificity is reported as similar or higher for cytology [50, 51].

Further molecular applications, such as coupling UroVysion™ FISH and FGFR3 mutational status are in investigation [54]. Although the following tests are not clinically used at this time, they represent a glimpse of future possibilities. Among these are the testing of epigenetic alterations in bladder carcinogenesis involving promoter hypermethylation and aberrant expression of microRNA [14]. Notably, aberrant expression of specific microRNAs is associated with the FGFR3 mutant bladder carcinogenesis pathway [14].

10.3 Other Assays for Urothelial Carcinoma

DNA ploidy has been used as an ancillary study in urine cytology [27, 31, 55–59]. Initially, DNA ploidy was determined using flow cytometry [60–63]. Later, DNA ploidy was performed using image analysis automated systems on Feulgen stained cytology preparations [55, 57, 58]. Of these methods, DNA ploidy by image analysis was found superior to DNA ploidy by flow cytometry [57]. This method also has some value in the follow-up detection of recurrent disease in patients with urinary diversion [55]. UroVysion™ is more specific than DNA ploidy image cytometry for the detection of aneuploid neoplastic cells, identifying twice as many abnormalities, and as a result has become a more popular ancillary test in the detection of urothelial carcinoma [52].

Other tests described in the literature are Bladder Tumor Antigen (BTA s*tat*®, and BTA TRAK®), nuclear matrix protein 22 (NMP22® BladderCheck®), urinary fibrinogen degradation products (FDP), ImmunoCyt™/uCyt+™, Quanticyt, Hb-dipstick, LewisX, Telomerase, Microsatellite LOH, cytokeratin 19 fragment enzyme link immunoabsorbent assay (CYFRA21-1 ELISA), urinary bladder cancer enzyme link immunoabsorbent assay (UBC ELISA), rt-PCR to determine the expression of cytokeratin 20, hyaluronic acid and hyaluronidase (HA-HAase), urine tissue polypeptide specific antigens (TPS), cDNA microarray and detection of certain microRNAs [13, 43, 64–70].

In addition to UroVysion™ FISH multiprobe (Abbot, DesPlaines, IL), BTA *stat*® and BTA-TRAK® (polyMedco, Radmond, WA), NMP22® BladderCheck® (Inverness Medical Innovation, Bedford, UK) and ImmunoCyt™/uCyt+™ (Scimedx, Denville, New Jersey) also have FDA approval for bladder cancer surveillance [68, 69, 71, 72].

ImmunoCyt™/uCyt+™ is an immunofluorescent test that uses three monoclonal antibodies labeled with fluorescent markers; two antibodies, M344 and LDQ10, react with a mucin glycoprotein and a third antibody, 19A211, reacts with a glycosylated form of carcinoembryonic antigen [73]. BTA *stat*® is an immunoassay using two different monoclonal antibodies to human complement factor H related protein (hCFHrp) [25, 72, 74–76]. NMP22® BladderCheck® is based on a lateral flow immunochromatographic method detecting a nuclear matrix protein 22 utilizing two different monoclonal antibodies, one as a capture antibody and one as a reporter antibody [71, 72, 77]. Although numerous other molecular studies have been published and are available, their use is still limited to research studies as their clinical relevance has not been established [13].

Recent advances in the knowledge of the molecular pathways and the pathogenesis of bladder cancer could make targeted therapy in urothelial carcinoma possible and the beginning of personalized or individualized therapy directed towards a specific molecular profile of the tumor [78]. The future in bladder carcinoma may involve the use of molecular studies to determine the diagnosis, individual therapy and prognosis [79, 80]. However, in bladder carcinoma, the era of personalized medicine is yet to begin.

10.4 The Molecular Diagnosis of Kidney Tumors

Currently, the molecular diagnosis of kidney tumors is still evolving. Studies mainly involve the molecular characterization of renal carcinomas to identify Xp11.2 translocations/TFE fusions. These carcinomas typically affect children and young adults and show papillary architecture with clear cells and nested patterns, but may also have cells with granular eosinophilic cytoplasm. Renal carcinomas with the *ASPL-TFE3* fusion contain cells with abundant clear to eosinophilic cytoplasm, discrete cell borders, prominent vesicular chromatin, and nucleoli. Psammoma bodies and hyaline nodules are usually present. Renal carcinomas with the *PRCC-TFE3* fusion reveal a more nested architecture with cells with a moderate amount of cytoplasm, hyaline nodules and fewer psammoma bodies. Using immunohistochemistry, these tumors have expression of the TFE3 protein, renal cell carcinoma marker antigen and CD10 and they may be cytokeratin and epithelial membrane antigen positive [76, 81]. The diagnosis of these tumors can be established based on morphology with confirmation by immunohistochemistry for TFE3. Tumors with the Xp11.2 translocation, all involving the *TFE3* gene [82, 83], include:

(a) t(X;1)(p11.2;q21) with the fusion of *PRCC* and *TFE3* genes
(b) t(X;17)(p11.2;p25) with the fusion of *ASPL (RCC17)* and *TFE3* genes

(c) t(X;1)(p11.2;p34) with the fusion of *PSF* and *TFE3* genes
(d) inv(X)(p11;q12) with the fusion of *NonO* (*p54*^{nrb}) and *TFE3* genes

These fusion proteins act as aberrant transcription factors. FISH and other molecular methods may be applied to confirm the specific molecular change in these tumors, although these tests are not widely available [82].

Molecular studies have shown some utility in pediatric tumors such as the cellular variant of congenital mesoblastic nephroma (but not the classic variant); this tumor shows the same t(12;15)(p13;q25) and *ETV6-NTRK3* genes fusion as infantile fibrosarcoma [84]. Rhabdoid tumor of the kidney shows a deletion of the hSNF5/INI1 gene [84]. As with molecular diagnostics for renal cell carcinoma, these tests are not in routine clinical use.

References

1. Johansson SL, Cohen SM (1997) Epidemiology and etiology of bladder cancer. Semin Surg Oncol 13(5):291–298
2. Cohen SM, Johansson SL (1992) Epidemiology and etiology of bladder cancer. Urol Clin North Am 19(3):421–428
3. Cohen SM, Shirai T et al (2000) Epidemiology and etiology of premalignant and malignant urothelial changes. Scand J Urol Nephrol Suppl 205:105–115
4. Czerniak B, Chaturvedi V et al (1999) Superimposed histologic and genetic mapping of chromosome 9 in progression of human urinary bladder neoplasia: implications for a genetic model of multistep urothelial carcinogenesis and early detection of urinary bladder cancer. Oncogene 18(5):1185–1196
5. Heney NM (1992) Natural history of superficial bladder cancer. Prognostic features and long-term disease course. Urol Clin North Am 19(3):429–433
6. Kaufman DS, Shipley WU et al (2009) Bladder cancer. Lancet 374(9685):239–249
7. Koch M, McPhee MS et al (1988) Five year follow-up of patients with cancer of the bladder – the Northern Alberta experience. Clin Invest Med 11(4):253–258
8. Holmang S, Hedelin H et al (1999) Recurrence and progression in low grade papillary urothelial tumors. J Urol 162(3 Pt 1):702–707
9. Millan-Rodriguez F, Chechile-Toniolo G et al (2000) Primary superficial bladder cancer risk groups according to progression, mortality and recurrence. J Urol 164(3 Pt 1):680–684
10. Holmang S, Andius P et al (2001) Stage progression in Ta papillary urothelial tumors: relationship to grade, immunohistochemical expression of tumor markers, mitotic frequency and DNA ploidy. J Urol 165(4):1124–1128, discussion 1128–1130
11. Cheng L, Davidson DD et al (2010) The origins of urothelial carcinoma. Expert Rev Anticancer Ther 10(6):865–880
12. Chuang S-T, Tracy RA et al (2010) Carcinogenetic pathway of superficial low-grade urothelial carcinoma. In: Coppola D (ed) Mechanisms of oncogenesis, vol 12. Springer, New York, pp 279–284
13. Cheng L, Zhang S et al (2010) Bladder cancer: translating molecular genetic insights into clinical practice. Hum Pathol 42(4):455–481
14. van der Kwast TH, Bapat B (2009) Predicting favourable prognosis of urothelial carcinoma: gene expression and genome profiling. Curr Opin Urol 19(5):516–521
15. Cordon-Cardo C, Cote RJ et al (2000) Genetic and molecular markers of urothelial premalignancy and malignancy. Scand J Urol Nephrol Suppl 205:82–93
16. Hartmann A, Rosner U et al (2000) Clonality and genetic divergence in multifocal low-grade superficial urothelial carcinoma as determined by chromosome 9 and p53 deletion analysis. Lab Invest 80(5):709–718

17. Marano A, Pan Y et al (2000) Chromosomal numerical aberrations detected by fluorescence in situ hybridization on bladder washings from patients with bladder cancer. Eur Urol 37(3):358–365
18. Obermann EC, Junker K et al (2003) Frequent genetic alterations in flat urothelial hyperplasias and concomitant papillary bladder cancer as detected by CGH, LOH, and FISH analyses. J Pathol 199(1):50–57
19. Tsukamoto M, Matsuyama H et al (2002) Numerical aberrations of chromosome 9 in bladder cancer. A possible prognostic marker for early tumor recurrence. Cancer Genet Cytogenet 134(1):41–45
20. Bubendorf L, Grilli B et al (2001) Multiprobe FISH for enhanced detection of bladder cancer in voided urine specimens and bladder washings. Am J Clin Pathol 116(1):79–86
21. Veltman JA, Fridlyand J et al (2003) Array-based comparative genomic hybridization for genome-wide screening of DNA copy number in bladder tumors. Cancer Res 63(11):2872–2880
22. Sokolova IA, Halling KC et al (2000) The development of a multitarget, multicolor fluorescence in situ hybridization assay for the detection of urothelial carcinoma in urine. J Mol Diagn 2(3):116–123
23. Dickinson SI (2010) Carcinogenetic pathway of urothelial carcinoma. In: Coppola D (ed) Mechanisms of oncogenesis, vol 12. Springer, New York, pp 285–293
24. Amling CL (2001) Diagnosis and management of superficial bladder cancer. Curr Probl Cancer 25(4):219–278
25. Nese N, Gupta R et al (2009) Carcinoma in situ of the urinary bladder: review of clinicopathologic characteristics with an emphasis on aspects related to molecular diagnostic techniques and prognosis. J Natl Compr Canc Netw 7(1):48–57
26. Caraway NP, Katz RL (2010) A review on the current state of urine cytology emphasizing the role of fluorescence in situ hybridization as an adjunct to diagnosis. Cancer Cytopathol 118(4):175–183
27. Koss LG, Deitch D et al (1985) Diagnostic value of cytology of voided urine. Acta Cytol 29(5):810–816
28. Bischoff CJ, Clark PE (2009) Bladder cancer. Curr Opin Oncol 21(3):272–277
29. Koss LG, Esposti L et al (1986) The role of cytology in the diagnosis, detection and follow-up of bladder cancer. Prog Clin Biol Res 221:97–108
30. Lokeshwar VB, Habuchi T et al (2005) Bladder tumor markers beyond cytology: international consensus panel on bladder tumor markers. Urology 66(6 Suppl 1):35–63
31. Murphy WM (1990) Current status of urinary cytology in the evaluation of bladder neoplasms. Hum Pathol 21(9):886–896
32. Shirodkar SP, Lokeshwar VB (2008) Bladder tumor markers: from hematuria to molecular diagnostics – where do we stand? Expert Rev Anticancer Ther 8(7):1111–1123
33. Bubendorf L (2011) Multiprobe fluorescence in situ hybridization (UroVysion) for the detection of urothelial carcinoma – FISHing for the right catch. Acta Cytol 55(2):113–119
34. Halling KC (2003) Vysis UroVysion for the detection of urothelial carcinoma. Expert Rev Mol Diagn 3(4):507–519
35. Tapia C, Glatz K et al (2011) Evaluation of chromosomal aberrations in patients with benign conditions and reactive changes in urinary cytology. Cancer Cytopathol 119(6):404–410
36. Murata S, Iseki M et al (2010) Molecular and immunohistologic analyses cannot reliably solve diagnostic variation of flat intraepithelial lesions of the urinary bladder. Am J Clin Pathol 134(6):862–872
37. Vrooman OP, Witjes JA (2009) Molecular markers for detection, surveillance and prognostication of bladder cancer. Int J Urol 16(3):234–243
38. Bergman J, Reznichek RC et al (2008) Surveillance of patients with bladder carcinoma using fluorescent in-situ hybridization on bladder washings. BJU Int 101(1):26–29
39. Halling KC, Kipp BR (2008) Bladder cancer detection using FISH (UroVysion assay). Adv Anat Pathol 15(5):279–286
40. Ferra S, Denley R et al (2009) Reflex UroVysion testing in suspicious urine cytology cases. Cancer 117(1):7–14

41. Savic S, Zlobec I et al (2009) The prognostic value of cytology and fluorescence in situ hybridization in the follow-up of nonmuscle-invasive bladder cancer after intravesical Bacillus Calmette-Guerin therapy. Int J Cancer 124(12):2899–2904
42. Galvan AB, Salido M et al (2011) A multicolor fluorescence in situ hybridization assay: a monitoring tool in the surveillance of patients with a history of non-muscle-invasive urothelial cell carcinoma: a prospective study. Cancer Cytopathol 119(6):395–403
43. Halling KC, King W et al (2002) A comparison of BTA stat, hemoglobin dipstick, telomerase and Vysis UroVysion assays for the detection of urothelial carcinoma in urine. J Urol 167(5):2001–2006
44. (2010) UroVysion Bladder Cancer Kit. Retrieved 31 July 2011, from http://www.abbottmolecular.com/us/products/oncology/fish/bladder-cancer-urovysion.html
45. (2005) FDA 510(k) #K050840: Duet™ System. BioView, Ltd., Retrieved 31 July 2011, from http://www.accessdata.fda.gov/cdrh_docs/pdf5/K050840.pdf
46. (2007) FDA 510(k) #K062577: Ikoniscope® oncoFISH™ Bladder Test System. Ikonisys, Inc., Retrieved 31 July 2011, from http://www.accessdata.fda.gov/cdrh_docs/pdf6/K062755.pdf
47. Marganski WA, El-Sirgany Costa V et al (2011) Digitized microscopy in the diagnosis of bladder cancer: analysis of >3000 cases during a 7-month period. Cancer Cytopathol 119(4):279–289
48. Smith GD, Bentz JS (2010) "FISHing" to detect urinary and other cancers: validation of an imaging system to aid in interpretation. Cancer Cytopathol 118(1):56–64
49. Smith GD, Riding M et al (2010) Integrating a FISH imaging system into the cytology laboratory. CytoJournal 7:3
50. Halling KC, King W et al (2000) A comparison of cytology and fluorescence in situ hybridization for the detection of urothelial carcinoma. J Urol 164(5):1768–1775
51. Karnwal A, Venegas R et al (2010) The role of fluorescence in situ hybridization assay for surveillance of non-muscle invasive bladder cancer. Can J Urol 17(2):5077–5081
52. Dalquen P, Kleiber B et al (2002) DNA image cytometry and fluorescence in situ hybridization for noninvasive detection of urothelial tumors in voided urine. Cancer 96(6):374–379
53. Yoder BJ, Skacel M et al (2007) Reflex UroVysion testing of bladder cancer surveillance patients with equivocal or negative urine cytology: a prospective study with focus on the natural history of anticipatory positive findings. Am J Clin Pathol 127(2):295–301
54. Wild PJ, Fuchs T et al (2009) Detection of urothelial bladder cancer cells in voided urine can be improved by a combination of cytology and standardized microsatellite analysis. Cancer Epidemiol Biomarkers Prev 18(6):1798–1806
55. Caraway NP, Khanna A et al (2007) Combination of cytologic evaluation and quantitative digital cytometry is reliable in detecting recurrent disease in patients with urinary diversions. Cancer 111(5):323–329
56. Giella JG, Ring K et al (1992) The predictive value of flow cytometry and urinary cytology in the follow up of patients with transitional cell carcinoma of the bladder. J Urol 148 (2 Pt 1):293–296
57. Koss LG, Wersto RP et al (1989) Predictive value of DNA measurements in bladder washings. Comparison of flow cytometry, image cytophotometry, and cytology in patients with a past history of urothelial tumors. Cancer 64(4):916–924
58. Mora LB, Nicosia SV et al (1996) Ancillary techniques in the follow up of transitional cell carcinoma: a comparison of cytology, histology and deoxyribonucleic acid image analysis cytometry in 91 patients. J Urol 156(1):49–54, discussion 54–55
59. Tribukait B, Gustafson H (1980) Impulse cytophotometric studies on DNA in bladder carcinoma. Onkologie 3(6):278–288
60. Bakhos R, Shankey TV et al (2000) Comparative analysis of DNA flow cytometry and cytology of bladder washings: review of discordant cases. Diagn Cytopathol 22(2):65–69
61. Jitsukawa S, Tachibana M et al (1987) Flow cytometry based on heterogeneity index score compared with urine cytology to evaluate their diagnostic efficacy in bladder tumor. Urology 29(2):218–222

62. Murphy WM, Emerson LD et al (1986) Flow cytometry versus urinary cytology in the evaluation of patients with bladder cancer. J Urol 136(4):815–819
63. Ring KS, Karp F et al (1990) Enhanced detection of bladder cancer using the epithelial surface marker epithelial membrane antigen: a preliminary report. J Occup Med 32(9):904–909
64. Dyrskjot L, Ostenfeld MS et al (2009) Genomic profiling of microRNAs in bladder cancer: miR-129 is associated with poor outcome and promotes cell death in vitro. Cancer Res 69(11):4851–4860
65. Dyrskjot L, Zieger K et al (2007) Gene expression signatures predict outcome in non-muscle-invasive bladder carcinoma: a multicenter validation study. Clin Cancer Res 13(12):3545–3551
66. Guo B, Che T et al (2011) Screening and identification of specific markers for bladder transitional cell carcinoma from urine urothelial cells with suppressive subtractive hybridization and cDNA microarray. Can Urol Assoc J 5(6):E129–E137
67. Klein A, Zemer R et al (1998) Expression of cytokeratin 20 in urinary cytology of patients with bladder carcinoma. Cancer 82(2):349–354
68. Tetu B (2009) Diagnosis of urothelial carcinoma from urine. Mod Pathol 22(Suppl 2):S53–S59
69. van Rhijn BW, van der Poel HG et al (2005) Urine markers for bladder cancer surveillance: a systematic review. Eur Urol 47(6):736–748
70. Zieger K (2008) High throughput molecular diagnostics in bladder cancer – on the brink of clinical utility. Mol Oncol 1(4):384–394
71. Chiong E, Gaston KE et al (2008) Urinary markers in screening patients with hematuria. World J Urol 26(1):25–30
72. Shariat SF, Karam JA et al (2008) Urine cytology and urine-based markers for bladder urothelial carcinoma detection and monitoring: developments and future prospects. Biomark Med 2(2):165–180
73. Olsson H, Zackrisson B (2001) ImmunoCyt a useful method in the follow-up protocol for patients with urinary bladder carcinoma. Scand J Urol Nephrol 35(4):280–282
74. Babjuk M, Kostirova M et al (2002) Qualitative and quantitative detection of urinary human complement factor H-related protein (BTA stat and BTA TRAK) and fragments of cytokeratins 8, 18 (UBC rapid and UBC IRMA) as markers for transitional cell carcinoma of the bladder. Eur Urol 41(1):34–39
75. Heicappell R, Wettig IC et al (1999) Quantitative detection of human complement factor H-related protein in transitional cell carcinoma of the urinary bladder. Eur Urol 35(1):81–87
76. Thomas L, Leyh H et al (1999) Multicenter trial of the quantitative BTA TRAK assay in the detection of bladder cancer. Clin Chem 45(4):472–477
77. Gray M, Sims TW (2004) NMP-22 for bladder cancer screening and surveillance. Urol Nurs 24(3):171–172, 177–179, 186
78. Voutsinas GE, Stravopodis DJ (2009) Molecular targeting and gene delivery in bladder cancer therapy. J BUON 14(Suppl 1):S69–S78
79. Mitra AP, Bartsch CC et al (2009) Strategies for molecular expression profiling in bladder cancer. Cancer Metastasis Rev 28(3–4):317–326
80. Mitra AP, Cote RJ (2009) Molecular pathogenesis and diagnostics of bladder cancer. Annu Rev Pathol 4:251–285
81. Argani P, Ladanyl M (2004) Renal carcinomas associated with Xp11.2 translocations/TFE gene fusions. In: Eble JN, Sauter G, Epstein JI, Sesterhenn IA (eds) Pathology and genetics of tumours of the urinary system and male genital organs, vol 6. IARC Press, Lyon, pp 37–38
82. Argani P, Antonescu CR et al (2001) Primary renal neoplasms with the ASPL-TFE3 gene fusion of alveolar soft part sarcoma: a distinctive tumor entity previously included among renal cell carcinomas of children and adolescents. Am J Pathol 159(1):179–192
83. Heimann P, El Housni H et al (2001) Fusion of a novel gene, RCC17, to the TFE3 gene in t(X;17)(p11.2;q25.3)-bearing papillary renal cell carcinomas. Cancer Res 61(10):4130–4135
84. Argani P, Ladanyi M (2003) Recent advances in pediatric renal neoplasia. Adv Anat Pathol 10(5):243–260

Chapter 11
Molecular-Genetic Testing in Penile, Scrotal, and Testicular Cancer

Nicholas A. Whitling, Sharon M. Hirsh, and Rodney E. Shackelford

Contents

N.A. Whitling • S.M. Hirsh • R.E. Shackelford (✉)
Department of Pathology and Laboratory Medicine, Tulane University School of Medicine, 1430 Tulane Avenue, SL-79, New Orleans, LA 70112-2699, USA
e-mail: rshackel@tulane.edu

D. Coppola (ed.), *Molecular Pathology and Diagnostics of Cancer*, Cancer Growth and Progression 16, DOI 10.1007/978-94-007-7192-5_11,

Abstract Malignant tumors of the penis, scrotum, and testes are rare, accounting for roughly 0.5 % of all male tumors. Presently the diagnosis of these tumors depends mainly on histologic examination, supplemented with immunohistochemistry. Over the past 20 years, however, many genetic changes have been identified that are largely specific to different tumors and tumor classes, such as 12p gains in testicular germ cell tumors. Although not commonly employed in the analysis of these tumors, molecular genetic testing is now available for many of these tumors and is becoming an increasingly important adjunct in their diagnosis and treatment. Here, we summarize what is known about the molecular pathology of these tumors and some of the molecular testing modalities currently available. We also briefly discuss the possible future molecular diagnostics of these tumors.

Keywords Germ cell tumor • Testes • Seminoma • Granulosa cell tumor • Leydig cell tumor • HPV • Genotyping • Cryptorchidism • Mesothelioma

Abbreviations

AAM	Aggressive angiomyxoma
AFP	α-fetoprotein
CGH	Comparative genomic hybridization
DSRCT	Desmoplastic small round cell tumor
FISH	Fluorescent in situ hybridization
hCG	Human chorionic gonadotropin
HPV	Human papilloma virus
ITGCNU	Intratubular germ cell neoplasia, unclassified
LCCSCT	Large cell calcifying Sertoli cell tumors
LCT	Leydig cell tumors
NOS	Not otherwise specified
PLAP	Placental-like alkaline phosphatase
RMS	Rhabdomyosarcoma
SCC	Squamous cell carcinoma
YST	Yolk sac tumors

11.1 Introduction

Penile cancer is an uncommon malignancy in the US and Europe, with approximately 1,400 cases reported each year in the US and 4,000 in Europe. This accounts for less than 0.5 % of all male cancers and has a peak incidence in men of over 70 years of age [1, 2]. The incidence of this malignancy shows considerable geographic variation, accounting for 10–20 % of male cancer in parts of Asia, Africa, and South America [3–5]. Multiple risk factors have been identified for penile cancer including tobacco use, human papilloma virus (HPV) infection, phimosis, balanitis, and poor hygiene [6–8]. Cessation of tobacco use and neonatal or early childhood, but not adult, circumcision lowers the incidence of penile cancer, most likely due to the elimination of chronic inflammation and toxic exposure [8–10]. Approximately 95 % of penile cancer is squamous cell carcinoma (SCC), with the remaining penile malignancies mainly being urothelial, basal, and adenocarcinomas, melanoma, and Kaposi sarcoma. Primary sarcomas of the penis, such as leiomyosarcoma, mesothelioma, and malignant fibrohistiocytic sarcomatous tumors are very rare [1–3, 8, 11–13].

11.2 HVP and Penile Cancer

Approximately 40 % of penile SCC is caused by HPV infection, with HPV types 16 and 18 accounting for ~70 % of penile SCCs [9, 11]. Interestingly, uncircumcised men exhibit a reduced clearance of HPV following infection and not surprisingly, the sex partners of uncircumcised men show an elevated cervical cancer incidence [14, 15]. More than 100 different HPV types have been identified, and it has been estimated that up to 200 types exist. Approximately 40 different HPV viruses infect the anogenital tract and other mucosal areas of the body, with infection being necessary, but not sufficient to cause nearly all (99 %) cervical cancers, and a large portion of anogential neoplasms and oral non-keratinizing SCCs. Significant subsets of 13–18 HPV types have been identified as conferring a probable or definite high-oncogenic risk. The molecular mechanisms by which HPV causes transformation are complex, involving host factors, such as chronic inflammation and immunosuppression, and viral-induced cell cycle progression, apoptosis inhibition, checkpoint ablation, and genomic instability induction [16–19]. Many of these events are mediated through the actions of the HPV E6 and E7 gene products, which bind and inactivate p53 and pRb, respectively [18, 19]. Interestingly, in most HPV infections, the viral genome remains episomal with the E6 and E7 proteins expressed at low levels. High-oncogenic risk HPV types, however, integrate into the epithelial basal cell genome and express high levels of E6 and E7, promoting malignancy [18, 19].

11.2.1 HPV Molecular Diagnostics

Although successful HPV vaccines have been developed, HPV infection remains common, with some 270,000 annual deaths worldwide from cervical cancer alone [1, 20–22]. Thus molecular diagnostics for HPV, especially the high-oncogenic risk types, is often clinically warranted. The detection and analysis of HPV types are largely done on cervical biopsies and cytological specimens, with very few studies examining HPV infection in men [16–19, 23, 24]. Like the analysis of cervical HPV infections, the detection of HPV proteins alone is not clinically significant, as many

HPV infections are benign and produce no significant pathology. Several methods have been employed to detect penile HPV. Here, we will review the most commonly used tests.

11.2.2 Histology

Cellular HPV infections produce specific cytologic changes that can often be seen by examination of hematoxylin-eosin stained slides. Although there is some variation with different anatomic sites, HPV infection are typically superficial, displaying enlarged, hyperchromatic nuclei, with irregular contours, and perinuclear cytoplasmic halos (koilocytotic atypia) [25, 26]. Although histologic analysis is relatively inexpensive and has a short turn-around time, interobserver variability is often high, leading to over-diagnosis of dysplasia over diagnosis in some biopsies, mainly due to non-viropathic changes that mimic koilocytic atypia (pseudokoilocytes) [27, 28].

11.2.3 Surrogate Markers for HPV Infection in Penile Cancer

Similar to the analysis of HPV-induced cervical dysplasia, p16INK4A and Ki-67 (MIB-1) have been used as surrogate markers for HPV-induced dysplasia in penile cancer [29–31]. Interestingly, Ki-67 nuclear staining correlates with penile cancer tumor grade and metastatic potential [31]. The utility of p16INK4A and Ki-67 as markers of dysplasia is covered in detail in the gynecologic malignancies chapter.

11.2.4 HPV PCR Testing

Due to the extremely high precision of nucleic acid hybridization and PCR amplification, both reactions are commonly used for HPV nucleic acid amplification and subtype identification. Although useful for detecting HPV nucleic acid, PCR amplification cannot distinguish between clinically inconsequential transient infections and infections related to significant pathology and oncogenesis [32–35]. For this reason, like all clinical testing modalities, PCR-based HPV analysis must be interpreted in the context of histologic findings and patient history and physical examination.

Flores et al. [36] employed a combination of PCR and hybridization to examine HPV status and type in 463 men between 18 and 40 years old, who had no current sexually transmissible infection and no history of genital warts. Samples were taken from six different anogenital regions, as well as from semen, urine, and venous blood. Samples were taken by genital swabbing, and the DNA was isolated using a QIAamp MiniKit. The samples were lysed and digested with proteinase K, and the DNA was eluted with nuclease-free water and stored at –20 °C until use. PCR was performed with a PGMY09/11 consensus primer pair for a portion of the HPV L1 gene using AmpliTaq Gold in 50 μL volume, with an amplification profile of 95 °C Hot start for 9 min, 95 °C denaturation for 1 min, annealing at 55 °C for 1 min, extension at 72 °C for 1 min for 40 cycles, followed by a final extension period of 5 min at 72 °C. Specimen adequacy was determined by co-amplifying human β-globin gene with B_PC04 and B_GH20 primers and a negative water-only control that lacked primers.

The resulting amplicons were biotin-labeled, denatured, hybridized to an HPV genotype strip, washed, probed with strepavidin-horseradish peroxidase conjugate, and washed. The hybridization/strepavidin binding was detected by a 5-min incubation in a mixture of hydrogen peroxide in sodium citrate buffer and tetramethylbenzidine in dimethylformamide. The genotype strip contained the β-globin gene control and L1 gene sequences for HPV types 6, 11, 16, 18, 26, 31, 33, 35, 39, 40, 42, 45, 51–56, 58, 59, 61, 62, 64, 66–73, 81–84, IS39, and CP6108. Strip interpretation was done by labeled overlay, with lines indicating the position of specific HPV probes types, relative to the reference mark. By this method, HPV was identified on the penile shaft, scrotum, and glands in 62.5 %, 50.0 %, and 44.8 % of the cases, respectively, with the oncogenic HPV types found in approximately ~10–20 % of the HPV-positive patients. The assay was highly reproducible, demonstrating that such testing can work on anatomic areas other than the cervix, and revealed a high rate of HPV infection rate in asymptomatic men.

11.2.5 Sanger and Pyrosequencing for HPV Genotyping

Both Sanger and pyrosequencing have been used to analyze cervical HPV infections but, so far, have not been applied to penile or scrotal patient samples. Due to the very low volume of these samples compared with the large number of cervical samples, clinical testing of penile and scrotal tissues for HPV by sequencing is unlikely to be implemented.

11.3 Scrotal/Paratesticular Cancer

Scrotal cancer is an uncommon malignancy, occurring in 1 per 1 million men in the US and Western Europe. SCC is most common (~27 %), with basal cell carcinoma (19 %), Bowen's disease (15 %), various sarcomas (13 %), extramammary Paget's disease (12 %), malignant melanoma (8 %), lymphoma (2 %), and mesothelioma (1 %) making up most of the remainder. The remaining 3 % are very rare tumors (see below, [36]). Percivall Pott carried out the initial epidemiological studies of scrotal cancer in 1775 and first described a strong correlation between being the profession of chimney sweep and scrotal cancer [37]:

> It is a disease which always makes its first attack on, and its first appearance in, the inferior part of the scrotum; where it produces a superficial, painful, ragged, ill-looking sore, with hard and rising edges. The trade call it the soot-wart. I never saw it under the age of puberty, which is, I suppose, one reason, why it is generally taken, both by patient and surgeon, for venereal, and being treated with mercurials, is thereby soon and much exasperated: in no great length of time, it pervades the skin, dartos, and membranes of the scrotum, and seizes the testicle, which it inlarges, hardens, and renders truly and thoroughly distempered; from whence it makes its way up the spermatic process into the abdomen, most frequently indurating, and spoiling the inguinal glands: when arrived within the abdomen, it affects some of the viscera, and then very soon becomes painfully destructive [sic].

Since this time, scrotal cancer has been related to many different environmental carcinogens, especially petrochemicals and HPV infection [36–39]. PCR combined with restriction-length polymorphism analysis for identifying the HPV type has been employed to analyze scrotal cancer; however, it is not commonly employed in clinical molecular diagnostics [39].

11.4 Rare Scrotal Tumors

A number of rare scrotal tumors show relatively specific molecular alterations. Due to the rarity of these tumors, clinical molecular diagnostics is not performed on them.

11.4.1 Aggressive Angiomyxoma (AAM)

In men, 38 % of aggressive angiomyxomas (AAMs) are derived from the pelviperineal interstitial tissue of the scrotum. Other sites of involvement include the spermatic cord (33 %), perineum (13 %), and intrapelvis organs, such as the urinary bladder (8 %) [41]. Despite this, AAMs primary to the scrotum are very rare, with only a few cases reported. AAMs are rare, locally aggressive, myxoid mesenchymal tumors found almost solely in adult females, usually arising in the soft tissues of the pelvis, perineum, buttocks, and vulva [40–45]. Due to the extreme rarity of scrotal AAM, the tumor is often misdiagnosed as entities such as a hernia sac or hydrocele [41, 46]. No studies have been performed on the molecular pathology underlying scrotal AAMs; however, one study revealed that vulvar AAMs carry a t(8;12)(p12;q15) that causes aberrant expression of the HMGIC transcription factor [47]. Testing for this translocation is not currently performed on AAMs, due to the rarity of this tumor. However, it has been suggested that this translocation might be useful in identifying residual disease [47].

11.4.2 Desmoplastic Small Round Cell Tumor (DSRCT)

Desmoplastic small round cell tumors (DSRCTs) are rare, highly aggressive tumors that confer a poor prognosis; they are found mainly in the pediatric age group and young adults. Nearly all cases are initially confined to the abdomen, with a low percentage found in other anatomic sites, including the scrotum. Histologically, DSRCTs are characterized by small round blue cells embedded within a densely fibrotic, desmoplastic stroma. These tumors are typically reactive for epithelial, mesenchymal, and neural markers [48]. Over 95 % of DSRCTs carry a t(11;22)(p13;q12) that fuse the EWS and WT1 genes [48–50]. Histologically the DSRCT can closely resemble several other rare small blue cell tumors, such as Ewing's sarcoma/primitive neuroectodermal tumor, and some rhabdomyosarcomas (RMS); thus molecular diagnostic testing is often useful in establishing a diagnosis [48–51].

Chromosomal translocation t(11;22)(p13;q12) has been detected by a variety of different molecular techniques. Most commonly, reverse transcriptase-PCR is employed to amplify the nucleic acids regions immediately surrounding the unique EWS and WT1 gene fusion point. Ladanyi et al. [50] isolated RNA from DSRCT snap-frozen tissue and reverse transcription was performed on 1 μg RNA for 30 min at 42 °C using a GeneAmp RNA PCR kit. The reverse transcriptase was denatured at 99 °C for 5 min, and the PCR reagents were added using a forward primer corresponding to EWS exon 7 (5′-TCCTACAGCCAAGCTCCAAGTC-3′) and two reverse primers corresponding to WT1 exons 8 and 9 (5′-ACCTTCGTTCACAGTCCTTTG-3′ and 5′-GACCAGGAGAACTTTCGCTGAC-3′). The fusion sequence was amplified by 40 cycles of 94 °C for 1 min, 60 °C for 1 min, and 72 °C for 30 s, followed by a final extension at 72 °C for 5 min. The resulting amplicons were analyzed by gel electrophoresis followed by transfer onto nitrocellulose and probing for the EWS/WT1 fusion product [50, 52].

11.4.3 Liposarcoma

Scrotal/paratesticular liposarcomas are rare malignancies usually found in men in the fourth to sixth decade and include different histologic subtypes, such as well differentiated, myxoid/round cell, pleomorphic, and dedifferentiated liposarcomas. Liposarcomas are usually diagnosed based on the clinical presentation, imaging studies, and histologic analysis [53]. In cases where these modalities do not allow a clear diagnosis, molecular diagnostics can be employed as many liposarcoma subtypes show unique molecular alterations. For example, the myxoid/round cell liposarcomas usually carry a t(12;16)(q13;p11) that can be analyzed by reverse transcriptase-PCR as is done for the EWS/WT1 fusion product [50, 52–54]. Other liposarcoma subtypes carry identifiable molecular alterations, such as 12q13-q21 amplification seen in well- and dedifferentiated liposarcomas [55].

11.4.4 Malignant Mesothelioma

Malignant mesothelioma is a rare tumor that arises in mesothelial-lined body cavities, most commonly in the pleura and peritoneum and far less commonly in the tunica vaginalis and pericardium. Malignant mesothelioma can exhibit a wide spectrum of histologic subtypes making diagnosis based on histology alone difficult. Although specific molecular alterations have been identified in malignant mesothelioma such as a unique microRNA expression pattern, immunohistochemical analysis is typically used in cases were a diagnosis is not possible based on histology alone [56, 57].

11.4.5 Rhabdomyosarcoma (RMS)

Rhabdomyosarcoma (RMS) can occur anywhere in the body, with ~7 % occurring in the paratesticular tissue. In this location, embryonal RMS is most common with other types, such as the alveolar and pleomorphic RMS types being less common [58–60]. Most RMSs occur in the pediatric group and in young adults, with a bimodal age distribution showing peaks at 5 and 16 years of age [60]. The diagnosis of RMS depends on the clinical presentation, histology, and immunohistochemistry [58–60]. Seventy to eighty percentage alveolar RMS carry t(2;13)(q35;q14) (~70 %) or t(1;13)(p36;q14) (~10 %) translocation fusing portions of the PAX3-FKHR or PAX7-FKHR genes, respectively. Analysis of these translocations usually involves reverse transcriptase-PCR employing primers spanning the gene fusion region [50, 52, 61, 62].

11.4.6 Leiomyosarcoma

Leiomyosarcomas rarely occur in the scrotal/paratesticular area [63]. Although these tumors often carry identifiable molecular changes, they are typically complex and do not lend themselves to clinical molecular analysis [64]. The diagnosis of these tumors typically depends on histologic analysis, supplemented with immunohistochemistry [63].

11.5 Testicular Germ Cell Tumors

Although uncommon, testicular neoplasms are the most common cancers among men aged 15–44 years, with 98 % being germ cell tumors. The highest incidence of testicular tumors (1.5/100,000) is found in individuals with Northern European ancestry, with the incidence in Denmark and Norway up to 10 times higher than in

African and Asian men [65–67]. In 2006, the American Cancer Society estimated that 8,250 US men developed testicular, with 370 men dying of these tumors. Although these tumors represent ~0.5 % of all Caucasian male cancer, they account for only ~0.1 % of cancer-related deaths, due to many of these tumors being curable. Interestingly, their incidence has increased substantially over the past four decades [66–68].

Roughly 90 % of testicular neoplasm arise from germ cells, with seminomas being most common, accounting for ~50 % of all testicular germ cell tumors and often making a large percentage of mixed germ cell tumors. With the exception of the spermatocytic seminoma, germ cell tumors typically arise from intratubular germ cell neoplasia, unclassified (ITGCNU) [69, 70]. The non-seminomatous germ cell tumors include embryonal carcinoma, yolk sac carcinoma, choriocarcinoma, teratomas, mixed germ cell tumors, spermatocytic seminomas, polyembryomas, and diffuse embryomas [71]. The genetics, histology, and usual clinical course of these cancers are diverse, with tumors, such as seminomas, having a relatively good prognosis (even when widely metastatic), while other tumors, such as choriocarcinoma, having a much poorer prognosis [72]. Several risk factors have been identified for testicular germ cell cancers. These are summarized below.

11.5.1 Genetic Inheritance

Having an effected father or brother with testicular cancer confers a relative risk for testicular cancer of 6–10, consistent with a heritable genetic predisposition [73]. The risk factor is higher in twins than in non-twins, as well as higher in dizygotic than in monozygotic twins, possibly due to higher maternal estrogen levels secondary to two placentas [74]. Several genetic loci conferring a testicular cancer predisposition have been identified. These include the phosphodiesterase 11A gene variants known to reduce the gene product's enzymatic activity and gr/gr deletions on the Y chromosome [75, 76]. Several genome-wide association studies have demonstrated that alterations at 12q22 (KITLG), 5q31.1 (SPRY4), 6p21.31 (BAK1), 5p15 (TERT), and 12p13 (ATF7IP) confer an increased risk for testicular cancer. Interestingly, spermatocytic seminoma, which does not arise from ITGCN, shows a different set of mutations involving DMRT1 and RET [77].

11.5.2 Cryptorchidism

Cryptorchidism (undescended testes) is closely associated with ITGCNU. The incidence of in situ testicular carcinoma is 2–3 % in cryptorchordic testes compared to 0.43 % in bilaterally descended testes – a 32-fold increased risk with cryptorchidism [78–80]. The highest risk is seen with intra-abdominal cryptorchidism, which develops cancer five-times more often than inguinal cryptorchidism

[78]. Additionally, bilateral undescended testicles develop in situ carcinoma at a higher rate than unilateral undescended testicles, and, interestingly, the descended testes in men with unilateral cryptorchidism show an elevated carcinoma incidence of 20–30 % compared to bilaterally descended testes [78, 81]. Delayed orchiopexy increases the risk for cancer, supporting a casual role for cryptorchidism leading to cancer [82, 83]. However, Kallmann syndrome, characterized by congenital hypogonadotropic hypogonadism and cryptorchidism, does not shown an elevated testicular cancer incidence [84]. Additionally, although different ethnic groups have roughly the same incidence of cryptorchidism, testicular cancer between different ethnic groups shows enormous differences [85]. Last, both conditions are associated with premature birth, low birth weight, and other gonadal abnormalities [86]. Presently, it is not clear whether cryptorchidism confers an increased cancer risk or whether cryptorchidism and cancer share common risk factors. They are however closely interrelated.

11.5.3 Sexual Development Disorders

Sexual development disorders are congenital conditions in which sexual development is atypical at the anatomic, gonadal, or chromosomal/genetic levels(s). Many show an elevated incidence of testicular cancer. The highest increased incidence is seen in testes-specific protein Y-encoded positive gonadal dysgenesis, which shows a 15–35 % increase in germ cell tumors. Individuals with this condition overexpress testes-specific protein Y-encoded, the main candidate for the so-called gonadoblastoma locus on Y chromosome. Testes-specific protein Y-encoded is highly expressed in ITGCNU and seminomas (coexpressing with placental-like alkaline phosphatase [PLAP], c-KIT, OCT4, Ki-67, and cyclin B), indicating a possible role in carcinogenesis, Additionally, its ectopic expression in cultured cells up-regulates pro-growth genes frequently overexpressed in ITGCNU [87, 88]. Other sexual development disorders, including partial androgen insensitivity syndrome, complete androgen insensitivity, and ovotesticular sexual development, show increased testicular cancer incidences of 15 %, 0.8 %, and 2.6 %, respectively [87, 88].

11.5.4 Other Factors

Many other factors may be involved in the pathogenesis of testicular cancer. These include low birth weight, exogenous hormone and disrupting endocrine chemical exposures, maternal age, impaired male fertility, height, body mass index, occupational exposure, childhood physical activity, and testicular trauma. For many of these factors, the evidence is either weak, or presently equivocal, and further studies are needed define the specific roles of these factors in testicular carcinogenesis [89].

11.5.5 *Molecular Testing for Testicular Germ Cell Neoplasms*

The diagnosis of most testicular tumors is accomplished by the histologic analysis of hematoxylin-eosin-stained slides, often supplemented with immunohistochemistry. In fact, only three laboratories in the US currently offer molecular diagnostic testing for testicular tumors [90]. Here, we will review some of the molecular techniques applied to each germ cell neoplasm type.

11.5.5.1 Intratubular Germ Cell Neoplasia Unclassified

ITGCNU is the precursor lesion for most germ cell neoplasms, with the exception of the spermatocytic seminoma, and is found at increased rates in conditions with an increased germ cell tumor incidence ([69–71], see above). Histologically, ITGCU is characterized by seminiferous tubules containing large atypical primitive appearing cells, with clear cytoplasm, enlarged vesicular nuclei, and prominent nucleoli. There is no spermatogenesis present, and the tubular lamina propria is often thickened and hyalinized. The cells typically stain for PLAP, CD117, OCT4, and p53. ITGCNU usually does not spontaneously regress and most cases will eventually progress to an invasive germ cell tumor. The treatment is typically radiotherapy or orchiectomy, with the former preserving testicular endocrine functions (but not fertility), and the latter providing the greatest success rates [71].

Very few molecular studies of ITGCNU have been performed, although comparative genomic hybridization (CGH) studies have demonstrated that ITGCNU carries many of the chromosomal alterations seen in seminomas and other germ cell tumors, including gains of material from chromosomes 1, 5, 7, 8, 12q, and X, with loss of material from chromosome 18. Interestingly, the commonly seen gains of 12p in seminomas and other germ cell tumors are not present, indicating that gains at 12p may be required for the progression of ITGCNU to invasive neoplasm [91, 92]. Presently, besides histologic analyses, immunohistochemistry is used to diagnose ITGCNU, where immunostains for p53, PLAP, OCT4, and CD117 are helpful is establishing a diagnosis, as is periodic acid-Schiff staining [71, 93].

11.5.5.2 Seminomas

Seminomas are the most common post-pubertal testicular germ cell neoplasms, with the World Health Organization recognizing a seminoma with syncytiotrophoblastic giant cells variant. Seminomas have several histologic variants characterized by different growth patterns including cribiform/microcystic, tubular, intertubular, and the anaplastic or atypical seminoma characterized by an increased mitotic rate, greater nuclear pleomorphism, and a lower number of associated infiltrating lymphocytes. Immunohistochemically, seminomas are PLAP, OCT4, and CD117 positive, focally/weakly positive for cytokeratin 40 % of the time, and negative for CD30, α-fetoprotein (AFP), and human chorionic gonadotropin (hCG) [71].

Histologically seminomas generally show a pattern of sheets of tumor cells with clear cytoplasm separated by fibrous trabeculae rich in T-lymphocytes. The tumor cells are large, uniform, round to polyhedral cells having distinct plasma membranes, clear cytoplasm, and large nuclei with "salt and pepper" chromatin and one to several prominent nucleoli. Mitotic activity is usually low, and about 10 % of seminomas will have a significant non-seminomatous component [61].

Although multiple genetic alterations have been identified in testicular seminomas, 12p overexpression often secondary to isochromosome formation is the only consistent change found in seminomas and other testicular germ cell neoplasms [94–96]. Analysis of ITGCNU following laser capture microdissection with degenerate oligonucleotide primed PCR reveal gains in 12p in ITGCNU adjacent to histologically identifiable invasive germ cell tumors, while ITGCNU without a nearby invasive component either had no 12p gains or only "diminutive" 12p gains. Thus, 12p gains appear to be required for the development of germ cell neoplasia invasion [97]. Comparative expressed sequence hybridization studies have revealed overexpressed genomic sequences at 12p11.2-p12.1, 4q12, and 12p13, with the KRAS2, CMAS, EKI1, LRMP, C12orf2, ITPR2, FLJ10637, TM7SF3, SURB7, CCND2, MLF2, PTMS, GLU3, HPH1, c-KIT, and LRP6 genes commonly overexpressed [98–100].

11.5.5.3 Germ Cell Tumor Molecular Testing

CGH array and fluorescent in situ hybridization (FISH) are presently the main molecular tests used to detect seminomas and other testicular germ cell tumors, with other testing modalities presently limited to research applications. Both of these techniques work well in the identification of 12p amplification and have utility in the analysis of testicular germ cell tumors where histology and immunohistochemistry give ambiguous results.

11.5.5.3.1 CGH

In CGH reference (normal) and test (tumor) tissues are compared to identify deleted or amplified genomic tumor regions in the test sample. The reference and test genomic DNAs are isolated and labeled with different fluorochromes. Care is taken such that the two fluorochromes do not have any spectral overlap. Additionally, the reference sample is always from healthy tissue, often from sources such as peripheral lymphocytes. The two labeled samples are then hybridized together on an array that covers the genomic area being interrogated. Typically, the sequences being interrogated are attached to a solid support, such as glass or nitrocellulose that does not interfere with hybridization. The hybridization is performed under maximally stringent temperature and buffer conditions to lessen non-Watson-Crick (non-specific) hybridizations as much as possible. Following hybridization and multiple washing steps, the signal intensity on the solid support is calculated using the background signal intensity against the intensity of each fluorochrome emission. The ratios of each fluorochrome on each specific hybridization spot is calculated and averaged over several replicate spots. The test to reference sample intensities are often standardized by dividing the median of all the hybridization spots in the sample. Often chromosomal areas, such as the X chromosome, known to not undergo amplification or loss, are used as an internal control [98–100]. CGH has high specificity and under the right conditions is an excellent testing modality. However, it can be more complex, costly, and time-consuming than other molecular tests.

11.5.5.3.2 FISH

FISH is also employed to identify 12p amplification in testicular germ cell neoplasms. Most often, FISH probes specifically designed to hybridize with the regions of 12p, commonly amplified, are used in conjunction with FISH probes to unamplified chromosomal regions. Each FISH probe carries a different fluorochrome. 12p amplification is identified by an increased ratio of 12p FISH probe hybridization to control probe hybridization. FISH assays are relatively easy to perform and over one million assays are done worldwide each year.

11.5.5.4 Testicular Choriocarcinomas

Choriocarcinoma is a rare tumor, representing only about 1 % of testicular tumors in its pure form and more commonly occurs as a component of a mixed tumor. Choriocarcinoma is typically clinically aggressive, often presenting with metastases to the lungs, liver, and brain. Histologically, choriocarcinomas are characterized by an attempt to replicate the architecture of immature placental villi, with a cap of syncytiotrophoblasts (large multinuclear cell with eosinophilic and vacuolated cytoplasm) surrounding cytotrophoblasts consisting of round cells with distinct cell borders, clear cytoplasm, and unremarkable, bland nuclei. Usually, the syncytiotrophoblasts are positive for hCG, HPL, and EMA [71]. Due to the rarity of these tumors, very little molecular testing is performed on them and their analysis rests upon histology, supplemented with immunohistochemistry.

11.5.5.5 Testicular Embryonal Carcinomas

Embryonal carcinoma is rare, accounting for about 2 % of testicular tumors in its pure form and is a component in about 85 % of non-seminomatous testicular germ cell tumors. About two thirds of embryonal carcinomas present with metastases, typically to the lungs. Histologically, embryonal carcinomas typically consist of sheets of epithelioid pleomorphic cells with indistinct cell borders, eosinophilic to amphophilic cytoplasm, with large pleomorphic nuclei having prominent nucleoli and overlapping nuclei. Often many apoptotic bodies and mitotic figures are present. Embryonal carcinomas are positive for CD30, PLAP, and OCT4 [71]. Like other testicular germ cell tumors, embryonal carcinomas often show 12p amplification [71]. Molecular testing is seldom performed on these tumors and when done is limited to 12p analysis.

11.5.5.6 Testicular Yolk Sac Tumors

Yolk sac tumors (YST), also known as endodermal sinus tumors, recapitulate primary embryonic yolk sac tissue and are usually a component of non-seminomatous testicular germ cell tumors in adults. In the pediatric age group, YST is the most common testicular tumor, with incidence peaking before 2 years old. About 95 % of individuals with a YST component in the tumor show elevated serum AFP. Histologically, YST shows many different architectural patterns, most commonly a "microcystic pattern" consisting of interconnecting cords and ribbons of tumor cells within a myxoid stroma. About 50 % of YCT have Schiller-Duvall bodies, a glomerulus-like structure pathognomonic for YSTs. The tumors cells usually show bland nuclei and eosinophilic hyaline globules that are α-1-antitrypsin and diastase-PAS staining positive, not usually seen in other testicular germ cell tumors. YSTs are usually positive for cytokeratin and AFP, showing diffuse cytoplasmic staining, while CD30 staining is variable. Like other testicular germ cell tumors, YSTs show 12p amplification, which is sometimes analyzed by molecular diagnostics testing [71, 98–101]. Interestingly, pediatric YSTs do not show 12p amplification, but show structural alterations of chromosomes 1, 3, and 6, and RUNX3 gene promoter hypermethylation [102, 103]. These molecular alterations are not commonly analyzed in the diagnosis of pediatric YSTs.

11.5.5.7 Spermatocytic Seminoma

Spermatocytic seminomas are testicular germ cell tumors that do not arise from ITGCN and are unrelated to seminomas. Spermatocytic seminomas are uncommon, representing 1–4 % of testicular tumors, occurring at an average age of 55 years. The histologic analysis of the spermatocytic seminoma lies in identifying three separate cell types: small, intermediate, and multinucleated giant cells. The small cells are 6–8 μm in diameter and have a narrow rim of eosinophilic cytoplasm. Intermediate cells are 15–18 μm in diameter, have round nuclei with filamentous chromatin and prominent nucleoli, and have a more voluminous eosinophilic cytoplasm. The giant cells are more pleomorphic, 50–100 μm in diameter, and can have multiple nuclei. Spermatocytic seminomas usually have a high mitotic index, and lack fibrous septae and lymphocytes. They are positive for CAM5.2 and are usually negative for keratin, EMA, PLAP, OCT4, HCG, CD30, and AFP [71]. Molecular-genetic analyses of spermatocytic seminomas have shown consistent gains on chromosome 9p, with DMRT1 (at 9p24.3) overexpression likely playing a role in spermatocytic seminoma development [71, 77, 98–100, 104]. Presently, molecular diagnostic testing is not performed on this rare tumor.

11.5.5.8 Other Malignant Testicular Germ Cell Tumors

Testicular teratomas, teratocarcinoma, and polyembryomas often show 12p amplification [71]. Due to the rarity of these tumors and their distinctive histology, molecular testing is seldom performed on them.

11.6 Testicular Sex Cord Tumors

Sex cord tumors make up ~5 % of all testicular tumors and are derived from cord-like masses which invaginate from the germinal epithelium during embryogenesis and give rise to the rete testes and seminiferous tubules [105]. In the testes, the sex cord tumors are the Sertoli, Leydig, Sertoli-Leydig, and granulosa cell tumors, which are named by the cell types from which they arise. For many of these tumors, specific subtypes exist that will be discussed in each section on a specific tumor [105–107]. Many of these tumors are very rare. For example, although the ovarian granulosa cell tumor is fairly common, its testicular counterpart is very rare, with only about 28 recorded cases [108]. Thus for most of these tumors, molecular diagnostics is not performed and the molecular alterations underlying these tumors are poorly understood.

11.6.1 Sertoli Cell Tumors

Sertoli cell tumors, also called androblastomas, include the Sertoli cell tumor not otherwise specified (NOS), Sclerosing Sertoli cell tumors, Sertoli-Leydig cell tumors, and large cell calcifying Sertoli cell tumors (LCCSCTs). The latter tumor can be associated with Peutz-Jeger and Carney syndromes. The Lipid-Rich Sertoli cell tumor is found almost exclusively in the ovary [107].

11.6.1.1 Sertoli Cell Tumor NOS

Sertoli cell tumors NOS of the testes make up approximately 1 % of all testicular tumors, appearing at a mean age of 45 years over a wide age range (15–80 years) [109, 110]. About 20 % are malignant and most typically present as a unilateral slowly enlarging well-circumscribed mass. Histologically, the tumor cells typically have moderate amount of pale to slightly eosinophilic cytoplasm, often with large cytoplasmic vacuoles. They exhibit minimal nuclear atypia, a low mitotic rate, and a general resemblance to Sertoli cells. The tumor cells form diffuse sheets or large nodular aggregates and may display a solid, trabecular, or tubular architecture that resemble immature seminiferous tubules [110].

Due to the relative rarity of Sertoli cell tumor NOS of the testes, little is known about the molecular alterations underlying these tumors. CGH studies have shown multiple molecular changes in Sertoli cell tumor NOS that typically varied from cases to case, indicating a high degree of tumor heterogeneity. Gains in the X chromosome were common. Less frequently, losses of all or portions of chromosome 2 and 19 are seen [111]. Additionally, animal studies have shown that increased β-catenin may play a role in the development of these tumors [112]. Presently, there is insufficient knowledge about the molecular alterations underlying the Sertoli cell tumors, and, due to the rarity of these tumors, clinical molecular testing is rarely performed on them.

11.6.1.2 Sclerosing Sertoli Cell Tumors

Sclerosing Sertoli cell tumors are very rare, with one overview recording only 14 cases reported in the literature [113]. Histologically these tumors resemble those of Sertoli cell tumors NOS, but exhibit extensive hypocellular, collagenous stroma separating clusters of Sertoli cells. The average age of presentation is about 35 years, are usually unilateral, and are rarely malignant [113, 114]. Due to the extreme rarity of these tumors, molecular analyses have not been performed on them.

11.6.1.3 Large Cell Calcifying Sertoli Cell Tumors (LCCSCT)

Large cell calcifying Sertoli cell tumors LCCSCTs are rare tumors with only about 60 cases recorded in the literature. Approximately 25 % of these tumors are malignant and may be associated with the Peutz-Jeghers syndrome (see Chap. 5, Colorectal Carcinoma) or the Carney complex. Histologically, LCCSCTs show large tumor cells with abundant eosinophilic cytoplasm, extensive amorphous calcifications, and tubule formation with focal areas of trabecular or solid differentiation [115]. Malignant tumors typically have two or more of the following features: (1) a size >4 cm, (2) greater than three mitoses/10 high power fields, (3) significant nuclear atypia, (4) necrosis, or (5) lymphovascular invasion [116].

About one third of males with the Carney complex will have LCCSCTs. The Carney complex was first described in 1985 by Carney et al. [117] and is characterized by abnormal skin pigmentation, usually pale brown to black lentigines that are often the presenting feature, myxomas of the heart, skin, breast, oropharynx, and female genital tract, primary pigmented nodular adrenocortical disease often causing Cushing syndrome, multiple thyroid adenomas, and psammomatous schwannomas in approximately 10 % of individuals. The Carney complex is usually diagnosed based on the clinical presentation; however, molecular testing is clinically performed. Approximately 62 % of individuals with Carneys complex have identifiable mutations at 17q23-24, where the tumor suppressor gene, the regulatory subunit type 1A (RIα) of cAMP-dependent protein kinase (PRKAR1A) gene is located [118]. Additionally, about 20 % of individuals with Carney complex have genetic alterations linked to 2p16, where loss of heterozygosity and copy number gains have been detected [119].

Molecular clinical testing for the Carney Complex usually involves PCR amplification of the 12 exons and proximal intronic regions of the PRKAR1A gene, followed by sequencing of the resulting amplicons. Bertherat et al. [118] analyzed 353 patients who met the diagnostic criteria for Carney complex, had primary pigmented nodular adrenocortical disease, or had previously identified PRKAR1A gene mutations; 62 % of the tested individuals carried detectable PRKAR1A gene mutations, of which 82 % resulted in no detectable protein expression due to nonsense mRNA mediated decay. Interestingly, a frequency of 491-492delTG was found to be associated with lentigines, cardiac myxomas, and thyroid tumors.

11.6.1.4 Sertoli-Leydeg Cell Tumor

The Sertoli-Leydeg cell tumor is exceptionally rare, with less than 10 cases described in the testes [120]. Little is known about the molecular alterations underlying these tumors.

11.6.2 Leydig Cell Tumors (LCT)

Leydig cell tumors (LCTs) represent approximately 0.8–3 % of all testicular tumors and are the most common interstitial neoplasms of the testes [105, 106]. LCTs may occur at any age, but are most commonly shown in those between the ages of 5 and 10 years and between 30 and 60 years. Roughly 10 % of LCTs are malignant, while almost all-pediatric LCTs are benign. Grossly, LCTs are sharply delineated solid masses within the testicular stroma. Microscopically the tumor cells form nest or sheets of large polygonal cells with abundant granular eosinophilic cytoplasm, with scattered lipofuscin pigment and Reinke crystals seen in less than 50 % of these tumors. LCT can be hormonally active, producing either androgens or less commonly estrogens, which lead to masculinizing or feminizing effects [105, 106, 121].

Leydig cell tumorigenesis appears to depend on alterations in the hypothalamic-pituitary-testicular axis leading to excessive Leydig cell stimulation by luteinizing hormone [122]. One study on three pediatric testicular LCTs showed three different mutations in the luteinizing hormone receptor, two of which increased receptor expression and one that increased basal cAMP production 28 ± 3-fold. All three mutations caused increased cell growth when transiently transfected into COS-7 cells. Additionally, a low percentage of adult LCTs show fumarate hydratase mutations [123]. Because little is known about the molecular alterations in LCTs and many of these alterations occur in a low percentage of these tumors [123], the diagnosis of LCTs is presently based on the clinical presentation and histology, supplemented with immunohistochemistry.

11.6.3 Granulosa Cell Tumors

Granulosa cell tumors of the testes are rare, with only 28 cases reported in the literature [108]. The tumor usually presents as a slowly growing testicular mass that histologically resembles its more common ovarian counterpart; usually being well-circumscribed with uniform to mildly pleomorphic cells with medium-sized ovoid or elongated nuclei with fine chromatin, inconspicuous nuclei, and scattered nuclear grooves. In the review by Hanson et al. [108], 21 % of testicular granulosa cell tumors metastasized. Due to the extreme rarity of these tumors, clinical molecular diagnostics is not performed on them. However, one study demonstrated that these tumors often have dysregulated WNT/CTNNB1 and PI3K/AKT signaling pathways [124].

11.7 Conclusion

Clinical molecular diagnostics are not commonly performed on penile, scrotal and testicular malignancies. This is partly due to the rarity of some of these tumors but also because diagnosis can usually be successfully rendered by the combination of clinical presentation, histology, and immunohistochemistry. This is especially true for germ cell tumors of the testes. As new molecular therapies are developed, the identification of specific molecular alterations will become necessary prior to the initiation of therapy.

References

1. Landis SH, Murray T, Bolden S, Wingo PA (1999) Cancer statistics, 1999. CA Cancer J Clin 49:8–31
2. Mosconi AM, Roila F, Gatta G, Theodorec C (2005) Cancer of the penis. Crit Rev Oncol Hematol 53:165–177
3. Persky L (1977) Epidemiology of cancer of the penis. Recent Results Cancer Res 60:97–109
4. Misra S, Chaturvedi A, Misra NC (2004) Penile carcinoma: a challenge for the developing world. Lancet Oncol 5:240–247
5. Favorito LA, Nardi AC, Ronalsa M, Zequi SC, Sampaio FJ, Glina S (2008) Epidemiologic study on penile cancer in Brazil. Int Braz J Urol 34:587–591, discussion 591–593
6. Harish K, Ravi R (1995) The role of tobacco in penile carcinoma. Br J Urol 75:375–377
7. Parkin DM, Bray F (2006) Chapter 2: The burden of HPV-related cancers. Vaccine 24(Suppl 3): S11–S25
8. Pow-Sang MR, Ferreira U, Pow-Sang JM, Nardi AC, Destefano V (2010) Epidemiology and natural history of penile cancer. Urology 76(2 Suppl 1):S2–S6
9. Daling JR, Madeleine MM, Johnson LG, Schwartz SM, Shera KA, Wurscher MA, Carter JJ, Porter PL, Galloway DA, McDougall JK, Krieger JN (2005) Penile cancer: importance of circumcision, human papillomavirus and smoking in in situ and invasive disease. Int J Cancer 116:606–616

10. Schoen EJ, Oehrli M, Colby C, Machin G (2000) The highly protective effect of newborn circumcision against invasive penile cancer. Pediatrics 105:E36
11. Hernandez BY, Barnholtz-Sloan J, German RR, Giuliano A, Goodman MT, King JB, Negoita S, Villalon-Gomez JM (2008) Burden of invasive squamous cell carcinoma of the penis in the United States, 1998–2003. Cancer 113(10 Suppl):2883–2891
12. Antunes AA, Nesrallah LJ, Goncalves PD, Ferreira YA, Campagnari JC, Srougi M (2005) Deep-seated sarcomas of the penis. Int Braz J Urol 31:245–250
13. Polsky EG, Lele SM, Holley P, Geissler R, Rowland RG (2003) Primary malignant mesothelioma of the penis: case report and review of the literature. Urology 62:551
14. Hernandez BY, Shvetsov YB, Goodman MT, Wilkens LR, Thompson P, Zhu X, Ning L (2010) Reduced clearance of penile human papillomavirus infection in uncircumcised men. J Infect Dis 201:1340–1343
15. Castellsague X, Bosch FX, Munoz N, Meijer CJ, Shah KV, de Sanjose S, Eluf-Neto J, Ngelangel CA, Chichareon S, Smith JS, Herrero R, Moreno V, Franceschi S, International Agency for Research on Cancer Multicenter Cervical Cancer Study Group (2002) Male circumcision, penile human papillomavirus infection, and cervical cancer in female partners. N Engl J Med 346:1105–1112
16. Walboomers JM, Jacobs MV, Manos MM, Bosch FX, Kummer JA, Shah KV, Snijders PJ, Peto J, Meijer CJ, Muñoz N (1999) Human papillomavirus is a necessary cause of invasive cervical cancer worldwide. J Pathol 189:12–19
17. Trottier H, Franco EL (2006) The epidemiology of genital human papillomavirus infection. Vaccine 24(Suppl 1):S1–S15
18. Buitrago-Pérez A, Garaulet G, Vázquez-Carballo A, Paramio JM, García-Escudero R (2009) Molecular signature of HPV-induced carcinogenesis: pRb, p53 and gene expression profiling. Curr Genomics 10:26–34
19. Lizano M, Berumen J, García-Carrancá A (2009) HPV-related carcinogenesis: basic concepts, viral types and variants. Arch Med Res 40:428–434
20. Parkin DM, Bray F, Ferlay J, Pisani P (2005) Global cancer statistics, 2002. CA Cancer J Clin 55:74–108
21. Roden RB, Ling M, Wu TC (2004) Vaccination to prevent and treat cervical cancer. Hum Pathol 35:971–982
22. Reisinger KS, Block SL, Lazcano-Ponce E, Samakoses R, Esser MT, Erick J, Puchalski D, Giacoletti KE, Sings HL, Lukac S, Alvarez FB, Barr E (2007) Safety and persistent immunogenicity of a quadrivalent human papillomavirus types 6, 11, 16, 18 L1 virus-like particle vaccine in preadolescents and adolescents: a randomized controlled trial. Pediatr Infect Dis J 26:201–209
23. Flores R, Abalos AT, Nielson CM, Abrahamsen M, Harris RB, Giuliano AR (2008) Reliability of sample collection and laboratory testing for HPV detection in men. J Virol Methods 149:136–143
24. Rombaldi RL, Serafini EP, Villa LL, Vanni AC, Baréa F, Frassini R, Xavier M, Paesi S (2006) Infection with human papillomaviruses of sexual partners of women having cervical intraepithelial neoplasia. Braz J Med Biol Res 39:177–187
25. Taichman LB, Reilly SS, LaPorta RF (1983) The role of keratinocyte differentiation in the expression of epitheliotropic viruses. J Invest Dermatol 81(1 Suppl):137s–140s
26. Koss LG, Durfee GR (1956) Unusual patterns of squamous epithelium of the uterine cervix: cytologic and histologic study of koilocytotic atypia. Ann N Y Acad Sci 63:1245–1261
27. Pirog EC, Baergen RN, Soslow RA, Tam D, DeMattia AE, Chen YT, Isacson C (2002) Diagnostic accuracy of cervical low-grade squamous intraepithelial lesions is improved with MIB-1 immunostaining. Am J Surg Pathol 26:70–75
28. Logani S, Lu D, Quint WG, Ellenson LH, Pirog EC (2003) Low-grade vulvar and vaginal intraepithelial neoplasia: correlation of histologic features with human papillomavirus DNA detection and MIB-1 immunostaining. Mod Pathol 16:735–741
29. Guerrero D, Guarch R, Ojer A, Casas JM, Ropero S, Mancha A, Pesce C, Lloveras B, Garcia-Bragado F, Puras A (2008) Hypermethylation of the thrombospondin-1 gene is associated with poor prognosis in penile squamous cell carcinoma. BJU Int 102:747–755

30. Senba M, Buziba N, Mori N, Wada A, Irie S, Toriyama K (2009) Detection of human papillomavirus and cellular regulators p16INK4a, p53, and NF-kappaB in penile cancer cases in Kenya. Acta Virol 53:43–48
31. Berdjis N, Meye A, Nippgen J, Dittert D, Hakenberg O, Baretton GB, Wirth MP (2005) Expression of Ki-67 in squamous cell carcinoma of the penis. BJU Int 96:146–148
32. Wheeler CM, Parmenter CA, Hunt WC, Becker TM, Greer CE, Hildesheim A, Manos MM (1993) Determinants of genital human papillomavirus infection among cytologically normal women attending the University of New Mexico student health center. Sex Transm Dis 20:286–289
33. Denny L, Kuhn L, Pollack A, Wainwright H, Wright TC Jr (2000) Evaluation of alternative methods of cervical cancer screening for resource-poor settings. Cancer 89:826–833
34. Bauer HM, Hildesheim A, Schiffman MH, Glass AG, Rush BB, Scott DR, Cadell DM, Kurman RJ, Manos MM (1993) Determinants of genital human papillomavirus infection in low-risk women in Portland, Oregon. Sex Transm Dis 20:274–278
35. Bosch FX, de Sanjose SS (2007) The epidemiology of human papillomavirus infection and cervical cancer. Dis Markers 23:213–227
36. Verhoeven RH, Louwman WJ, Koldewijn EL, Demeyere TB, Coebergh JW (2010) Scrotal cancer: incidence, survival and second primary tumours in the Netherlands since 1989. Br J Cancer 103:1462–1466
37. Brown JR, Thornton JL (1957) Percivall Pott (1714–1788) and chimney sweepers' cancer of the scrotum. Br J Ind Med 14:68–70
38. Burmer GC, True LD, Krieger JN (1993) Squamous cell carcinoma of the scrotum associated with human papillomaviruses. J Urol 149:374–377
39. Dianzani C, Calvieri S, Pierangeli A, Degener AM (2004) Identification of human papilloma viruses in male dysplastic genital lesions. New Microbiol 27:65–69
40. Chihara Y, Fujimoto K, Takada S, Hirayama A, Cho M, Yoshida K, Ozono S, Hirao Y (2003) Aggressive angiomyxoma in the scrotum expressing androgen and progesterone receptors. Int J Urol 10:672–675
41. Morag R, Fridman E, Mor Y (2009) Aggressive angiomyxoma of the scrotum mimicking huge hydrocele: case report and literature review. Case Rep Med 2009:157624
42. Durdov MG, Tomić S, Pisac VP, Spoljar MS (1998) Aggressive angiomyxoma of scrotum. Scand J Urol Nephrol 32:299–302
43. Sakata K, Ishikawa S, Tokue A, Hirota N (1997) Aggressive angiomyxoma of the scrotum. Urol Int 58:247–249
44. Murakami S, Ishiga N, Sho T, Sakai K, Fujii Y, Yamamoto Y (1996) Aggressive angiomyxoma occurring in the scrotum: report of a case. Surg Today 26:289–291
45. Iezzoni JC, Fechner RE, Wong LS, Rosai J (1995) Aggressive angiomyxoma in males. A report of four cases. Am J Clin Pathol 104:391–396
46. Wu CC, Yang SS, Chin DT, Hsieh CH, Hsueh YM, Tsai YC (2007) Scrotal aggressive angiomyxoma mimicking inguinal hernia. Asian J Androl 9:723–725
47. Kazmierczak B, Wanschura S, Meyer-Bolte K, Caselitz J, Meister P, Bartnitzke S, Van de Ven W, Bullerdiek J (1995) Cytogenic and molecular analysis of an aggressive angiomyxoma. Am J Pathol 147:580–585
48. Ordóñez NG (1998) Desmoplastic small round cell tumor: I: A histopathologic study of 39 cases with emphasis on unusual histological patterns. Am J Surg Pathol 22:1303–1313
49. Benjamine LE, Frederick WJ, Barr FC, Rauscher FJ III (1996) Fusion of the EWS1 and WT1 genes as a result of the t(11;22)(p13;q12) translocation in desmoplastic small round cell tumors. Med Pediatr Oncol 27:434–439
50. Ladanyi M, Gerald W (1994) Fusion of the EWS and WT1 genes in the desmoplastic small round cell tumor. Cancer Res 54:2837–2840
51. Gerald WL, Ladanyi M, de Alava E, Cuatrecasas M, Kushner BH, LaQuaglia MP, Rosai J (1998) Clinical, pathologic, and molecular spectrum of tumors associated with t(11;22)(p13;q12): desmoplastic small round-cell tumor and its variants. J Clin Oncol 16:3028–3036

52. Athale UH, Shurtleff SA, Jenkins JJ, Poquette CA, Tan M, Downing JR, Pappo AS (2001) Use of reverse transcriptase polymerase chain reaction for diagnosis and staging of alveolar rhabdomyosarcoma, Ewing sarcoma family of tumors, and desmoplastic small round cell tumor. J Pediatr Hematol Oncol 23:99–104
53. Montgomery E, Fisher C (2003) Paratesticular liposarcoma: a clinicopathologic study. Am J Surg Pathol 27:40–47
54. Panagopoulos I, Mandahl N, Ron D, Höglund M, Nilbert M, Mertens F, Mitelman F, Aman P (1994) Characterization of the CHOP breakpoints and fusion transcripts in myxoid liposarcomas with the 12;16 translocation. Cancer Res 54:6500–6503
55. Jain S, Xu R, Prieto VG, Lee P (2010) Molecular classification of soft tissue sarcomas and its clinical applications. Int J Clin Exp Pathol 3:416–428
56. Plas E, Riedl CR, Pfluger H (1998) Malignant mesothelioma of the tunica vaginalis: review of the literature and assessment of prognostic parameters. Cancer 83:2437–2446
57. Benjamin H, Lebanony D, Rosenwald S, Cohen L, Gibori H, Barabash N, Ashkenazi K, Goren E, Meiri E, Morgenstern S, Perelman M, Barshack I, Goren Y, Edmonston TB, Chajut A, Aharonov R, Bentwich Z, Rosenfeld N, Cohen D (2010) A diagnostic assay based on microRNA expression accurately identifies malignant pleural mesothelioma. J Mol Diagn 12:771–779
58. Weiss SW, Goldblum JR (2001) Rhabdomyosarcoma. Enzinger and Weiss's soft tissue tumors, 4th edn. Mosby, St. Louis, pp 785–835
59. Kishore B, Khare P, Gupta RJ, Gupta C, Khare V (2010) A rare case of paratesticular pleomorphic rhabdomyosarcoma diagnosed by fine needle aspiration: a case report. Diagn Cytopathol 38:121–126
60. Mason BJ, Kier R (1998) Sonographic and MR imaging appearances of paratesticular rhabdomyosarcoma. AJR Am J Roentgenol 171:523–524
61. Merlino G, Helman LJ (1999) Rhabdomyosarcoma – working out the pathways. Oncogene 185:340–348
62. Barr FG, Smith LM, Lynch JC, Strzelecki D, Parham DM, Qualman SJ, Breitfeld PP (2006) Examination of gene fusion status in archival samples of alveolar rhabdomyosarcoma entered on the Intergroup Rhabdomyosarcoma Study-III trial: a report from the Children's Oncology Group. J Mol Diagn 8:202–208
63. Rajkomar K, Mundy I (2007) Leiomyosarcoma of the scrotum – a rare tumour. N Z Med J 120:U2835
64. Guillou L, Aurias A (2010) Soft tissue sarcomas with complex genomic profiles. Virchows Arch 456:201–217
65. Ferlay J, Bray F, Pisani P, Parkin DM (2004) GLOBOCAN 2002: cancer incidence, mortality and prevalence worldwide, IARC cancer base No. 5 version 2.0. IARC Press, Lyon
66. Shah MN, Devesa SS, Zhu K, McGlynn KA (2007) Trends in testicular germ cell tumours by ethnic group in the United States. Int J Androl 30:206–213
67. Oosterhuis JW, Looijenga LH (2005) Testicular germ-cell tumours in a broader perspective. Nat Rev Cancer 5:210–222
68. Jemal A, Siegel R, Ward E, Murray T, Xu J, Smigal C, Thun MJ (2006) Cancer statistics, 2006. CA Cancer J Clin 56:106–130
69. Krag Jacobsen G, Barlebo H, Olsen J, Schultz HP, Starklint H, Søgaard H, Vaeth M (1984) Testicular germ cell tumours in Denmark 1976–1980: pathology of 1058 consecutive cases. Acta Radiol Oncol 23:239–247
70. Fischer CG, Waechter W, Kraus S, Fuentecilla PE, Weidner W, Dudeck J (1998) Urologic tumors in the Federal Republic of Germany: data on 56,013 cases from hospital cancer registries. Cancer 82:775–783
71. Bahrami A, Ro JY, Ayala AG (2007) An overview of testicular germ cell tumors. Arch Pathol Lab Med 131:1267–1280
72. Shintaku I, Satoh M, Okajima E, Fujimoto H, Kamoto T, Ogawa O, Kawai K, Akaza H, Tsukamoto T, Naito S, Miki T, Arai Y (2008) Survival of metastatic germ cell cancer patients assessed by international germ cell consensus classification in Japan. Jpn J Clin Oncol 38:281–287

73. Hopper JL, Carlin JB (1992) Familial aggregation of a disease consequent upon correlation between relatives in a risk factor measured on a continuous scale. Am J Epidemiol 136:1138–1147
74. Sharpe RM (2003) The 'oestrogen hypothesis' – where do we stand now? Int J Androl 26:2–15
75. Horvath A, Korde L, Greene MH, Libe R, Osorio P, Faucz FR, Raffin-Sanson ML, Tsang KM, Drori-Herishanu L, Patronas Y, Remmers EF, Nikita ME, Moran J, Greene J, Nesterova M, Merino M, Bertherat J, Stratakis CA (2009) Functional phosphodiesterase 11A mutations may modify the risk of familial and bilateral testicular germ cell tumors. Cancer Res 69:5301–5306
76. Nathanson KL, Kanetsky PA, Hawes R et al (2005) The Y deletion gr/gr and susceptibility to testicular germ cell tumor. Am J Hum Genet 77:1034–1043
77. Gilbert D, Rapley E, Shipley J (2011) Testicular germ cell tumours: predisposition genes and the male germ cell niche. Nat Rev Cancer 11:278–288
78. Giwercman A, Bruun E, Frimodt-Møller C, Skakkebaek NE (1989) Prevalence of carcinoma in situ and other histopathological abnormalities in testes of men with a history of cryptorchidism. J Urol 142:998–1001
79. Zöller G, Ringert RH, Hermann R (2005) Hodenhochstand im Kindesalter – oft zu spät behandelt. Dtsch Arztebl 102:A1750–A1752
80. Linke J, Loy V, Dieckmann KP (2005) Prevalence of testicular intraepithelial neoplasia in healthy males. J Urol 173:1577–1579
81. Martin DC (1982) Malignancy in the cryptorchid testis. Urol Clin North Am 9:371–376
82. Pettersson A, Richiardi L, Nordenskjold A, Kaijser M, Akre O (2007) Age at surgery for undescended testis and risk of testicular cancer. N Engl J Med 356:1835–1841
83. Tuazon E, Banks K, Koh CJ, De Filippo RE, Chang A, Hardy BE, Cortessis VK (2008) Re: Prepubertal orchiopexy for cryptorchidism may be associated with lower risk of testicular cancer. J Urol 180:783–784
84. Ginsburg J (1997) Unanswered questions in carcinoma of the testis. Lancet 349:1785–1786
85. Berkowitz GS, Lapinski RH, Godbold JH, Dolgin SE, Holzman IR (1995) Maternal and neonatal risk factors for cryptorchidism. Epidemiology 6:127–131
86. Moller H, Skakkebaek NE (1996) Risks of testicular cancer and cryptorchidism in relation to socioeconomic status and related factors: case–control studies in Denmark. Int J Cancer 66:287–293
87. Pleskacova J, Hersmus R, Oosterhuis JW, Setyawati BA, Faradz SM, Cools M, Wolffenbuttel KP, Lebl J, Drop SL, Looijenga LH (2010) Tumor risk in disorders of sex development. Sex Dev 4:259–269
88. Li Y, Tabatabai ZL, Lee TL, Hatakeyama S, Ohyama C, Chan WY, Looijenga LH, Lau YF (2007) The Y-encoded TSPY protein: a significant marker potentially plays a role in the pathogenesis of testicular germ cell tumors. Hum Pathol 38:1470–1481
89. McGlynn KA, Cook MB (2009) Etiologic factors in testicular germ-cell tumors. Future Oncol 5:1389–1402
90. http://www.amptestdirectory.org/directory/st_test_list.php?s_search_by=2
91. Summersgill B, Osin P, Lu YJ, Huddart R, Shipley J (2001) Chromosomal imbalances associated with carcinoma in situ and associated testicular germ cell tumours of adolescents and adults. Br J Cancer 85:213–220
92. Rodriguez E, Houldsworth J, Reuter VE, Meltzer P, Zhang J, Trent JM, Bosl GJ, Chaganti RS (1993) Molecular cytogenetic analysis of i(12p)-negative human male germ cell tumors. Genes Chromosomes Cancer 8:230–236
93. Moore BE, Banner BF, Golden M, Wada B, Liu Y, Ayala A, Jiang Z (2001) p53: a good diagnostic marker for intratubular germ cell neoplasia, unclassified. Appl Immunohistochem Mol Morphol 9:203–206
94. Atkin NB, Baker MC (1983) I(12p): specific chromosomal marker in seminoma and malignant teratoma of the testis? Cancer Genet Cytogenet 10:199–204
95. Rosenberg C, Van Gurp RJ, Geelen E, Oosterhuis JW, Looijenga LH (2000) Overrepresentation of the short arm of chromosome 12 is related to invasive growth of human testicular seminomas and nonseminomas. Oncogene 19:5858–5862

96. Summersgill B, Goker H, Weber-Hall S, Huddart R, Horwich A, Shipley J (1998) Molecular cytogenetic analysis of adult testicular germ cell tumours and identification of regions of consensus copy number change. Br J Cancer 77:305–313
97. Ottesen AM, Skakkebaek NE, Lundsteen C, Leffers H, Larsen J, Rajpert-De Meyts E (2003) High-resolution comparative genomic hybridization detects extra chromosome arm 12p material in most cases of carcinoma in situ adjacent to overt germ cell tumors, but not before the invasive tumor development. Genes Chromosomes Cancer 38:117–125
98. Rodriguez S, Jafer O, Goker H, Summersgill BM, Zafarana G, Gillis AJ, van Gurp RJ, Oosterhuis JW, Lu YJ, Huddart R, Cooper CS, Clark J, Looijenga LH, Shipley JM (2003) Expression profile of genes from 12p in testicular germ cell tumors of adolescents and adults associated with i(12p) and amplification at 12p11.2-p12.1. Oncogene 22:1880–1891
99. Goddard NC, McIntyre A, Summersgill B, Gilbert D, Kitazawa S, Shipley J (2007) KIT and RAS signalling pathways in testicular germ cell tumours: new data and a review of the literature. Int J Androl 30:337–348
100. Bourdon V, Naef F, Rao PH, Reuter V, Mok SC, Bosl GJ, Koul S, Murty VV, Kucherlapati RS, Chaganti RS (2002) Genomic and expression analysis of the 12p11-p12 amplicon using EST arrays identifies two novel amplified and overexpressed genes. Cancer Res 62:6218–6223
101. van Echten J, Oosterhuis JW, Looijenga LH, van de Pol M, Wiersema J, te Meerman GJ, Schaffordt Koops H, Sleijfer DT, de Jong B (1995) No recurrent structural abnormalities apart from i(12p) in primary germ cell tumors of the adult testis. Genes Chromosomes Cancer 14:133–144
102. van Echten J, Timmer A, van der Veen AY, Molenaar WM, de Jong B (2002) Infantile and adult testicular germ cell tumors: a different pathogenesis? Cancer Genet Cytogenet 135:57–62
103. Kato N, Tamura G, Fukase M, Shibuya H, Motoyama T (2003) Hypermethylation of the RUNX3 gene promoter in testicular yolk sac tumor of infants. Am J Pathol 163:387–391
104. Looijenga LH, Hersmus R, Gillis AJ, Pfundt R, Stoop HJ, van Gurp RJ, Veltman J, Beverloo HB, van Drunen E, van Kessel AG, Pera RR, Schneider DT, Summersgill B, Shipley J, McIntyre A, van der Spek P, Schoenmakers E, Oosterhuis JW (2006) Genomic and expression profiling of human spermatocytic seminomas: primary spermatocyte as tumorigenic precursor and DMRT1 as candidate chromosome 9 gene. Cancer Res 66:290–302
105. Dilworth JP, Farrow GM, Oesterling JE (1991) Non-germ cell tumors of testis. Urology 37:399–415
106. Conkey DS, Howard GC, Grigor KM, McLaren DB, Kerr GR (2005) Testicular sex cord-stromal tumours: the Edinburgh experience 1988–2002, and a review of the literature. Clin Oncol 17:322–327
107. Young RH (2005) Sex cord-stromal tumors of the ovary and testis: their similarities and differences with consideration of selected problems. Mod Pathol 18(Suppl 2):S81–S98
108. Hanson JA, Ambaye AB (2011) Adult testicular granulosa cell tumor: a review of the literature for clinicopathologic predictors of malignancy. Arch Pathol Lab Med 135:143–146
109. Abell MR, Holtz F (1968) Testicular and paratesticular neoplasms in patients 60 years of age and older. Cancer 21:852–870
110. Young RH, Koelliker DD, Scully RE (1998) Sertoli cell tumors of the testis, not otherwise specified: a clinicopathologic analysis of 60 cases. Am J Surg Pathol 22:709–721
111. Verdorfer I, Höllrigl A, Strasser U, Susani M, Hartmann A, Rogatsch H, Mikuz G (2007) Molecular-cytogenetic characterization of sex cord-stromal tumours: CGH analysis in Sertoli cell tumours of the testis. Virchows Arch 450:425–431
112. Chang H, Guillou F, Taketo MM, Behringer RR (2009) Overactive beta-catenin signaling causes testicular Sertoli cell tumor development in the mouse. Biol Reprod 81:842–849
113. Abbas F, Bashir NW, Hussainy AS (2005) Sclerosing Sertoli cell tumor of the testis. J Coll Physicians Surg Pak 15:437–438
114. Gravas S, Papadimitriou K, Kyriakidis A (1999) Sclerosing Sertoli cell tumor of the testis – a case report and review of the literature. Scand J Urol Nephrol 33:197–199
115. De Raeve H, Schoonooghe P, Wibowo R, Van Marck E, Goossens A (2003) Malignant large cell calcifying Sertoli cell tumor of the testis. Pathology 199:113–117

116. Kratzer SS, Ulbright TM, Talerman A, Srigley JR, Roth LM, Wahle GR, Moussa M, Stephens JK, Millos A, Young RH (1997) Large cell calcifying Sertoli cell tumor of the testis. Am J Surg Pathol 21(11):1271–1280
117. Carney JA, Gordon H, Carpenter PC, Shenoy BV, Go VL (1985) The complex of myxomas, spotty pigmentation, and endocrine overactivity. Medicine 64:270–283
118. Bertherat J, Horvath A, Groussin L, Grabar S, Boikos S, Cazabat L, Libe R, René-Corail F, Stergiopoulos S, Bourdeau I, Bei T, Clauser E, Calender A, Kirschner LS, Bertagna X, Carney JA, Stratakis CA (2009) Mutations in regulatory subunit type 1A of cyclic adenosine 5′-monophosphate-dependent protein kinase (PRKAR1A): phenotype analysis in 353 patients and 80 different genotypes. J Clin Endocrinol Metab 94:2085–2091
119. Stratakis CA, Carney JA, Lin JP, Papanicolaou DA, Karl M, Kastner DL, Pras E, Chrousos GP (1996) Carney complex, a familial multiple neoplasia and lentiginosis syndrome. Analysis of 11 kindreds and linkage to the short arm of chromosome 2. J Clin Invest 97:699–705
120. Gordon MD, Corless C, Renshaw AA, Beckstead J (1998) CD99, keratin, and vimentin staining of sex cord-stromal tumors, normal ovary, and testis. Mod Pathol 11:769–773
121. Al-Agha OM, Axiotis CA (2007) An in-depth look at Leydig cell tumor of the testis. Arch Pathol Lab Med 131:311–317
122. Holm M, Rajpert-De Meyts E, Andersson A-M, Skakkebk NE (2003) Leydig cell micronodules are a common finding in testicular biopsies from men with impaired spermatogenesis and are associated with decreased testosterone/LH ratio. J Pathol 199:378–386
123. Carvajal-Carmona LG, Alam NA, Pollard PJ, Jones AM, Barclay E, Wortham N, Pignatelli M, Freeman A, Pomplun S, Ellis I, Poulsom R, El-Bahrawy MA, Berney DM, Tomlinson IP (2006) Adult Leydig cell tumors of the testis caused by germline fumarate hydratase mutations. J Clin Endocrinol Metab 91:3071–3075
124. Boyer A, Paquet M, Laguë MN, Hermo L, Boerboom D (2009) Dysregulation of WNT/CTNNB1 and PI3K/AKT signaling in testicular stromal cells causes granulosa cell tumor of the testis. Carcinogenesis 30:869–878

Chapter 12
Molecular Pathology and Diagnostics of Gynecologic Malignancies

Rodney E. Shackelford, Masoumeh Ghayouri, Domenico Coppola, and Ardeshir Hakam

Contents

R.E. Shackelford
Department of Pathology and Laboratory Medicine, Tulane University School of Medicine, 1430 Tulane Avenue, SL-79, New Orleans, LA 70112, USA

M. Ghayouri • D. Coppola • A. Hakam, M.D. (✉)
Department of Pathology, H. Lee Moffitt Cancer Center and Research Institute, 12902 Magnolia Drive, Tampa, FL 33612, USA
e-mail: Ardeshir.Hakam@moffitt.org

D. Coppola (ed.), *Molecular Pathology and Diagnostics of Cancer*, Cancer Growth and Progression 16, DOI 10.1007/978-94-007-7192-5_12,

Abstract Gynecologic malignancies account for roughly 13 % of solid tissue tumors in women. Many of these malignancies, such as many ovarian tumors, first present at an advanced stage, making them difficult to treat. Until recently the analysis of these malignancies was largely limited to hematoxylin-eosin-stained slide examination, supplemented with immunohistochemical stains. Recently, molecular diagnostic techniques have been applied to these tumors with some success, especially with BRCA1/2 mutations and Lynch syndrome analyses. Here, we describe the present molecular diagnostic tests applied to gynecologic malignancies and discuss possible future developments in this field.

Keywords Gynecologic malignancies • HPV • BRCA1 • BRCA2 • Mole • Nampt • Ovary • Vulva • Fallopian tubes • Vagina • Lynch syndrome • Endometrium

Abbreviations

CDK	Cyclin-dependent protein kinase
dsDNA	Double-stranded DNA
EST	Endometrial stromal tumor
FDA	US Food and Drug Administration
HNPCC	Hereditary nonpolyposis colorectal cancer
HPV	Human papilloma virus
HRM	High-resolution melting analysis
MMMT	Malignant mixed mullerian tumor
Nampt	Nicotinamide phosphoribosyltransferase
PCR	Polymerase chain reaction
PJS	Peutz-Jeghers syndrome
UCCC	Uterine clear cell carcinoma
UEA	Uterine endometrial adenocarcinoma
USC	Uterine serous carcinoma

12.1 Introduction

Gynecologic malignancies include cervical, endometrial, uterine, vaginal, vulvar, ovarian, and fallopian tube cancers. Together, these malignancies account for 13 % of all solid tumors in women, following breast, lung, and colon cancers, with cervical, uterine, and ovarian cancers making up ~95 % of gynecologic malignancies [1–3]. Until recently, the diagnosis and analysis of prognostic indicator(s) in gynecologic malignancies largely depended on examination of hematoxylin-eosin-stained slides, supplemented with immunohistochemical analyses. Over the past 15 years, molecular genetic studies of gynecologic malignancies have significantly contributed to our understanding of the pathogenesis and molecular differences between different gynecologic malignancies.

Currently, molecular studies are employed in the diagnosis, prognosis, and management of some types of gynecologic malignancies and of heritable gynecologic cancer syndromes. As molecular testing becomes more common, the cost of testing falls, and its implementation will undoubtedly help our understanding of the molecular pathology underlying gynecologic malignancies [4].

12.2 Cervical Cancer

12.2.1 Epidemiology, HPV, and the Molecular Pathogenesis of Cervical Cancer

Cervical cancer is the second most common gynecologic cancer and the most common cause of cancer-related death in women world-wide, with some 400,000 new cases and 200,000 deaths yearly [2]. In the United States, roughly 12,000 new cases are diagnosed yearly with 4,000 women dying of the disease. In addition, the associated medical costs are now over $2 billion [1–3, 5]. Clinical, molecular, and epidemiologic studies show that cervical cancer is overwhelmingly caused by epitheliotropic human papilloma virus (HPV) infection, with other causes such as diethylstilbestrol exposure, counting for a minority of cases [6–8]. HPV consists of more than 150 related DNA viruses, many capable of infecting multiple sites within the body, including the cervix, vulva, anus, vagina, mouth, esophagus, penis, and more rarely, the lungs, larynx, and stomach [6, 7, 9, 10]. The cervix is most the commonly infected site, with HPV detected in up to 95 % of high-grade cervical dysplasias and cancers [11]. Different HPV types have been classified into two categories based on their potential tumorigenicity. For example, HPV types 16, 18, 31, 33, 35, 39, 45, 51, 52, 56, 58, 59, 68, 73, and 82 confer a high risk for cervical cancer, whereas types 6, 11, 40, 42, 43, 44, 54, 61, 70, 72, 81 and CP6 108 carry a low cancer risk, with infection by these associated with condylomatas. Types 16 and 18 are by far the most common high-risk HPV types [6].

In general, the presence of a high-risk HPV type is insufficient to cause cancer. For example, only ~10 % of women infected with high-risk HPV types progress to precancerous lesions, with 20–30 % of those developing invasive cancer [12]. In general, other factors need to be present for progression to cancer, including tobacco use (which interferes with the cervical physical barrier), the presence of other sexually transmitted diseases (for example, HIV or herpes virus), alterations of hormonal status, promiscuity, β-carotene deficiency, and immunodeficient conditions such as pregnancy, AIDS, steroid treatment, and certain malignancies [11–13].

HPV is a small double-stranded DNA (dsDNA) virus of 7,900 base pairs that infects differentiating basal cells, requiring minor epithelial trauma for initial infection. The virus replicates in terminally differentiated epithelial cells, exiting within infected cells as both extrachromosomic multicopy nuclear plasmids and as integrated viral genomes [14]. Functionally, the HPV genome is divided into the Long Control Region and the Open Reading Frames, with the former containing regulatory sequences (promoters and enhancers) and target sequences for transcription factors that regulate HPV gene expression. The Open Reading Frames code for "early" and "late region" proteins, with the early region consisting of six nonstructural proteins (E1, E2, E4, E5, E6, and E7) and the late region coding for two structural proteins (L1 and L2) [14].

The mechanisms by which HPV causes cancer are not completely understood. Viral integration into the host genome is required for keratinocyte immortality. Upon integration, E6 and E7 protein expression is increased, conferring a growth advantage usually resulting in clonal expansion [14–19]. E6 and E7 bind and inhibit p53 and pRb activities, respectively. p53 is a transcription factor required for G_1 checkpoint and apoptotic functions, and induction of p21 and GADD45, which delay S phase entry and promote DNA repair. pRb inhibition increases protein synthesis which promotes S-phase cell cycle entry and also inhibits apoptosis [14–18, 20]. Together, HPV E6 and E7 proteins promote genomic instability and cell cycle entry [20]. Additionally, HPV integration and replication induce DNA damage, resulting in chromosomal translocations and host genomic rearrangements adjacent to the HPV integration site [14–19]. Together, HPV-induced genomic damage, combined with E6 and E7 expression, lead to dysplasia and eventual invasive carcinoma [21].

12.2.2 HPV Testing Methods

12.2.2.1 Histology

HPV is detected in cervical, vaginal, and vulvar biopsies mainly via histologic examination of hematoxylin-eosin-stained slides. Typically, HPV-infected cells are superficial, displaying enlarged, hyperchromatic nuclei, with cytoplasmic halos (koilocytotic atypia) [22, 23]. Although histologic examination is inexpensive and relatively rapid, there is considerable interobserver variation in the diagnosis of these lesions, leading to overdiagnosis. For example, a review of cervical, vaginal, and vulvar biopsies histologically diagnosed as low-grade squamous intraepithelial lesions or condylomas, revealed a ~33 % over-diagnosis in all three mucosal sites, mainly due to mimics of koilocytotic atypia (pseudokoilocytes) [24, 25]. Based on this, ancillary HPV testing in equivocal cases would be useful, preventing overdiagnosis with its attendant unnecessary medical treatment and costs. Unfortunately, many HPV detection techniques such as in situ hybridization and immunohistochemistry for viral capsid proteins have low sensitivity. Additionally, as yet, no US

Food and Drug Administration (FDA)-approved HPV tests applicable to tissue sections exist. Lastly, while HPV polymerase chain reaction (PCR) testing is sensitive, the specificity of this testing is less so, especially in women under 30 years, due to the prevalence of transient clinically benign infections [26–29].

Due to these problems, several surrogate markers for HPV infection are now in use. Both have proven useful in lowering the number of false positives in low-grade squamous intraepithelial lesions.

12.2.2.2 Ki-67

Ki-67 is a commercial monoclonal antibody that binds an antigen on a nuclear protein referred to as Ki-67 or MKI67. *Ki-67* is located at 10q25 and has 15 exons, encoding several transcripts that are translated into proteins ranging from 320 to 359 kDa. It is readily detected in G_1, S, G_2, and M phase, but not in G_0, making Ki-67 a good immunohistochemical marker for proliferating cells [30, 31]. Antisense oligonucleotides to Ki-67 inhibit cell proliferation in a dose-dependent manner in IM-9 cells, indicating that Ki-67 expression is likely an absolute requirement for cell proliferation [32].

HPV infection increases cellular proliferative activity; hence, Ki-67 expression is often altered where HPV-related pathology exists. Ki-67 is normally expressed only in the parabasal nuclei in normal cervical squamous epithelium. With HPV infection, Ki-67 staining extends to the intermediate and superficial epithelial layers, with increased and more superficial staining seen in higher-grade lesions and condylomas. Interestingly, apoptosis is seen in the higher grade lesions (high-grade squamous intraepithelial lesions and squamous cell carcinomas) [33, 34]. The sensitivity and specificity of Ki-67 as a marker for low-grade and high-grade squamous intraepithelial lesions are high for cervical, vaginal, and vulvar lesions. This stain is especially useful in making a diagnosis in equivocal cases [24, 25, 35]. Ki-67 staining is not 100 % specific for dysplastic epithelium, as staining above the parabasal cell layer may be seen in immature and regenerating epithelium, the edge of ulcers, and in vulgar squamous cell hyperplasia [36]. Assessment of the histology of the specific lesion is important in differentiating between these conditions and HPV-induced neoplastic conditions.

12.2.2.3 p16

p16, also known as CDKN2A or MTS1, is located at 9p21.3 and consists of multiple exons that encode multiple transcripts of the 16.5-kDa p16 protein and by an alternative promoter and reading frame, another protein, INK4a. p16 belongs to a group of tumor suppressor genes that includes p15INK4b, p21waf1, and p27KIP1, all of which negatively regulate the G_1 phase of cell cycle [37]. Specifically, p16 binds the cyclin-dependent protein kinases CDK4 and CDK6, inhibiting their interactions with cyclin D1. As a result, pRb phosphorylation is inhibited and the E2F transcription factors are sequestered, blocking G1→S phase progression. p16 expression loss allows cells to escape G_1 arrest [20, 38]. The HPV E7 oncoprotein binds pRb causing E2F release, resulting in G1→S progression despite high p16 expression [39–41]. Thus high p16 expression is a sensitive marker for HPV E7 protein expression [42]. Cuschieri et al. [42] reviewed 9 studies, including 2,178 cases, and found that 7 % of nondysplastic, 54 % of CIN1 cases, 86 % of CIN2 cases, and 96 % of CIN3 and invasive cancers showed diffuse p16 expression, demonstrating high specificity and sensitivity of p16 staining as a measure of HPV infection. As with Ki-67, p16 staining is not entirely specific for a neoplastic process or HPV infection. For example, benign cervical tubal metaplasia shows p16 positivity [43].

12.2.2.4 Other Markers

The catalytic subunit of *telomerase* is located at 5p15.33 and functions as an endogenous human telomerase reverse trancriptase that employs its integral RNA as a template for adding repeats to chromosomal ends [44, 45]. The telomerase RNA component is located at 3q26.2 and primes 5′-TTAGGG-3′ telomere repeats. Telomerase is up-regulated and activated as part of carcinogenesis [46]. Kailash et al. used reverse transcriptase-PCR to measure telomerase RNA expression changes in cervical cytology samples and compared these changes to high-risk HPV viral expression [47]. There is an excellent correlation between high-risk HPV types 16 and 18 and telomerase RNA expression, with sensitivity of 88.1 % and 100 % for high-risk HPV and telomerase RNA expression, respectively. Telomerase RNA weak positivity was seen in 12.7 % of normal cervical epithelium samples, in 63.6 % of those of mild squamous dysplasia, in 100 % of cervical samples affected by moderate and severe squamous cell dysplasia, and in 100 % of cases of squamous cell carcinoma in situ. Thus, telomerase RNA expression may be used as an adjunct to cytology and HPV DNA testing in triaging women with cervical lesions. Support for the above work also comes from the observation that the human telomerase RNA gene is often up-regulated in cervical intraepithelial neoplasia and carcinoma [48].

E-cadherin is an adhesion molecule involved in normal tissue morphogenesis, differentiation, signaling, and proliferation [49]. Ancuta et al. found that, of cervical carcinomas with E-cadherin loss, 75 % relapsed within 5 years, while only 37.5 % of cervical carcinomas with positive E-cadherin staining relapsed within 5 years [49]. Interestingly, of all the relapsed patients, 62.1 % of those with E-cadherin loss died of their disease, while only 25 % of those who maintained E-cadherin expression died of their disease. Thus initial E-cadherin cervical carcinoma staining may have potential as a prognostic marker.

p63 is located at 3q27-29 and encodes a protein with strong homology to p53 and the related gene p73. p63 is expressed in many tissues, including the basal cells of the epidermis, prostate, urothelium, and cervix [50]. Shirendeb et al. found basal cell p63 expression in benign cervical tissue, with staining extending to the intermediate and superficial epithelial layers with CINI → III dysplastic progression [51]. The p63 staining may also be a useful adjunctive stain for histologically equivocal cases.

12.2.2.5 PCR HPV Testing–Emphasize Typing

The majority of DNA-based HPV testing PCR amplify a portion of the highly conserved major structural gene L1, limiting the test to the presence or absence of viral DNA. Such testing cannot distinguish between transient, clinically insignificant HPV infections and those related to HPV-induced pathology and transformation [26–29]. There is also good evidence that HPV16 and other high-risk category viruses confer a significantly higher probability for HPV-induced transformation than do other viral types [6, 52]. Additionally, factors such as co-infection with different viral subtypes and the viral load are significant in determining transformation risk [53]. The extreme precision of PCR makes it ideal for identification of different HPC types, as well as the specific amplification and analysis of different HPV gene expression patterns. This has been used in several different systems to aid in the diagnosis of HPV infections.

1. *Analysis of HPV Early Gene Expression* via *Real-Time Quantitative Reverse Transcriptase PCR:* Analysis of specific HPV transcripts likely to be up regulated in dysplastic/malignant cells may be more specific for HPV-related pathologic changes than the presence of the HPV viral genome. The HPV E7 RNA transcript is a good candidate for such testing, as it plays a central role in inducing dysregulated cell cycle progression and transformation. Lamarcq et al. [54] analyzed HPV 16 and 18 E7 RNA expression via real-time quantitative reverse transcriptase PCR. RNA was isolated in cervical cytology samples and reverse transcribed in DNA via random heximer priming, and the resulting DNA was amplified with primers specific for each viral 57 type. Labeled probes were employed to detect real-time amplification. Zero percent of cytologically normal cervical samples expressed E7 RNA, with 47 % and 5 % of the high-grade lesions expressing HPV types 16 and 18 E7 RNAs, respectively. The remaining 53 % of high-grade lesions were thought to harbor other HPV type infections. The authors concluded that the detection of the E7 transcripts may be more specific than HPV DNA detection and may therefore have use in triaging women with abnormal Pap smears.
2. *Pyrosequencing for HPV Genotyping:* DNA sequencing is often considered the gold standard in molecular testing, particularly for viral testing. One problem with employing sequencing technologies is that many specimens harbor multiple HPV types, often yielding non-specific and uninterruptible sequence data. This problem has been solved through the use of HPV type-specific multiple sequencing primers followed by sequencing. For example, Gharizadeh et al. [55] used such

primers to first specifically PCR-amplify sequences of the seven most prevalent HPV types (6, 11, 16, 18, 31, 33, and 45) and analyze the resulting amplicons via pyrosequencing. The resulting amplicons were both specific and nonspecific, allowing the identification of specific sequences by the use of multiple sequencing primers, which in turn allowed the identification of the specific sequence signal. This technique has the advantage of eliminating the need for nested PCR reactions, cloning, and very high stringency PCR techniques. The disadvantage is that it is relatively costly and complex for routine cervical HPV screening. It does have value, as with other molecular diagnostic tests, in identifying women at greater risk to the presence of high-risk HPV types.

3. *HPV DNA Testing by Hybrid Capture:* Hybrid capture assays involve the isolation of sample DNA, followed by denaturation, mixing, and hybridization with labeled multiple RNA probes, each specific for one HPV type. The resulting RNA/DNA hybrids are captured by a specific antibody attached to a solid support (often the wall of a 96 well plate), the sample is washed, and the bound RNA/DNA hybrids are reacted with an alkaline phosphatase-conjugated antibody directed against RNA-DNA hybrids. After extensive washing, a chemiluminescent substrate is added that emits when it reacts with alkaline phosphatase. The light produced is measured via a luminometer and expressed in relative light units, allowing semiquantitative determination of viral DNA quantity in the specimen. In general, as little as 1 pg viral DNA can be detected with this technique [56, 57]. The method is largely reproducible, relatively inexpensive, and accurate. As with most molecular testing methods, long-term specimen storage results in poorer results secondary to DNA degradation [57]. This technique is currently FDA approved for cytologic preparations and is available through Digene.

12.3 Adenoma Malignum, Ovarian Sex Cord Tumor with Annular Tubules, and Peutz-Jeghers Syndrome

Peutz-Jeghers Syndrome (PJS) is a rare autosomal dominate disease characterized by pigmented mucocutaneous lesions, hamartomatous polyps mainly seen in the small intestine, and increased malignancies in multiple organs. Women with PJS often have a high incidence of cervical adenoma malignum and ovarian sex cord tumor with annular tubules, two rare, well-differentiated neoplasms [58–60]. The diagnosis of PJS and these two well-differentiated neoplasms rests upon the clinical presentation and histology supplemented with immunohistochemical analyses, respectively [58–63]. Molecular diagnostic testing in PJS is employed for prenatal diagnosis, kindred testing, and clinical diagnosis confirmation. Molecular testing for PJS involves the analysis of two genes, *BMPR1A* and *SMAD4,* via multiple molecular techniques such as DNA sequencing and PCR-based denaturing gradient gel electrophoresis [64–66].

12.4 Ovarian Cancer

12.4.1 Epidemiology, Types, and Molecular Pathogenesis

Ovarian cancer is comprises 15 distinct tumor types, each with a different histology, prognosis, underlying molecular pathology, and often surgical-chemotherapeutic treatment options [67, 68]. Approximately 90 % of these neoplasms are epithelial derived, with ~70 % being high-grade serous carcinomas [69]. Ovarian cancer is the fifth leading cause of female cancer-related deaths, with its yearly treatment costing ~$2.2 billion/year in the US [67, 68, 70]. Each of the major ovarian malignancies is characterized by specific mutations, which also correlate with their histologic and their malignant progression. Some of the major molecular lesions for each of the major ovarian malignancies are summarized below.

12.4.2 Ovarian Endometrioid Adenocarcinoma

Endometrioid adenocarcinoma accounts for ~10 % of ovarian tumors; it is often associated with endometriosis and typically presents as stage I or II [71]. The most common mutations found in this tumor are *KRAS*, *BRAF*, *PTEN* and *β-catenin* (*CTNNB1*) mutations.

12.4.2.1 KRAS

KRAS is the human homologue of the Kirsten rat sarcoma virus. KRAS transduces signals from several surface growth factor receptors (EGF-, HGF- and IGF-1 receptors), activating down-stream signaling proteins, including Raf, Braf, mTOR, MEK, ERK, and PIK3CA. The resulting gene expression patterns promote cell growth and division, while exerting anti-apoptotic and pro-angiogenesis effects. KRAS is a GTPase that becomes inactive upon hydrolysis of bound GTP to GDP. Activating KRAS mutations typically ablate KRAS GTPase activity, resulting in constitutive KRAS activation and tumor promotion [72–77]. KRAS mutations are seen in ~10 % of these malignancies; interestingly, ovarian endometriosis, a precursor lesion of endometrioid adenocarcinoma, shows a higher frequency of chromosomal abnormalities than extragonadal endometriosis [78, 79].

12.4.2.2 BRAF

BRAF is a serine/threonine kinase which functions downstream of KRAS. Following phosphorylation and activation by KRAS, BRAF activity increases cyclins D1-3, mdm2, and c-myc expression, promoting cell cycle entrance, increasing cell growth potential, and inhibiting apoptosis [80–82]. Many of the BRAF mutations in endometrioid ovarian carcinoma are the common V600E (valine → glutamate substitution) activating mutation seen in other malignancies [83, 84]. BRAF mutations are seen in ~10 % of endometrioid adenocarcinomas [78].

12.4.2.3 PTEN

PTEN also known as *MMAC1* or *TEP1*, is a phosphatidylinositol 3,4,5-triphosphate phosphatase. Phosphatidylinositol 3,4,5-triphosphate activates the PI3K/AKT signaling pathway, promoting cell growth and survival [85]. Inactivating *PTEN* mutations activate the PI3K/AKT signaling pathway and are seen in ~20 % of endometrioid ovarian carcinomas [68]. They have also been described in typical and atypical endometriosis, possibly functioning as early events in carcinogenesis [86, 87].

12.4.2.4 β-Catenin

Beta-catenin is the mammalian homologue of *Drosophila armadillo* and is mutated in at least 60 % of endometrioid ovarian carcinomas [88]. β-*catenin* exists in two major cellular pools, each exerting a different function. First, it is found on the plasma membrane where it provides a mechanical link between E-cadherin and β-catenin, forming a trimer that binds the intracellular actin cytoskeleton, promoting intercellular adherens junctions formation and likely suppressing tumor invasion. Second, in tumors, β-catenin is often found in the cytoplasm and nucleus where it is part of a large protein complex that includes AXIN1, AXIN2, APC, CSNK1A1, and GSK3B. This complex phosphorylates β-catenin and leads to ubiquitination and proteasomal degradation, keeping β-catenin levels low in normal cells. In many tumors, β-catenin carries mutations in codons 32, 33, 37, and 41 of exon 3. These mutations inhibit β-catenin phosphorylation and degradation, resulting in association with TCF/LEF-1 family members and WNT, leading to the transcription of pro-mitotic proteins including c-Myc and cyclin D1, and promoting transformation [89–91]. Roughly 80 % of ovarian endometrioid adenocarcinomas show nuclear β-*catenin* accumulation [68]. Finally, the combinations of *PTEN*/*KRAS* and β-*catenin*/*PTEN* mutations have been demonstrated to be sufficient to induce ovarian endometrioid carcinoma in engineered mouse models, demonstrating the importance of these mutations in the carcinogenesis of these malignancies [92, 93].

Due to this malignancy commonly presenting at stage I or II and carrying a low mortality and morbidity burden, molecular diagnostics is seldom applied to these tumors outside of the research settings. Additionally, BRCA mutations are not seen in endometrioid ovarian carcinomas [68].

12.4.3 Ovarian Mucinous Carcinoma

Ovarian mucinous carcinoma accounts for only 3–4 % of ovarian malignancies [68]. KRAS codon 12 and 13 mutations have been found in up to 55.7–75 % of these tumors [94, 95]. Low frequency BRAF mutations are also found in this tumor type [83]. Last, 15–20 % of these tumors expressed estrogen and progesterone receptors, CA19-9, CA-125, and HER2, with the last two markers expressed in a small percentage of these tumors [96].

12.4.4 Ovarian Clear Cell Carcinoma

Clear cell carcinoma is a high-grade ovarian malignant tumor that accounts for ~10 % of ovarian malignancies and usually presents with low-stage disease [68]. Kuo et al. [97] examined 97 ovarian clear cell carcinomas for *PIK3CA*, *TP53*, *KRAS*, *PTEN*, *CTNNB1*, and *BRAF* sequence mutations, finding 33 %, 15 %, 7 %, 5 %, 3 %, and 1 % mutant sequences, respectively. Samples taken from tumors with *PIK3CA* mutations showed intense phosphorylated AKT immunoreactivity. Thus, although arising from endometriosis like the endometrioid adenocarcinoma, the low *CTNNB1* mutation levels combined with the high *PIK3CA* mutation levels differentiate this tumor from endometrioid adenocarcinomas. Interestingly, although clear cell carcinomas are high-grade, they have DNA copy number changes resembling those reported for low-grade ovarian serous tumors, suggesting a relatively high level of genomic stability in these tumors [98].

12.4.5 Dysgerminoma

Dysgerminomas account for less than 1 % of ovarian malignancies and, like its more common testicular counterpart seminoma, these tumors have high (~60 %) isochromosome 12p and c-kit mutations [99–102].

12.4.6 Ovarian Granulosa Cell Tumor

Granulosa cell tumors account for 1–2 % of ovarian tumors and ~2 % of ovarian malignancies [68]. Ninety-five percent or more of these tumors have been shown to harbor a G→C mutation at nucleotide 402 (Cys134Trp) in the *FOXl2* gene [103–105]. FOXl2 is a member of the Forkhead/Winged-Helix family of transcription factors associated with blepharophimosis ptosis epicanthus inversus syndrome and in its unmutated form is normally found in ovarian granulosa cell nuclei [106, 107].

12.4.7 Low and High-Grade Ovarian Serous Carcinoma

Ovarian serous carcinomas have recently been divided into low- and high-grade tumors. Interestingly, the two tumor types appear to have different precursor lesions, with the low-grade tumors arising from serous borderline ovarian tumors or adenofibromas, and high-grade tumors arising from the Fallopian tube epithelium. Low-grade serous carcinomas are relatively rare, making up about 2 % of ovarian carcinomas [68]. Typically ~60 % will harbor *KRAS* codons 12 and 13 or the V600E *BRAF* activating mutations with KRAS [78, 94, 95]. A lower level of ERBB2 mutation is also seen (~6 %) [108]. Since KRAS, BRAF, and ERBB2 all activate the RAS-MAPK pathway, activation of this pathway is likely required for low-grade serous ovarian carcinoma genesis and progression [108]. These tumor types also commonly express estrogen and/or progesterone receptors, are not associated with BRCA1 and BRCA2 mutations, and only rarely have p53 mutations [68, 109].

In contrast, high-grade serous ovarian carcinomas show nearly 100 % p53 mutations (96.7 %), with the remaining cases showing molecular evidence of p53 dysfunction via MDM2 or MDM4 amplifications [110]. Additionally, while *BRCA* mutations are strongly associated with hereditary ovarian cancers, more than 50 % of high-grade serous carcinomas carry some *BRCA1* and *BRCA2* abnormalities, including promoter hypermethylation and gene mutations [111–113].

12.4.8 Nicotinamide Phosphoribosyltransferase Expression in Ovarian Tumors

Interestingly, nicotinamide phosphoribosyltransferase (Nampt) is overexpressed in many ovarian tumors compared to benign ovarian tissue; including serous adenocarcinoma, clear cell carcinoma, endometrioid carcinoma, yolk sac tumor, and mucinous adenocarcinoma [114]. Nampt catalyzes the rate-limiting step of NAD^+ synthesis [115]. Although apparently not a specific ovarian tumor subtype, Nampt overexpression suggests an increased NAD^+ requirement by these neoplasms. Since a specific Nampt inhibitor, FK866, has shown promising results in the treatment of human malignancies, this inhibitor may eventually have use as an adjunctive treatment for ovarian malignancies [116, 117].

12.4.9 BRCA1/2 Testing

12.4.9.1 Background

Roughly 90 % of ovarian malignancies are sporadic, with 5–10 % due to hereditary causes [118]. Thirty to fifty percent of hereditary ovarian malignancies are due to germline mutations of BRCA1 and BRCA2 located at 17q21 and 13q12, respectively [118]. These mutations typically follow an autosomal dominant pattern and are highly penetrant, with 80–90 % or more of individuals carrying these mutations developing ovarian cancers without intervention [119, 120]. Often different mutations occur at different frequencies in various populations. For example, ~2.6 % of the Ashkenazi Jewish population carry one of three BRCA mutations: BRCA1-185delAG, BRCA1-5382insC, and BRCA2-6174delT. These mutations have a frequency of ~1 %, 0.13 %, and 1.52 %, respectively, and confer a 64 %, 67 %, and 43 % lifetime cancer risk [121].

12.4.9.2 BRCA1

BRCA1 or "breast cancer 1, early onset" is a 208-kDA nuclear phosphoprotein that plays an important role in maintaining genomic stability, functioning as a tumor suppressor gene. BRCA1 functions in conjunction with MSH2, MSH6, MLH1, ATM, BLM, PMS2, RAD50, MRE11, and NBS, forming a nuclear protein complex involved in the recognition and repair of aberrant DNA structures and DNA breaks [122]. More than 1,000 *BRCA1* mutations have been identified, many either producing an abnormally short, nonfunctional protein, or no protein expression. Other *BRCA1* mutations include deletions and missense and nonsense mutations. *BRCA1* mutations increase breast, ovarian, pancreatic, fallopian tube, and male breast cancer risk [123].

12.4.9.3 BRCA2

BRCA2 or "breast cancer 2, early onset" is a 384-kDa protein that functions in DNA break repair, homologous recombination, and the S phase checkpoint. More than 800 *BRCA2* mutations have been identified, largely consisting of insertions/deletions resulting in small, nonfunctional proteins. *BRCA2* mutations increase the risk for breast, ovarian, prostate, pancreatic, fallopian tube, male breast cancer, and melanoma [124].

12.4.9.4 BRCA Testing

Only 0.2 % of the general population carries *BRCA1* or *BRCA2* mutations; therefore, general screening on women for these mutations is not recommended [121]. Currently, although there are no standard criteria for recommending *BRCA1* or *BRCA2* mutation testing, testing should be considered for women with; (1) breast cancer in a male relative, (2) two first-degree relatives diagnosed with breast cancer, with one diagnosis at age 50 or younger, (3) three or more first-degree relatives diagnosed with breast cancer, regardless of age, (4) a first-degree relative diagnosed with bilateral breast cancer, (5) two or more first- or second-degree relatives diagnosed with ovarian cancer, regardless of age, (6) a first- or second-degree relative diagnosed with both breast and ovarian cancer, or (7) a combination of first- or second-degree relatives diagnosed with breast cancer and ovarian cancer, with one cancer type per person. Women of Ashkenazi Jewish descent should consider testing if they have any first-degree relative diagnosed with breast or ovarian cancer or if they have two second-degree relatives diagnosed with breast or ovarian cancer [125].

BRCA1 and BRCA2 testing has been based on several molecular techniques, such as direct sequencing, denaturing high-performance liquid chromatography, Southern blotting, and denaturing gradient gel electrophoresis. Each of these techniques has specific advantages, disadvantages, and limitations. Below are the ones currently most commonly used.

Due to the very high number of *BRCA1* and BRCA*2* mutations, *DNA sequencing* is the method of choice when no prior knowledge exists concerning any specific BRCA mutation. Typically, genomic DNA is obtained from whole blood, purified, measured, and amplified via PRC with specific primers. Due to the large size of the BRCA genes, many primer pairs are required to fully amplify all exons and flanking intronic sequences. For example, King et al. [126] employed 78 pairs of M13-tagged PCR primers to amplify *BRCA1*. The resulting amplicons are usually analyzed via a commercial DNA sequencer employing Sanger or pyrosequencing, with software programs employed to facilitate analysis.

DNA sequencing has the advantage of interrogating every nucleotide. It suffers the drawbacks of (1) being relatively costly, (2) missing the loss of gene protein expression secondary to epigenetic silencing, (3) missing nonfunctional regulatory region mutations that are not sequenced, (4) being time consuming, and (5) being unable to detect large genomic deletions/rearrangements. Other reasons for lack of BRCA detection include selection of the wrong proband or the existence of mutations in undiscovered genes [127].

High-Resolution Melting Analysis (HRM) allows mutation analysis to be conducted in the same tube or well in which the sequence was amplified. In HRM, selected portions of the gene being tested are PCR amplified with specific primer sets in the presence of a specific dye. The dye has several properties: (1) it does not interfere with PCR reactions, (2) it absorbs at one light frequency and emits at another when bound to dsDNA, and (3) it emits light relatively poorly in the presence of denatured/ssDNA. HRM has been commonly used in *BRCA1* and *–2* molecular testing. Takano et al. [128] used HRM to analyze two founder Ashkenazi Jewish *BCRA1* 185delAG and BRCA*2* 5382insC mutations, in exons 2 and 20, respectively. Following PCR amplification, the reactions containing the amplicons and dye were cooled and then slowly heated; multiple data acquisitions (usually ~25) are taken per degree of temperature increase [129]. As the temperature increases, the dsDNA denatures to ssDNA, lowering fluorescent signal intensity and producing a sigmoid curve. Amplified *BRCA1* and *–2* sequences with denaturation points different than the wild-type control are mutated [128]. HRM is quick to perform but is also relatively expensive and does not identify specific mutations [128, 129].

Although there are over 1,000 *BRCA1* and 800 *BRCA2* mutations, *BRCA* mutations are often relatively constant within specific ethnic/racial groups [121, 123, 124]. Since whole-gene sequencing is cumbersome and expensive, techniques have been developed for targeting specific mutations (*Targeted Mutation Testing*). Such techniques are comparatively inexpensive and have a rapid turn-around time compared to sequencing. One common method, referred to as allele-specific PCR, uses two primers, one with a 3′ end with nucleotides that match the wild-type gene sequence and the other primer with a 3′ end that matches the specific gene mutation. The *Taq* polymerase initiates the PCR poorly from mismatched template-primer 3′-termini, with a 10^{-3} to 10^{-6} lower amplification efficiency depending on the mismatch type [130]. Thus in a PCR involving two such primers, only one amplicon would be produced, either wild-type or mutant, as the 3′ primer-template mismatch would not initiate a PRC reaction. An amplicon type, mutant or wild type, can be indentified in a variety of ways. For example, Takano et al. [128] used differences in HRM to identify BRCA mutations specific to Ashkenazi Jews. Similarly, Abbaszadegan et al. [131] employed allele-specific PCR to identify BRCA mutations in the same population. Two primers, one wild-type and the other corresponding to the mutant sequence, were used; each primer was 5′ and 3′ labeled with different fluorescent reporters and quencher dyes. The 5′ nuclease activity of the *Taq* polymerase generates fluorescence by separating the quencher from the fluorescent reporter. As the wild-type and mutant primer were labeled with different dyes, the emission spectra of the released dye identifies the *BRCA* sequence. This testing is highly accurate, low cost, and has a rapid turn-around time.

The *BRCA Protein Truncation Test* has been employed in *BRCA* testing in many labs. In this system, RNA is extracted usually from nucleated peripheral blood cells of the individual being tested. The RNA is converted into DNA, typically via M-MLV reverse transcriptase with random heximers as primers. The resulting cDNA is amplified with specific *BRCA* primers covering portions of the gene suspected of harboring mutations. The amplicons are in turn transcribed and translated in proteins in a reticulocytelysate system. The proteins are often labeled with ^{35}S-labeled proteins in the reticulocytelysate system or can be visualized in a gel via various protein stains. *BRCA* mutations are detected by comparing the migration of the patient-translated product to that of an individual without *BRCA* mutations. A shorter, faster-migrating translated product indicates the presence of a truncated mutation and very likely a nonfunctional protein. Although whole proteins may be translated [132], *BRCA1* and BRCA*2* are sufficiently large so that translating smaller portion of either gene facilitates analysis [133]. This testing method only detects truncating mutations, rendering it less sensitive than many other *BRCA* mutation testing methods.

Denaturing High-Performance Liquid Chromatography has been shown to give accurate and reliable results in *BRCA1* testing [133]. Genomic DNA is isolated and PCR amplified. The unpurified amplicons are partially heat denatured and placed within a linear acetonitrile gradient. The amplicon DNA heteroduplexes that form have internal sequence variations that are identified by reduced column retention time(s) relative to their homoduplex counterparts. The elution profiles for such samples are distinct from those having homozygous sequences, making the identification of samples harboring polymorphisms/mutations relatively easy. This technique has been used in many studies and is especially useful in identifying novel *BRCA* mutations rapidly and efficiently [134–136].

To summarize, Gerhardus et al. [133] compared 12 different *BRCA1* testing methods and determined that protein truncation, single-strand conformation polymorphism, micronucleus, conformation-sensitive gel electrophoresis, and two-dimensional gene scanning testing lacked sufficient sensitivity for clinical testing. Additionally, fluorescence-based conformation-sensitive gel electrophoresis, restriction endonuclease fingerprinting-single strand conformation polymorphism, RNA-based sequencing, enzymatic mutation detection, and multiple-dye cleavase fragment length polymorphism testing all required further evaluation. Denaturing high-performance liquid chromatography outperformed most testing methods.

Other than *BRCA1* and *BRCA2* testing, molecular testing for different ovarian malignancies is uncommon. As our knowledge of the molecular pathology underlying these tumors increases, molecular diagnostic testing will likely play an increasingly important role in the clinical management of these tumors.

12.4.10 Management of Patients with BRCA *Mutations*

Women with identified *BRCA* mutations should be clinically followed. In addition, their relatives, who might have *BRCA* mutations, should receive genetic counseling and molecular testing specific for the identified *BRCA* mutation [125]. Specifically, the following tests should be considered.

12.4.10.1 Cancer Screening

Women with identified *BRCA* mutations should undergo regular cancer screening, including mammography and clinical breast exams. Magnetic resonance imaging may also be useful for the early detection of breast cancer. Additionally, ovarian cancer screening should be via blood testing for CA-125 and transvaginal ultrasound.

12.4.10.2 Prophylactic Surgery

Bilateral prophylactic risk-reducing mastectomy and salpingo-oophorectomy may lower cancer risk but not eliminate it. Some data suggest that these risk-reducing prophylactic surgeries may have different efficacies between *BRCA1* and *–2* mutation carriers [137].

12.4.10.3 Chemoprevention

Tamoxifen may lower the breast cancer risk in women with *BRCA1* and BRCA*2* mutations [145, 146]. Interestingly, tamoxifen reduced the risk of developing breast cancer in the opposite breast of women being treated for an initial breast cancer [138, 139].

12.4.10.4 Risk Avoidance

Although there is little evidence indicating that avoiding cancer risk factors lowers the risks for breast and ovarian cancers, the National Cancer Institute recommends that women with *BRCA* mutations avoid known risk factors for these malignancies, such as obesity and smoking [125].

12.5 Endometrial Cancer

12.5.1 Epidemiology and Types

Uterine cancer is the most common gynecologic malignancy in the United States, with ~40,100 women diagnosed with endometrial cancer in 2008 and 7,470 dying of the disease [2, 68, 140]. Although the disease presents at an early stage with vaginal bleeding and is usually diagnosed at an earlier stage than ovarian cancers, the mortality rate has not decreased in 15 years for women presenting with distant metastases [140, 141]. Additionally, a subset of endometrial histologic subtypes, such as the serous, clear cell, and malignant mixed Mullerian tumor (MMMT) carry a poor prognosis [142]. Bokhman examined 366 patients with endometrial carcinomas and broadly divided the malignancies into two types based on distinct clinicopathologic features [143].

Type 1 accounts for ~65 % of endometrial carcinomas arising from a background of obesity, hyperlipidemia, and signs of hyperestrogenism such as anovulatory bleeding, infertility, endometrial and ovarian stromal hyperplasia, and late onset menopause. These malignancies are estrogen dependent, usually highly or moderately differentiated tumors with superficial myometrial invasion, and have a favorable prognosis. The prototypic Type 1 endometrial malignancy is endometrioid carcinoma.

Type 2 accounts for ~35 % of endometrial malignancies and does not arise in the clinicophysiologic setting of type 1 malignancies. They are estrogen insensitive, occur in older women, are more likely to be poorly differentiated, deeply invade the myometrium, and have metastases to the pelvic lymph nodes. They have few known risk factors and overall carry a poorer prognosis.

12.5.2 Uterine Endometrial Adenocarcinoma (UEA)

Uterine endometrial adenocarcinoma (UEA) arises in a setting of unopposed estrogen and is typically well-differentiated and has a good prognosis. Tamoxifen has been found to mildly increase the risk of UEA secondary to its weak estrogenic effects on the endometrium. It also increases endometrial cell proliferation, endometrial polyps, and endometrial hyperplasia [144–146].

12.5.2.1 PTEN

Like the ovarian endometrial adenocarcinoma, *PTEN* is commonly mutated in UEA. In fact, up to 83 % of UEAs show inactivating *PTEN* mutations [147–149]. As in the ovary, *PTEN* activity loss results in the activation of the signaling pathway that promotes cell growth and survival [85]. As expected, endometrial hyperplasia also shows PTEN mutations, with complex atypical hyperplasia having ~22 % *PTEN* mutations. 88 % of PTEN mutations occur in exons 5, 7, and 8, with frameshift, nonsense, missense, and silent mutations identified. Some data indicate that PTEN mutation also confers a better prognosis [150–152].

12.5.2.2 PIK3CA

PIK3CA is found at 3q26.32 and is a phosphatidylinositol 3-kinase family member that promotes cell proliferation, motility, and cell invasion, via AKT and PDK1 activation [153–156]. *PIK3CA* is mutated in up to 36 % of UEAs, and, as in colon cancers, it can coexist with *PTEN* and *KRAS* mutations [150]. Interestingly, *PIK3CA* mutation combined with p53 mutation/loss results in malignant transformation and a shorter survival time than in individuals with p53 mutations only [157]. Commonly, *PIK3CA* has missense exon 9 mutations, with mutations in exon 20 correlating with more aggressive tumor behavior [157].

12.5.2.3 KRAS

KRAS mutations are detected in up to 10–30 % of UEAs, occurring with approximately the same frequency in endometrial hyperplasias [150, 158]. *KRAS* mutations do not correlate with age of onset, histology, differentiation, or clinical stage and appear to have no prognostic value [158].

12.5.2.4 β-Catenin

Beta-catenin is mutated in UEAs as is its ovarian counterpart, and its accumulation is easily identified with immunohistochemistry [150]. β-*catenin* is mutated in 31–47 % of UEAs, and 0–3 % of endometrial malignancies without endometrioid histology [149].

12.5.3 Uterine Serous Carcinoma

Uterine serous carcinoma (USC) is a Type 2 malignancy, accounting for 10 % of endometrial carcinomas and pursues an aggressive clinical course compared to UEAs [143, 150].

12.5.3.1 p53

At least 90 % of USCs carry p53 mutations, with p53 overexpression readily identified by immunohistochemistry. Interestingly, p53 overexpression is also often in benign-appearing endometrial glands. Molecular analyses have demonstrated that the specific p53 mutations found are the same as in nearby USC, likely indicating that p53 mutations precede USC [159, 160].

12.5.3.2 HER2/neu

HER2/neu is expressed in ~60 % of USC, often with moderate to strong expression [161].

12.5.3.3 WT1

Approximately 97 % of ovarian serous carcinomas are WT1 positive, while USCs are not. This immunohistochemical difference has been useful in identifying tumor origin in metastases [162].

12.5.3.4 Uterine Clear Cell Carcinoma

Uterine clear cell carcinoma (UCCC) accounts for ~5 % of endometrial carcinomas. *PTEN* and *p53* mutations have been identified in UCCC, although at low frequencies. UCCCs appear to be heterogeneous malignancies that arise by presently unknown molecular pathway(s) [163].

12.5.4 Malignant Mixed Mullerian Tumors

Malignant mixed mullerian tumor (MMMT), also known as a carcinosarcoma, is a highly aggressive Type 2 malignancy. MMMTs are biphasic, having both epithelial and sarcomatous components. MMMTs show high p53 mutation frequency in both tumor components [143, 164].

12.5.5 Endometrial Stromal Tumors

Endometrial stromal tumors (ESTs) are rare uterine malignancies comprising ~15 % of uterine sarcomas and ~1 % of uterine malignancies [165]. Molecular diagnostics plays almost no role in the analysis of these tumors. ESTs have a high degree of morphologic and cytogenetic heterogeneity, making diagnosis difficult in some cases. Approximately 50 % of low-grade ESTs carry a *JAZF1/JJAZ1* gene fusion [166]. Combined with other established methods, analysis of this gene fusion may have value in the diagnosis of difficult cases [166].

12.6 Lynch Syndrome or Hereditary Nonpolyposis Colorectal Cancer

Hereditary nonpolyposis colorectal cancer (HNPCC) is the most common cause of hereditary colorectal carcinoma [167]. HNPCC shows an autosomal dominant inheritance and results from the loss of one or more DNA mismatched repair genes (*MLH1, MSH2, MSH6n* and *PMS2*), resulting in a specific form of genomic instability [168, 169]. HNPCC-associated extracolonic tumors include endometrial, ovarian, sebaceous, gastric, small intestinal, pancreatic, brain, hepatobiliary tract, and upper urothelial cancers [167–169]. Interestingly, women with *MSH6* mutations have a higher rate of endometrial tumors than colorectal carcinoma [170]. Molecular diagnostic testing for HNPCC is covered in Chap. 5, regarding colorectal carcinoma

12.7 Vulva

Cancer of the vulva is often associated with HPV infection, with the HPV E6 and E7 proteins playing a role in carcinogenesis [10, 14–20]. Molecular diagnostics is seldom employed in the clinical management of vulvar malignancies. p53, CHK2, and PTEN mutations have been identified in subsets of vulvar carcinomas [171, 172]. Last, although aggressive angiomyxomas have translocations involving 12q14-15, this work is in its early phase and as yet is not used in the diagnosis of these rare tumors [173].

12.8 Vagina

Like the vulva, vaginal cancer is often HPV-related, with ~50 % of malignancies having detectable p53 mutations [10, 174, 175]. Molecular diagnostics is seldom used in the management of these malignancies.

12.9 Fallopian Tube

Malignancies of the fallopian tubes seldom require molecular diagnostics for their diagnosis and clinical management. The fallopian tubes appear to be a common location for precursor lesions of high-grade serous ovarian carcinoma [176].

12.10 Hydatidiform Moles

Two different hydatidiform mole types exist, with each one having a different appearance and etiology (partial or complete). Histologically, in the complete mole, the villi are typically cystic and embryonic development is usually absent. In the partial mole, embryonic development is seen and a range of normal and abnormal cystic villi are present. At the molecular level the complete mole is diploid, with all 46 chromosomes being of paternal origin. Partial moles are triploid. The extra haploid chromosome set can have either a maternal origin (digynic triploidy) or a paternal origin (diandric triploidy) [177].

The ability to distinguish between non-moles, complete-, and incomplete moles is important in the clinical management and accurate risk assessment for gestational trophoblastic disease. However, the diagnosis of hydatidiform moles based solely on morphology suffers from poor interobserver reproducibility; therefore, several ancillary techniques are employed to assist in the diagnosis of these tumors [177, 178]. Short tandem repeat genotyping can identify the parental source of polymorphic alleles, allowing a specific diagnosis [178]. Although currently not in widespread use, molar testing is being clinically employed.

12.11 Conclusion

Gynecologic malignancies account for ~13 % of solid tumors in women. Although the diagnosis of these malignancies is largely dependent on histologic examination of hematoxylin-eosin-stained slides, molecular studies are becoming increasingly important in establishing a diagnosis, determining prognosis, and clinically managing these malignancies. Additionally, molecular studies are required for the diagnosis, management, and genetic counseling of individuals with hereditary gynecologic malignancies, such as those secondary to BRCA1 mutations. As the field of molecular diagnostics continues to grow, the expenses associated with testing diminish, and a more complete understanding of the molecular pathology underlying gynecologic malignancies is attained, the role for molecular testing in this area will increase.

Acknowledgement We would like to thank Miss Jennifer Burton for her help in manuscript preparation and proof reading.

References

1. American Cancer Society (2000) Cancer facts and figures-2000. American Cancer Society, Atlanta
2. Parkin DM (2005) Global cancer statistics. CA J Clin 55:74–108
3. American Cancer Society (2006) The worldwide cancer burden. American Cancer Society, Atlanta
4. Allison M (2008) Is personalized medicine finally arriving? Nat Biotechnol 26:509–517

5. Brown ML, Lipscomb J, Snyder C (2001) The burden of illness of cancer: economic cost and quality of life. Annu Rev Public Health 22:91–113
6. Munoz N, Bosch FX, de Sanjose S, Herrero R, Castellsague X, Shah KV, Snijders PJ, Meijer CJ, International Agency for Research on Cancer Multicenter Cervical Cancer Study Group (2003) Epidemiologic classification of human papillomavirus types associated with cervical cancer. N Engl J Med 348:518–527
7. Bosch FX, de Sanjose S (2002) Human papillomavirus in cervical cancer. Curr Oncol Rep 4:175–183
8. Li S, Hursting SD, Davis BJ, McLachlan JA, Barrett JC (2003) Environmental exposure, DNA methylation, and gene regulation: lessons from diethylstilbesterol-induced cancers. Ann N Y Acad Sci 983:161–169
9. de Villiers EM, Fauquet C, Broker TR, Bernard HU, zur Hausen H (2004) Classification of papillomaviruses. Virology 324:17–27
10. Shukla S, Bharti AC, Mahata S, Hussain S, Kumar R, Hedau S, Das BC (2009) Infection of human papillomaviruses in cancers of different human organ sites. Indian J Med Res 130:222–233
11. Lorincz AT, Reid R, Jensen AB, Greenberg MD, Lancaster W, Kurman RJ (1992) Human papillomavirus infection of the cervix: relative risk associations of 15 common anogenital types. Obstet Gynecol 79:328–337
12. Wang SS, Zuna RE, Wentzensen N, Dunn ST, Sherman ME, Gold MA, Schiffman M, Wacholder S, Allen RA, Block I, Downing K, Jeronimo J, Carreon JD, Safaeian M, Brown D, Walker JL (2009) Human papillomavirus cofactors by disease progression and human papillomavirus types in the study to understand cervical cancer early endpoints and determinants. Cancer Epidemiol Biomarkers Prev 18:113–120
13. Szostek S, Zawilinska B, Kopec J, Kosz-Vnenchak M (2009) Herpesviruses as possible cofactors in HPV-16-related oncogenesis. Acta Biochim Pol 56:337–342
14. Howley PM, Lowy DR (2001) In: Knipe DM et al (eds) Papillomaviruses and their replication. Lippincott Williams & Wilkins, Philadelphia, pp 2197–2230
15. McGlennen RC (2000) Human papillomavirus oncogenesis. Clin Lab Med 20:383–406
16. Pett M, Coleman N (2007) Integration of high-risk human papillomavirus: a key event in cervical carcinogenesis? J Pathol 212:356–367
17. Jeon S, Allen-Hoffmann BL, Lambert PF (1995) Integration of human papillomavirus type 16 into the human genome correlates with a selective growth advantage of cells. J Virol 69:2989–2997
18. Romanczuk H, Howley PM (1992) Disruption of either the E1 or the E2 regulatory gene of human papillomavirus type 16 increases viral immortalization capacity. Proc Natl Acad Sci U S A 89:3159–3163
19. Romanczuk H, Thierry F, Howley PM (1990) Mutational analysis of cis elements involved in E2 modulation of human papillomavirus type 16 P97 and type 18 P105 promoters. J Virol 64:2849–2859
20. Shackelford RE, Kaufmann WK, Paules RS (1999) Cell cycle control, checkpoint mechanisms, and genotoxic stress. Environ Health Perspect 107(Suppl 1):5–24
21. Kadaja M, Isok-Paas H, Laos T, Ustav E, Ustav M (2009) Mechanism of genomic instability in cells infected with the high-risk human papillomaviruses. PLoS Pathog 5:e1000397
22. Taichman LB, Reilly SS, LaPorta RF (1983) The role of keratinocyte differentiation in the expression of epitheliotropic viruses. J Invest Dermatol 81(1 Suppl):137s–140s
23. Koss LG, Durfee GR (1956) Unusual patterns of squamous epithelium of the uterine cervix: cytologic and histologic study of koilocytotic atypia. Ann N Y Acad Sci 63:1245–1261
24. Pirog EC, Baergen RN, Soslow RA, Tam D, DeMattia AE, Chen YT, Isacson C (2002) Diagnostic accuracy of cervical low-grade squamous intraepithelial lesions is improved with MIB-1 immunostaining. Am J Surg Pathol 26:70–75
25. Logani S, Lu D, Quint WG, Ellenson LH, Pirog EC (2003) Low-grade vulvar and vaginal intraepithelial neoplasia: correlation of histologic features with human papillomavirus DNA detection and MIB-1 immunostaining. Mod Pathol 16:735–741

26. Wheeler CM, Parmenter CA, Hunt WC, Becker TM, Greer CE, Hildesheim A, Manos MM (1993) Determinants of genital human papillomavirus infection among cytologically normal women attending the University of New Mexico student health center. Sex Transm Dis 20:286–289
27. Denny L, Kuhn L, Pollack A, Wainwright H, Wright TC Jr (2000) Evaluation of alternative methods of cervical cancer screening for resource-poor settings. Cancer 89:826–833
28. Bauer HM, Hildesheim A, Schiffman MH, Glass AG, Rush BB, Scott DR, Cadell DM, Kurman RJ, Manos MM (1993) Determinants of genital human papillomavirus infection in low-risk women in Portland, Oregon. Sex Transm Dis 20:274–278
29. Bosch FX, de Sanjosé S (2007) The epidemiology of human papillomavirus infection and cervical cancer. Dis Markers 23:213–227
30. Fonatsch C, Duchrow M, Rieder H, Schlüter C, Gerdes J (1991) Assignment of the human Ki-67 gene (MK167) to 10q25-qter. Genomics 11:476–477
31. Gerdes J, Lemke H, Baisch H, Wacker H-H, Schwab U, Stein H (1984) Cell cycle analysis of a cell proliferation-associated human nuclear antigen defined by the monoclonal antibody Ki-67. J Immunol 133:1710–1715
32. Schlüter C, Duchrow M, Wohlenberg C, Becker MH, Key G, Flad HD, Gerdes J (1993) The cell proliferation-associated antigen of antibody Ki-67: a very large, ubiquitous nuclear protein with numerous repeated elements, representing a new kind of cell cycle-maintaining proteins. J Cell Biol 123:513–522
33. Payne S, Kernohan NM, Walker F (1996) Proliferation in the normal cervix and in preinvasive cervical lesions. J Clin Pathol 49:667–671
34. Isacson C, Kessis TD, Hedrick L, Cho KR (1996) Both cell proliferation and apoptosis increase with lesion grade in cervical neoplasia but do not correlate with human papillomavirus type. Cancer Res 56:669–674
35. Sahebali S, Depuydt CE, Segers K, Vereecken AJ, Van Marck E, Bogers JJ (2003) Ki-67 immunocytochemistry in liquid based cervical cytology: useful as an adjunctive tool? Clin Pathol 56:681–686
36. Scurry J, Beshay V, Cohen C, Allen D (1998) Ki67 expression in lichen sclerosus of vulva in patients with and without associated squamous cell carcinoma. Histopathology 32: 399–404
37. Serrano M, Hannon GJ, Beach D (1993) A new regulatory motif in cell cycle control causing specific inhibition of cycling D/CDK4. Nature 366:704–707
38. Cobrinik D, Dowdy SF, Hinds PW, Mittnacht S, Weinberg RA (1992) The retinoblastoma protein and the regulation of cell cycling. Trends Biochem Sci 17:312–315
39. Mantovani F, Banks L (2001) The human papillomavirus E6 protein and its contribution to malignant progression. Oncogene 20:7874–7887
40. Munger K, Basile JR, Duensing S, Eichten A, Gonzalez SL, Grace M, Zacny VL (2001) Biological activities and molecular targets of the human papillomavirus E7 oncoprotein. Oncogene 20:7888–7898
41. Khleif SN, DeGregori J, Yee CL, Otterson GA, Kaye FJ, Nevins JR, Howley PM (1996) Inhibition of cyclin D-CDK4/CDK6 activity is associated with an E2F-mediated induction of cyclin kinase inhibitor activity. Proc Natl Acad Sci U S A 93:4350–4354
42. Cuschieri K, Wentzensen N (2008) Human papillomavirus mRNA and p16 detection as biomarkers for the improved diagnosis of cervical neoplasia. Cancer Epidemiol Biomarkers Prev 17:2536–2545
43. Horree N, Heintz AP, Sie-Go DM, van Diest PJ (2007) p16 is consistently expressed in endometrial tubal metaplasia. Cell Oncol 29:37–45
44. Bryce LA, Morrison N, Hoare SF, Muir S, Keith WN (2000) Mapping of the gene for the human telomerase reverse transcriptase, hTERT, to chromosome 5p15.33 by fluorescence in situ hybridization. Neoplasia 2:197–201
45. Nakamura TM, Morin GB, Chapman KB, Weinrich SL, Andrews WH, Lingner J, Harley CB, Cech TR (1997) Telomerase catalytic subunit homologs from fission yeast and human. Science 277:955–959

46. Kim NW, Piatyszek MA, Prowse KR, Harley CB, West MD, Ho PL, Coviello GM, Wright WE, Weinrich SL, Shay JW (1994) Specific association of human telomerase activity with immortal cells and cancer. Science 266:2011–2015
47. Kailash U, Soundararajan CC, Lakshmy R, Arora R, Vivekanandhan S, Das BC (2006) Telomerase activity as an adjunct to high-risk human papillomavirus types 16 and 18 and cytology screening in cervical cancer. Br J Cancer 95(9):1250–1257, Epub 2006 Oct 24
48. Sui W, Ou M, Dai Y, Chen J, Lan H, Yan Q, Huang H (2009) Gain of the human telomerase RNA gene TERC at 3q26 is strongly associated with cervical intraepithelial neoplasia and carcinoma. Int J Gynecol Cancer 19:1303–1306
49. Ancuţa E, Ancuţa C, Cozma LG, Iordache C, Anghelache-Lupaşcu I, Anton E, Carasevici E, Chirieac R (2009) Tumor biomarkers in cervical cancer: focus on Ki-67 proliferation factor and E-cadherin expression. Rom J Morphol Embryol 50:413–418
50. Yang A, Kaghad M, Wang Y, Gillett E, Fleming MD, Dötsch V, Andrews NC, Caput D, McKeon F (1998) p63, a p53 homolog at 3q27–29, encodes multiple products with transactivating, death-inducing, and dominant-negative activities. Mol Cell 2:305–316
51. Shirendeb U, Hishikawa Y, Moriyama S, Win N, Thu MM, Mar KS, Khatanbaatar G, Masuzaki H, Koji T (2009) Human papillomavirus infection and its possible correlation with p63 expression in cervical cancer in Japan, Mongolia, and Myanmar. Acta Histochem Cytoc 42:181–190
52. Khan MJ, Castle PE, Lorincz AT, Wacholder S, Sherman M, Scott DR, Rush BB, Glass AG, Schiffman M (2005) The elevated 10-year risk of cervical precancer and cancer in women with human papillomavirus (HPV) type 16 or 18 and the possible utility of type-specific HPV testing in clinical practice. Natl Cancer Inst 97:1072–1079
53. Gravitt PE, Kovacic MB, Herrero R, Schiffman M, Bratti C, Hildesheim A, Morales J, Alfaro M, Sherman ME, Wacholder S, Rodriguez AC, Burk RD (2007) High load for most high risk human papillomavirus genotypes is associated with prevalent cervical cancer precursors but only HPV16 load predicts the development of incident disease. Int J Cancer 121:2787–2793
54. Lamarcq L, Deeds J, Ginzinger D, Perry J, Padmanabha S, Smith-McCune K (2002) Measurements of human papillomavirus transcripts by real time quantitative reverse transcription-polymerase chain reaction in samples collected for cervical cancer screening. J Mol Diagn 4:97–102
55. Gharizadeh B, Oggionni M, Zheng B, Akom E, Pourmand N, Ahmadian A, Wallin KL, Nyrén P (2005) Type-specific multiple sequencing primers: a novel strategy for reliable and rapid genotyping of human papillomaviruses by pyrosequencing technology. J Mol Diagn 7:198–205
56. Schiffman MH, Kiviat NB, Burk RD, Shah KV, Daniel RW, Lewis R, Kuypers J, Manos MM, Scott DR, Sherman ME et al (1995) Accuracy and interlaboratory reliability of human papillomavirus DNA testing by hybrid capture. J Clin Microbiol 33:545–550
57. Negri G, Rigo B, Vittadello F, Egarter-Vigl E, Mian C (2004) Human papillomavirus typing with hybrid capture II on archived liquid-based cytologic specimens: is HPV typing always reproducible? Am J Clin Pathol 122:90–93
58. Brosens LA, van Hattem WA, Jansen M, de Leng WW, Giardiello FM, Offerhaus GJ (2007) Gastrointestinal polyposis syndromes. Curr Mol Med 7:29–46
59. Boardman LA, Thibodeau SN, Schaid DJ, Lindor NM, McDonnell SK, Burgart LJ, Ahlquist DA, Podratz KC, Pittelkow M, Hartmann LC (1998) Increased risk for cancer in patients with the Peutz-Jeghers syndrome. Ann Intern Med 128:896–899
60. Giardiello FM, Welsh SB, Hamilton SR, Offerhaus GJ, Gittelsohn AM, Booker SV, Krush AJ, Yardley JH, Luk GD (1987) Increased risk of cancer in the Peutz-Jeghers syndrome. N Engl J Med 316:1511–1514
61. Karuman P, Gozani O, Odze RD et al (2001) The Peutz–Jegher gene product LKB1 is a mediator of p53-dependent cell death. Mol Cell 7:1307–1319
62. Gong L, Zhang WD, Liu XY, Han XJ, Yao L, Zhu SJ, Lan M, Li YH, Zhang W (2010) Clonal status and clinicopathological observation of cervical minimal deviation adenocarcinoma. Diagn Pathol 5:25

63. Young RH (2005) Sex cord-stromal tumors of the ovary and testis: their similarities and differences with consideration of selected problems. Mod Pathol 18(Suppl 2):S81–S98
64. Howe JR, Roth S, Ringold JC, Summers RW, Järvinen HJ, Sistonen P, Tomlinson IP, Houlston RS, Bevan S, Mitros FA, Stone EM, Aaltonen LA (1998) Mutations in the SMAD4/DPC4 gene in juvenile polyposis. Science 280:1086–1088
65. Calva-Cerqueira D, Chinnathambi S, Pechman B, Bair J, Larsen-Haidle J, Howe JR (2009) The rate of germline mutations and large deletions of SMAD4 and BMPR1A in juvenile polyposis. Clin Genet 75:79–85
66. Sweet K, Willis J, Zhou XP, Gallione C, Sawada T, Alhopuro P, Khoo SK, Patocs A, Martin C, Bridgeman S, Heinz J, Pilarski R, Lehtonen R, Prior TW, Frebourg T, Teh BT, Marchuk DA, Aaltonen LA, Eng C (2005) Molecular classification of patients with unexplained hamartomatous and hyperplastic polyposis. JAMA 294:2465–2473
67. Tavassoli FA, Devilee P (eds) (2003) World Health Organization classification of tumors: pathology and genetics. Tumours of the breast and female genital organs. IARC, Lyon
68. Gilks CB, Prat J (2009) Ovarian carcinoma pathology and genetics: recent advances. Hum Pathol 40:1213–1223
69. Auersperg N, Ota T, Mitchell GW (2002) Early events in ovarian epithelial carcinogenesis: progress and problems in experimental approaches. Int J Gynecol Cancer 12:691–703
70. Brown ML, Riley GF, Schussler N, Etzioni RD (2002) Estimated health care costs related to cancer treatment from SEER-Medicare data. Medical Care 40(8 Suppl):IV104–IV117
71. Gilks CB (2010) Molecular abnormalities in ovarian cancer subtypes other than high-grade serous carcinoma. J Oncol 2010:740968
72. Malumbres M, Barbacid M (2003) RAS oncogenes: the first 30 years. Nat Rev Cancer 3:459–465
73. Der CJ, Krontiris TG, Cooper GM (1982) Transforming genes of human bladder and lung carcinoma cell lines are homologous to the ras genes of Harvey and Kirsten sarcoma viruses. Proc Natl Acad Sci U S A 79:3637–3640
74. Graziani A, Gramaglia D, dalla Zonca P, Comoglio PM (1993) Hepatocyte growth factor/scatter factor stimulates the Ras-guanine nucleotide exchanger. J Biol Chem 268:9165–9168
75. Hu YP, Patil SB, Panasiewicz M, Li W, Hauser J, Humphrey LE, Brattain MG (2008) Heterogeneity of receptor function in colon carcinoma cells determined by cross-talk between type I insulin-like growth factor receptor and epidermal growth factor receptor. Cancer Res 68:8004–8013
76. Bos JL (1989) Ras oncogenes in human cancer: a review. Cancer Res 49:4682–4689
77. Yarden Y, Sliwkowski MX (2001) Untangling the ErbB signaling network. Nat Rev Mol Cell Biol 2:127–137
78. Singer G, Oldt R 3rd, Cohen Y, Wang BG, Sidransky D, Kurman RJ, Shih I-M (2003) Mutations in BRAF and KRAS characterize the development of low-grade ovarian serous carcinoma. J Natl Cancer Inst 95:484–486
79. Körner M, Burckhardt E, Mazzucchelli L (2006) Higher frequency of chromosomal aberrations in ovarian endometriosis compared to extragonadal endometriosis: a possible link to endometrioid adenocarcinoma. Mod Pathol 19:1615–1623
80. Barault L, Veyrie N, Jooste V, Lecorre D, Chapusot C, Ferraz JM, Lièvre A, Cortet M, Bouvier AM, Rat P, Roignot P, Faivre J, Laurent-Puig P, Piard F (2008) Mutations in the RAS-MAPK, PI(3)K (phosphatidylinositol-3-OH kinase) signaling network correlate with poor survival in a population-based series of colon cancers. Int J Cancer 122:2255–2259
81. Loupakis F, Ruzzo A, Cremolini C, Vincenzi B, Salvatore L, Santini D, Masi G, Stasi I, Canestrari E, Rulli E, Floriani I, Bencardino K, Galluccio N, Catalano V, Tonini G, Magnani M, Fontanini G, Basolo F, Falcone A, Graziano F (2009) KRAS codon 61, 146 and BRAF mutations predict resistance to cetuximab plus irinotecan in KRAS codon 12 and 13 wild-type metastatic colorectal cancer. Br J Cancer 101:715–721
82. Benvenuti S, Sartore-Bianchi A, Di Nicolantonio F, Zanon C, Moroni M, Veronese S, Siena S, Bardelli A (2007) Oncogenic activation of the RAS/RAF signaling pathway impairs the response of metastatic colorectal cancers to anti-epidermal growth factor receptor antibody therapies. Cancer Res 67:2643–2648

83. Mayr D, Hirschmann A, Löhrs U, Diebold J (2006) KRAS and BRAF mutations in ovarian tumors: a comprehensive study of invasive carcinomas, borderline tumors and extraovarian implants. Gynecol Oncol 103(3):883–887
84. Ueda M, Toji E, Noda S (2007) Germ line and somatic mutations of BRAF V599E in ovarian carcinoma. Int J Gynecol Cancer 17:794–797
85. Chen YL, Law PY, Loh HH (2005) Inhibition of PI3K/Akt signaling: an emerging paradigm for targeted cancer therapy. Curr Med Chem Anticancer Agents 5:575–589
86. Thomas EJ, Campbell IG (2000) Molecular genetic defects in endometriosis. Gynecol Obstet Invest 50:44–50
87. Obata K, Hoshiai H (2000) Common genetic changes between endometriosis and ovarian cancer. Gynecol Obstet Invest 50:39–43
88. Oliva E, Sarrio D, Brachtel EF, Sánchez-Estévez C, Soslow RA, Moreno-Bueno G, Palacios J (2006) High frequency of beta-catenin mutations in borderline endometrioid tumours of the ovary. J Pathol 208:708–713
89. Ilyas M, Tomlinson IP (1997) The interactions of APC, E-cadherin and beta-catenin in tumour development and progression. J Pathol 182:128–137
90. van Es JH, Barker N, Clevers H (2003) You Wnt some, you lose some: oncogenes in the Wnt signaling pathway. Curr Opin Genet Dev 13:28–33
91. Palacios J, Gamallo C (1998) Mutations in the beta-catenin gene (CTNNB1) in endometrioid ovarian carcinomas. Cancer Res 58:1344–1347
92. Dinulescu DM, Ince TA, Quade BJ, Shafer SA, Crowley D, Jacks T (2005) Role of K-ras and Pten in the development of mouse models of endometriosis and endometrioid ovarian cancer. Nat Med 11:63–70
93. Wu R, Hendrix-Lucas N, Kuick R, Zhai Y, Schwartz DR, Akyol A, Hanash S, Misek DE, Katabuchi H, Williams BO, Fearon ER, Cho KR (2007) Mouse model of human ovarian endometrioid adenocarcinoma based on somatic defects in the Wnt/beta-catenin and PI3K/Pten signaling pathways. Cancer Cell 11:321–333
94. Enomoto T, Weghorst CM, Inoue M, Tanizawa O, Rice JM (1991) K-ras activation occurs frequently in mucinous adenocarcinomas and rarely in other common epithelial tumors of the human ovary. Am J Pathol 139:777–785
95. Cuatrecasas M, Villanueva A, Matias-Guiu X, Prat J (1997) K-ras mutations in mucinous ovarian tumors: a clinicopathologic and molecular study of 95 cases. Cancer 79: 1581–1586
96. Karaferic A, Jovanovic D, Jelic S (2009) Expression of HER2/neu, estrogen and progesterone receptors, CA 125 and CA19-9 on cancer cell membrane in patients with serous and mucinous carcinoma of the ovary. J BUON 14:635–639
97. Kuo KT, Mao TL, Jones S, Veras E, Ayhan A, Wang TL, Glas R, Slamon D, Velculescu VE, Kuman RJ, Shih I-M (2009) Frequent activating mutations of PIK3CA in ovarian clear cell carcinoma. Am J Pathol 174:1597–1601
98. Kuo KT, Mao TL, Chen X, Feng Y, Nakayama K, Wang Y, Glas R, Ma MJ, Kurman RJ, Shih IM, Wang TL (2010) DNA copy numbers profiles in affinity-purified ovarian clear cell carcinoma. Clin Cancer Res 16:1997–2008
99. Cossu-Rocca P, Zhang S, Roth LM, Eble JN, Zheng W, Karim FW, Michael H, Emerson RE, Jones TD, Hattab EM, Cheng L (2006) Chromosome 12p abnormalities in dysgerminoma of the ovary: a FISH analysis. Mod Pathol 19:611–615
100. Hoei-Hansen CE, Kraggerud SM, Abeler VM, Kaern J, Rajpert-De Meyts E, Lothe RA (2007) Ovarian dysgerminomas are characterised by frequent KIT mutations and abundant expression of pluripotency markers. Mol Cancer 6:12
101. Tian Q, Frierson HF Jr, Krystal GW, Moskaluk CA (1999) Activating c-kit gene mutations in human germ cell tumors. Am J Pathol 154:1643–1647
102. Pauls K, Wardelmann E, Merkelbach-Bruse S, Büttner R, Zhou H (2004) c-KIT codon 816 mutation in a recurrent and metastatic dysgerminoma of a 14-year-old girl: case study. Virchows Arch 445:651–654

103. Benayoun BA, Caburet S, Dipietromaria A, Georges A, D'Haene B, Pandaranayaka PJ, L'Hôte D, Todeschini AL, Krishnaswamy S, Fellous M, De Baere E, Veitia RA (2010) Functional exploration of the adult ovarian granulosa cell tumor-associated somatic FOXL2 mutation p.Cys134Trp (c.402C>G). PLoS One 5:e8789
104. Kalfa N, Philibert P, Patte C, Ecochard A, Duvillard P, Baldet P, Jaubert F, Fellous M, Sultan C (2007) Extinction of FOXL2 expression in aggressive ovarian granulosa cell tumors in children. Fertil Steril 87:896–901
105. Shah SP, Kobel M, Senz J, Morin RD, Clarke BA et al (2009) Mutation of FOXL2 in granulosa-cell tumors of the ovary. N Engl J Med 360:2719–2729
106. Crisponi L, Deiana M, Loi A, Chiappe F, Uda M et al (2001) The putative forkhead transcription factor FOXL2 is mutated in blepharophimosis/ptosis/ epicanthus inversus syndrome. Nat Genet 27:159–166
107. Cocquet J, De Baere E, Gareil M, Pannetier M, Xia X, Fellous M, Veitia RA (2003) Structure, evolution and expression of the FOXL2 transcription unit. Cytogenet Genome Res 101:206–211
108. Anglesio MS, Arnold JM, George J, Tinker AV, Tothill R, Waddell N, Simms L, Locandro B, Fereday S, Traficante N, Russell P, Sharma R, Birrer MJ, AOCS Study Group, deFazio A, Chenevix-Trench G, Bowtell DD (2008) Mutation of ERBB2 provides a novel alternative mechanism for the ubiquitous activation of RAS-MAPK in ovarian serous low malignant potential tumors. Mol Cancer Res 6:1678–1690
109. Dehari R, Kurman RJ, Logani S, Shih IM (2007) The development of high-grade serous carcinoma from atypical proliferative (borderline) serous tumors and low-grade micropapillary serous carcinoma: a morphologic and molecular genetic analysis. Am J Surg Pathol 31:1007–1012
110. Ahmed AA, Etemadmoghadam D, Temple J, Lynch AG, Riad M, Sharma R, Stewart C, Fereday S, Caldas C, Defazio A, Bowtell D, Brenton JD (2010) Driver mutations in TP53 are ubiquitous in high grade serous carcinoma of the ovary. J Pathol 221:49–56
111. Esteller M, Silva JM, Dominguez G, Bonilla F, Matias-Guiu X, Lerma E, Bussaglia E, Prat J, Harkes IC, Repasky EA, Gabrielson E, Schutte M, Baylin SB, Herman JG (2000) Promoter hypermethylation and BRCA1 inactivation in sporadic breast and ovarian tumors. J Natl Cancer Inst 92:564–569
112. Pal T, Permuth-Wey J, Betts JA, Krischer JP, Fiorica J, Arango H, LaPolla J, Hoffman M, Martino MA, Wakeley K, Wilbanks G, Nicosia S, Cantor A, Sutphen R (2005) BRCA1 and BRCA2 mutations account for a large proportion of ovarian carcinoma cases. Cancer 104:2807–2816
113. Thrall M, Gallion HH, Kryscio R, Kapali M, Armstrong DK, DeLoia JA (2006) BRCA1 expression in a large series of sporadic ovarian carcinomas: a Gynecologic Oncology Group study. Int J Gynecol Cancer 16(Suppl 1):166–171
114. Shackelford RE, Bui MM, Coppola D, Hakam A (2010) Over-expression of nicotinamide phosphoribosyltransferase in ovarian cancers. Int J Clin Exp Pathol 3:522–527
115. Garten A, Petzold S, Körner A, Imai S, Kiess W (2009) Nampt: linking NAD biology, metabolism and cancer. Trends Endocrinol Metab 20:130–138
116. Hasmann M, Schemainda I (2003) FK866, a highly specific noncompetitive inhibitor of nicotinamide phosphoribosyltransferase, represents a novel mechanism for induction of tumor cell apoptosis. Cancer Res 63:7436–7442
117. Pogrebniak A, Schemainda I, Azzam K, Pelka- Fleischer R, Nüssler V, Hasmann M (2006) Chemopotentiating effects of a novel NAD biosynthesis inhibitor, FK866, in combination with antineoplastic agents. Eur J Med Res 11:313–321
118. Szabo CI, King MC (1995) Inherited breast and ovarian cancer. Hum Mol Genet 4:1811–1817
119. Neuhausen S, Gilewski T, Norton L, Tran T, McGuire P, Swensen J, Hampel H, Borgen P, Brown K, Skolnick M, Shattuck-Eidens D, Jhanwar S, Goldgar D, Offit K (1996) Recurrent BRCA2 6174delT mutations in Ashkenazi Jewish women affected by breast cancer. Nat Genet 13:126–128

120. Struewing JP, Abeliovich D, Peretz T, Avishai N, Kaback MM, Collins FS, Brody LC (1995) The carrier frequency of the BRCA1 185delAG mutation is approximately 1 % in Ashkenazi Jewish individuals. Nat Genet 11:198–200
121. Ferla R, Calò V, Cascio S, Rinaldi G, Badalamenti G, Carreca I, Surmacz E, Colucci G, Bazan V, Russo A (2007) Founder mutations in BRCA1 and BRCA2 genes. Ann Oncol 18(Suppl 6):vi93–vi98
122. Wang Y, Cortez D, Yazdi P, Neff N, Elledge SJ, Qin J (2000) BASC, a super complex of BRCA1-associated proteins involved in the recognition and repair of aberrant DNA structures. Genes Dev 14:927–939
123. http://ghr.nlm.nih.gov/gene/BRCA1
124. http://ghr.nlm.nih.gov/gene/BRCA2
125. http://www.cancer.gov/cancertopics/factsheet/Risk/BRCA
126. King MC, Wieand S, Hale K, Lee M, Walsh T, Owens K, Tait J, Ford L, Dunn BK, Costantino J, Wickerham L, Wolmark N, Fisher B, National Surgical Adjuvant Breast and Bowel Project (2001) Tamoxifen and breast cancer incidence among women with inherited mutations in BRCA1 and BRCA2: National Surgical Adjuvant Breast and Bowel Project (NSABP-P1) Breast Cancer Prevention Trial. JAMA 286:2251–2256
127. Bellosillo B, Tusquets I (2006) Pitfalls and caveats in BRCA sequencing. Ultrastruct Pathol 30:229–235
128. Takano EA, Mitchell G, Fox SB, Dobrovic A (2008) Rapid detection of carriers with BRCA1 and BRCA2 mutations using high resolution melting analysis. BMC Cancer 8:59
129. Franklin WA, Haney J, Sugita M, Bemis L, Jimeno A, Messersmith WA (2010) KRAS mutation: comparison of testing methods and tissue sampling techniques in colon cancer. J Mol Diagn 12:43–50
130. Huang MM, Arnheim N, Goodman MF (1992) Extension of base mispairs by Taq DNA polymerase: implications for single nucleotide discrimination in PCR. Nucleic Acids Res 20:4567–4573
131. Abbaszadegan MR, Struewing JP, Brown KM, Snider JV, Goodsaid F, Gore-Langton R, Hughes MR (1997) Automated detection of prevalent mutations in BRCA1 and BRCA2 genes, using a fluorogenic PCR allelic discrimination assay. Genet Test 1:171–180
132. Powell SM, Petersen GM, Krush AJ, Booker S, Jen J, Giardiello FM, Hamilton SR, Vogelstein B, Kinzler KW (1993) Molecular diagnosis of familial adenomatous polyposis. N Engl J Med 329:1982–1987
133. Gerhardus A, Schleberger H, Schlegelberger B, Gadzicki D (2007) Diagnostic accuracy of methods for the detection of BRCA1 and BRCA2 mutations: a systematic review. Eur J Hum Genet 15:619–627
134. Kadouri L, Bercovich D, Elimelech A, Lerer I, Sagi M, Glusman G, Shochat C, Korem S, Hamburger T, Nissan A, Abu-Halaf N, Badrriyah M, Abeliovich D, Peretz T (2007) A novel BRCA-1 mutation in Arab kindred from east Jerusalem with breast and ovarian cancer. BMC Cancer 7:14
135. Vidal-Millán S, Taja-Chayeb L, Gutiérrez-Hernández O, Ramírez Ugalde MT, Robles-Vidal C, Bargallo-Rocha E, Mohar-Betancourt A, Dueñas-González A (2009) Mutational analysis of BRCA1 and BRCA2 genes in Mexican breast cancer patients. Eur J Gynaecol Oncol 30:527–530
136. Ratajska M, Brozek I, Senkus-Konefka E, Jassem J, Stepnowska M, Palomba G, Pisano M, Casula M, Palmieri G, Borg A, Limon J (2008) BRCA1 and BRCA2 point mutations and large rearrangements in breast and ovarian cancer families in Northern Poland. Oncol Rep 19:263–268
137. Kauff ND, Domchek SM, Friebel TM, Robson ME, Lee J, Garber JE, Isaacs C, Evans DG, Lynch H, Eeles RA, Neuhausen SL, Daly MB, Matloff E, Blum JL, Sabbatini P, Barakat RR, Hudis C, Norton L, Offit K, Rebbeck TR (2008) Risk-reducing salpingo-oophorectomy for the prevention of BRCA1- and BRCA2-associated breast and gynecologic cancer: a multicenter, prospective study. J Clin Oncol 26:1331–1337

138. Narod SA, Brunet JS, Ghadirian P, Robson M, Heimdal K, Neuhausen SL, Stoppa-Lyonnet D, Lerman C, Pasini B, de los Rios P, Weber B, Lynch H, Hereditary Breast Cancer Clinical Study Group (2000) Tamoxifen and risk of contralateral breast cancer in BRCA1 and BRCA2 mutation carriers: a case–control study. Hereditary Breast Cancer Clinical Study Group. Lancet 356:1876–1881
139. Gronwald J, Tung N, Foulkes WD, Offit K, Gershoni R, Daly M, Kim-Sing C, Olsson H, Ainsworth P, Eisen A, Saal H, Friedman E, Olopade O, Osborne M, Weitzel J, Lynch H, Ghadirian P, Lubinski J, Sun P, Narod SA, Hereditary Breast Cancer Clinical Study Group (2006) Tamoxifen and contralateral breast cancer in BRCA1 and BRCA2 carriers: an update. Int J Cancer 118:2281–2284
140. Jemal A, Siegel R, Ward E, Hao Y, Xu J, Murray T, Thun MJ (2008) Cancer statistics, 2008. CA Cancer J Clin 58:71–96
141. Han SS, Cho JY, Park IA, Park SK, Jeon YT, Kim JW, Park NH, Kang SB, Lee HP, Song YS (2008) Feasibility of routine lymphadenectomy in clinical stage-I endometrial cancer. Med Sci Monit 14:CR183–CR189
142. Cho KR (2009) Ovarian cancer update: lessons from morphology, molecules, and mice. Arch Pathol Lab Med 133:1775–1781
143. Bokhman JV (1983) Two pathogenetic types of endometrial carcinoma. Gynecol Oncol 15:10–17
144. Deligdisch L, Kalir T, Cohen CJ, de Latour M, Le Bouedec G, Penault-Llorca F (2000) Endometrial histopathology in 700 patients treated with tamoxifen for breast cancer. Gynecol Oncol 78:181–186
145. Fisher B, Costantino JP, Wickerham DL, Redmond CK, Kavanah M, Cronin WM, Vogel V, Robidoux A, Dimitrov N, Atkins J, Daly M, Wieand S, Tan-Chiu E, Ford L, Wolmark N (1998) Tamoxifen for prevention of breast cancer: report of the National Surgical Adjuvant Breast and Bowel Project P-1 Study. J Natl Cancer Inst 90(18):1371–1388
146. Mourits MJ, Ten Hoor KA, van der Zee AG, Willemse PH, de Vries EG, Hollema H (2002) The effects of tamoxifen on proliferation and steroid receptor expression in postmenopausal endometrium. J Clin Pathol 55:514–519
147. Lax SF (2004) Molecular genetic pathways in various types of endometrial carcinoma: from a phenotypical to a molecular-based classification. Virchows Arch 444:213–223
148. Hecht JL, Mutter GL (2006) Molecular and pathologic aspects of endometrial carcinogenesis. J Clin Oncol 24:4783–4791
149. Bansal N, Yendluri V, Wenham RM (2009) The molecular biology of endometrial cancers and the implications for pathogenesis, classification, and targeted therapies. Cancer Control 16:8–13
150. Levine RL, Cargile CB, Blazes MS, van Rees B, Kurman RJ, Ellenson LH (1998) PTEN mutations and microsatellite instability in complex atypical hyperplasia, a precursor lesion to uterine endometrioid carcinoma. Cancer Res 58:3254–3258
151. Sun H, Enomoto T, Fujita M, Wada H, Yoshino K, Ozaki K, Nakamura T, Murata Y (2001) Mutational analysis of the PTEN gene in endometrial carcinoma and hyperplasia. Am J Clin Pathol 115:32–38
152. Samarnthai N, Hall K, Yeh IT (2010) Molecular profiling of endometrial malignancies. Obstet Gynecol Int 2010:162363
153. Samuels Y, Velculescu VE (2004) Oncogenic mutations of PIK3CA in human cancers. Cell Cycle 3:1221–1224
154. Wong KK, Engelman JA, Cantley LC (2010) Targeting the PI3K signaling pathway in cancer. Curr Opin Genet Dev 20:87–90
155. Liu P, Cheng H, Roberts TM, Zhao JJ (2009) Targeting the phosphoinositide 3-kinase pathway in cancer. Nat Rev Drug Discov 8:627–644
156. Cantley LC (2002) The phosphoinositide 3-kinase pathway. Science 296:1655–1657
157. Catasus L, Gallardo A, Cuatrecasas M, Prat J (2009) Concomitant PI3K-AKT and p53 alterations in endometrial carcinomas are associated with poor prognosis. Mod Pathol 22:522–529

158. Dobrzycka B, Terlikowski SJ, Mazurek A, Kowalczuk O, Niklińska W, Chyczewski L, Kulikowski M (2009) Mutations of the KRAS oncogene in endometrial hyperplasia and carcinoma. Folia Histochem Cytobiol 47:65–68
159. Kovalev S, Marchenko ND, Gugliotta BG, Chalas E, Chumas J, Moll UM (1998) Loss of p53 function in uterine papillary serous carcinoma. Hum Pathol 29:613–619
160. Zhang X, Liang SX, Jia L, Chen N, Fadare O, Schwartz PE, Kong B, Zheng W (2009) Molecular identification of "latent precancers" for endometrial serous carcinoma in benign-appearing endometrium. Am J Pathol 174:2000–2006
161. Santin AD, Bellone S, Van Stedum S, Bushen W, De Las Casas LE, Korourian S, Tian E, Roman JJ, Burnett A, Pecorelli S (2006) Determination of HER2/neu status in uterine serous papillary carcinoma: comparative analysis of immunohistochemistry and fluorescence in situ hybridization. Gynecol Oncol 98:24–30
162. Goldstein NS, Uzieblo A (2002) WT1 immunoreactivity in uterine papillary serous carcinomas is different from ovarian serous carcinomas. Am J Clin Pathol 117:541–545
163. An HJ, Logani S, Isacson C, Ellenson LH (2004) Molecular characterization of uterine clear cell carcinoma. Mod Pathol 17:530–537
164. Soong R, Knowles S, Hammond IG, Michael C, Iacopetta BJ (1999) p53 protein overexpression and gene mutation in mixed Müllerian tumors of the uterus. Cancer Detect Prev 23:8–12
165. Mansi JL, Ramachandra S, Wiltshaw E, Fisher C (1990) Endometrial stromal sarcomas. Gynecol Oncol 36:113–118
166. Hrzenjak A, Moinfar F, Tavassoli FA, Strohmeier B, Kremser ML, Zatloukal K, Denk H (2005) JAZF1/JJAZ1 gene fusion in endometrial stromal sarcomas: molecular analysis by reverse transcriptase-polymerase chain reaction optimized for paraffin-embedded tissue. J Mol Diagn 7:388–395
167. Hampel H, Frankel WL, Martin E, Arnold M, Khanduja K, Kuebler P, Clendenning M, Sotamaa K, Prior T, Westman JA, Panescu J, Fix D, Lockman J, LaJeunesse J, Comeras I, de la Chapelle A (2008) Feasibility of screening for Lynch syndrome among patients with colorectal cancer. J Clin Oncol 26:5783–5788
168. Lynch HT, Shaw MW, Magnuson CW, Larsen AL, Krush AJ (1966) Hereditary factors in cancer. Study of two large midwestern kindreds. Arch Intern Med 117:206–212
169. Umar A, Boland CR, Terdiman JP et al (2004) Revised Bethesda Guidelines for hereditary nonpolyposis colorectal cancer (Lynch syndrome) and microsatellite instability. J Natl Cancer Inst 96:261–268
170. Wijnen J, de Leeuw W, Vasen H, van der Klift H, Moller P, Stormorken A, Meijers-Heijboer H, Lindhout D, Menko F, Vossen S, Moslein G, Tops C, Brocker-Vriends A, Wu Y, Hofstra R, Sijmons R, Cornelisse C, Morreau H, Fodde R (1999) Familial endometrial cancer in female carriers of MSH6 germline mutations. Nat Genet 23:142–144
171. Holway AH, Rieger-Christ KM, Miner WR, Cain JW, Dugan JM, Pezza JA, Silverman ML, Shapter A, McLellan R, Summerhayes IC (2000) Somatic mutation of PTEN in vulvar cancer. Clin Cancer Res 6:3228–3235
172. Reddy A, Yuille M, Sullivan A, Repellin C, Bell A, Tidy JA, Evans DJ, Farrell PJ, Gusterson B, Gasco M, Crook T (2002) Analysis of CHK2 in vulval neoplasia. Br J Cancer 86:756–760
173. Kazmierczak B, Wanschura S, Meyer-Bolte K, Caselitz J, Meister P, Bartnitzke S, Van de Ven W, Bullerdiek J (1995) Cytogenic and molecular analysis of an aggressive angiomyxoma. Am J Pathol 147:580–585
174. Pillai MR, Halabi S, McKalip A, Jayaprakash PG, Rajalekshmi TN, Nair MK, Herman B (1996) The presence of human papillomavirus-16/-18 E6, p53, and Bcl-2 protein in cervicovaginal smears from patients with invasive cervical cancer. Cancer Epidemiol Biomarkers Prev 5:329–335
175. Skomedal H, Kristensen G, Helland A, Nesland JM, Kooi S, Børresen AL, Holm R (1995) TP53 gene mutations and protein accumulation in primary vaginal carcinomas. Br J Cancer 72:129–133

176. Gross AL, Kurman RJ, Vang R, Shih I-M, Visvanathan K (2010) Precursor lesions of high-grade serous ovarian carcinoma: morphological and molecular characteristics. J Oncol 2010:126295
177. Devriendt K (2005) Hydatidiform mole and triploidy: the role of genomic imprinting in placental development. Hum Reprod Update 11:137–142
178. Murphy KM, McConnell TG, Hafez MJ, Vang R, Ronnett BM (2009) Molecular genotyping of hydatidiform moles: analytic validation of a multiplex short tandem repeat assay. J Mol Diagn 11:598–605

Chapter 13
Molecular Pathology of Bone and Soft Tissue Neoplasms and Potential Targets for Novel Therapy

Evita B. Henderson-Jackson, Anthony Conley, and Marilyn M. Bui

Contents

Abstract Bone and soft tissue tumors encompass a rare but a heterogenous group of mesenchymal neoplasms ranging from benign to malignant. Frequently, the diagnosis of many bone and soft tissue tumors prove to be difficult due to the enormous variety of histologic subtypes, with some of them (especially the tumors of spindle cell morphology) presenting with similar clinical, microscopic, immunohistochemical, and/or radiographic characteristics. With continuous and more advanced understanding of the cytogenetic and molecular genetics of bone and soft tissue tumors, it is hopeful that, eventually, classifying bone and soft tissue tumor types can be based on molecular pathology rather than by traditional histogenesis. More importantly, the forecast for the prognosis or prediction to therapy can also be benefited from molecular pathology. Chapter 13 will review the most

E.B. Henderson-Jackson • M.M. Bui (✉)
Department of Anatomic Pathology, H. Lee Moffitt Cancer Center and Research Institute, University of South Florida, College of Medicine, 12902 Magnolia Drive, Tampa, FL 33612, USA
e-mail: Marilyn.bui@moffitt.org

A. Conley
Department of Sarcoma, H. Lee Moffitt Cancer Center and Research Institute, University of South Florida, College of Medicine, 12902 Magnolia Drive, Tampa, FL 33612, USA

D. Coppola (ed.), *Molecular Pathology and Diagnostics of Cancer*, Cancer Growth and Progression 16, DOI 10.1007/978-94-007-7192-5_13,

current molecular testing of bone and soft tissue tumors and the biomarkers that have the potential for targeted therapy with focus on the recent developments from the past 5 years.

Keywords Cytogenetic • Molecular pathology • Diagnostic, bone tumor (neoplasm) • Soft tissue tumor (neoplasm) • Genetic • Prognosis • Prediction • Biomarkers • Targeted therapy

Abbreviations

ASPS	Alveolar soft part sarcoma
DFSP	Dermatofibrosarcoma protuberans
FISH	Fluorescent in situ hybridization
GIST	Gastrointestinal stromal tumor
HMO	Hereditary multiple osteochondromas
HSP	Heat-shock protein
IGF1R	Insulin-like growth factor 1 receptor
NTRK3	Neurotrophin 3 receptor gene
PDGFRA	Platelet-derived growth factor receptor alpha
PIK3CA	Phosphotidylinosital-3 kinase catalytic alpha polypeptide
PNET	Primitive neuroectodermal tumor
PPARγ	Peroxisome proliferator-activated receptor-gamma
PVNS	Pigmented villonodular synovitis
RT-PCR	Reverse transcription-polymerase chain reaction
SNP	Single nucleotide polymorphism
VEGFR	Vascular endothelial growth factor receptor
WDLPS/ALT	Well-differentiated liposarcoma/atypical lipomatous tumor

13.1 Introduction

Bone and soft tissue tumors encompass a rare but heterogenous group of mesenchymal neoplasms ranging from benign to malignant. The etiology of most tumors is unknown. There are reported associations with radiation, viral infections, chemical carcinogens, and genetic syndromes. Currently, mesenchymal neoplasms are diagnosed and classified using the criteria published by World Health Organization in 2002 [1]. The tumors are mainly classified by their histogenesis and incorporated cytogenetic and molecular genetic information. Morphologically, they are divided into groups by cell morphology and matrix formation. Spindle, small round cell, epithelioid/polygonal, pleomorphic, myxoid, fatty, giant cell, and chondro-osseous tumors are the main groups. Immunohistochemical studies are important ancillary tools to facilitate a definitive diagnosis by providing information regarding tumor histogenesis, proliferation index, and some the status of certain predictive markers. However, there are no reliable histochemical markers to determine if the tumor is benign versus malignant.

Genetic analysis of mesenchymal neoplasms has revealed three distinct groups. The first group contains genetically unstable sarcomas associated with complex karyotypes without possessing characteristic chromosomal rearrangements. Osteosarcoma, fibrosarcoma, and leiomyosarcoma [2–4] are such examples. These sarcomas can arise from a less aggressive form and evolve into a more aggressive process with increasing genomic instability and complexity. They can also arise de novo as a high-grade sarcoma. The second group is characterized by specific and recurrent chromosomal numerical or structural abnormalities, such as translocations, deletions, additions, and ring or giant chromosomes. There are usually distinct histopathologic characteristics and clinical scenarios associated with the soft tissue neoplasms with recurrent chromosomal rearrangements [2–4]. The examples are Ewing's sarcoma and myxoid liposarcoma. The third group exhibits molecular abnormalities such as gene amplification, mutations, and loss of heterozygosity. An example includes gastrointestinal stromal tumor (GIST).

13.2 Soft Tissue Tumor-Specific Genetic and Molecular Abnormalities

There are approximately 60 sarcoma subtypes and 52 benign soft tissue tumors. The core mechanisms of the pathogenesis of soft tissue tumors have been elegantly described and illustrated in the review article by Taylor et al. published in *Nature Reviews* [5]. A taxonomy of soft tissue sarcomas illustrate the differences and similarities in lineage for subtypes of sarcomas. A summary of the recurrent translocations in soft tissue sarcomas illustrate the relationship between subtypes.

The most common and recent cytogenetic and molecular abnormalities of soft tissue neoplasms are summarized in Table 13.1. Small round blue cell tumors, a group of primitive appearing neoplasms, are often difficult to classify. However, most of the small round blue cell tumors have an associated tumor-specific chromosomal translocation, which is diagnostically valuable [1]. Ewing's sarcoma, the second most common primary bone sarcoma in children, is associated with the t(11;22)(q24;q12) translocation. This translocation results in the fusion of the *EWSR1* gene, on chromosome 22q12, to a member of the *ETS* gene family of transcription factors, Fli1, on chromosome 11q24 [6]. This translocation is detected in approximately 85 % of Ewing's sarcomas and primitive neuroectodermal tumors (PNET). A second translocation, t(21;22)(q22;q12) found in 5–10 % of Ewing's sarcomas, fuses the *EWSR1* gene to a different *ETS* gene, *ERG*, found on chromosome 21q22 [7]. Many other less frequent translocations involving the *EWSR1* gene and other *ETS* genes and rarely *FUS* gene have been reported [2, 4].

Table 13.1 Characteristic genetic alterations in soft tissue neoplasms

Neoplasm	Translocation	Gene/alteration
Alveolar rhabdomyosarcoma	t(2;13)(q35;q14)	*PAX3-FOXO1*
	t(1;13)(p36;q14)	*PAX7-FOXO1*
	t(X;2)(q13;q35)	*PAX3-AFX*
Alveolar soft part sarcoma	der(17)t(X;17)(p11;q25)	*ASPL-TFE3*
Angiomatoid fibrous histiocytoma	t(12;22)(q13;q12)	*EWSR1-ATF1*
	t(2;22)(q33;q12)	*EWSR1-CREB1*
	t(12;16)(q13;p11)	*FUS-ATF1*
Clear cell sarcoma	t(12;22)(q13;q12)	*EWSR1-ATF1*
	t(2;22)(q33;q12)	*EWSR1-CREB1*
Congenital/infantile fibrosarcoma	t(12;15)(p13;q25)	*ETV6-NTRK3*
DFSP	t(17;22)(q21;q13) derivative ring chromosomes	*COLIA1-PDGFB*
Desmoid tumor (fibromatosis)	Trisomy 8 or 20; loss of 5q21	*CTNNB1 or APC* mutation
Desmoplastic small round cell tumor	t(11;22)(p13;q12)	*EWS-WT1*
Epithelioid hemangioendothelioma	t(1;3)(p36;q25)	*WWTR1-CAMTA1*
Epithelioid sarcoma (proximal type)	Inactivation of INI1	*INI1*
Ewing's sarcoma/PNET family	t(11;22)(q24;q12)	*EWS1-FLI1*
	t(21;22)(q22;q12)	*EWS1-ERG*
	t(7;22)(p22;q12)	*EWSR1-ETV1*
	t(2;22)(q33;q12)	*EWSR1-FEV*
	t(17 ;22)(q12 ;q12)	*EWSR1-E1AF*
	inv(22)(q12 ;q12)	*EWSR1-ZSG*
	t(16 ;21)(p11 ;q22)	*FUS-ERG*
Extrarenal rhabdoid tumor	Inactivation of INI1	*INI1*
Extraskeletal myxoid chondrosarcoma	t(9;22)(q22;q12)	*EWSR1-NR4A3*
	t(9;17)(q22;q11)	*TAF2N-NR4A3*
	t(9;15)(q22;q21)	*TCF12-NR4A3*
	t(3;9)(q11;q22)	*TFG-NR4A3*
GIST (Sporadic and familial)	Activating kinase mutations	*KIT or PDGFRA*
		ETV1 overexpression
		BRAF mutation
Inflammatory myofibroblastic tumor	t(1;2)(q22;p23)	*TPM3-ALK*
	t(2:19)(p23;p13)	*TPM4-ALK*
	t(2;17)(p23;q23)	*CLTC-ALK*
	t(2;2)(p23;q13)	*RANBP2-ALK*
	t(2;11)(p23;p15)	*CARS-ALK*
	inv(2)(p23;q35)	*ATIC-ALK*
Leiomyosarcoma		*MYOCD* amplification
Lipoma	t(3;12)(q27-28,q14-15)	*HMGA2-LPP*
Low-grade fibromyxoid sarcoma	t(7;16)(q33;p11)	*FUS-CREB3L2*
	t(11;16)(p11;p11)	*FUS-CREB3L1*

(contined)

Table 13.1 (continued)

Neoplasm	Translocation	Gene/alteration
Myoepithelioma	t(1;22)(q23;q12)	*EWSR1-PBX1*
Myoepithelial carcinoma	t(19;22)(q13;q12)	*EWSR1-ZNF444*
Myxoid/round cell liposarcoma	t(12;16)(q13;p11)	*FUS-DDIT3*
	t(12:22)(q13;q12)	*EWSR1-DDIT3*
		PIK3CA mutation
Myxofibrosarcoma		*NF1* deletion, point mutation and indel
Pericytoma	t(7;12)(p22;q13)	*ACTB-GLI1*
Pleomorphic liposarcoma		*NF1* deletion, point mutation and indel
Synovial sarcoma	t(X;18)(p11;q11)	*SS18-SSX1*
	t(X;18)(p11;q11)	*SS18-SSX2*
	t(X;18)(p11;q11)	*SS18-SSX4*
TGCT/PVNS	t(1;2)(p13;q35)	*CSF1-COL6A3*
WDLPS/ALT and DDLPS	12q14-15 (supernumerary ring chromosomes ; giant marker chromosomes)	Amplification of *MDM2, CDK4, HMGA2, SAS, GLI* and *JUN*

DFSP dermatofibrosarcoma protuberans, *PNET* peripheral primitive neuroectodermal tumor, *GIST* gastrointestinal stromal tumor, *WDLPS* well-differentiated liposarcoma, *ALT* atypical lipomatous tumor, *DDLPS* dedifferentiated liposarcoma, *TGCT* tenosynovial giant cell tumor, *PVNS* pigmented villonodular synovitis

Cytogenetic analysis of alveolar rhabdomyosarcoma, a common soft tissue neoplasm of young children, has demonstrated two specific chromosomal translocations [8]: the t(2;13)(q35;q14) translocation, which is found in 60 % of cases, and a less common variant t(1;13)(p36;q14) [9, 10]. These involve the *FKHR* gene (*FOXO1A*) on chromosome 13q14 and either *Pax3* (2q35) or *Pax7* (1p36) genes [11]. The Pax7-FKHR tumors are often seen in younger patients and are associated with a lower rate of metastasis and better survival than Pax3-FKHR tumors [12]. There is no specific chromosomal abnormality identified involving the embryonal subtype of rhabdomyosarcoma [13].

Desmoplastic small round cell tumor demonstrates multilineage differentiation and characteristically possesses the t(11;22)(p13;q12) translocation that fuses the *EWSR1* gene to *WT1*, the Wilm's tumor suppressor gene, on chromosome 11p13 [4, 14].

Extraskeletal myxoid chondrosarcoma, an uncommon sarcoma of uncertain lineage, demonstrates the EWS-NR4A3 fusion generated from a t(9;22)(q22;q12) translocation [15]. A second translocation that may be encountered is t(9;17)(q22;q11) [16]. Of note, there is no immunohistochemistry profile that can reliably diagnosis this particular sarcoma, making molecular studies important for the diagnosis of extraskeletal myxoid chondrosarcoma [17].

In addition to the small round blue cell tumors, several spindle cell sarcomas are associated with recurrent translocations. Importantly, synovial sarcoma, an aggressive neoplasm of uncertain histogenesis, demonstrates a recurrent reciprocal t(X;18)(p11.2; q11.2) translocation [1, 18]. The translocation fuses the *SYT* gene on chromosome 18q11 to one of the three homologous genes on Xp11 (*SSX1*, *SSX2*, or *SSX4*), which is detectable in 95 % of synovial sarcomas [2, 19]. The SYT-SSX1 fusion transcript is reportedly associated with biphasic histology, whereas the SYT-SSX2 fusion transcript is associated with a monophasic histology as well as a better metastasis-free survival [20].

Dermatofibrosarcoma protuberans (DFSP), a low-grade spindle cell neoplasm, possesses a specific chromosomal rearrangement consisting of either supernumerary ring chromosomes or unbalanced derivatives of t(17;22)(q22;q13) translocation. Both aberrations have sequences encoding a COL1A1-PDGFB fusion transcript that is commonly identified by reverse transcription-polymerase chain reaction (RT-PCR) [21–23]. Reportedly, imatinib mesylate (Gleevec, STI571/Glivec) has clinical activity against DFSP with t(17;22); however, fibrosarcomatous variants of DFSP without the translocation may not show a response. Molecular testing would be important in identifying patients with DFSP who have the translocation because they would more likely respond to therapy [24].

Congenital fibrosarcoma, another spindle cell sarcoma, has a characteristic cytogenetic change, t(12;15)(p13;q25) translocation, not found in the adult fibrosarcomas. In addition, the chromosomal rearrangement is identical to that described for congenital mesoblastic nephroma, acute myeloblastic leukemia, and secretory carcinoma of the breast [25–27]. Fusion of the *ETV6* gene on 12p13 to the neurotrophin 3 receptor gene (*NTRK3* or *TRKC*) on chromosome 15q25 is often difficult to identify cytogenetically and is better detected by FISH or PCR [28, 29].

Low-grade fibromyxoid sarcoma, a rare variant of fibrosarcoma, is associated with the FUS-CREB3L2 gene fusion or less frequently the FUS-CREB3L1 gene fusion, the result of translocations t(7;16) or t(11;16), respectively [30, 31]. The chromosomal abnormalities may be detected with either FISH or RT-PCR [32].

Gastrointestinal stromal tumor (GIST), a spindle cell sarcoma, is unlike the previous spindle cell sarcomas discussed in that it is characterized by activating oncogenic mutations instead of specific translocations or fusion genes [3]. KIT mutations are a defining feature of most GISTs, and, to a lesser degree, mutations in platelet-derived growth factor receptor alpha (PDGFRA) can also occur in GIST. These activating mutations lead to constitutive activation of their respective kinases, leading to downstream effects that decrease apoptosis and promote cellular survival [33–36]. A majority of GISTs reveal a mutation in one of three sites: KIT exon 11, KIT exon 9, or PDGFRA exon 18 [35, 37]. These mutation types correlate with the anatomic location and have prognostic implications. The KIT exon 11 mutations include in-frame deletions, point mutations, and internal tandem duplications; however, patients with point mutations fare better prognostically than those with deletions [38]. Small intestinal GISTs usually demonstrate KIT 9 exon mutations, and patients appear to have a higher mortality with small intestinal versus gastric GISTs with KIT 9 exon mutations [36, 39]. PDGFRA mutations are primarily localized to the stomach and have an epithelioid morphology, and they frequently exhibit an indolent clinical course [40, 41]. GISTs have been successfully treated with tyrosine kinase inhibitors that specifically target c-Kit, such as imatinib mesylate and sunitinib, which further support molecular genotyping of these tumors because the genotype correlates with different treatment outcomes, including progression-free survival and overall survival [35, 42–44]. The majority of laboratories use PCR to amplify the most commonly mutated exons with subsequent direct sequencing analysis of the amplified exon [3].

There are a few notable chromosomal abnormalities and genetic aberrations involving lipomatous neoplasms. Myxoid-round cell liposarcoma is known for its characteristic t(12;16)(q13;p11) reciprocal translocation, resulting in the formation of *FUS-DDIT3* chimeric gene in 95 % of cases [4, 45, 46]. Myxoid-round cell liposarcoma is radiosensitive; with the use of molecular studies as an adjunct to histopathology, patients will be able to get neoadjuvant therapy and reduce the risk of an ablative procedure [32]. Recently, Barretina et al. [47]performed a high-throughput, integrative analysis of DNA, mRNA, and mutational data to show that 18 % of myxoid-round cell liposarcomas contain mutations in the phosphotidylinosital-3 kinase catalytic alpha polypeptide (PIK3CA). Compared to the wild-type version, tumors with PIK3CA exhibited a shorter progression-free survival, suggesting a more aggressive course. On the other hand, well-differentiated liposarcoma/atypical lipomatous tumor (WDLPS/ALT) cytogenetically shows supernumerary ring chromosomes, giant marker chromosomes, and double minutes in 80 % of cases, corresponding to the amplification of the 12q13-15 band [2]. Several tumor-associated genes are localized to that band region, including MDM2 and CDK4 [48]. Pleomorphic liposarcomas, a less common liposarcoma variant, does not exhibit a specific chromosomal translocation, but these tumors have been shown to exhibit mutations in TP53 and NF1 [47].

There are sarcomas of uncertain histogenesis with characteristic translocations. Clear cell sarcoma (malignant melanoma of soft parts) demonstrates t(12;22)(q13;q12) translocation involving the *ATF-1* gene on chromosome 12q13 and *EWSR1* [49, 50]. Alveolar soft part sarcoma (ASPS) has a recurrent der(17)t(X;17)(p11;q25) unbalanced translocation [51]. This translocation involves the fusion of *TFE3* transcription factor gene on Xp11 and the *ASPL* gene on chromosome 17q25 [52]. The *ASPSCR1-TFE* fusion protein has been associated with overexpression of MET, and inhibition of MET by RNA interference has resulted in decrease growth of ASPS cells lines [53].

Extrarenal (and renal) rhabdoid tumors, proximal-type epithelioid sarcoma, and a subset of pediatric undifferentiated soft tissue sarcomas have an inactivating oncogenic mutation, specifically an inactivation of the tumor suppressor gene *SMARCB* (*INI1*) [54–57]. Basically, there is either a loss of both alleles or loss of one allele with an inactivating mutation of the other, resulting in the inactivation of the tumor suppressor gene [3]. SMARCB molecular abnormalities may be detected using conventional karyotyping, FISH, and direct sequencing and more recently with multiplex ligation-dependent probe amplification of single nucleotide polymorphism-array analysis to identify small deletions, duplications, or single base pair mutations within the tumors [3, 58].

13.3 Bone Tumor-Specific Genetic and Molecular Abnormalities

Approximately 0.2 % of bone tumors are primary, which is less frequent than metastasis to the bone and less common than soft tissue counterparts (1:10). There are 19 main subtypes of benign bone tumors and 22 subtypes of bone sarcomas. Table 13.2 summarizes the most common and recent cytogenetic and molecular abnormality of bone neoplasms.

Bone tumors are primarily of mesenchymal origin. Tumors of the bone as classified by the World Health Organization may be cartilaginous, osteogenic, fibrogenic, fibrohistiocytic, vascular, myogenic, lipogenic, neural, or notochordal [1]. However, there are instances when bone is involved by tumors of neuroectodermal origin, such as Ewing Sarcoma, or by tumors of undefined histogenesis, such as aneurysmal bone cyst.

Cartilagenous tumors produce a chondroid matrix and may either be benign or malignant in nature. Osteochondroma, a cartilage capped bony projection arising on the external surface of bone containing a marrow cavity continuous with that of the underlying bone, may form as a solitary lesion or multiple lesions as in hereditary

Table 13.2 Characteristic genetic alterations in bone neoplasms

Neoplasm	Translocation	Gene/alteration
Aneurysmal bone cyst	t(16;17)(q22;p13)	*CDH11-USP6*
	t(1;17)(p34.3;p13)	*THRAP3-USP6*
	t(3;17)(q21;p13)	*CNBP-USP6*
	t(9;17)(q22;p13)	*OMD-USP6*
	t(17 ;17)(q21 ;p13)	*COL1A1-USP6*
Bizarre parosteal osteochondromatous proliferation (Nora lesion)	t(1;17)(q32 ;q21)	*RDC1*
Chondrosarcoma or chondroma		*IDH1 or IDH2* Point mutation
Ewing's sarcoma/PNET family	t(11;22)(q24;q12)	*EWS1-FLI1*
	t(21;22)(q22;q12)	*EWS1-ERG*
	t(7;22)(p22;q12)	*EWSR1-ETV1*
	t(2;22)(q33;q12)	*EWSR1-FEV*
	t(17;22)(q12;q12)	*EWSR1-E1AF*
	inv(22)(q12;q12)	*EWSR1-ZSG*
	t(16;21)(p11;q22)	*FUS-ERG*
Fibrous dysplasia	Activating oncogenic mutations	*GNAS1*
Mesenchymal chondrosarcoma	t(8;8)(q13;q21)	*HEY1-NCOA2*
Osteosarcoma, low grade (parosteal and intramedullary)	12q14-15 (ring chromosomes, giant marker chromosomes)	*Amplification of CDK4, MDM2, HMGA2, GLI and SAS*
Osteosarcoma or chordoma		Multiple structural rearrangements
Subungual exostosis	t(X;6)(q24-q26;q15-21)	*COL12A1-COL4A5*

multiple osteochondromas (HMO) [1]. Cytogenetic aberrations have been identified in the *EXT1* gene located at 8p22-24.1 in sporadic and hereditary osteochondromas. Specifically, germline mutations in the tumor suppressor genes *EXT1* located at 8q24 and *EXT2* located at 11p11-p12 have been found in HMO [59–61]. Enchondroma is a benign hyaline cartilage tumor of medullary bone commonly involving the hands and feet [1]. By conventional cytogenetic analysis, aberrations involving chromosome 12 have been detected [62, 63]. Chondromyxoid fibroma frequently occurs in the long bones, particularly the tibia. It is a benign tumor composed of lobules of spindle-shaped cells with abundant myxoid or chondroid intercellular material [1]. Structural rearrangements of chromosome 6 have been found to be non-random, specifically involving the long arm (q13 and q25) and short arm (p25) [64–68]. Chondrosarcoma is a malignant tumor of hyaline cartilage differentiation that may contain myxoid changes, calcifications, or areas of ossification [1]. There are several subtypes of chondrosarcoma, including conventional, periosteal, dedifferentiated, mesenchymal, and clear cell. Genetic alterations involving chondrosarcoma are heterogeneous. Comparative genomic hybridization studies have revealed extensive genetic alterations, including gains of whole chromosomes or chromosome arms at 20q, 20p, and 14q23 or partial losses [69]. Loss of genetic material from 13q was found to be an independent predictor of metastasis development, regardless of tumor grade or size [68, 70, 71]. Dedifferentiated chondrosarcoma, a subtype of chondrosarcoma composed of a well-differentiated cartilage tumor juxtaposed to a high-grade non-cartilaginous sarcoma; reportedly possesses frequent structural and numerical alterations of chromosome 1 and 9 [1, 66, 72–75]. Identical somatic deletion in exon 7 of p53 have been identified in the cartilaginous, as well as within the dedifferentiated part [1, 66]. Mesenchymal chondrosarcoma is a rare subtype characterized by a biphasic pattern composed of undifferentiated small round cells and islands of well-differentiated hyaline cartilage [1]. In two cases of mesenchymal chondrosarcoma a Robertsonian (13;21) translocation was observed [76].

Osteogenic tumors produce a bony matrix or what is referred to as ‘osteoid’ and, depending on their behavior, are considered either benign or malignant. However, rarely benign osteogenic tumors undergo malignant transformation [1]. Osteoid osteoma is a benign cortically based bone-forming tumor defined by its small size, limited growth potential (seldom exceeds 1.0 cm), and disproportionate pain. Reportedly, there have been two of three cases of osteoid osteoma in which a loss of the distal part of chromosome arm 17q was detected [77]. Osteosarcoma, a highly malignant bone tumor, commonly arises within the long bones of children; however, about 15 % arise in adults secondary to a pre-existing condition, such as Paget disease [1]. The classical or conventional osteosarcoma may histologically show a variable of features and be subtyped as either osteoblastic, chondroblastic, or fibroblastic. There are other more rare subtypes, including telangiectatic osteosarcoma, small cell osteosarcoma, parosteal osteosarcoma, periosteal osteosarcoma, high-grade surface osteosarcoma, and more. Most osteosarcomas possess complex chromosomal alterations. However, there appear to be certain chromosomal regions that display recurrent amplifications. Amplification at 1q21-23 and 17p, together with co-amplification of 12q13-15, are frequently reported [78–84]. The *MDM2* gene is amplified in 14–27 % of osteosarcomas [82, 85, 86]. Amplification of CDK4 gene is found in aggressive lesions [87–89]. Lastly, the *MYC* gene has been shown to be amplified in 44 % of osteosarcomas (8q24) [90]. Understandably, low-grade variants of osteosarcoma have not been found to harbor complex aberrations. For example, low-grade central osteosarcoma show recurrent gains in minimal common regions at 12q13-14, 12p, and 6p21 [91]. Parosteal osteosarcoma, another low-grade osteosarcoma that arises on the surface of bone, reportedly shows ring chromosomes with co-amplification of *SAS*, *CDK4*, and *MDM2* genes with a minimal common region at 12q13-15 [92–94]. As stated previously, osteosarcomas may arise secondary to a pre-existing condition (Paget disease) or after radiation therapy. In tumors forming after radiation therapy, chromosomal losses are more often observed than gains [95]; 1p is lost in 57 % of post-radiation osteosarcomas, in contrast to conventional osteosarcomas that demonstrate only a 3 % loss [95, 96]. Osteosarcomas arising secondary to Paget disease of the bone show a frequent loss of heterozygosity at 18q [97]. A unique and rare tumorous lesion with aggressive growth known as bizarre parosteal osteochondromatous proliferation (Nora's lesion) is an exception to the rule, in that this neoplasm possesses a unique recurrent aberration t(1;17)(q32;q21) not found in most bone-forming tumors [98].

Fibrogenic tumors do not produce a mineralized matrix, but form collagen. Desmoplastic fibroma of the bone is a rare, benign neoplasm composed of spindle cells with minimal atypia and abundant collagen [1]. The histomorphology is identical to fibromatosis of the soft tissue. Like its soft tissue counterpart, a subset of desmoplastic fibromas of the bone show trisomies of 8 and 20 [99].

Ewing's sarcoma, as previously mentioned above, demonstrates the same aberrations as seen in its soft tissue counterpart.

Giant cell tumor of the bone is a locally aggressive neoplasm. Histology reveals sheets of neoplastic ovoid mononuclear cells interspersed with uniformly distributed large osteoclast-like giant cells [1]. A frequent chromosomal aberration detected in giant cell tumor of the bone is a reduction in the length of telomeres. Most commonly affected telomeres are 11p, 13p, 14p, 15p, 19q, 20q, and 21p [100–105].

Chordoma is a neoplasm that arises from notochordal remnants. It usually occurs in the sacrum or clivus. Typically, chordomas display a lobular growth pattern and contain neoplastic cells with bubbly cytoplasm known as "physaliphorous cells" [1]. In 9 of 16 cases of chordomas, hypodiploidy was identified. Chromosomes 3, 4, 10, and 13 were frequently lost [68, 106]. A tumor suppressor gene is believed to exist on distal 1p due to loss of heterozygosity at band 1p36 [107].

Admantinoma, a malignant biphasic tumor characterized by an epithelial and osteofibrous component, may derive from their osteofibrous dysplasia-like counterparts. Osteofibrous dysplasia and adamantinoma show similar cytogenetic alterations such as trisomies of chromosomes 7, 8, 12, 19, and 21 [108–111].

As described in soft tissue tumors, there are also tumors of undefined histogenesis that occur in the bone. Primary aneurysmal bone cyst, a cystic lesion of bone composed of blood-filled spaces separated by connective tissue septa with fibroblasts, giant cells, and reactive woven bone, has been shown to harbor a recurrent translocation t(16:17) in several cases [1, 112]. However, rearrangements are absent in secondary aneurysmal bone cysts [113]. Over the years, additional translocations have been identified, all of which result in oncogenic activation of the USP6 gene on chromosome 17p13 [114–116]. Fibrous dysplasia, a benign medullary fibro-osseous lesion, may involve one (monostotic) or more bones (polyostotic) [1]. It is characterized by activating mutations in the GNAS1 gene located on chromosome 20q12–q13.3, encoding the alpha subunit of the stimulatory G protein [117].

13.4 Therapy for Soft Tissue Tumors

Benign tumors are generally treated with surgical excision. Malignant tumors (sarcomas) can be treated with combination therapy, including surgery, chemotherapy, targeted therapy, radiation therapy, hormonal therapy, and immunotherapy. Surgery achieves local control and removes tumor burden. Radiation therapy is applicable when the surgical margin is positive or used neoadjuvant to facilitate subsequent resection. Cytotoxic chemotherapy is used for metastatic disease, unresectable tumors, or sensitive histological types. Sensitivity to chemotherapy is variable among sarcomas, and, at this time, histology appears to be the best predictor of response. Chemotherapy-sensitive tumors include Ewing's sarcoma, rhabdomyosarcoma, myxoid/round cell liposarcoma, synovial sarcoma, uterine leiomyosarcoma, desmoid tumor (fibromatosis), desmoplastic small-round-cell tumor, and angiosarcoma. Resistant histologic types include ASPS, clear cell sarcoma, and extraskeletal myxoid chondrosarcoma. Dedifferentiated liposarcomas, epithelioid sarcomas, and perivascular epithelioid cell tumors are minimally sensitive to cytotoxic chemotherapy, whereas fibrosarcoma, high-grade undifferentiated sarcoma, malignant peripheral nerve sheath tumor, solitary fibrous tumor/hemangiopericytoma, and hemangioendothelioma exhibit intermediate sensitivity to chemotherapy. Although histology may be the best predictor of response, histologic grade is the greatest predictor of recurrence [118]. Unfortunately, there are many more high-grade sarcoma subtypes resistant to anthracycline-based therapies compared to chemotherapy-sensitive subtypes. Furthermore, most clinical trials from the 1970s to present often "lump" multiple histologic subtypes together to increase the total sample size at the expense of diluting the overall effect of the chemotherapeutic agent. Thus, endpoints such as response rate or survival are often modest in benefit, resulting in controversy among many sarcoma specialists. Clearly, there is a need to improve our understanding of the molecular pathology so that the survival of patients afflicted with these rare diseases can be improved.

An excellent example of molecular-based therapy involves GISTs. This rare mesenchymal tumor is postulated to arise from the interstitial cell of Cajal and commonly involves the stomach and small intestine of adults (peak age of 60), with less than 10 % of cases in individuals under age 40 years. They may occur in extra-gastrointestinal sites, including the retroperitoneum, mesentery, and omentum. Ninety percent of GISTs harbor a mutation within the KIT gene and/or PDGFRA gene (80 % and 10 %, respectively) [119]. Recently, V600E BRAF mutation was identified in adult patients with GIST lacking KIT and PDGFRA mutations [120, 121]. GIST mutational analysis is important in the evaluation of patients with GIST tumors to analyze prognosis, to make decisions regarding adjuvant treatment, to predict treatment response, and to select appropriate dosage. Different types of mutations involving different exons result in varying clinical prognosis, histologic appearance, and treatment decisions for patients. Internal tandem repeats involving exon 11 are associated with gastric GISTs and an indolent course, whereas deletions within exon 11 are associated with a shorter survival, higher risk of recurrence, and an aggressive course. Exon 9 mutations are associated with small intestinal GISTs and a clinically aggressive course. PDGFRA missense mutations in exon 18, exon 14, or exon 12 occur in GISTs involving the stomach, which have an epithelioid or mixed epithelioid/spindle cell histology [3, 122, 123]. Historically, treatment of advanced GIST is revolved around surgery, with few effective systemic therapeutic options; however, the introduction of imatinib mesylate (ST1571; Gleevec), a selective tryosine kinase inhibitor that targets KIT and PDGFRA, has changed the course of this disease.

Imatinib is an oral FDA-approved drug for use as an adjuvant therapy following complete gross resection of tumor and in the management of unresectable and metastatic disease. GIST tumors with exon 11 mutations are the most responsive to imatinib therapy and GISTs with exon 9 mutations may benefit from an increase dose (800 mg). Patients with wild-type GIST and wild-type PDGFRA rarely show a favorable or sustained response to treatment. In this situation, other less common gene mutations are likely involved, such as in the succinyl dehydrogenase gene, noted in patients with an inherited form of GIST that is often accompanied by the development of paragangliomas, and pulmonary hamartomas [124]. Other forms of wild-type KIT and wild-type PDGFRA GIST include tumors with activation the Ras pathway in NF1 patients or in tumors with insulin-like growth factor 1 receptor (IGF1R) amplification. Unfortunately, there are cases where patients with exon 9 and PDGFRA mutations have primary resistance to imatinib likely due to the structure of the ATP-binding loop, which results in decreased affinity for the drug [125]. Secondary resistance occurs and generally is due to additional mutations involving exon 11. Sunitinib malate (SU11248; Sutent) is a multi-targeted tyrosine kinase inhibitor that also inhibits vascular endothelial growth factor receptors (VEGFRs). It is used to treat patients with primary or secondary resistance to imatinib. Patients with exon 9 mutations or wild-type genotyping demonstrate a good response, although the overall response rate is noted to be less than 10 % [126]. As with imatinib, sunitinib resistance may evolve and thus represents an area of active investigation. Novel therapeutic strategies that target different aspects of the intracellular signaling pathway involving KIT and PDGFRA are being investigated, and potential options include the following: heat-shock protein (HSP)-90 inhibitor, everolimus, nilotinib, sorafenib, dasatinib, regorafenib, masitinib, PI3-kinase/mTOR dual inhibitors, and PI3-kinase inhibitors [127]. In a phase II efficacy study of sorafenib, partial response (13 %) and stable disease (58 %) were reported in 24 patients with resistance to imatinib or sunitinib. A multicenter phase II study of Masitinib revealed preliminary observations of objective partial response (50 %), stable disease (47 %), and primary refractory (3 %) with overall disease rate of 97 %. Phase III studies are underway comparing nilotinib and masitinib as single agents with imatinib in the first-line setting. The HSP-90 inhibitor inhibits HSP-90, a chaperone protein that aids in protein folding to stabilize KIT from degradation, to prevent stabilization of KIT, and to lead to its degradation [127].

Pigmented villonodular synovitis (PVNS; also known as diffuse-type giant cell tumor) is a potentially aggressive proliferative lesion involving synovial tissues of joints, tendon sheath, and bursa. The extra-articular form presents with an infiltrative soft tissue mass with or without involvement of the adjacent joint. PVNS affects young adults under age 40 years with a slight female predominance and occurs around the knee region a majority of the time [1, 128].

Translocation t(1;2)(p13;q35) [CSF1-COL6A3 fusion transcript] is found in a minority of cells in 63–77 % of patients with PVNS. This translocation leads to overexpression of CSF1, which plays a major role in the pathogenesis of PVNS. The mononuclear-histiocyte-like neoplastic cells and their proliferation is driven by expression of CSF1. Besides the autocrine stimulation, a paracrine effect is present with the recruitment of adjacent histocytes and oseoclast-like giant cells harboring the CSF1 receptor [128]. Treatment entails partial or complete excision of synovium and involved bones, and aggressive cases may be followed by low-dose radiotherapy; however, recurrences commonly occur and patients can undergo multiple surgeries. The possibility of targeted therapy with CSF1 inhibitors as an adjunct to surgery and radiation therapy may provide another avenue for patients to avoid multiple surgeries. CSF1 inhibitors include imatinib, sunitinib, and nilotinib. In a small case series and a case report, imatinib demonstrated clinical and radiologic responses in patients with PVNS. Prospective clinical trials are underway testing nilotinib [129–131].

Synovial sarcoma makes up about 5–10 % of soft tissue sarcomas affecting young adults, more commonly males. This neoplasm is unrelated to synovium; 80 % of cases occur in the deep soft tissue of the extremities, especially around the knee. Histologic variants identified in synovial sarcoma are biphasic type, monophasic type, calcifying type, and poorly differentiated (high grade) type. The translocation t(X;18)(p11.2;q11.2) is common to synovial sarcoma involving the SYT gene and either SSX1, SSX2 or SSX4 [1]. Synovial sarcoma has a survival rate ranging between 36 % and 76 % in 5 years and 20 % and 63 % in 10 years. The clinical course demonstrates a high rate of local recurrence and metastatic disease. About one fourth of patients have metastatic disease at initial diagnosis either to lung, lymph nodes, or bone. Unlike other sarcomas, this particular soft tissue sarcoma is known for its responsiveness to ifosfamide-based therapies. In at least one series, the overall response rate in patients treated with doxorubicin/ifosfamide was 58.6 %, and a separate study revealed a superior disease-specific survival for doxorubicin/ifosfamide-treated synovial sarcoma patients compared to those without this chemotherapy regimen [132, 133]. Unfortunately, the mechanisms by which ifosfamide-based regimens affect synovial sarcoma cells are poorly understood, primarily because ifosfamide requires hepatic activation. The VEGFR inhibitor, cediranib, inhibits tyrosine kinase activity of VEGFR-1 through VEGFR-3. A pediatric phase I study revealed objective responses in synovial sarcoma, Ewing's sarcoma, and osteosarcoma. mTOR inhibitors appear to be useful in possibly treating soft tissue neoplasms, including synovial sarcoma. Akt and mTOR are noted to be constitutively active in some synovial sarcomas, and their activation has correlated with metastasis. Bcl-2 inhibitors are another option to be studied in the treatment of synovial sarcoma. Bcl-2 is up-regulated in the common expression profile of synovial sarcoma and may be a major mechanism of chemoresistance. In vitro studies have proven successful at slowing growth and inducing apoptosis in cell lines in conjunction with cytotoxic agents [134–138].

WDLPS/ALT is one of the most common sarcomas of adulthood (age 40–60 years), commonly affecting the deep soft tissues of the proximal extremities and retroperitoneum. There are four subtypes: adipocytic, sclerosing, inflammatory, and spindle cell. Wide local excision is the choice of treatment. Although 15–53 % of these recur locally, this type of liposarcoma does not metastasize. The 5- and 10-year survival rates are 70–85 % and 50 %, respectively [1, 139, 140]. Dedifferentiation may occur especially in retroperitoneal lesions, which may metastasize. Dedifferentiated liposarcoma is composed of a well-differentiated liposarcoma and a non-lipomatous component. Ninety percent of dedifferentiated liposarcomas arise de novo, while the remaining 10 % occur in recurrences. Retroperitoneal location is a common site, making complete excision almost impossible. It has a metastatic rate between 10 % and 20 %, with an overall mortality of 50–75 %.

Both WDLPS/ALT and dedifferentiated liposarcoma demonstrate amplification of MDM2 and CDK4 on chromosome 12q13-15 due to ring and giant marker chromosomes [1, 141–143]. Besides surgery, potential molecularly targeted therapeutic entities include MDM2 and CDK4 inhibitors. MDM2 inhibitors aim to reactivate p53 and thus allow it to actively induce cell death in response to appropriate stressors. MDM2 antagonists have been shown to activate wild-type p53 and induce cell cycle arrest and apoptosis in cancer cell lines. Phase I trials with MDM2/p53 inhibitors (nutlin, RG7112) have shown signs of response in patients, with an induction of p53, p21, cell cycle arrest, and apoptosis. Phase I trials with CDK4 inhibitors are underway. Peroxisome proliferator-activated receptor-gamma (PPARγ) forms a heterodimeric complex with the retinoid X receptor. This complex regulates transcription of adipocyte-specific genes by binding sites on DNA. Agonist ligands for the PPARγ receptor have been shown to induce terminal differentiation of normal preadipocytes in human liposarcoma cells in vitro. Phase II trial with Troglitazone showed histologic/biochemical differentiation in three patients with high-grade liposarcoma; however, in a study of 12 patients treated with Rosiglitazone, which belongs to the same class of drugs (thiazolidinediones) as Troglitazone, results were not as promising, with median progression-free survival of 5.5 months.

Leiomyosarcomas exhibit smooth muscle differentiation and arise in the uterus, gastrointestinal tract, and in the lining of blood vessels. These tumors exhibit complex cytogenetics and no specific oncogenic event has been identified. This may be further complicated by the fact that this phenotype may be organ-specific [144]. Mutations in the p53 gene have been identified, resulting in decreased protein expression. Other molecular events associated with decreased protein expression include the inactivation of DAP kinase, p16, and RASSF1A. As with dedifferentiated liposarcomas, overexpression of CDK4 and MDM2 has been observed [144]. The most notable molecular aberration of therapeutic interest is the inactivation of PTEN. Mouse models with homozygous deletion of PTEN have been observed to develop leiomyosarcomas within the abdomen [145]. Furthermore, inhibition of the mTOR pathway by everolimus appeared to decrease tumor growth and improve survival of the affected mice. Standard cytotoxic chemotherapy is utilized for the treatment of metastatic disease with variable response. As with other sarcomas, better therapeutics are needed.

13.5 Therapy for Bone Tumors

Ewing's sarcoma/PNET is a small blue round cell sarcoma with varying degrees of neuroectodermal differentiation commonly occurring in individuals younger than 30 years, with a male predilection. Ewing's sarcoma/PNET often arises in the diaphysis/metaphyseal-diaphyseal portion of long bones, pelvis, and ribs. However, this sarcoma may occur in soft tissue, although rarely in visceral organs [1, 140]. Several recurrent translocations have been identified in Ewing's sarcoma/PNET. The translocation t(11;22)(q24;q12) EWSR1-FLI-1 fusion and t(21;22)(q22;q12) EWSR1-ERG fusion are found in Ewing's sarcoma/PNET in 85 % and 5–10 % of cases, respectively. Translocations not involving the EWS gene occur such as t(16;21)(p11;q24) [1, 146]. Treatment involves chemotherapy along with adjunctive surgical resection with or without radiotherapy for local control. With the available treatment, survival for localized disease is 65–70 %; however, for those with metastatic disease at the time of diagnosis, a survival of between 25 % and 30 % has been reported [134]. Other possible therapies could include a more molecularly targeted approach. The IGF1R signaling pathway has been implicated in the cancer biology of several tumors, including Ewing's sarcoma. Ewing's sarcoma clinical studies using IGF1R inhibitors (antibody-based therapy) are underway: Ganitumab (AMG479), Figitumumab (CP-751), and Cixutumumab (ADVL0821). mTOR inhibitors (rapamycin) have demonstrated the ability to arrest ES cell proliferation and downregulate levels of EWS/FLI-1 proteins. Finally, in studies of combined IGF1R and mTOR inhibition, response in patients was demonstrated [134, 147, 148]. Other therapeutic avenues include immunotherapy; in one reported case, complete remission of residual tumor was reported following autologous SCT and pulsed vaccination with dendritic cells. NK cell therapy is also being studied. Chemotherapy and radiation-induced tissue injury on malignant tissue may increase expression of NK-activating ligands, thus sensitizing tumor cells to NK killing. With NK cell infusion following chemoradiation, the NK cells should migrate to the site of disease and kill tumor tissue. Toxicity has been shown against ES cells in

Table 13.3 Promising targeted agents

Hallmarks	Mechanism of inhibition	Targeted agents	Sarcomas of therapeutic interest
Sustaining proliferation	AKT inhibitors	MK2206, Perifosine	Leiomyosarcoma (LMS), Gastrointestinal stromal tumor (GIST)
	EGFR inhibitors	Lapatinib	Chordoma
	ER inhibitors	Anastrozole, Letrozole	Endometrial stromal sarcoma (ESS)
	IGF1R inhibitors	IMC-A12, SCH 717454	Ewing's Sarcoma, Solitary Fibrous Tumor/ Hemangiopericytoma (SFT/HPC)
	KIT inhibitors	Imatinib, Nilotinib, Sunitinib	GIST
	mTOR inhibitors	Everolimus, Rapamycin	LMS
	PDGFR inhibitors	Axitinib, imatinib, Pazopanib, Sorafenib	Chordomas, Desmoid, DFSP
	PI3K inhibitors	BEZ235, LY249002	GIST, LMS, Myxoid liposarcoma
Evading growth suppressors	CDK inhibitors	Dinacliclib, Flavopiridol, PD0332991	Dedifferentiated Liposarcoma, Osteosarcoma
	y-secretase inhibitors	R04929097	Liposarcoma, Osteosarcoma
	MDM2 inhibitors	R05045337	Dedifferentiated Liposarcoma
	Notch inhibitors	GDC0449	Liposarcoma, Osteosarcoma
	Weel inhibitors	MK-1775	Osteosarcoma
Avoiding immune destruction	Anti-CTLA-4 antibody	Ipilimumab	N/A
Replicative immortality	Telomerase inhibitor	GRN163L	Liposarcoma, Malignant fibrous histiocytoma
Tumor-promoting inflammation	COX2 inhibition	Celecoxib	Epithelioid hemangioendothelioma (EHE)
Activating invasion & metastasis	c-MET inhibitors	Cabozantinib, Crizotinib	Alveolar soft part sarcoma (ASPS)
Inducing angiogenesis	VEGF inhibitors	Bevacizumab	Angiosarcoma, HPC/SFT
	VEGFR inhibitors	Pazopanib, Sunitinib, Sorafenib, Vandetanib	Angiosarcoma, ASPS, EHE, HPC/SFT
Genomic instability & mutation	HDAC inhibitors	Vorinostat, Panobinostat	ESS, Conventional Chondrosarcoma, LMS
	PARP inhibitors	Olaparib	Ewing's sarcoma
Resisting cell death	BH3 mimetics	ABT-263, ABT-737	GIST, Osteosarcoma
	TRAIL antibodies	Apo2L/TRAIL	Conventional chondrosarcoma
Deregulating cellular energetics	IHD1/2 inhibition	N/A	Conventional chondrosarocoma

vitro and in vivo (mice) [149, 150]. Lastly, angiogenesis inhibitors that bind to vascular endothelial growth factor, inhibiting the proliferation of endothelial cells and the formation of new blood vessels, could reduce interstitial pressure in tumors, aiding in the effective delivery of chemotherapy and improving the oxygenation of tumors, leading to better radiation effectiveness. Vascular endothelial growth factor is upregulated in Ewing's sarcoma/PNET. The Children's Oncology Group completed a clinical trial (COG-AEWS0521) of vincristine, cyclophosphamide, and topotecan with or without bevacizumab in patients with their first episode of recurrent ES [151]. Preliminary results have yet to be published [151].

13.6 Targeted Therapy for Bone and Soft Tissue Tumors

It is obvious that understanding the molecular pathology of sarcoma is an arduous task, given the number of histologic subtypes and the unique biology of each entity. Therefore, it is no surprise to assume that one therapy does not work for all. Targeted therapies offer patients a chance of better response for their disease process, especially when chemotherapy may not be effective. Although the scope of this chapter is the molecular pathology of sarcomas and some of these points have already been discussed, a summary of promising targeted agents have been framed in the context of the recently revised hallmarks of cancer [152] (see Table 13.3). Clearly, we need to further refine our diagnostic skills and improve upon our therapeutic approach to best optimize the care of our sarcoma patients.

References

1. Fletcher C, Uni K, Mertens F (eds) (2002) Pathology and genetics of tumours of soft tissue and bone, vol 5, World Health Organization classification of tumours. IARC Press, Lyon
2. Igbokwe A, Lopez-Terrada D (2011) Molecular testing of solid tumors. Arch Pathol Lab Med 135:67–82
3. Bridge J, Cushman-Vokoun A (2011) Molecular diagnostics of soft tissue tumors. Arch Pathol Lab Med 135:588–601
4. Ordonez J, Osuna D, Garcia-Dominguez D, Amaral A, Otero-Motta A, Mackintosh C, Sevillano M, Barbado M, Hernandez T, Alva E (2010) The clinical relevance of molecular genetics in soft tissue sarcomas. Adv Anat Pathol 17:162–181
5. Taylor B, Barretina J, Maki R, Antonescu C, Singer S, Ladanyi M (2011) Advances in sarcoma genomics and new therapeutic targets. Nat Rev 11:541–557
6. Sandberg A, Bridge J (2000) Updates on cytogenetics and molecular genetics of bone and soft tissue tumors: Ewing sarcoma and peripheral primitive neuroectodermal tumors. Cancer Genet Cytogenet 123(1):1–26
7. Sorensen P, Lessnick S, Lopez-Terrada D, Liu X, Triche TJ, Denny CT (1994) A second Ewing's sarcoma translocation, t(21;22), fuses the EWS gene to another ETS family transcription factor, ERG. Nat Genet 6(2):146–151
8. Parham D (2001) Pathologic classification of rhabdomyosarcomas and correlations with molecular studies. Mod Pathol 14(5):506–514

9. Douglass E, Shapiro D, Valentine M (1993) Alveolar rhabdomyosarcoma with the t(2;13): cytogenetic findings and clinicopathologic correlations. Med Pediatr Oncol 21(2):83–87
10. Wachtel M, Dettling M, Koscielniak E (2004) Gene expression signatures identify rhabdomyosarcoma subtypes and detect a novel t(2;2)(q35;p23) translocation fusing PAX3 to NCOA1. Cancer Res 64(16):5539–5545
11. Barr F, Galili N, Holick J, Biegel J, Rovera G, Emanuel B (1993) Rearrangement of PAX3 paired box gene in the paediatric solid tumour alveolar rhabdomyosarcoma. Nat Genet 3(2):113–117
12. Sorensen P, Lynch J, Qualman S (2002) PAX3-FKHR and PAX7-FKHR gene fusions are prognostic indicators in alveolar rhabdomyosarcoma: a report from the children's oncology group. J Clin Oncol 20:2672–2679
13. Bridge J, Liu J, Qualman S (2002) Genomic gains and losses are similar in genetic and histologic subsets of rhabdomyosarcoma, whereas amplification predominates in embryonal with anaplasia and alveolar subtypes. Genes Chromosomes Cancer 33(3):310–321
14. Ladanyi M, Gerald W (1996) Specificity of the EWS/WT1 gene fusion for desmoplastic small round cell tumor. J Pathol 180(4):462
15. Antonescu C, Argani P, Erlandson R (1998) Skeletal and extraskeletal myxoid chondrosarcoma: a comparative clinicopathologic, ultrastructural, and molecular study. Cancer 83:1504–1521
16. Panagopoulos I, Mertens F, Isaksson M (2002) Molecular genetic characterization of the EWS/CHN and RBP56/CHN fusion genes in extraskeletal myxoid chondrosarcoma. Genes Chromosomes Cancer 35:340–352
17. Tanas M, Goldblum J (2009) Fluorescence in-situ hybridization in the diagnosis of soft tissue neoplasms: a review. Adv Anat Pathol 16:383–391
18. Enzinger F, Weiss S (2001) Soft tissue tumors, 4th edn. Mosby, St. Louis
19. de Leeuw B, Balemans M, Olde Weghuis D, Geurts van Kessel A (1995) Identification of two alternative fusion genes, SYT-SXX1 and SYT-SSX2, in t(X;18)(p11.2;q11.2)-positive synovial sarcomas. Hum Mol Genet 4(6):1097–1099
20. Kawai A, Woodruff J, Healey J, Brennan M, Antonescu C, Ladanyi M (1998) SYT-SSX gene fusion as a determinant of morphology and prognosis in synovial sarcoma. N Engl J Med 338(3):153–160
21. Patel K, Szabo S, Hernandez V (2008) Dermatofibrosarcoma protuberans COL1A1-PDGFB fusion is identified in virtually all dermatofibrosarcoma protuberans cases when investigated by newly developed multiplex reverse transcription polymerase chain reaction and fluoresence in situ hybridization assays. Hum Pathol 39(2):184–193
22. Naeem R, Lux M, Huang S, Naber S, Corson J, Fletcher J (1995) Ring chromosomes in dermatofibrosarcoma protuberans are composed of interspersed sequences from chromosomes 17 and 22. Am J Pathol 147(6):1553–1558
23. Terrier-Lacombe M, Guillou L, Maire G (2003) Dermatofibrosarcoma protuberans, giant cell fibroblastoma, and hybrid lesions in children: clinicopathologic comparative analysis of 28 cases with molecular data–a study from the French Federation of Cancer Centers Sarcoma Group. Am J Surg Pathol 27(1):27–39
24. Rutkowski P, Van Glabbeke M, Rankin C (2010) Imatinib mesylate in advanced dermatofibrosarcoma protuberans: pooled analysis of two phase II clinical trials. J Clin Oncol 28(10):1772–1779
25. Knezevish S, McFadden D, Tao W, Lim J, Sorensen P (1998) A novel ETV6-NTRK3 gene fusion in congenital fibrosarcoma. Nat Genet 18(2):184–187
26. Knezevish S, Garnett M, Pysher T, Beckwith J, Grundy P, Sorensen P (1998) ETV6-NTRK3 gene fusions and trisomy 11 establish a histogenetic link between mesoblastic nephroma and congenital fibrosarcoma. Cancer Res 58(22):5046–5048
27. Tognon C, Knezevich S, Huntsman D (2002) Expression of the ETV6-NTRK3 gene fusion as a primary event in human secretory breast carcinoma. Cancer Cell 2:367–376
28. Schofield D, Fletcher J, Grier H, Yunis E (1994) Fibrosarcoma in infants and children: application of new techniques. Am J Surg Pathol 18(1):14–24

29. Argani P, Fritsch M, Kadkol S, Schuster A, Beckwith J, Perlman E (2000) Detection of the ETV6-NTRK3 chimeric RNA of infantile fibrosarcoma/cellular congenital mesoblastic nephroma in paraffin-embedded tissue: application to challenging pediatric renal stromal tumors. Mod Pathol 13(1):29–36
30. Storlazzi C, Mertens F, Nascimento A (2003) Fusion of the FUS and BBF2H7 genes in low grade fibromyxoid sarcoma. Hum Mol Genet 12:2349–2358
31. Mertens F, Fletcher C, Antonescu C (2005) Clinicopathologic and molecular genetic characterization of low-grade fibromyxoid sarcoma, and cloning of a novel FUS/CREB3L1 fusion gene. Lab Invest 85:408–415
32. Flanagan A, Delaney D, O'Donnell P (2010) The benefits of molecular pathology in the diagnosis of musculoskeletal disease: part 1 of a two part review: soft tissue tumors. Skeletal Radiol 39:105–115
33. Hirota S, Isozaki K, Moriyama Y (1998) Gain-of-function mutations of c-kit in human gastrointestinal stromal tumors. Science 279(5350):577–580
34. Hirota S, Ohashi A, Nishida T (2003) Gain-of-function mutations of platelet-derived growth factor receptor alpha gene in gastrointestinal stromal tumors. Gastroenterology 125(3):660–667
35. Debiec-Rychter M, Sciot R, Le C (2006) KIT mutations and dose selection for imatinib in patients with advanced gastrointestinal stromal tumours. Eur J Cancer 42(8):1093–1103
36. Lasota J, Miettinen M (2008) Clinical significance of oncogenic KIT and PDGFRA mutations in gastrointestinal stromal tumors. Histopathology 53(3):245–266
37. Andersson J, Bumming P, Meis-Kindblom JM (2006) Gastrointestinal stromal tumors with KIT exon 11 deletions are associated with poor prognosis. Gastroenterology 130(6):1573–1581
38. Miettinen M, Sobin L, Lasota J (2005) Gastrointestinal stromal tumors of the stomach: a clinicopathologic, immunohistochemical, and molecular genetic study of 1765 cases with long-term follow-up. Am J Surg Pathol 29(1):52–68
39. Antonescu C, Sommer G, Sarran L (2003) Association of KIT exon 9 mutations with nongastric primary site and aggressive behavior: KIT mutation analysis and clinical correlates of 120 gastrointestinal stromal tumors. Clin Cancer Res 9(9):3329–3337
40. Lasota J, Corless C, Heinrich M (2008) Clinicopathologic profile of gastrointestinal stromal tumors (GISTs) with primary KIT exon 13 or exon 17 mutations: a multicenter study on 54 cases. Mod Pathol 21(4):476–484
41. Lasota J, Dansonka-Mieszkowska A, Sobin L, Miettinen M (2004) A great majority of GISTs with PDGFRA mutations represent gastric tumors of low or no malignant potential. Lab Invest 84(7):874–883
42. Heinrich M, Corless C, Blanke C (2006) Molecular correlates of imatinib resistance in gastrointestinal stromals tumors. J Clin Oncol 24(29):4764–4774
43. Debiec-Rychter M, Dumez H, Judson I (2004) Use of c-KIT/PDGFRA mutational analysis to predict the clinical response to imatinib in patients with advanced gastrointestinal stromal tumours entered on phase I and II studies of the EORTC Soft Tissue and Bone Sarcoma Group. Eur J Cancer 40(5):689–695
44. Heinrich M, Corless C, Demetri G (2005) Kinase mutations and imatinib response in patients with metastatic gastrointestinal stromal tumor. J Clin Oncol 21(23):4342–4349
45. Sandberg A (2004) Updates on the cytogenetics and molecular genetics of bone and soft tissue tumors: liposarcoma. Cancer Genet Cytogenet 155(1):1–24
46. Powers M, Wang W-L, Hernandez V (2010) Detection of myxoid liposarcoma-associated FUS-DDIT3 rearrangement variants including a newly identified breakpoint using an optimized RT-PCR assay. Mod Pathol 23(10):1307–1315
47. Barretina J, Taylor BS, Banerji S, Ramos AH, Lagos-Quintana M, Decarolis PL, Shah K, Socci ND, Weir BA, Ho A, Chiang DY, Reva B, Mermel CH, Getz G, Antipin Y, Beroukhim R, Major JE, Hatton C, Nicoletti R, Hanna M, Sharpe T, Fennell TJ, Cibulskis K, Onofrio RC, Saito T, Shukla N, Lau C, Nelander S, Silver SJ, Sougnez C, Viale A, Winckler W, Maki RG, Garraway LA, Lash A, Greulich H, Root DE, Sellers WR, Schwartz GK, Antonescu CR,

Lander ES, Varmus HE, Ladanyi M, Sander C, Meyerson M, Singer S (2010) Subtype-specific genomic alterations define new targets for soft-tissue sarcoma therapy. Nat Genet 42(8):715–721
48. Binh M, Sastre-Garau X, Guillou L (2005) MDM2 and CDK4 immunostainings are useful adjuncts in diagnosing well-differentiated and dedifferentiated liposarcoma subtypes: a comparative analysis of 559 soft tissue neoplasms with genetic data. Am J Surg Pathol 29(10):1340–1347
49. Bridge J, Sreekantaiah C, Neff J, Sandberg A (1991) Cytogenetic findings in clear cell sarcoma of tendons and aponeuroses: malignant melanoma of soft parts. Cancer Genet Cytogenet 52(1):101–106
50. Zucman J, Delattre O, Desmaze C (1993) EWS and ATF-1 gene fusion induced by t(12;22) translocation in malignant melanoma of soft parts. Nat Genet 4(4):341–345
51. Heimann P, Devalck C, Debusscher C, Sariban E, Vamos E (1998) Alveolar soft part sarcoma: further evidence by FISH for the involvement of chromosome band 17q25. Genes Chromosomes Cancer 23(2):194–197
52. Ladanyi M, Lui M, Antonescu C (2001) The der(17)t(X;17)(p11;q25) of human alveolar soft part sarcoma fuses the TFE3 transcription factor gene to ASPL, a novel gene at 17q25. Oncogene 20(1):48–57
53. Mitton B, Federman N (2012) Alveolar soft part sarcomas: molecular pathogenesis and implications for novel targeted therapies. Sarcoma 2012:428789
54. Biegel J, Allen C, Kawasaki K (1996) Narrowing the critical region for a rhabdoid tumor locus in 22q11. Genes Chromosomes Cancer 16(2):94–105
55. Versteege I, Sevenet N, Lange J (1998) Truncating mutations of hSNF5/INI1 in aggressive paediatric cancer. Nature 394(6689):203–206
56. Modena P, Lualdi E, Facchinetti F (2005) SMARCB1/INI1 tumor suppressor gene is frequently inactivated in epithelioid sarcomas. Cancer Res 65(10):4012–4019
57. Kreiger P, Judkins A, Russo P (2009) Loss of INI1 expression defines a unique subset of pediatric undifferentiated soft tissue sarcomas. Mod Pathol 22(1):142–150
58. Jackson E, Sievert A, Gai X (2009) Genomic analysis using high-density single nucleotide polymorphism-based oligonucleotide arrays and multiplex ligation-dependent probe amplification provides a comprehensive analysis of INI1/SMARCB1 in malignant rhabdoid tumors. Clin Cancer Res 15(6):1923–1930
59. Bovee J, Cleton-Jansen A, Wuyts W, Caethoven G, Taminiau A, Bakker E, Van Hul W, Cornelisse C, Hogendoorn P (1999) EXT-mutation analysis and loss of heterozygosity in sporadic and hereditary osteochondromas and secondary chondrosarcomas. Am J Hum Genet 65(3):689–698
60. Mertens F, Rydholm A, Kreicbergs A, Willen H, Jonsson K, Heim S, Mitelman F, Mandahl N (1994) Loss of chromosome band 8q24 in sporadic osteocartilaginous exostoses. Genes Chromosomes Cancer 9:8–12
61. Bridge J, Nelson M, Orndal C, Bhatia P, Neff J (1988) Clonal karyotypic abnormalities of the hereditary multiple exostoses chromosomal loci 8q24.1 (EXT1) and 11p11-12 (EXT2) in patients with sporadic and hereditary osteochondromas. Cancer 82:1657–1663
62. Gunawan B, Weber M, Bergmann F, Wildberger J, Niethard F, Fuzesi L (2000) Clonal chromosome abnormalities in enchondromas and chondrosarcomas. Cancer Genet Cytogenet 120:127–130
63. Bridge J, Persons D, Neff J, Bhatia P (1992) Clonal karyotypic aberrations in enchondromas. Cancer Detect Prev 16:215–219
64. Halbert A, Harrison W, Hicks M, Davino N, Cooley L (1998) Cytogenetic analysis of a scapular chondromyxoid fibroma. Cancer Genet Cytogenet 104:52–56
65. Safar A, Nelson M, Neff J, Maale G, Bayani J, Squire J, Bridge J (2000) Recurrent anomalies of 6q25 in chondromyxoid fibroma. Hum Pathol 31:306–311
66. Sawyer J, Swanson C, Lukacs J, Nicholas R, North P, Thomas J (1998) Evidence of an association between 6q13-21 chromosome aberrations and locally aggressive behavior in patients with cartilage tumors. Cancer 82:474–483

67. Granter S, Renshaw A, Kozakewich H, Fletcher J (1998) The pericentromeric inversion, inv (6)(p25q13), is a novel diagnostic marker in chondromyxoid fibroma. Mod Pathol 11:1273–1276
68. Tallini G, Dorfman H, Brys P, Dal Cin P, de Wever I, Fletcher C, Jonson K, Mandahl N, Mertens F, Mitelman F, Rosai J, Rydholm A, Samson I, Sciot R, van den Berghe H, Vanni R, Willen H (2002) Correlation between clinicopathological features and karyotype in 100 cartilaginous and chordoid tumors. A report from the chromosomes and morphology (CHAMP) collaborative study group. J Pathol 196:194–203
69. Schrage Y, Bovee J (2005) Bone tumors: an overview. Atlas Genet Cytogenet Oncol Haematol. http://documents.crevues.inist.fr/bitstream/2042/38197/1-03205
70. Bridge J, Bhatia P, Anderson J, Neff J (1993) Biologic and clinical significance of cytogenetic and molecular cytogenetic abnormalities in benign and malignant cartilaginous lesions. Cancer Genet Cytogenet 69:79–90
71. Mandahl N, Gustafson P, Mertens F, Akerman M, Baldetorp B, Gisselsson D, Knuutila S, Bauer H, Larsson O (2002) Cytogenetic aberrations and their prognostic impact in chondrosarcoma. Genes Chromosomes Cancer 33:188–200
72. Bridge J, DeBoer J, Travis J, Johansson S, Elmberger G, Noel S, Neff J (1994) Simultaneous interphase cytogenetic analysis and fluorescence immunophenotyping of dedifferentiated chondrosarcoma. Implications for histopathogenesis. Am J Pathol 144:215–220
73. Bovee J, Cleton-Jansen A, Rosenberg C, Taminiau A, Cornelisse C, Hogendoorn P (1999) Molecular genetic characterization of both components of a dedifferentiated chondrosarcoma, with implications for its histogenesis. J Pathol 189:454–462
74. O'Malley D, Opheim K, Barry T, Chapman D, Emond M, Conrad E, Norwood T (2001) Chromosomal changes in a dedifferentiated chondrosarcoma: a case report and review of the literature. Cancer Genet Cytogenet 124:105–111
75. Swarts S, Neff J, Johansson S, Bridge J (1996) Cytogenetic analysis of dedifferentiated chondrosarcoma. Cancer Genet Cytogenet 89:49–51
76. Naumann S, Krallman P, Unni K, Fidler M, Neff J, Bridge J (2002) Translocation der(13;21)(q10;q10) in skeletal and extraskeletal mesenchymal chondrosarcoma. Mod Pathol 15:572–576
77. Baruffi M, Volpon J, Neto J, Casartelli C (2001) Osteoid osteomas with chromosome alterations involving 22q. Cancer Genet Cytogenet 124:127–131
78. Knuutila S, Autio K, Aalto Y (2000) Online access to CGH data of DNA sequence copy number changes. Am J Pathol 157:689
79. Forus A, Florenes V, Maelandsom G, Fodstad O, Myklebost O (1994) The protooncogene CHOP/GADD153, involved in growth arrest and DNA damage response, is amplified in a subset of human sarcomas. Cancer Genet Cytogenet 78:165–171
80. Khatib Z, Matsushime H, Valentine M, Shapiro D, Sherr C, Look A (1993) Coamplification of the CDK4 gene with MDM2 and GLI in human sarcomas. Cancer Res 53:5535–5541
81. Momand J, Zambetti G, Olson D, George D, Levine A (1992) The mdm-2 oncogene product forms a complex with the p53 protein and inhibits p53-mediated transactivation. Cell 69:1237–1245
82. Oliner J, Kinzler K, Meltzer P, Gerorge D, Vogelstein B (1992) Amplification of a gene encoding a p53-associated protein in human sarcomas. Nature 358:80–83
83. Roberts W, Douglass E, Peiper S, Houghton P, Look A (1989) Amplification of the gli gene in childhood sarcomas. Cancer Res 49:5407–5413
84. Smith S, Weiss S, Jankowski S, Coccia M, Meltzer P (1992) SAS amplification in soft tissue sarcomas. Cancer Res 52:3746–3749
85. Atiye J, Wolf M, Kaur S, Monni O, Böhling T, Kivioja A, Tas E, Serra M, Tarkkanen M, Knuutila S (2005 Feb) Gene amplifications in osteosarcoma – CGH microarray analysis. Genes Chromosomes Cancer 42(2):158–163
86. Ladanyi M, Cha C, Lewis R, Jhanwar S, Huvos A, Healey J (1993) MDM2 gene amplification in metastatic osteosarcoma. Cancer Res 53:16–18

87. Berner J, Forus A, Elkahloun A, Meltzer P, Fodstad O, Myklebost O (1996) Separate amplified regions encompassing CDK4 and MDM2 in human sarcomas. Genes Chromosomes Cancer 17:254–259
88. Forus A, Florenes V, Maelandsom G, Fodstad O, Myklebost O (1994) 12q13-14 amplica in human sarcomas without MDM2 include CDK4, SAS and GADD153/CHOP. Cancer Genet Cytogenet 77:200
89. Maelandsom G, Berner J, Florenes V, Forus A, Hovig E, Fodstad O, Myklebost O (1995) Homozygous deletion frequency and expression levels of the CDKN2 gene in human sarcoma – relationship to amplification and mRNA levels of CDK4 and CCND1. Br J Cancer 72:393–398
90. Stock C, Kager L, Fink F, Gadner H, Ambros P (2000) Chromosomal regions involved in the pathogenesis of osteosarcomas. Genes Chromosomes Cancer 28:329–336
91. Tarkkanen M, Bohling T, Gamberi G, Ragazzini P, Benassi M, Kivioja A, Kallio P, Elomaa I, Picci P, Knuutila S (1998) Comparative genomic hybridization of low-grade central osteosarcoma. Mod Pathol 11:421–426
92. Mertens F, Mandahl N, Orndal C, Baldetorp B, Bauer H, Rydholm A, Wiebe T, Willen H, Akerman M, Heim S, Mitelman F (1993) Cytogenetic findings in 33 osteosarcomas. Int J Cancer 55:44–50
93. Sinovic J, Bridge J, Neff J (1992) Ring chromosome in parosteal osteosarcoma. Clinical and diagnostic significance. Cancer Genet Cytogenet 62:50–52
94. Szymanska J, Mandahl N, Mertens F, Tarkkanen M, Karaharju E, Knuutila S (1996) Ring chromosomes in parosteal osteosarcoma contain sequences from 12q13-15: a combined cytogenetic and comparative genomic hybridization study. Genes Chromosomes Cancer 16:31–34
95. Mertens F, Larramendy M, Gustavsson A, Gisselsson D, Rydholm A, Brosjo O, Mitelman F, Knuutila S, Mandahl N (2000) Radiation-associated sarcomas are characterized by complex karyotypes with frequent rearrangements of chromosome are 3p. Cancer Genet Cytogenet 116(89–96)
96. Tarkkanen M, Wiklund T, Virolainen M, Larramendy M, Mandahl N, Mertens F, Blomqvist C, Tukiainen E, Miettinen M, Elomaa I, Knuutila S (2001) Comparative genomic hybridization of postirradiation sarcomas. Cancer 92:1992–1998
97. Nellissery M, Padalecki S, Brkanac Z, Singer F, Roodman G, Unni K, Leach R, Hansen M (1998) Evidence for a novel osteosarcoma tumor-suppressor gene in the chromosome 18 region genetically linked with Paget disease of bone. Am J Hum Genet 63:817–824
98. Nilsson M, Domanski H, Mertens F, Mandahl N (2004) Molecular cytogenetic characterization of recurrent translocation breakpoints in bizarre parosteal osteochondromatous proliferation (Nora's lesion). Hum Pathol 35(9):1063–1069
99. Bridge J, Swarts S, Buresh C, Nelson M, Degenhardt J, Spanier S, Maale G, Meloni A, Lynch J, Neff J (1999) Trisomies 8 and 20 characterize a subgroup of benign fibrous lesions arising in both soft tissue and bone. Am J Pathol 154:729–733
100. Schwartz H, Dahir G, Butler M (1993) Telomere reduction in giant cell tumor of bone and with aging. Cancer Genet Cytogenet 71:132–138
101. Bridge J, Neff J, Mouron B (1992) Giant cell tumor of bone. Chromosomal analysis of 48 specimens and review of the literature. Cancer Genet Cytogenet 58:2–13
102. Panagopoulos I, Mertens F, Domanski H, Isaksson M, Brosjo O, Gustafson P, Mandahl N (2001) No EWS/FLI1 fusion transcripts in giant-cell tumors of bone. Int J Cancer 93:769–772
103. Sciot R, Dorfman H, Brys P, Dal Cin P, De Wever I, Fletcher C, Jonson K, Mandahl N, Mertens F, Mitelman F, Rosai J, Rydholm A, Samson I, Tallini G, Van den Berghe H, Vanni R, Willen H (2000) Cytogenetic-morphologic correlations in aneurysmal bone cyst, giant cell tumor of bone and combined lesions. A report from the CHAMP study group. Mod Pathol 13:1206–1210
104. Tarkkanen M, Kaipanien A, Karaharju E, Bohling T, Szymanska J, Helio H, Kivioja A, Elomaa I, Knuutila S (1993) Cytogenetic study of 249 consecutive patients examined for a bone tumor. Cancer Genet Cytogenet 68:1–21

105. Zheng M, Siu P, Papadimitriou J, Wood D, Murch A (1999) Telomeric fusion is a major cytogenetic aberration of giant cell tumors of bone. Pathology 31:373–378
106. Scheil S, Bruderlein S, Liehr T, Starke H, Herms J, Schulte M, Moller P (2001) Genome-wide analysis of sixteen chordomas by comparative genomic hybridization and cytogenetics of the first human chordoma cell line, U-CH1. Genes Chromosomes Cancer 32:203–211
107. Miozzo M, Dalpra L, Riva P, Volonta M, Macciardi F, Pericotti S, Tibiletti M, Cerati M, Rohde K, Larizza L, Fuhrman Conti A (2000) A tumor suppressor locus in familial and sporadic chordoma maps to 1p36. Int J Cancer 87:68–72
108. Hazelbag H, Van den Broek L, Fleuren G, Taminiau A, Hogendoorn P (1997) Distribution of extracellular matrix components in adamantinoma of long bones suggests fibrous-to-epithelial transformation. Hum Pathol 28:183–188
109. Kanamori M, Antonescu C, Scott M, Bridge R, Neff J, Spanier S, Scarborough M, Vergara G, Rosenthal H, Bridge J (2001) Extra copies of chromosomes 7, 8, 12, 19, and 21 are recurrent in adamantinoma. J Mol Diagn 3:16–21
110. Mandahl N, Heim S, Rydholm A, Willen H, Mitelman F (1989) Structural chromosome aberrations in an adamantinoma. Cancer Genet Cytogenet 42:187–190
111. Sozzi G, Miozzo M, Di Palma S, Minelli A, Calderone C, Danesino C, Pastorino U, Pierotti M, Della Porta G (1990) Involvement of the region 13q14 in a patient with adamantinoma of the long bones. Hum Genet 85:513–515
112. Panoutsakopoulos G, Pandis N, Kyriazoglou I, Gustafson P, Mertens F, Mandahl N (1999) Recurrent t(16;17)(q22;p13) in aneurysmal bone cysts. Genes Chromosomes Cancer 26:265–266
113. Oliveira A, Perez-Atayde A, Inwards C, Medeiros F, Derr V, Hsi B (2004) USP6 and CDH11 oncogenes identify the neoplastic cell in primary aneurysmal bone cysts and are absent in so-called secondary aneurysmal bone cysts. Am J Pathol 165(5):1773–1780
114. Oliveira A, Hsi B, Weremowicz S, Rosenberg A, Dal Cin P, Joseph N (2004) USP6 (Tre2) fusion oncogenes in aneurysmal bone cyst. Cancer Res 64(6):1920–1923
115. Oliveira A, Perez-Atayde A, Dal Cin P, Gebhardt M, Chen C, Neff J (2005) Aneurysmal bone cyst variant translocations upregulate USP6 transcription by promoter swapping with the ZNF9, COL1A1, TRAP150, and OMD genes. Oncogene 24:3419–3426
116. Oliveira A, Chou M, Perez-Atayde A, Rosenberg A (2006) Aneurysmal bone cyst: a neoplasm driven by upregulation of the USP6 oncogene. J Clin Oncol 24(1):e1
117. Bianco P, Rimminucci M, Majolagbe A, Kuznetsov S, Collins M, Mankani M (2000) Mutations of the GNAS1 gene, stromal cell dysfunction, and osteomalacic changes in non-McCune-Albright fibrous dysplasia of bone. J Bone Miner Res 15(1):120–128
118. Pisters PW, Leung DH, Woodruff J, Shi W, Brennan MF (1996) Analysis of prognostic factors in 1,041 patients with localized soft tissue sarcomas of the extremities. J Clin Oncol 14(5):1679–1689
119. Kumar V, Abbas A, Fausto N, Aster J (2010) Robbins & Cotran pathologic basis of disease, 8th edn. Elsevier, Philadelphia
120. Agaram N, Wong G, Guo T (2008) Novel V600E BRAF mutations in imatinib-naive and imatinib-resistant gastrointestinal stromal tumors. Genes Chromosomes Cancer 47:853–859
121. Agaimy A, Terracciano T, Dirnhofer S (2009) V600E BRAF mutations are alternative early molecular events in a subset of IT/PDGFRA wild-type gastrointestinal stromal tumors. J Clin Pathol 62:613–616
122. Judson I (2010) Targeted therapies in soft tissue sarcomas. Ann Oncol 21(Suppl 7):277–280
123. Wardelmann E, Schildhaus H, Merkelbach-Bruse S (2010) Soft tissue sarcoma: from molecular diagnosis to selection of treatment. Pathological diagnosis of soft tissue sarcoma amid molecular biology and targeted therapies. Ann Oncol 21(Suppl 7):265–269
124. Janeway KA, Kim SY, Lodish M, Nose V, Rustin P, Gaal J, Dahia PL, Liegl B, Ball ER, Raygada M, Lai AH, Kelly L, Hornick JL, O'Sullivan M, de Krijger RR, Dinjens WN, Demetri GD, Antonescu CR, Fletcher JA, Helman L, Stratakis CA (2011) Defects in succinate dehydrogenase in gastrointestinal stromal tumors lacking KIT and PDGFRA mutations. Proc Natl Acad Sci U S A 108(1):314–318

125. Kelly-Downs E, Rubin B (2011) Gastrointestinal stromal tumors: molecular mechanisms and targeted therapies. Pathol Res Int 2011:7
126. Demetri GD, van Oosterom AT, Garrett CR, Blackstein ME, Shah MH, Verweij J, McArthur G, Judson IR, Heinrich MC, Morgan JA, Desai J, Fletcher CD, George S, Bello CL, Huang X, Baum CM, Casali PG (2006) Efficacy and safety of sunitinib in patients with advanced gastrointestinal stromal tumour after failure of imatinib: a randomised controlled trial. Lancet 368(9544):1329–1338
127. Quek R, George S (2010) Update on the treatment of gastrointestinal stromal tumors (GISTs): role of imatinib. Biologics Targets Ther 4:19–31
128. Weiss S, Goldblum J (eds) (2008) Enzinger and Weiss's soft tissue tumors. Mosby Elsevier, St. Louis
129. Blay J, El Sayadi H, Thiesse P (2008) Complete response to imatinib in relapsing pigmented villonodular synovitis/tenosynovial giant cell tumor (PVNS/TGCT). Ann Oncol 19:821–822
130. Cassier P, Stacchiotti S, Gelderblom H (2010) Imatinib mesylate for the treatment of locally advanced and/or metastatic pigmented villonodular synovitis/tenosynovial giant cell tumor (PVNS/TGCT). In: ASCO annual meeting; 2010, Chicago. J Clin Oncol 28:15s (suppl; abstr 10012)
131. Ravia V, Wang W, Lewis V (2011) Treatment of tenosynovial giant cell tumor and pigmented villonodular synovitis. Curr Opin Oncol 23:361–366
132. Spurrell EL, Fisher C, Thomas JM, Judson IR (2005) Prognostic factors in advanced synovial sarcoma: an analysis of 104 patients treated at the Royal Marsden Hospital. Ann Oncol 16(3):437–444
133. Canter RJ, Qin LX, Maki RG, Brennan MF, Ladanyi M, Singer S (2008) A synovial sarcoma-specific preoperative nomogram supports a survival benefit to ifosfamide-based chemotherapy and improves risk stratification for patients. Clin Cancer Res 14(24):8191–8197
134. Subbiah V, Kurzrock R (2011) Phase 1 clinical trials for sarcomas: cutting edge. Curr Opin Oncol 23:352–360
135. Sleijfer S, Ray-Coquard I, Papai Z (2009) Pazopanib, a multikinase angiogenesis inhibitor, in patients with relapsed or refractory advanced soft tissue sarcoma: a phase II study from the European Organization for Research and Treatment of Cancer-Soft Tissue and Bone Sarcoma Group (EORTC study 62043). J Clin Oncol 27(19):3126–3132
136. Dobashi Y, Suzuki S, Sato E (2009) EGFR-dependent and independent activation of Akt/mTOR cascade in bone and soft tissue tumors. Mod Pathol 22(10):128–140
137. Mancuso T, Mezzelani A, Riva C (2000) Analysis of SYT-SSX fusion transcripts and bcl-2 expression and phosphorylation status in synovial sarcoma. Lab Invest 80(6):805–813
138. Joyner D, Albritton K, Bastar J (2006) G3139 antisense oligonucleotide directed against antiapoptotic bcl-2 enhances doxorubicin cytotoxicity in the FU-SY-1 synovial sarcoma line. J Orthop Res 24(3):474–480
139. Weiss S (2002) Soft tissue sarcomas: lessons from the past, challenges for the future. Mod Pathol 15(1):77–86
140. Mills S, Carter D, Greenson J (eds) (2009) Sternberg's diagnostic surgical pathology, 5th edn. Lippincott Williams & Wikins, Philadelphia
141. Henricks W, Chu Y, Goldblum J, Weiss S (1997) Dedifferentiated liposarcoma: a clinicopathological analysis of 155 cases with a proposal for an expanded definition of dedifferentiation. Am J Surg Pathol 21(3):271–281
142. McCormick D, Mentzel T, Beham A, Fletcher C (1994) Dedifferentiated liposarcoma: clinicopathologic analysis of 32 cases suggesting a better prognostic subgroup among pleomorphic sarcomas. Am J Surg Pathol 18(12):1213–1223
143. Singer S, Antonescu C, Riedel E, Brennan M, Pollock R (2003) Histologic subtype and margin of resection predict pattern of recurrence and survival for retroperitoneal liposarcoma. Ann Surg 238(3):358–371
144. Yang J, Du X, Chen K, Ylipaa A, Lazar AJ, Trent J, Lev D, Pollock R, Hao X, Hunt K, Zhang W (2009) Genetic aberrations in soft tissue leiomyosarcoma. Cancer Lett 275(1):1–8

145. Hernando E, Charytonowicz E, Dudas ME, Menendez S, Matushansky I, Mills J, Socci ND, Behrendt N, Ma L, Maki RG, Pandolfi PP, Cordon-Cardo C (2007) The AKT-mTOR pathway plays a critical role in the development of leiomyosarcomas. Nat Med 13(6):748–753
146. Longtin R (2003) Ewing's sarcoma: a miracle drug waiting to happen? J Natl Cancer Inst 95(21):1574–1576
147. Pinto A, Dickman P, Parham D (2011) Pathobiologic markers of the Ewing sarcoma family of tumors: state of the art and prediction of behaviour. Sarcoma 2011:15
148. Pappo A, Pater S (2010) Activity of R1507, a monoclonal antibody to the insulin-like growth factor-1 receptor (IGF1R), in patients with recurrent or refractory Ewing's sarcoma family of tumors (ESFT): results of a phase II SARC study. In: Proceedings of the ASCO annual meeting. June 4–8, Chicago, IL
149. Cho D, Shook D, Shimasaki N, Chang Y, Fujisaki H, Campana D (2010) Cytotoxicity of activated natural killer cells against pediatric solid tumors. Clin Cancer Res 16(15):3901–3909
150. Ahn Y, Weigel B, Verneris M (2010) Killing the killer: natural killer cells to treat Ewing's sarcoma. Clin Cancer Res 16:3819–3821
151. Karosas A (2010) Ewing's sarcoma. Am J Health Syst Pharm 67(19):1599–1605
152. Hanahan D, Weinberg RA (2011) Hallmarks of cancer: the next generation. Cell 144(5):646–674

Chapter 14
Molecular Pathology and Diagnostics of Pancreatic Endocrine Neoplasms

Aejaz Nasir, Jonathan R. Strosberg, Larry K. Kvols, Jalil Muhammad, Nelly A. Nasir, Omie Mills, and Domenico Coppola

Contents

A. Nasir, M.D., M.Phil., FCAP (✉)
Diagnostic & Experimental Pathology & Tailored Therapeutics Program,
Eli Lilly & Company, Indianapolis, IN 46285, USA
e-mail: nasirae@lilly.com

J.R. Strosberg • L.K. Kvols
GI Tumor Program, Neuroendocrine Research Division,
H. Lee Moffitt Cancer Center and Research Institute, Tampa, FL, USA

J. Muhammad
School of Medicine, George Mason University, Falls Church, VA, USA

N.A. Nasir
Department of Pathology & Laboratory Medicine, Sir Mortimer Jewish General Hospital,
McGill University, Montreal, Canada

D. Coppola (ed.), *Molecular Pathology and Diagnostics of Cancer*,
Cancer Growth and Progression 16, DOI 10.1007/978-94-007-7192-5_14,

Abstract Pancreatic Endocrine Neoplasms (PENs) are a group of rare tumors thought to arise from the endocrine cells of the pancreas. These tumors may be functional (hormone producing), or non functional. They have a wide range of presenting symptoms. Recent research efforts have shown the complex biology of these tumors, and have started to uncover the molecular alterations responsible for the genesis of these neoplasms. In this chapter we give an overview of the molecular tests available to detect such alterations, and of their diagnostic and prognostic significance.

Keywords Pancreatic endocrine neoplasms • Pancreatic endocrine tumors/carcinomas • Classifications of PENS • Molecular genetic • Islets of Langerhans

Abbreviations

AP1	Activator protein-1
bFGF	Basic fibroblast growth factor
CLP-PET	Clinically localized pancreatic endocrine tumors
CPGs	Candidate progression genes
EFR1	Estrogen receptor gene
FHIT	Fragile histidine triad
hMLH1	Human MutL homologue
IGF	Insulin-like growth factor
IGFBP-3	Insulin-like growth factor binding protein 3
IHC	Immunohistochemistry
LOH	Loss of heterozygosity
MAG	Metastasis-associated gene
MECC	Monohormonal endocrine cell clusters
MEN1	Multiple endocrine neoplasia type 1
MP	Metastatic primary
mTOR	Mammalian target of rapamycin
NF1	Neuofibromatosis type 1

O. Mills
Department of Pathology & Cell Biology, College of Medicine, University of South Florida, Tampa, FL, USA

D. Coppola
Department of Anatomic Pathology, H. Lee Moffitt Cancer Center and Research Institute, Tampa, FL, USA

GI Tumor Program, Neuroendocrine Research Division, H. Lee Moffitt Cancer Center and Research Institute, Tampa, FL, USA

Department of Pathology & Cell Biology, College of Medicine, University of South Florida, Tampa, FL, USA

NGF	Nerve growth factor
PECAs	Pancreatic endocrine carcinomas
PENS	Pancreatic endocrine neoplasm
PETs	Pancreatic endocrine tumors
PRAD-1	Parathyroid adenoma-related protein
SDHD	Succinate dehydrogenase subunit D
SST	Somatostatin
SSTRs	G-protein-coupled transmembrane receptors
TGF	Transforming growth factor
TSC1, TSC2	Tuberous sclerosis genes 1 & 2
VHL	von Hippel-Lindau genes

14.1 Introduction

The endocrine pancreas is composed of groups of endocrine cells known as islets of Langerhans, which are scattered throughout the organ and in the vicinity of pancreatic ducts [1–3]. The pancreatic islet cell population consists of alpha (α) cells, beta (β) cells, pancreatic polypeptide (PP) cells and delta (δ) cells [4]. Pancreatic endocrine neoplasms (PENs) are characterized by diverse clinical presentation and outcome and complex biology. PENs comprise about 2 % of all pancreatic neoplasms [5]. Every year, about 2,500 new PENs are diagnosed [6, 7]. The incidence of PENs is <1 per 100,000 person-years, although autopsy incidence ranges from 0.8 % to 10 % as they often remain clinically silent and undiagnosed [8]. PENs are associated with a better prognosis than exocrine pancreatic cancers, with an overall 5-year patient survival rate of 35–60 % [9]. There has been no strong association between environmental risk and the development of PENs. A recent study found no association with first-hand tobacco exposure or alcohol use [8].

14.2 Functional and Pathologic Classification of PENs

PENs are categorized as functional or nonfunctional. Functional tumors secrete polypeptide hormones such as insulin, gastrin, glucagon, somatostatin, vasoactive intestinal peptide, adrenal corticotrophic hormone, parathyroid hormone-related peptide, growth hormone, calcitonin, melanocyte-stimulating hormone, vasopressin, and norephinephrine, and elicit a clinically recognizable, hormone-related syndrome. Nonfunctional tumors secrete biologically inactive peptides and do not produce hormone-associated symptoms [10]. Approximately half of all PENs are nonfunctional [7].

Pathologic classification of PENs based on tumor size, proliferative activity (Ki-67 index), angioinvasion, invasion of adjacent organs, the presence or absence of distant metastases, hormone activity and clinical syndromes has been shown to be of some use in predicting the clinical behavior of these neoplasms [7, 11]. However, a better understanding of the molecular diagnostic aspects of these unpredictable neoplasms will contribute to improved diagnostic and therapeutic strategies and better patient outcome.

Current molecular techniques have shown that the biology of PENs is complex, without a particular biologic pathway driving these clinically challenging neoplasms. These tumors appear to develop in stages with multiple sequential mutations that contribute to ultimate progression to malignancy [12]. Several factors interact in complex ways to influence development, differentiation, secretion and the interaction of PENs with the tumor microenvironment [13]. Major events involved in pancreatic endocrine neoplasm initiation, progression and distant metastasis include basic fibroblast growth factor (bFGF), fragile histidine triad (FHIT), multiple endocrine neoplasia type 1 (MEN1), neurofibromatosis type 1 (NF1, neurofibromin), nerve growth factor (NGF), parathyroid adenoma–related protein (PRAD-1), transforming growth factor (TGF), tuberous sclerosis genes 1 and 2 (TSC1, TSC2), vascular endothelial growth factor (VEGF) and von Hippel-Lindau (VHL) genes.

14.3 Hereditary Syndromes Associated with PENs

The multiple endocrine neoplasia syndromes associated with PENs include multiple endocrine neoplasia type 1 (MEN1 gene), von Hippel-Lindau disease (vHL gene), neurofibromatosis (NF-1 gene), and tuberous sclerosis (TSC1 and TSC2 genes).

14.3.1 Multiple Endocrine Neoplasia Syndrome, Type 1

Multiple endocrine neoplasia syndrome, type 1 (MEN-1) is an autosomal dominant familial syndrome first described by Moldawer et al. [14] and Wermer [15]. Clinically, it is characterized by parathyroid adenomas, pancreatic endocrine neoplasms, and pituitary hyperplasia or neoplasia [16]. Other rarer neoplasms include bronchial and thymic carcinoids, adrenocortical tumors and cutaneous lipomas and collagenomas [17]. While hyperparathyroidism is the most common endocrine manifestation of MEN-1, PENs are the second most common endocrine manifestation and occur in about 60 % or more of MEN-1 patients. The majority of PENs in MEN1 are non-functional. However, most common functional entero-pancreatic endocrine tumors in MEN-1 patients are gastrinomas [18, 19], which often occur in the wall of the duodenum and in peri-pancreatic lymph nodes, and also insulinomas. Clustering of subvariants of MEN-1 such as insulinomas [20, 21] and aggressive gastrinomas [22] within small MEN-1 families suggest specific MEN-1 mutations may correlate with specific clinical variants. PENs in MEN-1 syndrome are invariably multifocal and may be widely dispersed in the pancreas and duodenum [18].

Consequently, the role of surgical management becomes particularly challenging and controversial [23, 24]. PENs in MEN-1 may also present as multiple clinically silent entero-pancreatic macroadenomas, which may be found at surgery or at autopsy in almost 100 % of MEN-1 patients older than 40 years [20, 25, 74]. Approximately 80 % of MEN1 cases are familial, whereas 20 % appear to be associated with new mutations based on negative familial history [26].

The MEN1 gene is a tumor suppressor gene [25, 27] mapped to a specific region on the long arm of chromosome 11 (11q13). The gene encodes a nuclear protein called menin, which interacts with several other proteins including junD, a member of the activator protein-1 (AP1) transcription factor family, SMAD1, SMAD3, SMAD5, PEM, NM23, nuclear factor kB and runx2 [28–35]. Mutations in MEN1 gene are the principal genetic abnormality in MEN1 syndrome, seen in most PENs in MEN1 patients and in about one third of sporadic PENs, as an early event in the neoplastic process.

The tumorigenesis in MEN-1 patients is thought to be a two-step inactivation of the MEN1 gene, in which both copies of the MEN1 gene must be inactivated in order for tumorigenesis to occur. A "two-hit" hypothesis has been proposed whereby germline inactivation of one allele is followed by somatic inactivation of the second allele in a predisposed cell, leading to clonal proliferation [36]. Virtually all first hits at the MEN1 gene are small mutations involving one to several bases [37, 38]. Most MEN1 gene mutations occur in the locus of exon 2 [39]. However, hundreds of unique germline and somatic mutations, broadly distributed across the MEN1 open reading frame, have been found [16, 38, 40]. Most of the first-hit mutations predict premature truncation of the menin protein, while other mutations predict missense mutations or replacement of one to three amino acids, all of which result in inactivation or absence of menin protein. The second step in MEN-1 tumorigenesis always occurs in somatic tissue, usually as a postnatal event. The second-hit mutations are usually large chromosomal or subchromosomal rearrangements with a resultant deletion that includes the remaining normal MEN1 gene.

14.3.2 Loss of Heterozygosity at 11q13

Loss of heterozygosity (LOH) is used mainly to show loss of the normal copy of the MEN1 gene. In MEN-1 patients, LOH at 11q13 was found in almost 100 % of gastrinomas and other pancreatic endocrine tumors, as well as non-pancreatic endocrine neoplasia [41, 42]. Some sporadic endocrine tumors of the type found in MEN-1 show frequent LOH at 11q13. An underlying mutation at 11q13 has been traced to the MEN1 gene in about 50 % of sporadic MEN-1 like tumors with 11q13 LOH. Somatic mutations of the MEN1 gene occur in about 20 % of sporadic solitary PENs [26, 30, 43]. Therefore, MEN1 gene mutations are among the most common mutations in sporadic PENs. Among functional PENs, MEN1 gene mutations occur in about 25 % gastrinomas, 10–20 % insulinomas and 50 % VIPomas [44–47].

14.3.3 Events Following Inactivation of MEN1 Gene

After MEN1 gene inactivation, other unknown genes or undetected mutations in MEN1 gene may contribute to MEN-1 tumor development. Studies suggest that the tumorigenic pathway of MEN-1 overlaps and interacts with other homeostatic cell pathways [48–51]. Multifocal microadenoma is an early monoclonal or oligoclonal islet cell lesion in MEN-1, which may represent a hyperplastic precursor stage to subsequent neoplastic development [52]. Monohormonal endocrine cell clusters (MECCs) develop most frequently within normal pancreatic islets but also in exocrine pancreatic ducts and hyperplastic islets through 11q13 LOH. MECCs progress to microadenomas (MA) with disruption of the normal islet structure and transformation into neoplastic process. Evidence in support of microadenomas in MEN1 patients includes hyperplastic foci of gastrin cells seen by light microscopy in the duodenum of gastrinoma specimens from MEN-1 but not from sporadic gastrinomas [53]. Furthermore, in the heterozygous knockout of the MEN1 gene in mice, giant hyperplastic islets precede the development of insulinoma, suggesting that subtle islet hyperplasia may be an unrecognized precursor lesion in MEN-1 of humans despite the presence of one normal MEN1 allele. One could speculate that hyperplasia is an expression of MEN1 heterozygosity [54, 55].Further studies are needed to link these findings with an as yet undiscovered genetic basis of tumor development.

14.3.4 Von Hippel-Lindau Syndrome

Von Hippel-Lindau syndrome (VHL) is an autosomal dominant disorder characterized by hemangioblastomas of the central nervous system, renal cell carcinomas, retinal angiomas, visceral cysts, pheochromocytomas and PENs, which occur in10–20 % of VHL patients [56–59]. The VHL gene, mapped to chromosome 3p25.3 [60], is a tumor suppressor gene that has an inhibitory effect on transcription elongation and facilitates the proteasome-mediated degradation of the hypoxia-inducible factor 1 (HIF-1) protein [16, 61]. The alpha subunit of HIF-1 is highly sensitive to tissue oxygen levels. In the presence of normal oxygen levels, it is bound by the VHL protein complex and covalently linked to ubiquitin in order to be targeted for degradation. In the absence of the VHL protein, HIF-1 alpha levels increase, leading to overproduction of hypoxia-associated cytokines, including erythropoietin, vascular endothelial growth factor (VEGF), and platelet-derived growth factor [5, 62–67]. These cytokines have been implicated in tumor growth. However, the precise mechanism of tumorigenesis is unknown. Other factors contributing to tumor pathogenesis may include matrix metalloproteinases such as MMP1 [68, 69]. VEGF inhibition, with resultant inhibition of angiogenesis, is currently under investigation as a potential therapeutic strategy for PENs [70, 71].

The majority of patients present with a germline mutation of the gene from the affected parent and a normal copy of the gene from the unaffected parent. Tumor develops when both alleles are inactivated, usually as the result of a deletion [5]. In one study 12.3 % of 155 patients with VHL went on to develop PENs [72]. Majority of these neoplasms tend to be nonfunctional, and are frequently composed of cells with foamy, clear cytoplasm, similar to clear cells typical of renal cell carcinomas in VHL [41, 73]. LOH of the VHL gene was found in 100 % of PENs (6 of 6 tumors) analyzed by PCR-single strand conformational polymorphism and fluorescent in situ hybridization. All the tumors in this study were nonfunctional [41]. These findings support a role for VHL gene mutation in the formation of VHL-associated PENs. In patients with sporadic PENs, no mutations were found in the VHL gene, although allelic loss on chromosome 3p was found in 33 % of 43 patients with sporadic PENs [74].

14.3.5 Neurofibromatosis Type 1

Neurofibromatosis type 1 (NF-1) is a neurocutaneous syndrome characterized by neurofibromas, Lisch nodules on the iris, dermal café-au-lait spots, as well as a variety of endocrine neoplasms, including somatostatin-producing neuroendocrine tumors of the duodenal wall, pheochromocytomas, hyperparathyroidism, hypothalamic or optic nerve tumors [16] and rarely somatostatinomas of the pancreas [5, 75, 76]. NF-1 is caused by a mutation of the NF-1 gene, a tumor suppressor gene located on chromosome 17q11 that code for the protein neurofibromin. Mutations cause the premature truncation of neurofibromin. The precise role of the NF-1 gene in the development of PENs still remains to be elucidated.

14.3.6 Tuberous Sclerosis

Tuberous sclerosis is a rare autosomal dominant syndrome associated with the development of hamartomas and benign tumors in multiple organs, including skin, brain, and kidney. Two gene mutations have been described: TSC1 on 9q34 encoding hamartin [77] and TSC2 on 16p13.3 encoding tuberin, with identification of the tuberous sclerosis gene on chromosome 16 [78]. Together, these proteins function as a tumor suppressor gene complex and control the activity of mammalian target of rapamycin (mTOR) [16]. A complex of hamartin and tuberin is thought to regulate cell-cycle progression, possibly through upregulation of the mTOR cell-signaling pathway [79, 80]. mTOR is an intracellular protein that is key in the control of cell growth, protein synthesis, and autophagy [71] and is involved in the regulation of β-catenin stability and activity [5]. One to five percent of patients with tuberous sclerosis can develop PENs that demonstrate LOH on 16p13.3 or lack of tuberin immunoreactivity [5, 81–83]. Based on these findings, the RADIANT 1 (RAD In

Advanced Neuroendocrine Tumors) trial, a phase II study, focused on the evaluation of everolimus, an mTOR inhibitor, in patients with advanced PENs who have failed cytotoxic chemotherapy [71].

14.4 Molecular Genetic Analyses in Sporadic PENs

The majorities of PENs are sporadic and lack any association with germline mutations. The genetic aberrations implicated in sporadic PENs are poorly understood. Oncogenes and tumor suppressor genes that are mutated in common human malignancies (p53, APC, Rb, K-ras) do not appear to be associated with PENs [84–86]. Both within genetic syndromes characterized by PENs and in sporadic PENs, genomic studies have identified specific molecular patterns that characterize individual PENs. In the case of MEN1 associated insulinoma, these molecular abnormalities include gain of function in dlk1, PCNA, TERT, ASK and NFkB [93, 257, 262, 283], and loss of function of menin, p27, p18, JunD and FANCD2 [87–89]. Sporadic insulinomas are characterized by gain in function of cyclD/CDK4, Akt1, Abl, TGFa/EGFR and Bcl2 [193, 194, 263, 263, 264, 265, 266, 277, 280] and loss of function of several proteins, including PTEN, p16, p15 and RKIP [168, 190, 260, 261, 270, 271]. Several of these genes and markers have also been studied in other PENs with variable findings.

14.5 Comparative Genomic Hybridization Studies in PENs

Several studies have used comparative genomic hybridization (CGH) to identify chromosomal aberrations in PENs. One of the most consistent chromosomal alteration is loss of 11q, which harbors the MEN1 gene [90]. Zikusoka et al. [81] compared six studies using comparative genomic hybridization to detect gains and losses in various chromosomes in PENs. The most frequent gains were on chromosomes 7 and 20. The most frequent losses were on chromosomes 2, 6q, 21q, and Y. Chromosomal aberrations associated most frequently with malignant behavior and metastasis included gains of chromosomes 7, 14q, 4, and Xq, as well as losses of chromosomes 6p, 3p, 6q, and 21q [91–93]. Male patients with malignant insulinomas have been reported to show loss of Y chromosome and gain of Xp [75, 91]. Similarly, PENs in females have been shown to exhibit loss of X chromosome [75]. Furthermore, loss of sex chromosome has been associated with metastatic disease, local invasion and poor patient survival [75]. Other chromosomal aberrations identified in PENs include gains of chromosomes 19, 5, 14p, 12q, 17, 20q, 15, 18, 9q, and 17p, as well as losses of chromosomes 1p, 6, 11q, 3q, 11p, and Xq [91, 92, 94–97]. Overall, nonfunctional PENs contained more genetic aberrations than functional PENs [91], metastases had a higher average number of chromosomal aberrations than matched primaries [94] and 11q losses and 7q gains were reported in multiple studies, supporting their role in the development of PENs.

14.6 Loss of Heterozygosity (LOH) Studies in PENs

LOH analysis is a powerful molecular tool used to identify tumor suppressor gene loci that are involved in the formation and progression of neoplasms, including PENs. An LOH frequency greater than 35 % at a specific chromosomal locus exceeds the rates of random genomic instability and strongly suggests a relevant tumor suppressor gene at that locus [98, 99]. A technical advantage with LOH is that it can detect even smaller chromosomal deletions that could be missed by CGH. Several chromosomal aberrations have been identified in sporadic PENs. Using LOH, most common abnormalities are found in chromosomes 1, 3 and 6. LOH at chromosome 1 was found in 34 % of PETs and was found to be more common in tumors with hepatic metastasis [100, 101]. Chen et al. [102] identified chromosome 1 LOH on 1q31–32 and 1q21–23 in almost half of the gastrinomas studied and found an association with aggressive growth, liver metastasis and post-surgical recurrence of liver metastasis, suggesting a worse prognosis for patients with chromosome 1 aberrations. Overall, 56 % of 273 metatsatic PENs analyzed in several different studies were found to show various chromosomal aberrations, especially in chromosomes 1, 3, 6, X and Y, as opposed to 39 % of 264 non-metastatic PENs [75, 91, 98, 100, 102–109]. These data point toward a potential association between chromosomal aberrations and progression of PENs.

Chromosome 3 is the location of the vHL gene (3p25.3) [60], which has been associated with vHL syndrome-associated PENs. Recent studies have shown LOH at loci proximal to vHL locus [103] and LOH at 3p14.2–3p21 loci occur more often in malignant insulinomas than in benign insulinomas. Barghorn et al. [104] found highly statistically significant increased frequency of LOH at 3p25.3–p23 in malignant as compared to benign PENs, and in metastasizing as compared to non-metastasizing PENs. Additionally, a strong correlation was found between the loss of alleles on chromosome 3p and clinically metastatic PENs. These findings suggest a tumor suppressor gene at 3p25.3–p23 that may be associated with sporadic PEN development and that losses of larger centromeric regions are associated with metastatic progression. In another study, LOH at 3q was found in half of sporadic PENs with hepatic metastases, while PENs without hepatic metastasis showed no LOH at this location [105]. Microsatellite markers demonstrate the smallest common deleted region at 3q27-qter, the region of p51 (a member of the p53 tumor suppressor family) [110]. These findings are suggestive of a late event in the molecular pathogenesis of PENs, consistent with advanced stage of tumor development [81].

LOH detected chromosomal loss at 6q in 6 % of sporadic PENs overall and in 100 % of insulinomas, suggesting a chromosomal aberration specific to insulinomas [91]. Additional findings were smallest regions of allelic deletions at 6q22 (50 %) and 6q23–24 (41.2–56.3 %). Also, more chromosome 6 aberrations were detected by FISH in metastatic relative to benign PENs [106]. Thus, chromosome 6 alterations may play a specific role in the molecular pathogenesis and progression of insulinomas. LOH at chromosomal arm 9p, the home of p16, is a frequent finding in PENs. However, Moore et al. [111] found a p16 mutation in only one insulinoma out of 41 PENs, none of which showed methylation. Current studies seem to indicate that p16 inactivation by promoter methylation may be restricted to functional gastrinomas. Rare homozygous p16 gene deletions have also been reported in PENs [107]. Using CGH, Speel et al. [93] found 9q gain to be the most common gain in insulinomas (50 %).

The tumor suppressor gene, PTEN, is located at chromosome 10q23 [112] performed a mutation analysis of the entire coding region of PTEN in 33 PENs and found only one tumor with a somatic mutation in exon 6. However, 10q23 region LOH was detected in more than half of malignant and in none of 7 benign PENs. All samples with LOH at 10q23 were malignant PENs. This suggests that allelic loss of this region could be associated with malignant behavior. In non-neoplastic pancreatic islet cells, immunohistochemical expression of PTEN protein is localized to the nucleus. PTEN expression was lost in the single malignant PEN with two structural hits; however, all of the PENs with LOH remained PTEN-immunoreactive but PTEN was localized predominately in the cytoplasm and cell membrane in 23 of 24 (96 %) PENs. No increase in malignant behavior is associated with this shifting of PTEN from the nucleus but is associated with the neoplastic state in general. Based on the above findings [112] it was proposed that inappropriate compartmentalization of PTEN (cytoplasmic as opposed to nuclear localization of PTEN) could be an initiating event in the genesis of PENs, whereas physical loss of 10q leads to progressive malignancy.

Chromosome 11q13, discussed previously, is associated with *MEN1* and the development of most MEN1-associated PENs as well as some sporadic PENs. Chromosome 11p13–15 was studied in a comparative genomic hybridization investigation of 25 PENs from 23 patients. 11p13–15 loss was found in 24 % of cases, likely representing uncharacterized tumor suppressor genes in this region [94]. Chromosome 11q23 harbors the tumor suppressor gene *succinate dehydrogenase subunit D (SDHD)* [113]. A number of studies have shown significant allelic loss of 11q extending to 11q23, or distal to 11q13, and have thus postulated that a previously unrecognized tumor suppressor in this region plays a role in PEN development [47, 91, 108]. Chromosome 12p12 is the location of the K-ras gene, which is commonly mutated in pancreatic ductal adenocarcinomas but is found only rarely in PENs [111], supporting the idea that exocrine and endocrine pancreatic neoplasms involve different genetic pathways. Chromosome 17p13 is home to TP53, which plays a significant role in the tumorigenesis of pancreatic ductal carcinomas, but not PENs. A study by Moore et al. [114] supported previous suggestions that the presence of a tumor suppressor gene other than TP53 on chromosomal arm 17p is involved in the molecular pathogenesis of nonfunctional PENs.

Chromosome 18q21 mutations may play a role in the molecular pathogenesis of nonfunctional PENs, whereas select functional tumors lack this change [115]. 18q21 is the location of the *DPC4/Smad4 gene*, a cell cycle regulator [116]. However, in another series of PENs, these chromosomal aberrations were not detected in any of the 19 nonfunctional PENs analyzed [117]. Chromosome 22 was studied in gastrinomas, insulinomas, VIPomas, and nonfunctional PENs, and LOH was found on chromosome 22q in 22 of 23 tumors [109]. Another study found LOH in 57 % of insulinomas at 22q12.1–q12.2 [118]. This site is the location of the hSNF5/INI1 gene, implicated in medulloblastoma and other pediatric central nervous system tumors [119]. Further studies could not find an alteration in this gene suggesting it is not the cause of tumor development [81, 118]. X chromosome losses were seen in patients with functional and nonfunctional PENs and were associated with shorter patient survival [8] and clinically aggressive behavior [75, 98, 120]. Y chromosome losses were found frequently in PENs from males (36 %) and were associated with metastasis, local invasion, and high proliferation rates [75].

14.7 Cell Cycle Regulars in Sporadic PENs

Regulation of the cell cycle keeps cell death (apoptosis) in balance with cell growth (proliferation). Loss of cell cycle regulation is one of the hallmarks of neoplasia. Understanding the regulatory mechanisms of the cell cycle are complex, as multiple, often repetitive pathways may be involved. A number of studies have shown that common cell cycle regulators are involved in the molecular pathogenesis of PENs.

P27KIP1 is a cell kinase inhibitor that opposes cell cycle progression and is located on chromosome 12p12–p13.1 [121]. A study by Guo et al. [122] found overexpression of P27KIP in sporadic PENs. An elevation of P27KIP1 expression was found to be inversely related to Ki-67 in a study of 109 gastroenteropancreatic NETs, suggesting that P27KIP1 may inhibit proliferation in these tumors [123].

Loss of p16INK4/p14ARF, a tumor suppressor gene located on 9p21 [124] 1, leads to tumorigenesis as a result of deregulation of p53 and cyclin-dependent kinase/retinoblastoma pathways [125]. Reports found inactivating p16INK4 gene alterations (such as homozygous deletion and methylation at the 5′CpG islands of promoter regions) in 92 % of gastrinomas and nonfunctional PENs. Loss of expression of genes in the 9p21 region was found in 57 % of nonfunctional PENs, 30 % of insulinomas, and 22 % of gastrinomas. This study also found CpG promoter methylation of the p16 gene [126].

Cyclin D1, on chromosome 11q13 [127, 128], plays an important role in cell cycle regulation. Nuclear expression of Cyclin D1 was found to be increased in almost half of the PENs [129]. Sporadic PENs were specifically studied and Cyclin D1 overexpression was found in 65 % (20 out of 31) of the PENs studied compared to normal pancreatic tissue [130]. Pathways associated with Cyclin D1, specifically the P38/mitogen-activated protein kinase and Akt/PKB pathways, were activated in PENs, whereas down-regulation of the extracellular signal-regulated kinase pathway was also found with overexpression of Cyclin D1 [131–133].

Other cell cycle regulators have been studied with controversial results, including the retinoblastoma tumor suppressor gene initially found to be deleted in insulinomas [134, 135] but without further confirmation [74, 136, 137] and, as mentioned previously DPC4/Smad4 on chromosome 18q21 [116].

Cell cycle regulators studied and found not to be important contributors to PEN development to date include P53 located on chromosome 17p13.1 [114, 138–140], β-catenin located on chromosome 3p21 [141, 142], phospholipase CB3 located on chromosome 11q13 [143], and retinoic acid receptor β located on chromosome 3p24 [144, 145].

14.8 Other Molecular Genetic Abnormalities in Sporadic PENs

PI3K-Akt/PKB pathway participates in the mediation of β-cell mass up-regulation [146–148]. This pathway activates downstream messengers and transcription factors such as PDX-1, Ngn-3, Isl-1, NeuroD/Beta2, and Nkx2.2, known to act during pancreatic embryogenesis. Glucose and insulin-like growth factor (IGF) induce activation of the PI3K-Akt/PKB pathway and promote in vitro proliferation of insulinoma cells [147]. A persistent stimulus that promotes proliferation is seen in other tumors, including the persistence of achlorhydria inducing gastrinomas. Mouse studies found that up-regulation of the PI3K-Akt/PKB pathway is not sufficient for neoplastic transformation [146].

K-RAS2, on chromosome 12p12.1 [149], is an important oncogene that transduces cell growth signals, mutations of which lead to growth factor-independent stimulation of cell proliferation [150]. K-RAS2 mutations were not detected in PENs in a study by Yashiro et al. [151]. Another study found strong K-RAS2 immunoreactivity and mutations in 4 of 6 insulinomas studied [152].

Somatostatin (SST) and G-protein-coupled transmembrane receptors (SSTRs) seem to play a role as regulators of islet cell proliferation [1]. Loss of SST/SSTR signaling may contribute to the genesis of PENs. In support of this theory, MEN-1 studies showed decreased expression of SST and islet amyloid polypeptide in MEN syndrome type 1 [153], providing a link between loss of menin, suppression of SST and islet amyloid polypeptide expression and oncogenesis.

The dominant effect of the protooncogene c-Myc is apoptosis of the islet cells. However, increased expression of c-Myc has been demonstrated in glucose-induced hyperplasia of pancreatic islets. Thus, the effects of this gene depend on the environmental effects and the influences of other genes and proteins. Pelengaris and Khan [154] proposed a model of accumulating mutations leading to progression from hyperplasia to neoplasia. c-Myc is thought to be an early event in hyperplastic islets. c-Myc expression was found to be increased in hyperplastic islets and benign and malignant insulinomas.

RIP-Tag2 oncogene expression in transgenic mice leads to islet cell hyperplasia and neoplasia. Tag oncoprotein inactivates tumor suppressor proteins p53 and pRb. Decreased apoptosis is also seen due to overexpression of antiapoptotic protein Bcl-XL and Bcl-2. These antiapoptotic proteins counteract the effects of proapoptotic c-Myc [154, 155].

HER-2 neu, found on chromosome 11q21 [156], is a well-known oncogene that is overexpressed in some cases of breast carcinoma and is associated with increased malignant behavior, proliferation, and metastasis [157]. HER-2 neu has been studied in gastrinomas, where its overexpression was found in a minority of these tumors, and was associated with liver metastasis [158].

The CpG island methylation of the estrogen receptor gene (ESR1), located on chromosome 6q24 [159], has also been described in breast carcinoma and has significant therapeutic implications, indicating tamoxifen resistance [160]. Estrogen receptor gene methylation was found in 64 % of PENs in one study [144].

14.9 Molecular Biologic Aspects of PENs

Human MutL homologue 1 (hMLH1), found on chromosome 3p21.3 [161], is a mismatch repair gene. One study found hMLH1 to be hypermethylated in 23 % of PENs with evidence of microsatellite instability [162]. Promoter hypermethylation (gene silencing) was associated with an improved 5-year survival (100 % vs. 56 %).

Telomerase, on chromosome 5p15.33 [163], is an enzyme that maintains the chromosomal telomere. Telomere degradation is a normal part of the cell cycle, but aberrations of telomerase can lead to tumorigenesis [81]. Telomerase activity may predict an unfavorable outcome in PENs [8, 164].

Thrombomodulin, an endothelial anticoagulant, when overexpressed, reduces cellular proliferation and promotes cellular adhesion in vitro, while expression of thrombomodulin in vivo is inversely correlated with metastatic spread [165, 166].

E-cadherin functions to promote cell-cell adhesion. Loss of E-cadherin is associated with invasion and metastasis in many malignancies. Chetty et al. [13] found aberrant E-cadherin expression in more than 50 % of PENs, which strongly correlated with lymph node and liver metastasis. In addition, nuclear E-cadherin was seen in 18/57 cases when stained with antibodies detecting the cytoplasmic fragment of E-cadherin. This is a previously undescribed staining pattern in PENs.

Cell signaling pathways influence tumor growth and hormonal activity. Neuroendocrine cells can express the insulin-like growth factor (IGF) and its receptor (IGFR) [167]. Cell line studies indicate that IGF-1 can act in autocrine and paracrine fashion to inhibit apoptosis and stimulate secretion of chromogranins, possibly by activating the P13K-AKT pathway. VEGF is also expressed by neuroendocrine tumors, and elevated levels of VEGF have been associated with tumor progression [168, 169].

14.10 Gene Expression Profiling Studies in PENs

Pancreatic endocrine tumors/carcinomas (PETs/PECAs) are clinically challenging neoplasms. Based on the presence or absence of metastases and/or gross invasion of adjacent organs, they are classified as pancreatic endocrine carcinomas (PECAs) or pancreatic endocrine tumors (PETs) [WHO-2004] [10]. In the presence of negative metastatic work-up at the time of first tissue diagnosis, it is difficult to predict which of these tumors will become metastatic ('malignant') or remain localized to the pancreas ('benign'). Standard histologic criteria, including grade, tumor size and Ki-67 index, often fail to predict malignant behavior [170]. Patients who develop metastases are rarely cured and 5-year survival rates diminish significantly. Therefore, discovery of molecular markers of prognosis is vitally important in order to quantify the risk of metastatic recurrence in patients with resected primary tumors.

The broad heterogeneity that characterizes neuroendocrine tumors has always posed problems regarding their correct classification [171]. In recent years, several refined histopathologic classification, grading and staging schemes have been proposed for PETs and, to some extent, validated to categorize these heterogeneous neoplasms into various diagnostic and prognostic subgroups [10, 11, 172–179]. However, due primarily to the diverse biology of these rare neoplasms, there is no single internationally acceptable prognostic scheme that would allow accurate determination of prognosis in a particular case.

In order to identify newer diagnostic, prognostic markers and therapeutic targets, lately there has been an increasing application of high-throughput technologies, including gene expression profiling, to the study of pancreatic endocrine tumors [153, 180–185]. Genes that have been associated with malignant behavior in human PENs include VEGF-C [186], met proto-oncogene, insulin-like growth factor binding protein 3 (IGFBP-3) [187], MEN-1 gene [188], c-N-ras , HER-2/neu [158] and c-myc, TGF-alpha, c-K-ras and p53 [152]. Most of these studies were conducted on small numbers of specimens and have not been fully validated. In a recent study [182], gene expression profiles of primary PECAs and their hepatic metastases were found to be similar, suggesting that most genetic abnormalities accumulate at the level of primary PETs. Therefore, identification of a set of genes and/or their protein products in the primary tumor tissue in clinically localized pancreatic endocrine tumors (CLP-PET), may have significant prognostic and therapeutic implications. Clinical utility of a metastasis-associated gene (MAG) signature as a predictor of future metastases has been shown in breast [189] and prostate [190] cancers and in medulloblastoma [191]. However, molecular markers of progression in primary pancreatic endocrine tumors are largely unknown.

Gene expression profiling using microarray analysis has identified a number of genes typical of PENs [153, 182, 186, 187, 192]. Similarly, histologically normal pancreatic islets were compared with PENs, showing overexpression of 66 genes, especially IGFBP3 (a growth factor), fibronectin (a cell migration/adhesion molecule), and oncogenes like MLLT10/AF10. One hundred and nineteen genes were under-expressed, including p21CIP1 (a cell cycle regulator), JunD (a transcription factor), and NME3 (a metastasis suppressor gene). Another gene expression study compared normal islet cells and three neuroendocrine tumor cell lines; 667 genes were up-regulated, and 323 were down-regulated [182, 192].

Recently, we selected pathologically well-characterized subsets of frozen PEN tissues and adjacent histologically normal pancreatic islets, and used a comprehensive genome-wide expression profiling approach and discovered a novel set of candidate progression genes (CPGs) that were differentially expressed in surgically resected metastatic primary (MP)-PECAs relative to clinically localized primary

(CLP)-PETs [193–195]. Many of these genes, including RUNX1T, palladin, insulin receptor, CD24 antigen and NRCAM had not previously been associated with progression in PENs. We have successfully validated two of our leading candidate progression genes (RUNX1T1, palladin) at the protein level using immunohistochemistry (IHC) on larger independent test sets of MP-PECAs and CLP-PETs [196, 197]. We are now focused to advance our discovery of novel molecular markers (CPGs) to the next step of larger scale clinical validation, using the roadmaps proposed in recent literature with regard to the discovery and validation of gene-based biomarkers. Although gene expression profiling studies have identified newer candidate genes that are providing newer insights into the molecular pathology and biology of PENs, comparison among these published studies continues to be a challenge due to variations in study designs, patient populations investigated, and tumor samples analyzed.

14.11 Summary

A large number of studies have contributed significantly to our current understanding of molecular pathology and diagnosis of pancreatic endocrine neoplasms. PENs exhibit a diverse spectrum of molecular genetic aberrations similar to their broad clinical presentation. Nonfunctional PENs exhibit more molecular aberrations than functional PENs. Also, malignant behavior seems to be associated with increasing genetic aberrations, suggesting specific genes may be associated with metastases in PENs. Genome wide studies have identified several genetic abnormalities in PENs, some of which predict malignant behavior in various subtypes of PENs and adverse clinical outcome while others provide molecular evidence in support of earlier stages of neoplastic transformation of PENs. Comparative genomic hybridization studies found that most frequent chromosomal gains were on chromosomes 7 and 20. The most frequent losses were on chromosomes 2, 6q, 21q, and Y. The chromosome aberrations most frequently associated with metastasis included gains of chromosomes 7, 14q, 4, and Xq, as well as losses of chromosomes 6p, 3p, 6q, and 21q. LOH analyses have identified multiple tumor suppressor gene loci that contribute to the pathogenesis of PENs. Genetic syndromes, which include PENs as one of their components, allow for the identification of genes associated with the genesis of PENs, including MEN1, vHL, NF-1, TSC1 and TSC2. Gene expression profiling using microarray analyses has identified a large number of genes differentially expressed in PENs when compared with normal islets, suggesting their involvement in initiation or progression of PENs. These include IGFBP3, fibronectin, oncogene MLLT10/AF10, p21C1P1, JunD, NME3, RUNX1T1, paladin and p21. While these studies are providing critical scientific evidence to refine our understanding of the molecular complexity of these neoplasms, pooling of large data sets and comparison among these molecular studies is challenging because of variations in study designs, patient populations, and tumor samples (fresh-frozen versus archival) and variation in the technical platforms used. A number of interesting lines of investigation are lending credence to various hypotheses regarding the molecular pathogenesis, progression and therapeutic responsiveness of PENs. Some the recent studies have focused on cathepsins, CD44, NESP-55, hMLH1, telomerase, thrombomodulin, and E-cadherin expression/activity. Advanced molecular testing, is currently making it more feasible to pursue newer lines of genetic studies to unravel an increasing number of chromosomal aberrations associated with PENs. Multiple molecular alterations, involving cell migratory, cell cycle and angiogenic functions have been found to promote PEN development, growth, invasion, and metastases. As a result of these studies, phase III trials of novel therapies targeting cell regulators such as mTOR, VEGF and other targets have been completed. Focused investigation of various mediators/mechanisms implicated in the molecular pathogenesis and progression of PENs will contribute to novel diagnostic, therapeutic and preventive strategies. These efforts need to be integrated with the development and validation of robust assays for prognostic and predictive biomarkers that can be used in the clinic. All of these efforts will ultimately translate into more efficacious, safer and cost-effective therapeutic and monitoring options for patients with PENs.

Acknowledgments The authors would like to acknowledge the excellent support from Brenda Barrow and Rasa Hamilton of Moffitt Cancer Center, Tampa, FL, USA.

References

1. Ballian N, Hu M, Liu SH, Brunicardi FC (2007) Proliferation, hyperplasia, neogenesis, and neoplasia in the islets of Langerhans. Pancreas 35(3):199–206
2. Pour PM, Pandey KK, Batra SK (2003) What is the origin of pancreatic adenocarcinoma? Mol Cancer 2:13
3. Schmied BM, Ulrich AB, Friess H, Buchler MW, Pour PM (2001) The patterns of extrainsular endocrine cells in pancreatic cancer. Teratog Carcinog Mutagen 21(1):69–81
4. Grube D, Bohn R (1983) The microanatomy of human islets of Langerhans, with special reference to somatostatin (D-) cells. Arch Histol Jpn 46(3):327–353
5. Mittendorf EA, Shifrin AL, Inabnet WB, Libutti SK, McHenry CR, Demeure MJ (2006) Islet cell tumors. Curr Probl Surg 43(10):685–765
6. Rindi G, Capella C, Solcia E (2000) Introduction to a revised clinicopathological classification of neuroendocrine tumors of the gastroenteropancreatic tract. Q J Nucl Med 44(1):13–21
7. Goldin SB, Aston J, Wahi MM (2008) Sporadically occurring functional pancreatic endocrine tumors: review of recent literature. Curr Opin Oncol 20(1):25–33
8. Halfdanarson TR, Rubin J, Farnell MB, Grant CS, Petersen GM (2008) Pancreatic endocrine neoplasms: epidemiology and prognosis of pancreatic endocrine tumors. Endocr Relat Cancer 15(2):409–427
9. Tomassetti P, Campana D, Piscitelli L, Casadei R, Santini D, Nori F et al (2005) Endocrine pancreatic tumors: factors correlated with survival. Ann Oncol 16(11):1806–1810
10. Heitz P, Komminoth P, Perren A, Klimstra D, Dayal Y, Bordi C et al (2004) Tumors of the endocrine pancreas. IARC Press, Lyon
11. Heymann MF, Joubert M, Nemeth J, Franc B, Visset J, Hamy A et al (2000) Prognostic and immunohistochemical validation of the capella classification of pancreatic neuroendocrine tumours: an analysis of 82 sporadic cases. Histopathology 36(5):421–432
12. Calender A (2000) Molecular genetics of neuroendocrine tumors. Digestion 62(Suppl 1):3–18
13. Chetty R (2008) An overview of practical issues in the diagnosis of gastroenteropancreatic neuroendocrine pathology. Arch Pathol Lab Med 132(8):1285–1289

14. Moldawer MP, Nardi GL, Raker JW (1954) Concomitance of multiple adenomas of the parathyroids and pancreatic islets with tumor of the pituitary: a syndrome with a familial incidence. Am J Med Sci 228(2):190–206
15. Wermer P (1954) Genetic aspects of adenomatosis of endocrine glands. Am J Med 16(3):363–371
16. Kronenberg H, Melmeds S, Polonsky K, Larson P (2008) Williams textbook of endocrinology, 11th edn. Saunders/Elsevier, Philadelphia
17. Brandi ML, Gagel RF, Angeli A, Bilezikian JP, Beck-Peccoz P, Bordi C et al (2001) Guidelines for diagnosis and therapy of MEN type 1 and type 2. J Clin Endocrinol Metab 86(12):5658–5671, Epub 2001/12/12
18. Marx SJ, Agarwal SK, Kester MB, Heppner C, Kim YS, Skarulis MC et al (1999) Multiple endocrine neoplasia type 1: clinical and genetic features of the hereditary endocrine neoplasias. Recent Prog Horm Res 54:397–438, discussion –9. Epub 1999/11/05
19. Pipeleers-Marichal M, Somers G, Willems G, Foulis A, Imrie C, Bishop AE et al (1990) Gastrinomas in the duodenums of patients with multiple endocrine neoplasia type 1 and the Zollinger-Ellison syndrome. N Engl J Med 322(11):723–727, Epub 1990/03/15
20. Skogseid B, Eriksson B, Lundqvist G, Lorelius LE, Rastad J, Wide L et al (1991) Multiple endocrine neoplasia type 1: a 10-year prospective screening study in four kindreds. J Clin Endocrinol Metab 73(2):281–287
21. Gaitan D, Loosen PT, Orth DN (1993) Two patients with Cushing's disease in a kindred with multiple endocrine neoplasia type I. J Clin Endocrinol Metab 76(6):1580–1582
22. Burgess JR, Greenaway TM, Parameswaran V, Challis DR, David R, Shepherd JJ (1998) Enteropancreatic malignancy associated with multiple endocrine neoplasia type 1: risk factors and pathogenesis. Cancer 83(3):428–434
23. Norton JA, Fraker DL, Alexander HR, Venzon DJ, Doppman JL, Serrano J et al (1999) Surgery to cure the Zollinger-Ellison syndrome. N Engl J Med 341(9):635–644, Epub 1999/08/26
24. Thompson NW (1998) Current concepts in the surgical management of multiple endocrine neoplasia type 1 pancreatic-duodenal disease. Results in the treatment of 40 patients with Zollinger-Ellison syndrome, hypoglycaemia or both. J Intern Med 243(6):495–500
25. Majewski JT, Wilson SD (1979) The MEA-I syndrome: an all or none phenomenon? Surgery 86(3):475–484
26. Agarwal SK, Burns AL, Sukhodolets KE, Kennedy PA, Obungu VH, Hickman AB et al (2004) Molecular pathology of the MEN1 gene. Ann N Y Acad Sci 1014:189–198, Epub 2004/05/22
27. Knudson AG (1996) Hereditary cancer: two hits revisited. J Cancer Res Clin Oncol 122(3):135–140
28. Thepot D, Weitzman JB, Barra J, Segretain D, Stinnakre MG, Babinet C et al (2000) Targeted disruption of the murine JunD gene results in multiple defects in male reproductive function. Development 127(1):143–153, Epub 2000/02/02
29. Agarwal SK, Guru SC, Heppner C, Erdos MR, Collins RM, Park SY et al (1999) Menin interacts with the AP1 transcription factor JunD and represses JunD-activated transcription. Cell 96(1):143–152
30. Hendy GN, Kaji H, Sowa H, Lebrun JJ, Canaff L (2005) Menin and TGF-beta superfamily member signaling via the Smad pathway in pituitary, parathyroid and osteoblast. Horm Metab Res 37(6):375–379
31. Kaji H, Canaff L, Lebrun JJ, Goltzman D, Hendy GN (2001) Inactivation of menin, a Smad3-interacting protein, blocks transforming growth factor type beta signaling. Proc Natl Acad Sci U S A 98(7):3837–3842
32. Lemmens IH, Forsberg L, Pannett AA, Meyen E, Piehl F, Turner JJ et al (2001) Menin interacts directly with the homeobox-containing protein Pem. Biochem Biophys Res Commun 286(2):426–431
33. Heppner C, Bilimoria KY, Agarwal SK, Kester M, Whitty LJ, Guru SC et al (2001) The tumor suppressor protein menin interacts with NF-kappaB proteins and inhibits NF-kappaB-mediated transactivation. Oncogene 20(36):4917–4925
34. Agarwal S, Scecheri P, Rice T, Kennedy P, Ozawa A, Burgess-Hickman A et al (2006) MEN1 gene: mutation and pathophysiology. Ann Endocrinol (Paris) 67(Suppl 4):IS12–IS13

35. Agarwal SK, Impey S, McWeeney S, Scacheri PC, Collins FS, Goodman RH et al (2007) Distribution of menin-occupied regions in chromatin specifies a broad role of menin in transcriptional regulation. Neoplasia 9(2):101–107
36. Thakker RV, Bouloux P, Wooding C, Chotai K, Broad PM, Spurr NK et al (1989) Association of parathyroid tumors in multiple endocrine neoplasia type 1 with loss of alleles on chromosome 11. N Engl J Med 321(4):218–224, Epub 1989/07/27
37. Agarwal SK, Debelenko LV, Kester MB, Guru SC, Manickam P, Olufemi SE et al (1998) Analysis of recurrent germline mutations in the MEN1 gene encountered in apparently unrelated families. Hum Mutat 12(2):75–82
38. Kishi M, Tsukada T, Shimizu S, Futami H, Ito Y, Kanbe M et al (1998) A large germline deletion of the MEN1 gene in a family with multiple endocrine neoplasia type 1. Jpn J Cancer Res 89(1):1–5
39. Agarwal SK, Kester MB, Debelenko LV, Heppner C, Emmert-Buck MR, Skarulis MC et al (1997) Germline mutations of the MEN1 gene in familial multiple endocrine neoplasia type 1 and related states. Hum Mol Genet 6(7):1169–1175
40. Kumar V, Fausto N (eds) (2005) Pathologic basis of disease, 7th edn. Elsevier/Saunders, Philadelphia
41. Lubensky IA, Pack S, Ault D, Vortmeyer AO, Libutti SK, Choyke PL et al (1998) Multiple neuroendocrine tumors of the pancreas in von Hippel-Lindau disease patients: histopathological and molecular genetic analysis. Am J Pathol 153(1):223–231
42. Debelenko LV, Zhuang Z, Emmert-Buck MR, Chandrasekharappa SC, Manickam P, Guru SC et al (1997) Allelic deletions on chromosome 11q13 in multiple endocrine neoplasia type 1-associated and sporadic gastrinomas and pancreatic endocrine tumors. Cancer Res 57(11):2238–2243
43. Eubanks PJ, Sawicki MP, Samara GJ, Gatti R, Nakamura Y, Tsao D et al (1994) Putative tumor-suppressor gene on chromosome 11 is important in sporadic endocrine tumor formation. Am J Surg 167(1):180–185, Epub 1994/01/01
44. Zhuang Z, Vortmeyer AO, Pack S, Huang S, Pham TA, Wang C et al (1997) Somatic mutations of the MEN1 tumor suppressor gene in sporadic gastrinomas and insulinomas. Cancer Res 57(21):4682–4686
45. Wang EH, Ebrahimi SA, Wu AY, Kashefi C, Passaro E Jr, Sawicki MP (1998) Mutation of the MENIN gene in sporadic pancreatic endocrine tumors. Cancer Res 58(19): 4417–4420
46. Goebel SU, Heppner C, Burns AL, Marx SJ, Spiegel AM, Zhuang Z et al (2000) Genotype/phenotype correlation of multiple endocrine neoplasia type 1 gene mutations in sporadic gastrinomas. J Clin Endocrinol Metab 85(1):116–123
47. Gortz B, Roth J, Krahenmann A, de Krijger RR, Muletta-Feurer S, Rutimann K et al (1999) Mutations and allelic deletions of the MEN1 gene are associated with a subset of sporadic endocrine pancreatic and neuroendocrine tumors and not restricted to foregut neoplasms. Am J Pathol 154(2):429–436
48. Williamson C, Pannett AA, Pang JT, Wooding C, McCarthy M, Sheppard MN et al (1997) Localisation of a gene causing endocrine neoplasia to a 4 cM region on chromosome 1p35-p36. J Med Genet 34(8):617–619
49. Kytola S, Makinen MJ, Kahkonen M, Teh BT, Leisti J, Salmela P (1998) Comparative genomic hybridization studies in tumours from a patient with multiple endocrine neoplasia type 1. Eur J Endocrinol 139(2):202–206
50. Franklin DS, Godfrey VL, O'Brien DA, Deng C, Xiong Y (2000) Functional collaboration between different cyclin-dependent kinase inhibitors suppresses tumor growth with distinct tissue specificity. Mol Cell Biol 20(16):6147–6158
51. Pestell RG, Albanese C, Reutens AT, Segall JE, Lee RJ, Arnold A (1999) The cyclins and cyclin-dependent kinase inhibitors in hormonal regulation of proliferation and differentiation. Endocr Rev 20(4):501–534
52. Perren A, Anlauf M, Henopp T, Rudolph T, Schmitt A, Raffel A et al (2007) Multiple endocrine neoplasia type 1 (MEN1): loss of one MEN1 allele in tumors and monohormonal endocrine cell

clusters but not in islet hyperplasia of the pancreas. J Clin Endocrinol Metab 92(3):1118–1128, Epub 2006/12/21

53. Anlauf M, Perren A, Meyer CL, Schmid S, Saremaslani P, Kruse ML et al (2005) Precursor lesions in patients with multiple endocrine neoplasia type 1-associated duodenal gastrinomas. Gastroenterology 128(5):1187–1198, Epub 2005/05/12
54. Crabtree JS, Scacheri PC, Ward JM, Garrett-Beal L, Emmert-Buck MR, Edgemon KA et al (2001) A mouse model of multiple endocrine neoplasia, type 1, develops multiple endocrine tumors. Proc Natl Acad Sci U S A 98(3):1118–1123
55. Crabtree JS, Scacheri PC, Ward JM, McNally SR, Swain GP, Montagna C et al (2003) Of mice and MEN1: insulinomas in a conditional mouse knockout. Mol Cell Biol 23(17):6075–6085
56. Frosch M, Anthony D, Girolami U (2005) Robin's and Cotran's pathologic basis of disease, 7th edn. Elsevier/Saunders, Philadelphia
57. Binkovitz LA, Johnson CD, Stephens DH (1990) Islet cell tumors in von Hippel-Lindau disease: increased prevalence and relationship to the multiple endocrine neoplasias. AJR Am J Roentgenol 155(3):501–505
58. Hough DM, Stephens DH, Johnson CD, Binkovitz LA (1994) Pancreatic lesions in von Hippel-Lindau disease: prevalence, clinical significance, and CT findings. AJR Am J Roentgenol 162(5):1091–1094
59. Neumann HP, Dinkel E, Brambs H, Wimmer B, Friedburg H, Volk B et al (1991) Pancreatic lesions in the von Hippel-Lindau syndrome. Gastroenterology 101(2):465–471
60. LaForgia S, Lasota J, Latif F, Boghosian-Sell L, Kastury K, Ohta M et al (1993) Detailed genetic and physical map of the 3p chromosome region surrounding the familial renal cell carcinoma chromosome translocation, t(3;8)(p14.2;q24.1). Cancer Res 53(13):3118–3124
61. Pugh CW, Ratcliffe PJ (2003) Regulation of angiogenesis by hypoxia: role of the HIF system. Nat Med 9(6):677–684, Epub 2003/06/05
62. Maxwell PH, Pugh CW, Ratcliffe PJ (2001) The pVHL-hIF-1 system. A key mediator of oxygen homeostasis. Adv Exp Med Biol 502:365–376
63. Ratcliffe PJ, O'Rourke JF, Maxwell PH, Pugh CW (1998) Oxygen sensing, hypoxia-inducible factor-1 and the regulation of mammalian gene expression. J Exp Biol 201(Pt 8):1153–1162
64. Kim WY, Kaelin WG (2004) Role of VHL gene mutation in human cancer. J Clin Oncol 22(24):4991–5004
65. Lamberts SW, Krenning EP, Reubi JC (1991) The role of somatostatin and its analogs in the diagnosis and treatment of tumors. Endocr Rev 12(4):450–482
66. Na X, Wu G, Ryan CK, Schoen SR, di'Santagnese PA, Messing EM (2003) Overproduction of vascular endothelial growth factor related to von Hippel-Lindau tumor suppressor gene mutations and hypoxia-inducible factor-1 alpha expression in renal cell carcinomas. J Urol 170(2 Pt 1):588–592
67. Wang XC, Xu SY, Wu XY, Song HD, Mao YF, Fan HY et al (2004) Gene expression profiling in human insulinoma tissue: genes involved in the insulin secretion pathway and cloning of novel full-length cDNAs. Endocr Relat Cancer 11(2):295–303
68. Petrella BL, Lohi J, Brinckerhoff CE (2005) Identification of membrane type-1 matrix metalloproteinase as a target of hypoxia-inducible factor-2 alpha in von Hippel-Lindau renal cell carcinoma. Oncogene 24(6):1043–1052, Epub 2004/12/14
69. Petrella BL, Brinckerhoff CE (2006) Tumor cell invasion of von Hippel Lindau renal cell carcinoma cells is mediated by membrane type-1 matrix metalloproteinase. Mol Cancer 5:66, Epub 2006/12/05
70. Konno H, Arai T, Tanaka T, Baba M, Matsumoto K, Kanai T et al (1998) Antitumor effect of a neutralizing antibody to vascular endothelial growth factor on liver metastasis of endocrine neoplasm. Jpn J Cancer Res 89(9):933–939
71. Yao JC, Hoff PM (2007) Molecular targeted therapy for neuroendocrine tumors. Hematol Oncol Clin North Am 21(3):575–581
72. Hammel PR, Vilgrain V, Terris B, Penfornis A, Sauvanet A, Correas JM et al (2000) Pancreatic involvement in von Hippel-Lindau disease. The Groupe Francophone d'Etude de la Maladie de von Hippel-Lindau. Gastroenterology 119(4):1087–1095

73. Hoang MP, Hruban RH, Albores-Saavedra J (2001) Clear cell endocrine pancreatic tumor mimicking renal cell carcinoma: a distinctive neoplasm of von Hippel-Lindau disease. Am J Surg Pathol 25(5):602–609
74. Chung DC, Smith AP, Louis DN, Graeme-Cook F, Warshaw AL, Arnold A (1997) A novel pancreatic endocrine tumor suppressor gene locus on chromosome 3p with clinical prognostic implications. J Clin Invest 100(2):404–410
75. Missiaglia E, Moore PS, Williamson J, Lemoine NR, Falconi M, Zamboni G et al (2002) Sex chromosome anomalies in pancreatic endocrine tumors. Int J Cancer 98(4):532–538
76. Tan CC, Hall RI, Semeraro D, Irons RP, Freeman JG (1996) Ampullary somatostatinoma associated with von Recklinghausen's neurofibromatosis presenting as obstructive jaundice. Eur J Surg Oncol 22(3):298–301
77. van Slegtenhorst M, de Hoogt R, Hermans C, Nellist M, Janssen B, Verhoef S et al (1997) Identification of the tuberous sclerosis gene TSC1 on chromosome 9q34. Science 277(5327):805–808, Epub 1997/08/08
78. European Chromosome 16 Tuberous Sclerosis C (1993) Identification and characterization of the tuberous sclerosis gene on chromosome 16. Cell 75(7):1305–1315, Epub 1993/12/31
79. Sandsmark DK, Pelletier C, Weber JD, Gutmann DH (2007) Mammalian target of rapamycin: master regulator of cell growth in the nervous system. Histol Histopathol 22(8):895–903, Epub 2007/05/16
80. Castro AF, Rebhun JF, Clark GJ, Quilliam LA (2003) Rheb binds tuberous sclerosis complex 2 (TSC2) and promotes S6 kinase activation in a rapamycin- and farnesylation-dependent manner. J Biol Chem 278(35):32493–32496, Epub 2003/07/05
81. Zikusoka MN, Kidd M, Eick G, Latich I, Modlin IM (2005) The molecular genetics of gastroenteropancreatic neuroendocrine tumors. Cancer 104(11):2292–2309
82. Mak BC, Takemaru K, Kenerson HL, Moon RT, Yeung RS (2003) The tuberin-hamartin complex negatively regulates beta-catenin signaling activity. J Biol Chem 278(8):5947–5951
83. Verhoef S, van Diemen-Steenvoorde R, Akkersdijk WL, Bax NM, Ariyurek Y, Hermans CJ et al (1999) Malignant pancreatic tumour within the spectrum of tuberous sclerosis complex in childhood. Eur J Pediatr 158(4):284–287
84. Swenne I (1982) The role of glucose in the in vitro regulation of cell cycle kinetics and proliferation of fetal pancreatic B-cells. Diabetes 31(9):754–760
85. Bonner-Weir S, Deery D, Leahy JL, Weir GC (1989) Compensatory growth of pancreatic beta-cells in adult rats after short-term glucose infusion. Diabetes 38(1):49–53
86. Paris M, Bernard-Kargar C, Berthault MF, Bouwens L, Ktorza A (2003) Specific and combined effects of insulin and glucose on functional pancreatic beta-cell mass in vivo in adult rats. Endocrinology 144(6):2717–2727, Epub 2003/05/15
87. Jonkers YM, Ramaekers FC, Speel EJ (2007) Molecular alterations during insulinoma tumorigenesis. Biochim Biophys Acta 1775(2):313–332
88. Balogh K, Racz K, Patocs A, Hunyady L (2006) Menin and its interacting proteins: elucidation of menin function. Trends Endocrinol Metab 17(9):357–364, Epub 2006/09/26
89. Jin S, Mao H, Schnepp RW, Sykes SM, Silva AC, D'Andrea AD et al (2003) Menin associates with FANCD2, a protein involved in repair of DNA damage. Cancer Res 63(14):4204–4210
90. Gumbs AA, Moore PS, Falconi M, Bassi C, Beghelli S, Modlin I et al (2002) Review of the clinical, histological, and molecular aspects of pancreatic endocrine neoplasms. J Surg Oncol 81(1):45–53, discussion 4. Epub 2002/09/05
91. Speel EJ, Richter J, Moch H, Egenter C, Saremaslani P, Rutimann K et al (1999) Genetic differences in endocrine pancreatic tumor subtypes detected by comparative genomic hybridization. Am J Pathol 155(6):1787–1794
92. Zhao J, Moch H, Scheidweiler AF, Baer A, Schaffer AA, Speel EJ et al (2001) Genomic imbalances in the progression of endocrine pancreatic tumors. Genes Chromosomes Cancer 32(4):364–372
93. Speel EJ, Scheidweiler AF, Zhao J, Matter C, Saremaslani P, Roth J et al (2001) Genetic evidence for early divergence of small functioning and nonfunctioning endocrine pancreatic tumors: gain of 9Q34 is an early event in insulinomas. Cancer Res 61(13):5186–5192

94. Stumpf E, Aalto Y, Hoog A, Kjellman M, Otonkoski T, Knuutila S et al (2000) Chromosomal alterations in human pancreatic endocrine tumors. Genes Chromosomes Cancer 29(1):83–87
95. Tonnies H, Toliat MR, Ramel C, Pape UF, Neitzel H, Berger W et al (2001) Analysis of sporadic neuroendocrine tumours of the enteropancreatic system by comparative genomic hybridisation. Gut 48(4):536–541
96. Terris B, Meddeb M, Marchio A, Danglot G, Flejou JF, Belghiti J et al (1998) Comparative genomic hybridization analysis of sporadic neuroendocrine tumors of the digestive system. Genes Chromosomes Cancer 22(1):50–56
97. Kytola S, Hoog A, Nord B, Cedermark B, Frisk T, Larsson C et al (2001) Comparative genomic hybridization identifies loss of 18q22-qter as an early and specific event in tumorigenesis of midgut carcinoids. Am J Pathol 158(5):1803–1808
98. Pizzi S, D'Adda T, Azzoni C, Rindi G, Grigolato P, Pasquali C et al (2002) Malignancy-associated allelic losses on the X-chromosome in foregut but not in midgut endocrine tumours. J Pathol 196(4):401–407
99. Brown MR, Kohn EC, Hutter RV (2000) The new millennium: applying novel technology to the study of the cancer cell in situ. Cancer 88(1):2–5, Epub 2000/01/05
100. Ebrahimi SA, Wang EH, Wu A, Schreck RR, Passaro E Jr, Sawicki MP (1999) Deletion of chromosome 1 predicts prognosis in pancreatic endocrine tumors. Cancer Res 59(2):311–315
101. Guo SS, Arora C, Shimoide AT, Sawicki MP (2002) Frequent deletion of chromosome 3 in malignant sporadic pancreatic endocrine tumors. Mol Cell Endocrinol 190(1–2):109–114
102. Chen YJ, Vortmeyer A, Zhuang Z, Huang S, Jensen RT (2003) Loss of heterozygosity of chromosome 1q in gastrinomas: occurrence and prognostic significance. Cancer Res 63(4):817–823
103. Lott ST, Chandler DS, Curley SA, Foster CJ, El-Naggar A, Frazier M et al (2002) High frequency loss of heterozygosity in von Hippel-Lindau (VHL)-associated and sporadic pancreatic islet cell tumors: evidence for a stepwise mechanism for malignant conversion in VHL tumorigenesis. Cancer Res 62(7):1952–1955
104. Nikiforova MN, Nikiforov YE, Biddinger P, Gnepp DR, Grosembacher LA, Wajchenberg BL et al (1999) Frequent loss of heterozygosity at chromosome 3p14.2-3p21 in human pancreatic islet cell tumours. Clin Endocrinol (Oxf) 51(1):27–33
105. Guo SS, Wu AY, Sawicki MP (2002) Deletion of chromosome 1, but not mutation of MEN-1, predicts prognosis in sporadic pancreatic endocrine tumors. World J Surg 26(7):843–847
106. Barghorn A, Speel EJ, Farspour B, Saremaslani P, Schmid S, Perren A et al (2001) Putative tumor suppressor loci at 6q22 and 6q23-q24 are involved in the malignant progression of sporadic endocrine pancreatic tumors. Am J Pathol 158(6):1903–1911
107. Muscarella P, Melvin WS, Fisher WE, Foor J, Ellison EC, Herman JG et al (1998) Genetic alterations in gastrinomas and nonfunctioning pancreatic neuroendocrine tumors: an analysis of p16/MTS1 tumor suppressor gene inactivation. Cancer Res 58(2):237–240
108. Rigaud G, Missiaglia E, Moore PS, Zamboni G, Falconi M, Talamini G et al (2001) High resolution allelotype of nonfunctional pancreatic endocrine tumors: identification of two molecular subgroups with clinical implications. Cancer Res 61(1):285–292
109. Wild A, Langer P, Celik I, Chaloupka B, Bartsch DK (2002) Chromosome 22q in pancreatic endocrine tumors: identification of a homozygous deletion and potential prognostic associations of allelic deletions. Eur J Endocrinol 147(4):507–513
110. Ikawa S, Nakagawara A, Ikawa Y (1999) p53 family genes: structural comparison, expression and mutation. Cell Death Differ 6(12):1154–1161
111. Moore PS, Orlandini S, Zamboni G, Capelli P, Rigaud G, Falconi M et al (2001) Pancreatic tumours: molecular pathways implicated in ductal cancer are involved in ampullary but not in exocrine nonductal or endocrine tumorigenesis. Br J Cancer 84(2):253–262
112. Perren A, Komminoth P, Saremaslani P, Matter C, Feurer S, Lees JA et al (2000) Mutation and expression analyses reveal differential subcellular compartmentalization of PTEN in endocrine pancreatic tumors compared to normal islet cells. Am J Pathol 157(4):1097–1103
113. Hirawake H, Taniwaki M, Tamura A, Amino H, Tomitsuka E, Kita K (1999) Characterization of the human SDHD gene encoding the small subunit of cytochrome b (cybS) in mitochondrial succinate-ubiquinone oxidoreductase. Biochim Biophys Acta 1412(3):295–300

114. Moore PS, Missiaglia E, Antonello D, Zamo A, Zamboni G, Corleto V et al (2001) Role of disease-causing genes in sporadic pancreatic endocrine tumors: MEN1 and VHL. Genes Chromosomes Cancer 32(2):177–181
115. Bartsch D, Hahn SA, Danichevski KD, Ramaswamy A, Bastian D, Galehdari H et al (1999) Mutations of the DPC4/Smad4 gene in neuroendocrine pancreatic tumors. Oncogene 18(14):2367–2371
116. Hahn SA, Schutte M, Hoque AT, Moskaluk CA, da Costa LT, Rozenblum E et al (1996) DPC4, a candidate tumor suppressor gene at human chromosome 18q21.1. Science 271(5247):350–353
117. Perren A, Saremaslani P, Schmid S, Bonvin C, Locher T, Roth J et al (2003) DPC4/Smad4: no mutations, rare allelic imbalances, and retained protein expression in pancreatic endocrine tumors. Diagn Mol Pathol 12(4):181–186
118. Wild A, Langer P, Ramaswamy A, Chaloupka B, Bartsch DK (2001) A novel insulinoma tumor suppressor gene locus on chromosome 22q with potential prognostic implications. J Clin Endocrinol Metab 86(12):5782–5787
119. Biegel JA, Fogelgren B, Zhou JY, James CD, Janss AJ, Allen JC et al (2000) Mutations of the INI1 rhabdoid tumor suppressor gene in medulloblastomas and primitive neuroectodermal tumors of the central nervous system. Clin Cancer Res 6(7):2759–2763, Epub 2000/07/29
120. Chen YJ, Vortmeyer A, Zhuang Z, Gibril F, Jensen RT (2004) X-chromosome loss of heterozygosity frequently occurs in gastrinomas and is correlated with aggressive tumor growth. Cancer 100(7):1379–1387
121. Ponce-Castaneda MV, Lee MH, Latres E, Polyak K, Lacombe L, Montgomery K et al (1995) p27Kip1: chromosomal mapping to 12p12-12p13.1 and absence of mutations in human tumors. Cancer Res 55(6):1211–1214
122. Guo SS, Wu X, Shimoide AT, Wong J, Sawicki MP (2001) Anomalous overexpression of p27(Kip1) in sporadic pancreatic endocrine tumors. J Surg Res 96(2):284–288
123. Canavese G, Azzoni C, Pizzi S, Corleto VD, Pasquali C, Davoli C et al (2001) p27: a potential main inhibitor of cell proliferation in digestive endocrine tumors but not a marker of benign behavior. Hum Pathol 32(10):1094–1101
124. Mao L, Merlo A, Bedi G, Shapiro GI, Edwards CD, Rollins BJ et al (1995) A novel p16INK4A transcript. Cancer Res 55(14):2995–2997
125. Liggett WH Jr, Sidransky D (1998) Role of the p16 tumor suppressor gene in cancer. J Clin Oncol 16(3):1197–1206
126. Lubomierski N, Kersting M, Bert T, Muench K, Wulbrand U, Schuermann M et al (2001) Tumor suppressor genes in the 9p21 gene cluster are selective targets of inactivation in neuroendocrine gastroenteropancreatic tumors. Cancer Res 61(15):5905–5910
127. Schuuring E, Verhoeven E, Mooi WJ, Michalides RJ (1992) Identification and cloning of two overexpressed genes, U21B31/PRAD1 and EMS1, within the amplified chromosome 11q13 region in human carcinomas. Oncogene 7(2):355–361
128. Arnold A, Motokura T, Bloom T, Rosenberg C, Bale A, Kronenberg H et al (1992) PRAD1 (cyclin D1): a parathyroid neoplasia gene on 11q13. Henry Ford Hosp Med J 40(3–4):177–180
129. Chung DC, Brown SB, Graeme-Cook F, Seto M, Warshaw AL, Jensen RT et al (2000) Overexpression of cyclin D1 occurs frequently in human pancreatic endocrine tumors. J Clin Endocrinol Metab 85(11):4373–4378
130. Guo SS, Wu X, Shimoide AT, Wong J, Moatamed F, Sawicki MP (2003) Frequent overexpression of cyclin D1 in sporadic pancreatic endocrine tumours. J Endocrinol 179(1):73–79
131. Gille H, Downward J (1999) Multiple Ras effector pathways contribute to G(1) cell cycle progression. J Biol Chem 274(31):22033–22040
132. Lavoie JN, L'Allemain G, Brunet A, Muller R, Pouyssegur J (1996) Cyclin D1 expression is regulated positively by the p42/p44MAPK and negatively by the p38/HOGMAPK pathway. J Biol Chem 271(34):20608–20616
133. Weber JD, Raben DM, Phillips PJ, Baldassare JJ (1997) Sustained activation of extracellular-signal-regulated kinase 1 (ERK1) is required for the continued expression of cyclin D1 in G1 phase. Biochem J 326(Pt 1):61–68

134. Iwamura Y, Futagawa T, Kaneko M, Nakagawa K, Kawai K, Yamashita K et al (1992) Co-deletions of the retinoblastoma gene and Wilms' tumor gene and rearrangement of the Krev-1 gene in a human insulinoma. Jpn J Clin Oncol 22(1):6–9
135. Nakamura T, Iwamura Y, Kaneko M, Nakagawa K, Kawai K, Mitamura K et al (1991) Deletions and rearrangements of the retinoblastoma gene in hepatocellular carcinoma, insulinoma and some neurogenic tumors as found in a study of 121 tumors. Jpn J Clin Oncol 21(5):325–329
136. Chung DC, Smith AP, Louis DN, Graeme-Cook F, Warshaw AL, Arnold A (1997) Analysis of the retinoblastoma tumour suppressor gene in pancreatic endocrine tumours. Clin Endocrinol (Oxf) 47(5):523–528
137. Kawahara M, Kammori M, Kanauchi H, Noguchi C, Kuramoto S, Kaminishi M et al (2002) Immunohistochemical prognostic indicators of gastrointestinal carcinoid tumours. Eur J Surg Oncol 28(2):140–146
138. Nishikura K, Watanabe H, Iwafuchi M, Fujiwara T, Kojima K, Ajioka Y (2003) Carcinogenesis of gastric endocrine cell carcinoma: analysis of histopathology and p53 gene alteration. Gastric Cancer 6(4):203–209
139. Weckstrom P, Hedrum A, Makridis C, Akerstrom G, Rastad J, Scheibenpflug L et al (1996) Midgut carcinoids and solid carcinomas of the intestine: differences in endocrine markers and p53 mutations. Endocr Pathol 7(4):273–279
140. Oberg K, Eriksson B (2005) Endocrine tumours of the pancreas. Best Pract Res Clin Gastroenterol 19(5):753–781, Epub 2005/10/29
141. Kraus C, Liehr T, Hulsken J, Behrens J, Birchmeier W, Grzeschik KH et al (1994) Localization of the human beta-catenin gene (CTNNB1) to 3p21: a region implicated in tumor development. Genomics 23(1):272–274
142. Gerdes B, Ramaswamy A, Simon B, Pietsch T, Bastian D, Kersting M et al (1999) Analysis of beta-catenin gene mutations in pancreatic tumors. Digestion 60(6):544–548
143. Sinke RJ, Geurts van Kessel AG (1995) Localization of the human phosphatidylinositol-specific phospholipase c beta 3 gene (PLCB3) within chromosome band 11q13. Genomics 25(2):568–569
144. Chan AO, Kim SG, Bedeir A, Issa JP, Hamilton SR, Rashid A (2003) CpG island methylation in carcinoid and pancreatic endocrine tumors. Oncogene 22(6):924–934
145. Mattei MG, de The H, Mattei JF, Marchio A, Tiollais P, Dejean A (1988) Assignment of the human hap retinoic acid receptor RAR beta gene to the p24 band of chromosome 3. Hum Genet 80(2):189–190
146. Bernal-Mizrachi E, Wen W, Stahlhut S, Welling CM, Permutt MA (2001) Islet beta cell expression of constitutively active Akt1/PKB alpha induces striking hypertrophy, hyperplasia, and hyperinsulinemia. J Clin Invest 108(11):1631–1638
147. Hugl SR, White MF, Rhodes CJ (1998) Insulin-like growth factor I (IGF-I)-stimulated pancreatic beta-cell growth is glucose-dependent. Synergistic activation of insulin receptor substrate-mediated signal transduction pathways by glucose and IGF-I in INS-1 cells. J Biol Chem 273(28):17771–17779
148. Jetton TL, Lausier J, LaRock K, Trotman WE, Larmie B, Habibovic A et al (2005) Mechanisms of compensatory beta-cell growth in insulin-resistant rats: roles of Akt kinase. Diabetes 54(8):2294–2304
149. McBride OW, Swan DC, Tronick SR, Gol R, Klimanis D, Moore DE et al (1983) Regional chromosomal localization of N-ras, K-ras-1, K-ras-2 and myb oncogenes in human cells. Nucleic Acids Res 11(23):8221–8236
150. McCormick F (1995) Ras-related proteins in signal transduction and growth control. Mol Reprod Dev 42(4):500–506
151. Yashiro T, Fulton N, Hara H, Yasuda K, Montag A, Yashiro N et al (1993) Comparison of mutations of ras oncogene in human pancreatic exocrine and endocrine tumors. Surgery 114(4):758–763, discussion 63–4
152. Pavelic K, Hrascan R, Kapitanovic S, Karapandza N, Vranes Z, Belicza M et al (1995) Multiple genetic alterations in malignant metastatic insulinomas. J Pathol 177(4):395–400, Epub 1995/12/01

153. Dilley WG, Kalyanaraman S, Verma S, Cobb JP, Laramie JM, Lairmore TC (2005) Global gene expression in neuroendocrine tumors from patients with the MEN1 syndrome. Mol Cancer 4(1):9, Epub 2005/02/05
154. Pelengaris S, Khan M (2001) Oncogenic co-operation in beta-cell tumorigenesis. Endocr Relat Cancer 8(4):307–314
155. Hager JH, Hanahan D (1999) Tumor cells utilize multiple pathways to down-modulate apoptosis. Lessons from a mouse model of islet cell carcinogenesis. Ann N Y Acad Sci 887:150–163
156. Muleris M, Almeida A, Malfoy B, Dutrillaux B (1997) Assignment of v-erb-b2 avian erythroblastic leukemia viral oncogene homolog 2 (ERBB2) to human chromosome band 17q21.1 by in situ hybridization. Cytogenet Cell Genet 76(1–2):34–35
157. Bacus SS, Zelnick CR, Plowman G, Yarden Y (1994) Expression of the erbB-2 family of growth factor receptors and their ligands in breast cancers. Implication for tumor biology and clinical behavior. Am J Clin Pathol 102(4 Suppl 1):S13–S24
158. Goebel SU, Iwamoto M, Raffeld M, Gibril F, Hou W, Serrano J et al (2002) Her-2/neu expression and gene amplification in gastrinomas: correlations with tumor biology, growth, and aggressiveness. Cancer Res 62(13):3702–3710
159. Gosden JR, Middleton PG, Rout D (1986) Localization of the human oestrogen receptor gene to chromosome 6q24–q27 by in situ hybridization. Cytogenet Cell Genet 43(3–4):218–220
160. Altundag O, Altundag K, Gunduz M (2004) DNA methylation inhibitor, procainamide, may decrease the tamoxifen resistance by inducing overexpression of the estrogen receptor beta in breast cancer patients. Med Hypotheses 63(4):684–687
161. Kolodner RD, Hall NR, Lipford J, Kane MF, Morrison PT, Finan PJ et al (1995) Structure of the human MLH1 locus and analysis of a large hereditary nonpolyposis colorectal carcinoma kindred for mlh1 mutations. Cancer Res 55(2):242–248
162. House MG, Herman JG, Guo MZ, Hooker CM, Schulick RD, Cameron JL et al (2003) Prognostic value of hMLH1 methylation and microsatellite instability in pancreatic endocrine neoplasms. Surgery 134(6):902–908, discussion 9
163. Wick M, Zubov D, Hagen G (1999) Genomic organization and promoter characterization of the gene encoding the human telomerase reverse transcriptase (hTERT). Gene 232(1):97–106
164. Vezzosi D, Bouisson M, Escourrou G, Laurell H, Selves J, Seguin P et al (2006) Clinical utility of telomerase for the diagnosis of malignant well-differentiated endocrine tumours. Clin Endocrinol (Oxf) 64(1):63–67
165. House MG, Schulick RD (2006) Endocrine tumors of the pancreas. Curr Opin Oncol 18(1):23–29
166. Iino S, Abeyama K, Kawahara K, Yamakuchi M, Hashiguchi T, Matsukita S et al (2004) The antimetastatic role of thrombomodulin expression in islet cell-derived tumors and its diagnostic value. Clin Cancer Res 10(18 Pt 1):6179–6188
167. von Wichert G, Jehle PM, Hoeflich A, Koschnick S, Dralle H, Wolf E et al (2000) Insulin-like growth factor-I is an autocrine regulator of chromogranin A secretion and growth in human neuroendocrine tumor cells. Cancer Res 60(16):4573–4581, Epub 2000/09/02
168. Terris B, Scoazec JY, Rubbia L, Bregeaud L, Pepper MS, Ruszniewski P et al (1998) Expression of vascular endothelial growth factor in digestive neuroendocrine tumours. Histopathology 32(2):133–138, Epub 1998/04/17
169. La Rosa S, Uccella S, Finzi G, Albarello L, Sessa F, Capella C (2003) Localization of vascular endothelial growth factor and its receptors in digestive endocrine tumors: correlation with microvessel density and clinicopathologic features. Hum Pathol 34(1):18–27, Epub 2003/02/28
170. Alexiev BA, Drachenberg CB, Papadimitriou JC (2007) Endocrine tumors of the gastrointestinal tract and pancreas: grading, tumor size and proliferation index do not predict malignant behavior. Diagn Pathol 2:28, Epub 2007/08/10
171. Bajetta E, Catena L, Procopio G, Bichisao E, Ferrari L, Della Torre S et al (2005) Is the new WHO classification of neuroendocrine tumours useful for selecting an appropriate treatment? Ann Oncol 16(8):1374–1380, Epub 2005/06/09

172. Falconi M, Plockinger U, Kwekkeboom DJ, Manfredi R, Korner M, Kvols L et al (2006) Well-differentiated pancreatic nonfunctioning tumors/carcinoma. Neuroendocrinology 84(3):196–211, Epub 2007/02/22
173. Bettini R, Boninsegna L, Mantovani W, Capelli P, Bassi C, Pederzoli P et al (2008) Prognostic factors at diagnosis and value of WHO classification in a mono-institutional series of 180 non-functioning pancreatic endocrine tumours. Ann Oncol 19(5):903–908, Epub 2008/01/23
174. Pape UF, Jann H, Muller-Nordhorn J, Bockelbrink A, Berndt U, Willich SN et al (2008) Prognostic relevance of a novel TNM classification system for upper gastroenteropancreatic neuroendocrine tumors. Cancer 113(2):256–265, Epub 2008/05/29
175. Kloppel G, Rindi G, Anlauf M, Perren A, Komminoth P (2007) Site-specific biology and pathology of gastroenteropancreatic neuroendocrine tumors. Virchows Arch 451(Suppl 1):S9–S27, Epub 2007/08/09
176. Solcia E, Rindi G, Paolotti D, La Rosa S, Capella C, Fiocca R (1999) Clinicopathological profile as a basis for classification of the endocrine tumours of the gastroenteropancreatic tract. Ann Oncol 10(Suppl 2):S9–S15, Epub 1999/07/10
177. Wick MR, Graeme-Cook FM (2001) Pancreatic neuroendocrine neoplasms: a current summary of diagnostic, prognostic, and differential diagnostic information. Am J Clin Pathol 115(Suppl):S28–S45, Epub 2002/05/08
178. Hochwald SN, Zee S, Conlon KC, Colleoni R, Louie O, Brennan MF et al (2002) Prognostic factors in pancreatic endocrine neoplasms: an analysis of 136 cases with a proposal for low-grade and intermediate-grade groups. J Clin Oncol 20(11):2633–2642, Epub 2002/06/01
179. Rindi G, Kloppel G, Alhman H, Caplin M, Couvelard A, de Herder WW et al (2006) TNM staging of foregut (neuro)endocrine tumors: a consensus proposal including a grading system. Virchows Arch 449(4):395–401, Epub 2006/09/13
180. Maitra A, Hansel DE, Argani P, Ashfaq R, Rahman A, Naji A et al (2003) Global expression analysis of well-differentiated pancreatic endocrine neoplasms using oligonucleotide microarrays. Clin Cancer Res 9(16 Pt 1):5988–5995, Epub 2003/12/17
181. Bloomston M, Durkin A, Yang I, Rojiani M, Rosemurgy AS, Enkmann S et al (2004) Identification of molecular markers specific for pancreatic neuroendocrine tumors by genetic profiling of core biopsies. Ann Surg Oncol 11(4):413–419, Epub 2004/04/09
182. Capurso G, Lattimore S, Crnogorac-Jurcevic T, Panzuto F, Milione M, Bhakta V et al (2006) Gene expression profiles of progressive pancreatic endocrine tumours and their liver metastases reveal potential novel markers and therapeutic targets. Endocr Relat Cancer 13(2):541–558, Epub 2006/05/27
183. Couvelard A, Hu J, Steers G, O'Toole D, Sauvanet A, Belghiti J et al (2006) Identification of potential therapeutic targets by gene-expression profiling in pancreatic endocrine tumors. Gastroenterology 131(5):1597–1610, Epub 2006/10/27
184. Duerr EM, Mizukami Y, Ng A, Xavier RJ, Kikuchi H, Deshpande V et al (2008) Defining molecular classifications and targets in gastroenteropancreatic neuroendocrine tumors through DNA microarray analysis. Endocr Relat Cancer 15(1):243–256, Epub 2008/03/04
185. Shida T, Furuya M, Kishimoto T, Nikaido T, Tanizawa T, Koda K et al (2008) The expression of NeuroD and mASH1 in the gastroenteropancreatic neuroendocrine tumors. Mod Pathol 21(11):1363–1370, Epub 2008/07/01
186. Hansel DE, Rahman A, Hermans J, de Krijger RR, Ashfaq R, Yeo CJ et al (2003) Liver metastases arising from well-differentiated pancreatic endocrine neoplasms demonstrate increased VEGF-C expression. Mod Pathol 16(7):652–659
187. Hansel DE, Rahman A, House M, Ashfaq R, Berg K, Yeo CJ et al (2004) Met proto-oncogene and insulin-like growth factor binding protein 3 overexpression correlates with metastatic ability in well-differentiated pancreatic endocrine neoplasms. Clin Cancer Res 10(18 Pt 1): 6152–6158, Epub 2004/09/28
188. Vortmeyer AO, Lubensky IA, Skarulis M, Li G, Moon YW, Park WS et al (1999) Multiple endocrine neoplasia type 1: atypical presentation, clinical course, and genetic analysis of multiple tumors. Mod Pathol 12(9):919–924, Epub 1999/09/25

189. Van't Veer LJ, Dai H, van de Vijver MJ, He YD, Hart AA, Mao M et al (2002) Gene expression profiling predicts clinical outcome of breast cancer. Nature 415(6871):530–536, Epub 2002/02/02
190. Singh D, Febbo PG, Ross K, Jackson DG, Manola J, Ladd C et al (2002) Gene expression correlates of clinical prostate cancer behavior. Cancer Cell 1(2):203–209, Epub 2002/06/28
191. Pomeroy SL, Tamayo P, Gaasenbeek M, Sturla LM, Angelo M, McLaughlin ME et al (2002) Prediction of central nervous system embryonal tumour outcome based on gene expression. Nature 415(6870):436–442, Epub 2002/01/25
192. Metz DC, Jensen RT (2008) Gastrointestinal neuroendocrine tumors: pancreatic endocrine tumors. Gastroenterology 135(5):1469–1492
193. Nasir A, McCarthy S, Agrawal D, Bloom G, Zeringer E, Chen D, et al. (eds) (2008) Novel progression genes in pancreatic endocrine neoplasms. In: Annual meeting of the American Society of Clinical Oncology, Chicago
194. Nasir A, McCarthy S, Zeringer E, Bloom G, Eschrich S, Chen D, et al. (eds) (2008) Discovery and validation of progression-associated genes in primary pancreatic endocrine tumors. In: North American Neuroendocrine Tumor Society (NANETS) symposium, South Hampton, Bermuda
195. Nasir A, Helm J, Strosberg J, Henderson-Jackson E, Turner L, Hafez N, et al. (eds) (2009) Molecular markers outclass pathologic criteria of malignancy in predicting liver metastases in primary pancreatic endocrine neoplasms. In: International meeting of the European Neuroendocrine Tumor Society (ENETS) meeting, Granada
196. Nasir A, Helm J, Turner L, Chen DT, Strosberg J, Hafez N et al (2011) RUNX1T1: a novel predictor of liver metastasis in primary pancreatic endocrine neoplasms. Pancreas 40(4):627–633, Epub 2011/04/19
197. Henderson-Jackson EB, Helm J, Strosberg J, Nasir NA, Yeatman TJ, Kvols LK et al (2011) Palladin is a marker of liver metastasis in primary pancreatic endocrine carcinomas. Anticancer Res 31(9):2957–2962, Epub 2011/08/27

Chapter 15
Molecular Pathology and Diagnostics of Childhood Tumors

Enid Gilbert-Barness and Kristen Eisbrenner

Contents

E. Gilbert-Barness (✉)
Department of Pathology and Cell Biology, Pediatrics and Obstetrics and Gynecology,
University of South Florida College of Medicine at Tampa General Hospital,
Tampa, FL, USA
e-mail: egilbert@tgh.org

K. Eisbrenner
University of South Florida College of Medicine at Tampa General Hospital,
Tampa, FL, USA

D. Coppola (ed.), *Molecular Pathology and Diagnostics of Cancer*,
Cancer Growth and Progression 16, DOI 10.1007/978-94-007-7192-5_15,

Abstract Neoplasms in the fetus and infant are discussed in reference to types, incidence, clinical features, behavior, and response to treatment. Tumors that occur predominately in the first year of life have certain features of embryonic growth, including Wilms' tumors, neuroblastomas, embryonic sarcomas, yolk sac tumors of the testis, hepatoblastomas, and medulloblastomas of the brain, as well as sacrococcygeal tumors that have an overgrowth of embryonic components. Chromosome translocations, tumor suppressor genes, and some syndromes and congenital malformations associated with childhood tumors are discussed.

Keywords Childhood tumors • Molecular • Genetic • Chromosome abnormalities

Abbreviations

ARMS	Alveolar rhabdomyosarcoma
BWS	Beckwith-Wiedemann syndrome
CHEK2	Checkpoint kinase 2
CN	Cystic nephroma
CNS	Central nervous system
ERMS	Embryonal rhabdomyosarcoma
EWS	Ewing sarcoma
FAP	Familial adenomatous polyposis
FISH	Fluorescent in situ hybridization
GIST	Gastrointestinal stromal tumors
HPV	Human papilloma virus
IGF2	Insulin-like growth factor II
MEN1	Multiple endocrine neoplasia type 1
MEN2	Multiple endocrine neoplasia type 2
NF1	Neurofibromatosis type 1
NF2	Neurofibromatosis type 2
PDGF	Platelet-derived growth factor
PNET	Primitive neuroectodermal tumor
PTCH	Patch
RT-PCR	Reverse transcription-polymerase chain reaction
SHH	Sonic hedgehog
SMO	Smoothened
VHL	Von Hippel-Lindau
WAGR syndrome	Wilms' tumor, aniridia, genitourinary abnormalities and mental retardation
WT-1	Wilms' tumor-1 gene product

15.1 Introduction

Neoplasms in the fetus and infant are not entirely the same as those in the adult; differences include the types, incidence, clinical features, behavior, and response to treatment [1–13].

Continued growth without maturation of certain cells that are normally present during embryonic development, but that usually mature after birth, is responsible for many malignant congenital tumors. Wilms' tumors are derived from the metanephric blastema that has lost its propensity for differentiation but not for growth. Neuroblastomas of the adrenal gland occur from cells that arise in the neural crest and wander into the gland early in embryonic life. Normally, these cells differentiate into chromaffin tissue, but occasionally the transformation fails to take place, and a proliferation without differentiation produces a neuroblastoma.

Other tumors that occur predominantly in the first year of life and have certain features of embryonic growth include embryonic sarcomas, yolk sac tumors of the testis, hepatoblastomas, and medulloblastomas of the brain. Some teratomas of the sacrococcygeal and retroperitoneal regions can be included with those having an overgrowth of embryonic components that fail to mature. The cells of many sarcomas resemble immature fibroblasts and are also a result of failure of maturation coupled with an excessive stimulus for growth.

15.2 Incidence

The most common malignancies noted at birth are, in order, neuroblastoma, leukemia, sarcomas, and brain tumors [1, 11, 13–15]. Leukemia-lymphoma, brain tumors, neuroblastoma, and soft tissue sarcomas, in decreasing order of occurrence, are the more common neoplasms noted in older children and adolescents under 15 years of age [16].

15.3 Mechanisms in Carcinogenesis

Cancer is an uncontrolled growth of cells resulting from an alteration in cell DNA that produces a deregulation of normal growth [17]. A malignant cell becomes independent of normal regulatory control, and multiplies, producing a clone of cancer cells that subsequently develops into a neoplasm. There are several mechanisms, occurring as single or multiple events, by which the DNA of a normal cell becomes transformed into a cancer cell; this process is termed carcinogenesis. The known mechanisms include point mutations in DNA (the replacement of a single base pair within a gene by an incorrect one), gene deletions (loss of a large amount of DNA resulting in loss of all or part of the gene), and chromosomal translocations with gene rearrangements (the broken ends of the DNA from two different chromosomes may be joined incorrectly, resulting in parts of each chromosome being exchanged) [17].

15.4 Chromosome Translocations

Lejeune's recognition of trisomy 21 in Down syndrome predicted the many steps at which altered gene expression can produce abnormal tissue growth (neoplasia) or development (congenital anomalies). The similarities between molecular embryology and molecular oncology are strengthened by anomaly patterns (syndromes) that include cancer predisposition (e.g., Beckwith-Wiedemann syndrome [BWS], neurofibromatosis-1),

Table 15.1 Examples of chromosomal abnormalities associated with childhood tumors

Chromosomal defect	Childhood tumor
1p del, 1p32-p36 del, double minutes	Neuroblastoma
11p13 del, trisomy 18	Wilms' tumor
13q14 del	Retinoblastoma
	Osteosarcoma
Trisomy 21 (Down syndrome)	Leukemia
Monosomy 7	Leukemia and myelodysplasia syndrome
t(11q23), t(1;22), t(9;11)	Leukemia
t(1:22) (p13;q13)	Leukemia
Gonadal dysgenesis (46,XY; 45X/46,XY)	Gonadoblastoma, Germinoma
Klinefelter síndrome (XXY)	Teratoma
t(11;22)(q24;q12) t(21;22)	Ewing sarcoma/PNET
t(11;22)(p13;q12)	Intra-abdominal desmoplastic small round cell tumor
t(2;13)	Alveolar rhabdomyosarcoma
del 1p	Astrocytoma

From: Isaacs [18]

the dual roles of many proto-oncogene/tumor suppressor genes as developmental genes (e.g., PAX/C-KIT genes in Waardenburg syndrome/Piebald trait), and the stepwise progression from primary mutation, environmental factor, and epigenetic change to multifactorial (e.g., HOX genes in human leukemias and limb defects). Chromosomal abnormalities associated with neoplasia are shown in Table 15.1.

The number of chromosomal rearrangements and gene mutations associated with tumors is now so great that almost every cancer patient undergoes some sort of molecular or cytogenetic testing. The same progression from chromosome anomaly to causative breakpoint to cancer/tumor suppressor gene (Table 15.2) can now be followed for most developmental anomalies, and epigenesis is a central factor in both neoplasia and development [20, 21].

Chromosome analysis is now merging with DNA chips to provide telomere or array analyses, capable of defining subtle deletion/duplication of any chromosome segment by its altered fluorescent pattern.

15.5 Controlling Gene Expression

Increasing gene expression occurs by increasing the number of DNA copies of that gene (gene amplification). Human folate-resistant cell cultures are seen in aggressive neuroblastomas that amplify N-Myc. The new controlling mechanisms offer novel means for understanding and manipulating developmental gene regulation.

Table 15.2 Tumor suppressor genes involved in human neoplasms

Gene	Chromosomal location	Neoplasms associated with somatic mutations	Neoplasms associated with inherited (germ-line) mutations
WT-1	11p13	Wilms' tumor	Wilms' tumor
p53	17p13.1	Most human cancers	Li-Fraumeni syndrome: carcinomas of breast and adrenal cortex; sarcomas; leukemias; brain tumors
APC	5q21	Carcinomas of colon, stomach and pancreas	Familial adenomatous polyposis coli; carcinomas of colon
DCC	18q21	Carcinomas of colon and stomach	Unknown
VHL	3p25	Renal cell carcinoma	von Hippel-Lindau disease: retinal and cerebellar hemangioblastomas; renal cell carcinomas; angiomas and cysts of many visceral organs
NF-1	17q11	Schwannomas	Neurofibromatosis type 1; neural tumors
NF-2	22q12	Schwannomas and meningiomas	Neurofibromatosis type 2; central (acoustic) schwannomas; meningiomas
Rb	13q14	Retinoblastoma; osteo- sarcoma; carcinomas of breast, bladder, prostate, and lung	Retinoblastoma; osteosarcoma

From: Isaacs [19]

The relevance of new, non-classical pathways that control gene expression is reinforced by progressive DNA expansions/contractions and a myriad of possible gene rearrangements characteristic of most cancers.

15.6 DNA Methylation

Methylation of DNA contributes to cell differentiation, since the changes in DNA structure and expression will be transmitted to all daughter cells of a progenitor cell. Methylation of promoters probably plays a major role in cellular differentiation during embryogenesis: cells eliminate the transcription of unwanted genes by methylating their promoters.

Methylation inhibits (and occasionally activates) a very large number of genes, including some proto-oncogenes [22]. In cancers, there is often a decreased expression of DNA methyltransferase which leads to a nonspecific demethylation of 5-methylcytosine. This demethylation can reactivate the expression of proto-oncogenes, which thus act as unregulated growth-promoting agents (e.g., oncogenes, telomerases). Reactivated expression of genes involved in cell migration may lead to the emergence of more aggressive clones (clonal evolution). Abnormal methylation (hence inactivation) of anti-oncogenes similarly plays a major role in cancer development.

15.7 Zinc-Fingers

Transcription factors are those with a zinc-finger motif; zinc molecules cause these proteins to have a tertiary structure resembling fingers. The "fingers" bind the promoters of the genes under their control, to activate or inhibit them. Zinc finger proteins have multiple domains, allowing them to coordinate multiple different expression pathways. WT-1 (the Wilms' tumor-1 gene product), the fly developmental gene hunchback, and certain hormone and retinoic acid receptors belong to the zinc-finger class of transcription factors.

15.8 Loss of Imprinting and Cancer

Genomic imprinting was discovered in the 1980s and is now recognized to be very important clinically [23–25]. Imprinting is characterized by the differential activation of alleles according to their parental origin, associated with different patterns of DNA methylation.

Mammals are diploid organisms, meaning that all somatic cells possess two copies of the genome. Each autosomal gene is therefore represented by two copies, or alleles, with one copy inherited from each parent at fertilization. For the vast majority of autosomal genes, expression may occur from either allele. However, a small proportion (<1 %) of genes are imprinted, meaning that expression occurs from only one allele. Imprinting, therefore, is defined as the parental allele-specific expression of a very limited set of genes. This is an epigenetic phenomenon whereby the DNA of the two alleles of a gene is differentially modified so that only one parental allele is normally expressed [26]. The expressed allele is dependent on its parental origin. For example, the gene encoding insulin-like growth factor II (IGF2) is only expressed from the allele inherited from the father. Similarly, human triploidy with two paternal genomes produces fetal and placental tissue (hydatidiform mole), whereas triploidy with two maternal genomes biases toward fetal tissues only (ovarian teratomas). This regulation on an epigenetic marking of parental alleles occurs during gametogenesis. Mis-regulation of imprinted gene expression or loss of imprinting refers to loss of monoallelic gene regulation and concomitant biallelic expression.

In Beckwith-Wiedemann syndrome (BWS), partial moles, complete moles, and many cancers, this equilibrium is altered, leading to loss of imprinting and IGF2 over-expression. This has been documented in Wilms' tumor, Ewing sarcoma, rhabdomyosarcoma, adrenocortical tumors, hepatoblastoma, hepatocellular carcinoma, and pheochromocytoma. Conversely, the incidence of these tumors is greatly increased in BWS, and placentas of BWS fetuses can show mole-like changes. IGF2 is also overexpressed in choriocarcinoma, leukemias, and germ cell tumors, as well as in bladder, breast, cervical, esophageal, gastric, colorectal, pulmonary, ovarian, prostatic, renal cell and other carcinomas and tumors.

15.9 Intercellular Signaling in Development: Sonic Hedgehog

Embryonic cellular signaling pathways can be extremely complex, with core molecules that influence the development of multiple organs. A prototype is the sonic hedgehog (SHH; a member of the hedgehog gene family). In the absence of SHH protein, the Patch (PTCH) plasma membrane protein inhibits smoothened (SMO) protein. Binding of SHH with PTCH lifts this inhibition, allowing SMO to activate the SHH cascade, including GL12, GL13, CBP, and SUFU molecules [27, 28]. Mutations involving this cascade can result in a wide range of diseases, including tremors, holoprosencephaly, Greig cephalopolysyndactyly, Pallister-Hall syndrome, Rubinstein-Taybi syndrome, the nevoid basal cell carcinoma syndrome, basal cell carcinoma (syndromic and sporadic forms), medulloblastoma, meningiomas, primitive neuroectodermal tumors, breast adenocarcinomas, trichoepitheliomas, squamous cell carcinomas, esophageal carcinomas, fetal rhabdomyomas, and rhabdomyosarcomas [27].

15.9.1 Examples: Sequential Gene Expression in Growth and Neoplasia

Molecular analysis has defined many growth-related molecules through their alteration in tumors [27, 29–35]. The definition of molecular changes that fulfill Knudson's two-hit or two-stage hypothesis has also been reviewed [36]. Although Knudson's explanation involved one abnormal RB1 allele from the germline (predisposition or first hit), followed by somatic RB1 gene mutations in susceptible tissue (second hit in retina), epigenetic changes can also be placed on this pathway to neoplasia. This is reflected in the fact that most germline RB1 mutations originate on the paternal chromosome, implying a role for genomic imprinting/DNA methylation. Characterization of the RB1 gene as a cell cycle regulatory element places it within cell proliferation/cell death pathways.

15.10 Handling of Pediatric Tumor Specimens

Many pediatric tumors require immunostaining, molecular investigation, and electron microscopy for a definitive diagnosis and prognosis. All diagnostic pediatric tumor specimens should be submitted to the laboratory as fresh tissue immediately following biopsy when possible. The specimen should be divided into samples for formalin fixation and paraffin embedding, glutaraldehyde fixation for electron microscopy, snap freezing or storage in RNA protection medium for molecular studies such as reverse transcription-polymerase chain reaction (RT-PCR), with

Table 15.3 Staging system for Wilms' tumor cancer oncology group

Stage I	Limited to kidney and completely resected, renal capsule intact Fine needles aspiration or percutaneous core needle biopsy does not upstage the tumor The presence of necrotic tumor or chemotherapy-induced change in the renal sinus and/or within perirenal fat should not be regarded as a reason for upstaging a tumor providing it is completely excised and does not reach the resection margins
Stage II	Tumor infiltrates beyond kidney but is completely resected (a) The tumor extends beyond the kidney or penetrates through the renal capsule and/or fibrous pseudocapsule into perirenal fat but is completely resected (resection margins clear) (b) Tumor infiltrates the renal sinus and/or blood and/or lymphatic vessels outside the renal parenchyma but is completely resected (c) Tumor infiltrates adjacent organs or ureter but is completely resected
Stage III	Gross or microscopic residual tumor confined to abdomen (a) Incomplete excision of the tumor which extends beyond resection margins (gross or microscopic tumor remains postoperatively) (b) Any abdominal lymph nodes are involved (c) Tumor rupture before or intraoperatively (d) The tumor has penetrated through the peritoneal surface (e) Tumor implants are found on the peritoneal surface (f) Tumor thrombi present at resection margins of vessel or ureter transected or removed piecemeal by surgeon (g) The tumor has been surgically biopsied (wedge biopsy) prior to preoperative chemotherapy or surgery
Stage IV	Hematogenous metastasis or lymph node metastasis outside the abdominal and pelvic region
Stage V	Bilateral renal tumors at diagnosis. Each side should be sub-staged according to the above classification

imprints ("dabs") fixed for fluorescent in situ hybridization (FISH) in methanol, cytogenetic studies, or frozen for storage and subsequent analysis if required. Many molecular techniques such as FISH and RT-PCR may also be performed on routinely fixed paraffin-embedded material.

15.10.1 Wilms' Tumor (Nephroblastoma)

Wilms' tumor (Table 15.3) is a malignant embryonal neoplasm derived from nephrogenic blastemal cells. Several lines of differentiation are commonly seen and often replicate the histology of developing kidneys. Approximately 10 % of patients with Wilms' tumor also have congenital abnormalities and malformation syndromes. The most common malformations are hemihypertrophy and genitourinary anomalies. The common syndromes associated with Wilms' tumor include BWS, WAGR syndrome (Wilms' tumor, aniridia, genitourinary abnormalities and mental retardation), and Denys-Drash syndrome (mesangial sclerosis, pseudohermaphroditism and nephroblastoma) [37–41]. Abnormalities involving the Wilms' tumor locus, 11p13, are consistently found in the tumors of patients with WAGR and Denys-Drash syndrome. The 11p13 Wilms' tumor locus encodes two coordinately regulated zinc-finger transcripts, WT-1 and WIT-1. These genes are highly expressed in the developing urogenital system [42–44]. The WT-1 protein binds to several sites on promoters of an IGF2 gene as well as to a promoter of the platelet-derived growth factor (PDGF) A-chain gene [45, 46]. The gene controls mesenchymal-epithelial transition during renal development. Furthermore, WT-1 expression induces transcription of one of the seven proapoptotic genes, *Bak,* and blocks cellular proliferation and DNA synthesis [47]. Interference with these normal regulatory influences of WT-1 may be an important factor in the genesis of nephroblastoma, which typically express high levels of IGF2 [48] and may also overproduce PDGF [49]. The expression patterns of WT-1 and Pax-2 in the metanephros overlap to a considerable extent; however, expression of WT-1 peaks as that of Pax-2 is decreasing. Therefore, it is possible that WT-1 represses Pax-2, and Pax-2 expression fails to down-regulate in the epithelial component of Wilms' tumor and in nephroblastomatosis, the putative precursor of nephroblastoma [50]. Despite the strong association of WT1 mutations with Wilms' tumor predisposition, WT-1 is mutated in only a minority of sporadic Wilms' tumors [51]. This low prevalence of WT-1 abnormalities in sporadic Wilms' tumor led to the recognition of other genes involved in pathogenesis. Evidence supporting this is provided by the linkage of familial BWS to a locus at chromosome 11p15, designated WT-2 [52, 53]. Approximately 1 % of the patients with Wilms' tumor have a positive family history for the same neoplasm. Most of the pedigrees suggest autosomal dominant transmission with variable penetrance and expressivity. This suggests that genetic loci other than WT-1 and WT-2 are responsible for the pathogenesis of many familial as well as sporadic Wilms' tumors [54, 55].

In gross examination, the most important factors to document are capsular invasion and hilar and sinus involvement along with adequate sampling of the tumor. Histology blocks should include at least one block per centimeter of the largest tumor diameter, tumor-kidney interface, capsule, hilar area, macroscopically normal kidney (at least two), and other areas of pathological significance. Some cases may be markedly cystic; in these, the tumor must be carefully examined for the presence of nodular solid areas. Particular attention should be paid to assessment of the capsule, hilar vessels, including the cut end, and renal sinus.

A triphasic Wilms' tumor includes epithelial, stromal, and blastemal elements microscopically. Relative proportions of the epithelial components may vary widely such that one is markedly dominant (Fig. 15.1). The stromal component may vary widely from areas of stellate cells within a myxoid background to spindle cells recapitulating primitive mesenchyme. Smooth and striated muscle are the most common differentiated stromal cell types. Occasionally, a wide range of other stromal components may be present, including cartilage, osteoid, and even glial tissues.

Post-chemotherapy features include necrosis, fibrosis, and foamy and hemosiderin-laden macrophages. Rapidly dividing cells, such as those of the blastemal or primitive epithelial components, tend to respond to chemotherapy, whereas the stromal

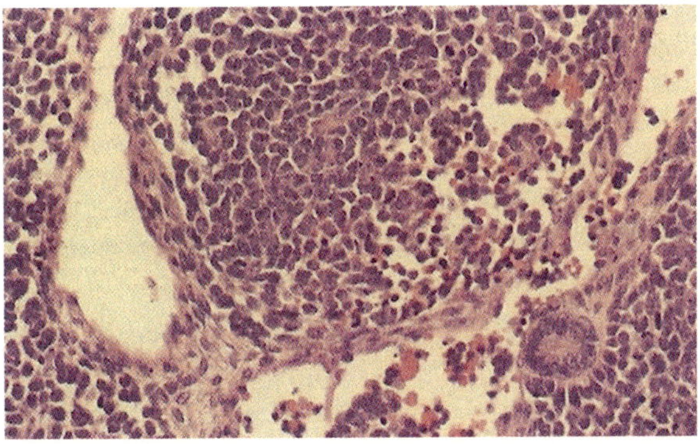

Fig. 15.1 Nephroblastemal elements in Wilms' tumor (From Gilbert-Barness [56])

elements will not. Thus, tumors with significant stromal differentiation may not reduce much in size during chemotherapy. Also, stromal components may appear to be more prominent in a post-chemotherapy specimen. The tumor that remains predominantly viable following chemotherapy and in which the main component is blastema is associated with an adverse prognosis.

15.10.2 Unfavorable Histology in Wilms' Tumor (Anaplasia)

Nuclear anaplasia in the context of Wilms' tumor has very specific criteria required for its definition, such as nuclear hyperchromasia, nuclear enlargement in which affected nuclei are at least three times the size of adjacent non-anaplastic nuclei, and abnormal multipolar mitoses. Using such criteria, anaplasia is present in approximately 5–10 % of Wilms' tumors, occurring more commonly in those diagnosed in later childhood and in black patients. Anaplasia may either be focal or diffuse. Focally, one or a few, well-circumscribed, localized regions of anaplasia are found within the primary tumor that is completely excised, with the majority of tumor containing no significant nuclear atypia. Diffuse anaplasia occurs in multiple fields or outside the primary tumor and is associated with a poor response to chemotherapy. Anaplasia is of major clinical significance when present in tumors, which are potentially incompletely excised. Focal anaplasia or anaplasia in stage I cases may be of importance. Anaplasia is identified as an adverse prognostic factor. Transcription profiling indicates that a cluster of genes separates anaplastic from non-anaplastic Wilms' tumor.

Immunohistochemical staining is often extremely useful in the diagnosis of Wilms' tumor from a needle core biopsy. A core biopsy may simply demonstrate small round blue cells, which could represent the blastema of Wilms' tumor or several other embryonal tumors of infancy and childhood. The most useful immunohistochemical marker is WT-1. Areas of stromal differentiation, and well-differentiated epithelial structures, may not express nuclear WT-1. Cytokeratin staining may help with the identification or confirmation of epithelial differentiation. CD56 is also useful, since primitive renal blastema is diffusely and strongly CD56 positive. Nuclear p53 is expressed in 75 % of anaplastic nephroblastomas. At present, there are no diagnostic or prognostic markers useful for the evaluation of Wilms' tumor.

15.10.3 Nephrogenic Rests and Nephroblastomatosis

Nephrogenic rests are classically divided into perilobar and intralobar types. Perilobar rests are more common and are found in subcapsular peripheral locations with well-demarcated margins on low power. Intralobar rests present anywhere within the kidney and often have a more irregular and intermixed margin. The clinical relevance is their potential increased risk for subsequent development of Wilms' tumor. Wilms' tumors in association with intralobar rests develop at a younger age on average. The risk appears highest for intralobar rests in patients under 1 year of age. When a Wilms' tumor develops within a nephrogenic rest, there is a superimposed nodular growth of the proliferating component and formation of a fibrous pseudocapsule around the tumor with the compressed rest at the periphery.

15.10.4 Cystic Nephroma and Cystic Partially Differentiated Nephroblastoma

Cystic nephroma (CN) is predominantly seen in children under 5 years of age. Its characteristic imaging appearance is of a well-circumscribed mass distinct from the surrounding kidney and predominantly cystic with thin septa. In CN, the septa contain no solid nodules and only mature elements. In cystic partially differentiated nephroblastoma, the septa also contain embryonal elements that do not form solid nodules, thus conforming to the outlines of the septa. If classical components of Wilms' tumor are present, forming nodular structures that distort the septal contours, the lesion should be classified as cystic Wilms' tumor. Both CN and cystic partially differentiated nephroblastoma are adequately treated by resection alone with an excellent prognosis and no chemotherapy required. Predominantly, cystic Wilms' tumor, although almost always stage I and therefore with a correspondingly good prognosis, should be treated as an appropriately staged Wilms' tumor. There is an association between CN and pleuropulmonary blastoma [57].

The classical pattern of CN demonstrates nests of ovoid cells separated by fibrovascular septa. Cord cells may be ovoid, epithelioid, or spindled with bland nuclei without prominent nucleoli. Septa demonstrate a marked regularly branching "chicken wire" pattern of capillaries. A wide variety of other patterns have been described. These include myxoid, sclerosing, cellular epithelioid, palisaded, spindled, storiform, and anaplastic variants. Most cases are composed of a mixture of such patterns.

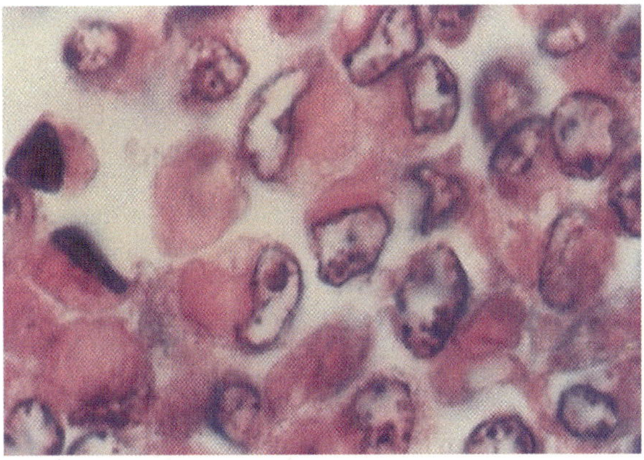

Fig. 15.2 Rhabdoid tumor cells with variable presence of intracytoplasmic inclusions (From Gilbert-Barness [56])

15.10.5 Clear Cell Carcinoma of the Kidney

Clear cell carcinoma of the kidney comprises 3 % of malignant pediatric renal tumors. The average age at diagnosis is 3 years. There are no specific diagnostically or prognostically useful genetic features. Metastatic disease is present in 5 % of cases and up to 60 % of those have bone metastases. The tumor is solid, cystic, and cream to tan in color. Immunohistochemical stains vimentin and bcl2 are usually positive. Cytokeratin, WT1, and CD99 staining is negative [57]. The vimentin staining is unlike the dot-like pattern characteristic of renal rhabdoid tumors.

15.10.6 Renal Rhabdoid Tumor

Rhabdoid tumors are rare, comprising 2 % of pediatric renal malignancies. These tumors are predominantly shown in young children, with average age at diagnosis of 1 year. This tumor is exceptionally rare in children over 5 years of age.

In patients with renal rhabdoid tumors, genetic abnormalities of the *hsNF5/INI1* tumor suppressor gene on chromosome 22 are characteristic. The gene is important for chromatin remodeling, and inactivation is tumorigenic. Mutations, deletions, and chromosome losses inactivating INI1 vary widely; therefore, a single readily available RT-PCR-based assay is not available.

Patients with renal rhabdoid tumors have an increased risk of malignant embryonal tumors of the posterior fossa; approximately 10–20 % develop a posterior fossa tumor. Rhabdoid tumors are aggressive, and the majority of patients (up to 80 %) present with metastatic disease. Grossly, rhabdoid tumors have large, solid and cystic areas with extensive areas of hemorrhage and necrosis. They are poorly defined and locally infiltrative. Microscopically, rhabdoid tumors contain eccentric nuclei and eosinophilic intracytoplasmic inclusions (Fig. 15.2). Vimentin immunostaining demonstrates characteristic strong dot-like perinuclear cytoplasmic staining in a significant proportion of cells. INI1 immunostaining is characteristically absent in the nucleus of rhabdoid tumor cells. INI1 nuclear staining is positive in the nucleus of almost all other pediatric tumors, although, renal medullary carcinoma and some cells of synovial sarcoma may also be INI1 negative.

15.10.7 Congenital Mesoblastic Nephroma

Congenital mesoblastic nephroma is a low-grade spindle cell neoplasm affecting the renal medulla. Representing 2–5 % of pediatric tumors, congenital mesoblastic nephroma is also the most common congenital renal neoplasm. A vast majority of cases present in the first year of life (90 %). Some patients may develop hypertension. Congenital mesoblastic nephroma demonstrates a t(12;15)(p13;q25) ETV6-NTRK3 translocation, also found in congenital/infantile fibrosarcoma and secretory carcinoma of the breast. RT-PCR may be useful diagnostically [58]. Overall, 95 % of patients have an event-free survival; however, prognosis is worse with stage III with cellular congenital mesoblastic nephroma in patients 3 months or older. Grossly, the tumor has a cystic and solid whorled fibrous appearance resembling a fibroid. The cellular subtype may appear softer and more hemorrhagic.

Microscopic subtypes are classical, cellular, and mixtures and may be identified on the basis of molecular characterization and morphological features. The cellular subtype represents 40–60 % of cases and is morphologically indistinguishable from an infantile fibrosarcoma. There is increased cellularity with mitoses and focal necrosis. Mixed subtypes comprise less than 10 % of cases. The presence of incomplete excision is the main cause of local recurrence. The majority of cases with recurrence have been the cellular subtype with an abnormal gene fusion product present.

15.10.8 Renal Cell Carcinoma in Childhood

Renal cell carcinoma is uncommon in childhood and comprises 2–5 % of pediatric renal tumors. It usually occurs in children 10–15 years of age. Genetic changes are similar to adult cases. A range of familial and syndromic conditions may be associated with renal cell carcinoma development such as Von Hippel-Lindau (VHL) syndrome, hereditary papillary renal carcinoma syndrome, hereditary leiomyomatosis and renal cell cancer, Birt-Hogg-Dubé syndrome, and tuberous sclerosis. Twenty percent have metastases at diagnosis. The tumor may have a predominant clear cell, cystic papillary, or chromophobe pattern. Renal cell carcinoma is cytokeratin positive in all tumors and CD10 positive in greater than 90 %. EMA, vimentin, and CEA staining may also be positive.

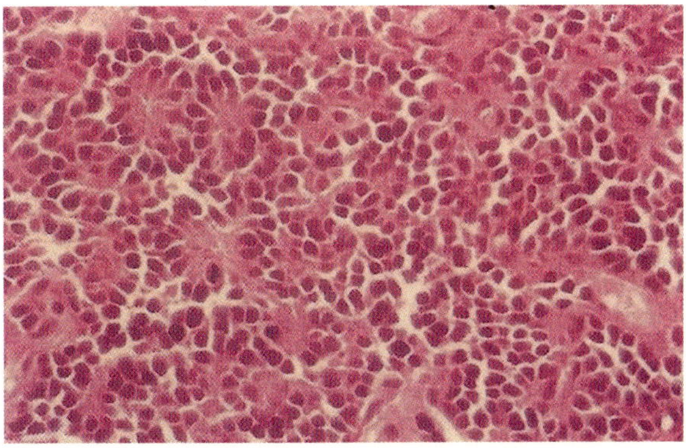

Fig. 15.3 Homer-Wright rosettes in neuroblastoma (From Gilbert-Barness [56])

15.10.9 Neuroblastoma

The incidence of neuroblastoma is 1 per 100,000 [59]. Seventy percent of patients have metastatic disease at presentation [60]. Age, clinical stage, molecular findings, and an undifferentiated subtype all influence overall survival [61]. The International Neuroblastoma Pathology Classification system [62] is as follows:

1. Neuroblastoma, undifferentiated: No ganglion cell differentiation of neuroblasts, no definite neurofibrillary stroma on light microscopy, sheets of small round to ovoid cells.
2. Neuroblastoma, poorly differentiated: Nests of neuroblasts within neurofibrillary background stroma, usually identifiable on routine light microscopy, <5 % of neuroblasts show ganglion cell differentiation (Fig. 15.3).
3. Neuroblastoma, differentiating: >5 % of neuroblasts show ganglion cell differentiation, nuclei have a prominent nucleolus. The cell has abundant eosinophilic/amphophilic cytoplasm, and the cell diameter must be more than twice nuclear diameter.
4. Ganglioneuroblastoma, intermixed: Well-defined nests of neuroblasts within neurofibrillary background stroma that are scattered throughout the lesion. Usually presents differentiating neuroblasts within the nests of cells (Fig. 15.4). No discreet identifiable nodules are present. Less than 50 % of the lesion is represented by neuroblastoma cells. Greater than 50 % of the lesion is represented by Schwannian stroma and mature ganglion cells.
5. Ganglioneuroblastoma, nodular: There is a macroscopic, hemorrhagic nodule within a larger bland lesion. The surrounding areas are stroma-rich or stroma dominant areas with mature or maturing ganglion cells; the well-demarcated nodule has Schwannian stroma, poor neuroblastomatous tissue; may be multiple, nodules morphologically those of neuroblastoma. Outcome of ganglioneuroblastoma, nodular is based on prognostic features of the neuroblastoma component [64], including all molecular/biological markers.

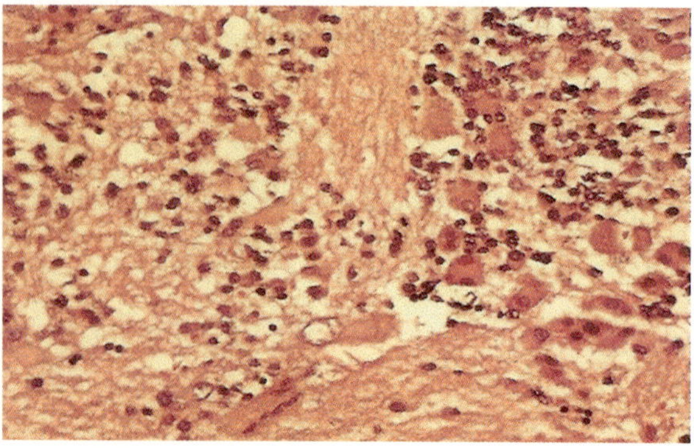

Fig. 15.4 Neuroblasts and variable ganglion cell differentiation in ganglioneuroblastoma (From Gilbert-Barness [63])

Table 15.4 Neuroblastoma prognostic categories

Mitosis karyorrhexis index (MKI)	
Low MKI	Fewer than 100 mitotic and karyorrhectic cells/5,000 tumor cells, or less than 2 % of tumor consisting of mitotic and karyorrhectic cells
Intermediate MKI	100–200 mitotic and karyorrhectic cells/5,000 tumor cells, or 2–4 % of tumor consisting of mitotic and karyorrhectic cells
High MKI	More than 200 mitotic and karyorrhectic cells/5,000 tumor cells, or greater than 4 % of tumor consisting of mitotic and karyorrhectic cells
International neuroblastoma staging system	
Stage 1	Localized tumor with complete gross excision, with or without microscopic residual disease; representative ipsilateral lymph nodes negative for tumor microscopically (nodes attached to and removed with the primary tumor may be positive)
Stage 2A	Localized tumor with incomplete gross excision; representative ipsilateral nonadherent lymph nodes negative for tumor microscopically
Stage 2B	Localized tumor with or without complete gross excision, with ipsilateral nonadherent lymph nodes positive for tumor; enlarged contralateral lymph nodes must be negative microscopically
Stage 3	Unresectable unilateral tumor infiltrating across the midline, with or without regional lymph node involvement or localized unilateral tumor with contralateral regional lymph node involvement; or localized unilateral tumor with contralateral regional lymph node involvement, or midline tumor with bilateral extension by infiltration (unresectable) or by lymph node involvement. The midline is defined as the vertebral column. Tumors originating on one side and crossing the midline must infiltrate to or beyond the opposite side of the vertebral column
Stage 4	Any primary tumor with dissemination to distant lymph nodes, bone marrow, liver, skin, and/or other organs (except as defined for stage 4A)
Stage 4S	Localized primary tumor (as defined for stage 1, 2A, or 2B), with dissemination limited to skin, liver, and/or bone marrow (limited to infants less than 1 year of age). Marrow involvement should be minimal (less than 10 % of total nucleated cells identified as malignant by bone biopsy or by bone marrow aspirate). More extensive bone marrow involvement would be considered stage 4 disease. The results of the MBG scan (if performed) [57] should be negative for disease in the bone marrow

Molecular studies are mandatory for risk assessment and management in neuroblastic tumors, and it is important for optimal specimen handling to allow FISH and other molecular studies. Current biological markers associated with adverse prognosis are N-MYC amplification, DNA diploidy, 1p deletion and 17q gain. Mitosis karyorrhexis index is calculated per 5,000 neuroblasts, usually within 6–8 high-power fields in cellular tumors in a 3 μm-thick evenly stained section. The mitosis karyorrhexis index is not carried out on small needle biopsy specimens or post-treatment specimens.

Specimens are assigned to 1 of 3 prognostic categories (see Table 15.4). On immunohistochemical staining CD56 is positive and also highlights neurofibrillary stroma. NB84 is positive. CD44 is positive and associated with a better prognosis. Schwannian stroma is S100 positive.

15.10.10 Rhabdomyosarcoma

This is a malignant mesenchymal tumor with skeletal muscle differentiation. In childhood, there are two main types: embryonal (ERMS) and alveolar (ARMS). The pleomorphic type affects adults.

15.10.10.1 Embryonal Rhabdomyosarcoma

This is the most common pediatric soft tissue sarcoma. Most develop in children less than 10 years old, 50 % in those less than 5 years old, and 5 % in those less than 1 year old. 11p15 loss is reported; however, it is not diagnostically useful, and there is no characteristic fusion transcript. Despite skeletal muscle differentiation, only 5 % arise in the skeletal muscle of extremities. Fifty percent develop in the head and neck, whereas 30 % are genitourinary including paratesticular. The remainder are from a wide range of sites including bile ducts and retroperitoneum.

Microscopically there are sheets of immature round to ovoid to spindle mesenchymal cells (rhabdomyoblasts). Cellularity is variable within a loose stroma. The degree of morphological skeletal muscle differentiation varies and includes strap cells, tadpole cells, and spider cells (Fig. 15.5). Differentiation is especially prominent post-chemotherapy. The spindle cell variant consists predominantly of spindle cells with fascicles, whorls, or a storiform pattern. The Botryoid variant consists of ERMS affecting the wall beneath an epithelial surface in vagina, bladder, or bile ducts. There is an intraluminal polypoid growth pattern macroscopically. The microscopic cambium layer is a layer of neoplastic cells immediately beneath the epithelium in loose myxoid stroma. The anaplastic/pleomorphic variant has nuclear enlargement, hyperchromasia, and anaplasia.

Immunohistochemical staining with vimentin is positive. Desmin positivity is cytoplasmic, whereas myogenin positivity is nuclear. All rhabdomyosarcomas show myogenin expression with more widespread expression in ARMS (usually greater

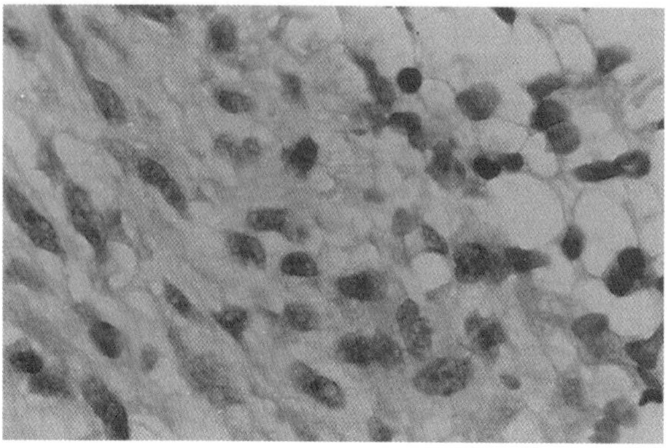

Fig. 15.5 Atypical cells with skeletal muscle differentiation in rhabdomyosarcoma (From Gilbert-Barness [56])

than 70 % positive) than in ERMS (usually less than 30 % positive). Myogenin may be very focal in a limited sample such as core biopsy. MyoD1 is positive in nuclei in cases with myogenin staining. Myoglobin is positive in well-differentiated cells. Other markers may highlight aberrant expression.

15.10.10.2 Alveolar Rhabdomyosarcoma

Clinically, this tumor is the more aggressive variant of rhabdomyosarcoma. Alveolar architecture is not always present. The characteristic gene fusion transcript is present in the majority of cases, detectable by molecular techniques including FISH with FKHR break-apart probes and RT-PCR for fusion transcript deletion. Approximately 60 % have the PAX3-FKHR translocation, 20 % have PAX7-FKHR translocation, and 20 % are fusion-negative [57]. Clinical features include a rapidly growing mass with almost any site involved, and 40 % are located in the extremities. ARMS may present with disseminated disease with or without an identifiable primary site. Bone marrow metastases occur. The classic alveolar pattern consists of fibrovascular septa, tumor cell nests that may be dyscohesive (Fig. 15.6). The solid variant has sheets of round tumor cells and no septae surrounding or stroma formation. The histological features show a limited correlation with PAX/FKHR fusion status. Only totally solid alveolar architecture is associated with absence of PAX/FKHR fusion products. No morphological features predict any particular fusion type.

15.10.11 Hepatoblastoma

Hepatoblastoma is the most common hepatic malignancy of childhood and comprises 1 % of pediatric malignancies. Ninety percent occur in the first 5 years of life and less than 5 % are congenital. Fifty-fold have increased risk of birth weight of

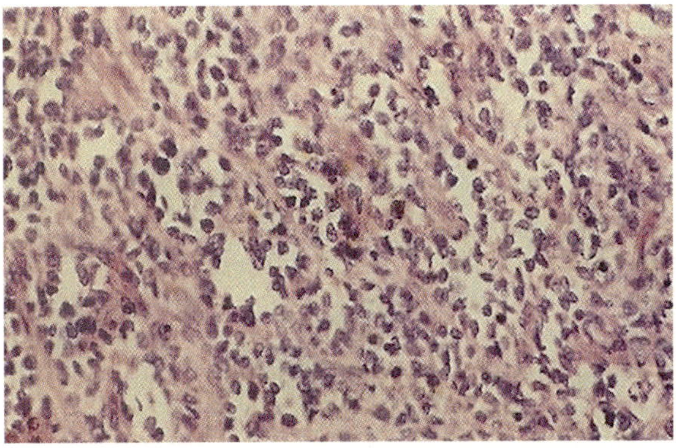

Fig. 15.6 Dyscohesion of cells resulting in the characteristic alveolar growth pattern of alveolar rhabdomyosarcoma (From Gilbert-Barness [56])

less than 1,000 g. There are rare predisposing syndromes in 5 % of cases such as BWS, trisomies, and familial adenomatous polyposis (FAP). Ten percent of sporadic hepatoblastomas have APC gene mutations.

In 80 % of cases, there is a single mass, whereas 20 % have multiple lesions. Anemia is present in 70 % and thrombocytosis in 50 %. Greater than 90 % of cases show elevated serum AFP concentration. Forty to 60 % are unresectable at diagnosis, but 85 % are resectable post-chemotherapy. Ten to 20 % of cases have lung metastases at diagnosis. The overall survival rate is 70 %.

Histopathologically, the tumor has a mixture of features that may be highly variable in both fetal and embryonal epithelial cells, stroma of connective tissue, osteoid, skeletal muscle or rare other epithelial types as well as teratoid features. Extramedullary hematopoiesis may be present. Immunohistochemical staining is especially useful other than to exclude other tumors.

15.10.12 Desmoplastic Small Round Cell Tumor

Desmoplastic small round cell tumor affects children and young adults, with more males affected than females. Characteristic and diagnostic is the t(11;22)(p13;q12), Ewing sarcoma (EWS)-WT1 fusion. The patient usually presents with disseminated abdominal disease. Presentation depends on the site; if aggressive, the patient has a poor prognosis. Histopathological features include infiltrative growth with desmoplastic spindle cell stroma that is variably vascular. Tumor cells are uniform, ovoid, and hyperchromatic with scant cytoplasm. Intracytoplasmic inclusions may be present. The cells are arranged in nests of variable shapes and sizes. Mitoses and necrosis may be present.

The tumor has polyphenotypic expression with CK, EMA, desmin, vimentin, and NSE staining. Anticarboxyterminus WTI is nuclear positive, and myogenin and MyoD1 are negative. Molecular techniques are required for confirmation of diagnosis.

15.10.13 Extrarenal Malignant Rhabdoid Tumor

This tumor occurs in infants and children. Congenital tumors are reported. There is an association with family history of a range of malignancies and posterior fossa tumors. Like renal rhabdoid tumors, there are abnormalities of the *hSNF5/INI1* gene on chromosome 22 [57]. Clinical features consist of mass lesions at almost any site. The tumor is aggressive and has a poor prognosis; however, this has improved with current chemotherapy regimes. Histopathological features include sheets of malignant cells with vesicular nuclei, prominent nucleoli, eosinophilic cytoplasm, mitoses, and necrosis. There is a variable extent of intracytoplasmic inclusions, which are often easier to identify at the periphery or in myxoid areas. The small cell variant has cells with scant cytoplasm. Some tumors may have a markedly myxoid stroma. On immunohistochemical staining, there is co-expression of CK and vimentin. Perinuclear "dot-like" expression highlights inclusions that are composed of intermediate filaments by electron microscopy. There is variable non-diagnostic expression of other antibodies. Negative INI1 nuclear expression is essentially diagnostic.

15.10.14 Ewing Sarcoma/Primitive Neuroectodermal Tumor

EWS and primitive neuroectodermal tumor (PNET) are primary malignant small round cell tumors of bone and soft tissue. Because they have a similar phenotype and share an identical chromosome translocation, they are viewed as the same tumor, differing from each other only in their degree of neural differentiation. Tumors that demonstrate neural differentiation by light microscopy, immunohistochemistry, or electron microscopy have been traditionally labeled PNET, and those that are undifferentiated by these analyses are diagnosed as EWS. These tumors account for approximately 6–10 % of primary malignant bone tumors. Most patients are 10–15 years old, and approximately 80 % are younger than 20 years. Boys are affected more frequently than girls, although the disease occurs much more often in girls than boys during the first 3 years of life. There is a striking predilection for whites; blacks are rarely afflicted.

In EWS/PNET, approximately 85 % have a t(11;22)(q24;q12) translocation, 5–10 % of cases have a t(21;22)(q22;q12) translocation, and in less than 1 % of tumors, a t(7;22)(p22;q12) translocation is present. The fusion gene (EWS-FLI1) generated from the translocation plays a vital role in the molecular genesis of this neoplasm [57]. The aberrant gene acts as a dominant oncogene, and the resultant chimeric proteins function as aberrant transcription factors that stimulate cell proliferation.

EWS/PNET can arise in any portion of the skeleton but usually develops in the diaphysis or metadiaphysis of long tubular bones and the flat bones of the pelvis. In young children, the pelvis, ribs, and proximal long bones are preferentially affected. The tumor typically presents as a painful enlarging mass, and the affected site is frequently tender, warm, and swollen. Systemic findings that mimic infection include fever, elevated sedimentation rate, anemia, and leukocytosis.

Arising in the medullary cavity, EWS/PNET usually transgresses the cortex and periosteum, producing a soft tissue mass. The tumor is tan-white or fish flesh-like in appearance and frequently contains areas of hemorrhage and necrosis. The cells grow in sheets or irregular islands with an organoid growth pattern within which Homer-Wright rosettes may be present. Occasionally, tumor cells are larger, have irregular nuclear contours, and prominent nucleoli. Mitoses are easily identified, and necrosis may be extensive. Special histochemical stains demonstrate glycogen in up to 75 % of tumors. In a minority of cases dense core neurosecretory granules are seen by electron microscopy.

EWS/PNET cells express vimentin, CD99 (MIC-2), FLI-1, C-kit and one or more neural markers including NSE, Leu-7, S100, neurofilament, and keratin in approximately 20 % of cases [57]. EWS/PNET is usually treated with a combination of chemotherapy and surgery. The chemotherapy is given preoperatively, and chemotherapy-induced necrosis of 90 % or greater is considered a good response. Radiotherapy is reserved for tumors that are surgically inaccessible, inadequately excised tumors, and patient palliation. Effective chemotherapy has dramatically improved the prognosis to a 75 % 5-year survival of which at least 50 % are long-term cures.

15.10.15 Testicular and Paratesticular Tumors

Most germ cell tumors are seminomas in young adults; however, in younger children, they are usually teratomas and yolk sac tumors.

Seminomas. Seminomas are composed of sheets of uniform round to ovoid cells with minimal pleomorphism; in most cases, they are associated with lymphoid infiltrates. PLAP and CD117 are positive in almost all cases [57].

Embryonal Carcinoma. Embryonal carcinoma is composed of sheets, papillae, and cysts with poorly differentiated cells containing overlapping polygonal, vesicular nuclei and prominent nucleoli. CD30, CK and focal PLAP stains are positive.

Yolk Sac Tumor. This is the most common malignant germ cell tumor in infancy. Ninety percent are associated with elevated serum AFP levels and contain ovoid vacuolated cells with scattered hyaline globules. Yolk sac tumors are mitotically active. There are numerous growth patterns, and most cases contain many of the patterns: microcystic/reticular, macrocytic, solid, alveolar, endodermal sinus (Schiller-Duval bodies), papillary, myxomatous, polyvesicular/vitelline, hepatoid, and enteric (Fig. 15.7). They are cytokeratin and AFP focally positive.

Choriocarcinoma. This tumor is very rare in childhood even as a component of mixed malignant germ cell tumor. Choriocarcinoma is positive for cytokeratin, inhibin, and hCG.

Teratoma. Teratoma occurs in infancy and is composed of tissues recapitulating all three germ layers. It is well-demarcated. Malignant areas may be present including focal PNET. It has a benign behavior in infancy.

Mixed Germ Cell Tumor. Normal immature fetal germ cells express PLAP and CD117. Infantile/congenital testicular tumors are most likely juvenile granulosa cell tumors rather than germ cell tumors.

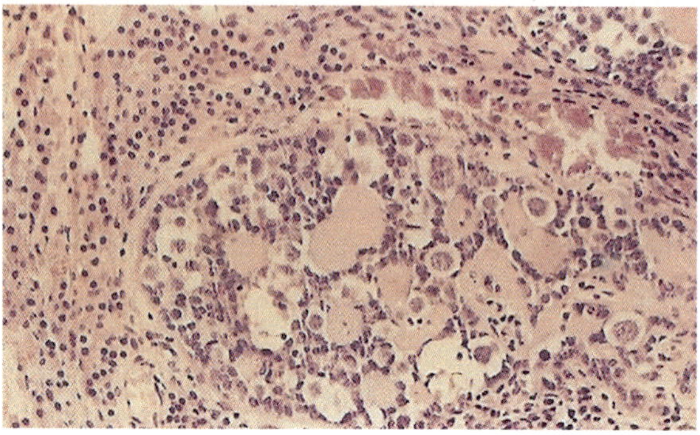

Fig. 15.7 Organoid structures in a yolk sac tumor (From Gilbert-Barness [56])

15.10.16 Testicular Sex-Cord Stromal Tumors

Leydig Cell Tumors. This comprises less than 5 % of pediatric testicular tumors. Leydig cell tumors occur in children between ages 3 and 9 years, presenting as a painless unilateral testicular enlargement. Endocrine features may be present, including gynecomastia and precocious puberty. The tumor is a well-circumscribed, yellow-brown nodule. Histopathologically, it is composed of diffuse sheets of large polygonal cells with eosinophilic cytoplasm; Reinke crystals are present in less than 40 %. The cells have regular nuclei with prominent nucleoli. Malignant behavior occurs in 10 % of tumors, particularly tumors greater than 5 cm in diameter and those containing cytological atypia, mitoses, necrosis and vascular invasion. The cells are vimentin and inhibin positive [57].

Sertoli Cell Tumors. Sertoli cell tumors are very rare in childhood. The histopathological appearance is sheets of bland ovoid cells with tubular formations. Malignancy is associated with pleomorphism, mitoses, and invasion. It is vimentin positive and variably inhibin positive.

Large Cell Calcifying Sertoli Cell Tumor. Large cell calcifying Sertoli cell tumor is a variant occurring in childhood. The average age at diagnosis is 16 years. It may be sporadic and is associated with Carney and Peutz-Jeghers syndromes. Twenty percent are malignant and 40 % are bilateral. It is composed of nests/cords of polygonal cells with eosinophilic cytoplasm with myxoid/hyaline stroma. Foci of calcification may be present.

Juvenile Granulosa Cell Tumor. Juvenile granulose cell tumors are the most frequent congenital testicular neoplasm. It presents as a testicular mass. Twenty percent are associated with ambiguous genitalia. It is composed of a cystic and solid mass with focal areas of hemorrhage. Cysts with inner granulosa-like cells and outer theca-like cells are present. There are intervening solid areas with plump ovoid-spindle cells. The tumor cells are vimentin, cytokeratin, and S100 negative. Inhibin is positive.

Gonadoblastoma. Usually, gonadoblastoma occurs in gonadal dysgenesis patients who have a Y chromosome present. This tumor has been rarely reported in otherwise normal males. It is composed of Sertoli-like cells surrounding seminoma-like germ cells. Hyaline nodules and basement membrane-like material may be calcified.

Testicular Involvement. The testes may be involved in hematopoietic neoplasms, especially acute lymphoblastic leukemia.

15.10.17 Juvenile Laryngeal Papillomatosis

This is a human papilloma virus (HPV)-related lesion, especially types 6 and 11. HPV types 11 and 16 are associated with a more aggressive course. Presenting usually during the first 5 years of life, it affects around 1 % of children born to mothers with vaginal condyloma. Clinically, there are multiple laryngeal papillomatous lesions. Extralaryngeal spread also occurs in 30 % of patients, and bronchial/pulmonary involvement occurs in 5 %. There is rare esophageal involvement. The mortality rate is 5–15 %. Complications include infection, asphyxia, secondary pulmonary complications, and malignant transformation to squamous cell carcinoma (rare). HPV-11 is especially associated with more severe disease, including tracheal involvement and pulmonary disease. Papillomatous lesions are covered by non-keratinizing squamous epithelium. There may be koilocytosis and dyskeratosis. Usually pleomorphism is absent.

15.10.18 Thyroid Carcinoma

Children with thyroid carcinoma tend to present with more advanced disease than adults, with lymph node and lung metastases. They have higher recurrence rates but better overall survival.

Papillary Carcinoma of Thyroid. This tumor presents as a single thyroid nodule/mass lesion. The mass is usually solid and unencapsulated, and it may appear multifocal. Lymphatic spread may occur but metastases rarely occur outside the lymph node. There is follicular architecture of cells with characteristic overlapping nuclei that are enlarged, oval, optically clear or ground glass, and have nuclear grooves. There are variable areas of papillary architecture with central vascular stromal cores; some nuclear features are present. Psammoma bodies with concentric lamination and calcification are present. There are several variants of papillary thyroid carcinoma: follicular, macrofollicular, oncocytic, clear cell, diffuse sclerosing, tall cell, columnar, solid, and microcarcinoma (less than 1 cm). Immunohistochemical staining shows CK19, cytokeratin, and TTF-1 positivity, whereas thyroglobulin and chromogranin are negative [57]. Five-year survival is greater than 95 %.

Follicular Carcinoma of Thyroid. This is mainly found in adults and is rare in children. It is a thyroid mass lesion. The tumor is usually solid and encapsulated or infiltrating with vascular and lymphatic spread. There is a follicular architecture without the characteristic grooved nuclei of papillary carcinoma. Variants include minimally invasive, widely invasive, oncocytic, and clear cell. The immunohistochemical staining pattern is: cytokeratin, thyroglobulin, TTF-1, CK19, bcl2, beta-catenin positive, and chromogranin negative.

Medullary Thyroid Carcinoma. Children are affected when associated with multiple endocrine neoplasia types 2A (MEN2A), 2B (MEN2B), and familiar medullary thyroid carcinoma syndromes. It may even present in infancy in these syndromes. RET germline mutations are present. These patients may have other MEN2 features and have distant metastases. Calcitonin levels are high, and they may present with other unusual endocrine paraneoplastic features. Immunohistochemical staining includes positive CEA, with strong expression associated with a worse prognosis. Calcitonin, chromogranin, synaptophysin, and TTF1 stains are positive, and there are variably S100 positive sustentacular cells present peripherally.

Thyroid C-cell Hyperplasia. Thyroid C-cell hyperplasia is a precursor of medullary carcinoma of thyroid. It is calcitonin and chromogranin positive. This may be a difficult diagnosis, and some cases may represent microinvasive medullary carcinoma.

15.10.19 Adrenal Cortical Carcinoma

Clinical features include mass effect and excess hormone production, including androgen-virilization, glucocorticoid-related Cushing syndrome, and mineralocorticoid effect, resulting in hypertension. There are sheets and trabeculae of cells morphologically resembling normal adrenal cortex. Clear and eosinophilic cytoplasm exists with variable nuclear atypia and a high mitotic rate. The main features suggesting malignant behavior are diameter greater than 5 cm, fibrous bands, necrosis, capsular invasion, muscular invasion, and a high mitotic rate. Adrenal cortical carcinoma is alpha-inhibin positive and chromogranin negative. The tumor may be only weakly positive for cytokeratin, and EMA and CEA negative. It may be related to a germline point mutation of p53 even without a positive family history, acting in a tissue-specific manner. It may be associated with Li-Fraumeni or BWS. Overall, children have a better prognosis than adults.

15.10.20 Pheochromocytoma

This is a tumor of chromaffin cells from the adrenal medulla. Ninety percent are benign and 10 % are malignant. Ten percent are associated with neurofibromatosis type 1 (NF1), MEN2, VHL, and/or familial cases. Many abnormalities are reported, including RET defect, but currently this is non-diagnostic. Clinical features include catecholamine secretion effect, especially episodic hypertension. This tumor is solid with areas of hemorrhage/necrosis. The tumor has a nested architecture (zellballen) with surrounding sustentacular cells. The neoplastic cells show granular cytoplasm and variable nuclear pleomorphism. Scattered melanin containing cells and ganglion cells may be present. Features of malignancy are metastatic disease, capsular invasion, vascular invasion, local extension into periadrenal tissue, necrosis, increased cellularity, pleomorphism, spindle cell phenotype, atypical and increased mitoses, loss of S100 positive sustentacular cells, and an increased proliferation index (MIB-1). Chromogranin is positive, and EMA is negative.

15.10.21 Other Predisposing Conditions Associated with Pheochromocytoma and Other Endocrine Tumors

15.10.21.1 Multiple Endocrine Neoplasia Type 2

Autosomal dominant activating germline mutations of the RET gene at 10q11.2 cause this syndrome. Specific codon mutations within RET correlate with disease phenotype and severity [65]. MEN2 pheochromocytomas may be preceded by diffuse medullary adrenal hyperplasia. Nodules are less than 1 cm in diameter and are more commonly bilateral and multiple. Less than 5 % of MEN2 pheochromocytomas are malignant. Parathyroid hyperplasia occurs when all glands become enlarged and hypercellular with mainly cytologically bland chief cells, histologically identical to sporadic cases. MEN2 is rarely associated with Hirschsprung disease. In view of the risk of medullary carcinoma, prophylactic thyroidectomy is performed in children less than 6 years of age in MEN2a and less than 2 years of age in MEN2b. Screening for pheochromocytoma should start at the age of 6 years.

15.10.21.2 Multiple Endocrine Neoplasia Type 1

This is an autosomal dominant inherited disorder due to mutation of the MEN1 gene, which codes for a protein called menin. Presentation occurs in late adolescence to adulthood, and 50 % have hyperparathyroidism by 20 years of age. Neuroendocrine tumors develop in parathyroid, pancreas, pituitary, adrenal, and other locations. Gastrinoma/Zollinger-Ellison syndrome occurs in about 50 % of cases.

15.10.22 Breast Carcinoma

Breast carcinoma is rare in children and may affect both females and males. The secretory subtype is most common, and it may be solid and tubular. The ovoid neoplastic cells have pale eosinophilic granular cytoplasm and intracytoplasmic lumina. Secretory breast carcinoma is associated with a balanced translocation, t(12;15), creating a ETV6-NTRK3 gene fusion [57]. This same translocation is also seen in congenital fibrosarcoma and congenital cellular mesoblastic nephroma [66]. Prognosis is good in children.

15.10.23 *Juvenile Papillomatosis*

This is a mass lesion in the breast that usually occurs in young adults but is also reported in children and rarely in infant boys [57]. There is an increased risk of familial breast cancer. The unencapsulated macrocystic lesion with fibrous stroma consists of multiple cysts, dilated ducts with apocrine metaplasia, duct ectasia, sclerosing adenosis-like changes, epithelial hyperplasia, and microcalcifications.

15.10.24 *Phyllodes Tumor*

This is a biphasic lesion similar to fibroadenoma that occurs only rarely in children. Most are benign, but local recurrence and metastases have been reported. There is a 2 % mortality, and 10–20 % have local recurrence [67]. Microscopically, epithelial structures are surrounded by stromal overgrowth. The stroma is more cellular than in fibroadenoma. Frankly malignant mesenchymal change may occur. The epithelium forms broad leaf-like areas with epithelial hyperplasia/metaplasia. Malignant behavior is based on the degree of hypercellularity, pleomorphism, mitotic count, and stromal overgrowth. Local relapse is associated with positive margins and fibroproliferation in surrounding tissue and necrosis [68].

15.10.25 *Osteosarcoma*

Osteosarcoma is a malignant mesenchymal tumor producing osteoid. All ages are affected, with a peak incidence between ages 10 and 20 years. Males are more often affected than females. Osteosarcoma usually presents in the metaphysis of the long bones, and pathological fractures occur in 5–10 %. Aggressive behavior results in metastases especially to the lungs and bones. There is a 60–80 % survival rate. Response to preoperative chemotherapy is the best predictor of outcome. After chemotherapy, necrosis greater than 90 % indicates a 80–90 % survival rate. A minority of patients have predisposing syndromes, mainly in older patients, including retinoblastoma syndrome, Li-Fraumeni syndrome, Paget disease of the bone, fibrous dysplasia (McCune-Albright syndrome), and previous radiotherapy. Children with a high dose of radiotherapy are at the highest risk for osteosarcoma to develop in adulthood.

Subtypes of osteosarcoma include osteoblastic, fibroblastic, and chondroblastic types. CD99 staining is positive, diffuse, and cytoplasmic. Osteopontin/osteonectin staining is positive. It may be focally CK positive or SMA positive. Response to chemotherapy is of vital importance. The operative specimen must have formal mapping in order to estimate the response to chemotherapy.

15.10.25.1 Telangiectatic Osteosarcoma

Pathological fractures occur more commonly than in the classical type. A destructive, lytic lesion usually involves a long bone. Cystic blood-filled spaces are separated by thin septa, which contain the malignant osteoid-producing cells [57].

15.10.25.2 Low-Grade Central Osteosarcoma

This is a well-differentiated intramedullary tumor. The long bones are preferentially affected, especially the femur. The tumor has a firm, solid, gray-white, fibroblastic stroma with focal osteoid production. The stroma contains malignant cells that are less pleomorphic, and it appears less cellular. There are bony spicules with intervening spindle cell stroma.

15.10.25.3 Parosteal Osteosarcoma

This tumor is usually seen in young adults. It affects females more than males. It is low-grade with good survival. Long bones are affected, especially the femur. It arises on the bone surface with well-formed trabeculae.

15.10.26 Malignant Skin Tumors in Childhood

15.10.26.1 Basal Cell Carcinoma

Basal cell carcinoma (BCC) is extremely rare in children. It occurs in association with xeroderma pigmentosum, nevus sebaceous, multiple nevoid BCC (Gorlin syndrome), and other predisposing genodermatoses, as well as in previous radiotherapy fields. The histopathological features consist of asymmetric aggregates of basaloid cells with peripheral palisading. Some aggregates of cells are separated from the stroma by retraction clefts. The stroma may be edematous and contain mucin. Every pattern of BCC may be found in children.

15.10.26.2 Squamous Cell Carcinoma

This is rare in children and occurs in association with xeroderma pigmentosum, pre-existing dermatoses, dystrophic epidermolysis bullosa, old burn scars, dyskeratosis, congenital (Fanconi) anemia, congenital immune defects, and immunosuppressive treatment. The most common sites are the face, hands, and forearms. Squamous cell carcinoma presents as a superficial erythematous nodule with ulceration covered by crusts. Histopathological features consist of irregular nests of epidermal cells that proliferate downwards and invade the dermis. There is dyskeratosis and keratin pearls with varying degrees of differentiation. Prognosis depends on the extent of invasion and the degree of differentiation.

15.10.26.3 Dermatofibrosarcoma Protuberans

This is an infiltrative fibrohistiocytic tumor that is locally aggressive. There is a t(17;22) translocation of the COL1A1 and PDGF receptor genes. Dermatofibrosarcoma protuberans is closely related to giant cell fibroblastoma. Spindled-shaped fibrohistiocytic cells are arranged in short interweaving fascicles. Mitoses are rare. Immunostaining for CD34 is positive, and some cells are positive for Factor XIIIa. CD34 is only focally positive in a minority of dermatofibrosarcoma protuberans cases.

15.10.27 Pediatric Pulmonary Tumors

15.10.27.1 Inflammatory Myofibroblastic Tumor

This tumor comprises 80 % of benign lung tumors in children. It is most common in the second decade but can occur in the first year of life. Cough, fever, hemoptysis, and chest pain are the usual symptoms. The recurrence rate is approximately 14 %. It is usually a solitary lesion in the lung periphery that is firm and white on cut surface and may be gritty. The lesion contains two main components: a proliferation of spindle cells in fascicles and a variable admixed lymphoplasmacytic infiltrate. Central scarring is common. There may also be multinucleated giant cells, granulomas, ossification, calcification, and vascular invasion. Spindle cells express vimentin and smooth muscle actin. ALK-1 is positive in 40 % of cases. Those with extension beyond the lung may recur in approximately 50 % of cases.

15.10.27.2 Pleuropulmonary Blastoma

This is a malignant tumor of early childhood. It is associated with trisomy 8 in some cases, but this is nonspecific. It may be multifocal and may be associated with neoplasia in other family members. Particularly common is the association with cystic nephroma. It presents with chest pain, cough, fever, respiratory distress, and pneumothorax. It is classified into types I, II and III based on the macroscopic and microscopic features [57].

Type I. This is the least common. It occurs in children under 2 years of age with median age of 9 months. The muscle cells stain with vimentin, desmin and myogenin.

Type II. This accounts for about 45 % of cases. It occurs in slightly older children than type I, with median age of 31 months. It is cystic either grossly or microscopically with solid areas. Solid areas are composed of malignant connective tissue elements, rhabdomyosarcoma, blastema, and/or spindle cell sarcoma. The cystic lining is benign.

Type III. This type is present in 40 % of cases, in a slightly older group than type II, with median age of 42 months. It is a solid tumor with no cysts. It is large and attached to the pleura and invades the lung. It may obliterate a lobe or an entire lung, and it is hemorrhagic and friable. The histological appearance is similar to the solid areas of type II. It may contain immature or frankly malignant cartilage, and it may metastasize to the brain, bone, liver or other sites.

15.10.27.3 Primary Pulmonary Carcinoid

This lesion is second in frequency to pleuropulmonary blastoma as a primary malignant lung tumor of childhood. WHO classifies carcinoids into typical and atypical based on mitotic count and presence of necrosis [57]. It is intrabronchial or peripheral.

15.10.27.4 Mucoepidermoid Tumor

Symptoms are related to bronchial obstruction, such as recurrent pneumonia, pyrexia, hemoptysis, or cough. It is centrally located in the proximal bronchial tree. Less than 5 % metastasize to local nodes, and it generally follows an indolent course. Mucoepidermoid tumors are usually an endobronchial tumor with a yellow color with extension through the bronchial wall. Low-grade tumors predominate in children and have solid and cystic areas; solid areas consist mainly of epithelium [57]. Necrosis is uncommon, and there are infrequent mitotic figures. Non-keratinizing squamous epithelium may be present. The stroma may show edema, fibrosis, hyalinization, and calcification.

15.10.27.5 Teratoma

In the lung, teratomas are most common in the left upper lobe. Symptoms include chest pain, hemoptysis, and cough. Chest x-rays show cysts with calcification. Teratomas are cystic and contain all three germinal layers. Large bronchi may be involved [57]. Most are mature and benign.

15.10.27.6 Cardiac Teratoma

Nearly two-thirds of cases present in infants, usually within the pericardial cavity and attached to the heart near the great arteries. The tumor may be intramural. The presentation may be cardiac failure, pericardial effusion, or cardiac tamponade. These tumors are rarely malignant.

15.10.27.7 Askin Tumor/Small Round Cell Tumor of the Thoracopulmonary Region

This is identical to a soft tissue PNET at other sites. Usually presenting in the second decade, it is more common in females with a ratio of 3:1. The tumor arises in the chest wall with variable involvement of the pleura and lung. Grossly, tumors up to 15 cm in diameter are round or multinodular and non-encapsulated. The cut surface is grayish-white with foci of necrosis and hemorrhage. Both the histological features and molecular characteristics are similar to PNET at other sites [57].

15.10.27.8 Bronchogenic Carcinoma

This is rare in children but has been reported. Histological appearances are similar to adult types.

15.10.27.9 Pulmonary Metastatic Disease

For some tumors such as adrenocortical carcinoma, alveolar soft part sarcoma, and osteosarcoma, surgical removal of the metastatic tumor is necessary for patient survival. In Wilms' tumor and EWS/PNET, which are radiation sensitive, the value of surgical removal of the metastatic tumor is not proven. In the case of neuroblastoma, differentiated thyroid cancer and rhabdomyosarcoma, secondary tumors in the lung are rarely removed. Histopathological features are identical to the primary site. They may show superimposed post-chemotherapy changes.

15.10.28 Familial Adenomatous Polyposis

FAP includes greater than 100 polyps throughout the colon. There is an increased risk of hepatoblastoma and endocrine tumors. Adenomas usually develop in teens, but FAP may also present in childhood with desmoid/Gardner fibromatoses or congenital hypertrophy of retinal pigment epithelium. Colorectal carcinoma develops at an average age of 40 years and rarely in childhood. Prophylactic colectomy should be performed. Other soft tissue lesions may occur, including juvenile nasopharyngeal angiofibroma and rhabdomyosarcoma. In the stomach, cystic polyps occur in one-fourth to three-fourths of cases. Histologically there is a mixture of normal mucosa and cystic glands lined by mucus-secreting epithelium, parietal cells, and chief cells. These lesions in the stomach are generally regarded as hamartomas with a very low risk of malignancy. However, gastric adenomas do occur in about 10 % of cases of FAP, but malignant transformation is uncommon. Duodenal adenomas are much more common, and these can develop into the usual adult type carcinoma.

15.10.29 Burkitt's Lymphoma

This is one of the most common malignant tumors of the intestine in children. It is either endemic and associated with EBV infection or sporadic and not associated with EBV. Symptoms are associated with bowel obstruction, perforation, or intussusception. Burkitt's lymphoma is very sensitive to chemotherapy. Grossly, there is an ulcerating mass in the ileocecal area with infiltration of the bowel wall. There are sheets of monotonous lymphoid cells microscopically with a starry-sky pattern. The mitotic count is high, and greater than 95 % of cells are positive with Ki67 staining (proliferation index). Antigens expressed include CD19, CD20, CD22, and CD79a. Many cells express CD10 [57]. The tumor cells dissect among the smooth muscle cells of the muscularis propria without destroying them.

15.10.30 Mesenchymal Gastrointestinal Tumors

These are infiltrating lesions composed of bland spindle cells with no significant atypia. Leiomyomas are desmin and caldesman positive, although CD34 and CD117 are negative.

15.10.31 Gastrointestinal Stromal Tumors

Gastrointestinal stromal tumors (GIST) consist of spindle and epithelioid cells and are associated with KIT gene mutations and PDGF receptor-alpha activating mutations. They are treated with imatinib. Different mutations/mechanisms of tyrosine kinase activation occur in childhood cases; they may have no detectable common mutations. CD117 stains are positive with strong diffuse membranous and cytoplasmic staining. CD34 stains are positive in greater than 70 % of cases. Desmin is negative, with one-third of cases focally positive for smooth muscle actin. Familial cases have been reported. The carney triad is composed of gastric GIST, pulmonary chondroma, and extra-adrenal paraganglioma with increased risk of association with NF1.

Gastrointestinal autonomic nerve tumors (GANT) are morphologically spindle and epithelioid tumors which present similar to GIST and are now known to be a GIST variant.

15.10.32 Pancreatoblastoma

This is the most common malignant pediatric pancreatic tumor but is rare nonetheless. The patient is usually less than 10 years of age with a median age of 2–4 years. One-third of pancreatoblastomas occur in adults. Congenital cases have been reported [69]. Most cases are sporadic, and some are associated with BWS, especially congenital cases. Pancreatoblastoma may present as an extracolonic manifestation of FAP. There is an increased risk in Asians. Allelic loss on chromosome 11p occurs in 90 %. Molecular alterations in the APC/beta-catenin pathway occur in 70 % of patients [57]. Clinical features include a non-specific abdominal mass and a solitary solid pancreatic lesion in the head or tail of the pancreas. Metastases have occurred by presentation in 20–35 % of cases, with one-third of patients having increased alphafetoprotein levels. The prognosis is good if localized but poor if metastases are present. Histological features include a solid or cystic mass that is well circumscribed with hemorrhage and necrosis. It has a nested and organoid pattern with epithelial islands separated by fibrous bands. Epithelial components are nests of polygonal cells with bland nuclei and granular cytoplasm plus squamoid nests of variable size. Areas with ductal differentiation are rare. The stroma consists of fibrous tissue that may be hypercellular with rare foci of metaplastic bone or cartilage. There may be primitive mesenchymal areas. Immunohistochemical staining shows a variable expression of trypsin, chymotrypsin, lipase, chromogranin, synaptophysin, CEA, and cytokeratin. Nuclear and cytoplasmic beta-catenin expression is present in 80 % of cases, especially in the squamoid areas [57].

15.10.33 Brain Tumors

Gangliocytomas are rare tumors that have been described in patients with neurofibromatosis and Peutz-Jeghers syndrome. Seventy percent of these tumors are in the temporal lobe. Gangliocytoma consists of dysplastic neurons with loss of cytological organization, including perimembranous Nissl substance, cytomegaly, abnormal clustering, abnormal localization, and multinucleation. There are intermixed reactive glial cells and perivascular reticulin deposition.

Ganglioglioma consists of dysplastic neurons and neoplastic glial cells, which resemble a diffuse or pilocytic astrocytoma; this tumor rarely contains a clear cell (oligodendroglial-like) component. Rosenthal fibers, eosinophilic granular bodies, and perivascular lymphocyte cuffing may be present. The stroma is often microcystic and myxoid but may be fibrillary and calcified. Necrosis is usually absent. Microvascular proliferation may be seen. The ganglion cells stain with a range of routine neuronal markers. Coarse synaptophysin and strong chromogranin staining are in contrast to the weak staining of most native neurons. The glial component stains with GFAP. The tumor and peritumoral parenchyma stains with CD34 in approximately 70 % of cases. Ki67 is positive but stains less than 3 % of cells.

15.10.33.1 Desmoplastic Infantile Astrocytoma and Ganglioglioma

These tumors usually occur in the first 1–2 years of life, but occasional cases may occur later. They are WHO grade I. Seizures or neurological deficit may occur.

It has a very good prognosis. Desmoplastic infantile ganglioglioma will contain dysplastic ganglion cells. The poorly differentiated neuroepithelial component contains small round cells. The desmoplastic component stains positive for vimentin and GFAP. The small cell component stains positive for GFAP and MAP2. Neuronal markers are negative. It may express desmin. Cytokeratin and EMA are negative. Ki67 may be increased, but there is poor correlation with the clinical outcome.

15.10.33.2 Dysembryoplastic Neuroepithelial Tumor

This tumor is classified as WHO grade I. The age at presentation is highly variable, but typically it occurs in teenagers and young adults. There is a relatively uniform population of small round cells. A metachromatic stroma with scattered ganglion cells with calcification may be seen. Oligodendrocyte-like cells are small round cells with finely granular chromatin and indistinct cytoplasm. Floating neurons are present in pools of mucinous material. Calcification and hemosiderin may be present. The mucinous material is positive for Alcian blue. Oligodendrocyte-like cells are typically GFAP negative and S100 positive. Floating neurons will stain with standard neuronal markers (for example, NeuN, neurofilament). CD34 may be positive and Ki67 proliferation index is low.

15.10.33.3 Central and Extraventricular Neurocytoma

Neurocytomas are WHO grade I. Most show no genetic predisposition. Clinical features include occurrence at any age, but these tumors are uncommon in childhood. Extraventricular neurocytomas have a similar morphology but can occur anywhere in the central nervous system (CNS). Raised intracranial pressure is the commonest clinical finding.

Central Neurocytoma. Histological features include uniform round nuclei with salt and pepper chromatin, and they are usually cytologically bland. There is patchy fibrillary stroma with neuropil islands. Other patterns may include oligodendroglioma-like pattern, rosettes resembling pineocytomatous rosettes, Homer-Wright rosettes, perivascular pseudorosettes, ganglion cell differentiation, and arborizing vessels resembling a neuroendocrine tumor. Calcification is present.

Atypical Neurocytoma. Atypical features include increased mitotic activity, microvascular proliferation, and necrosis. Histological atypia is poorly predictive of clinical behavior. Ki67 is greater than 2–3 %.

On immunohistochemical staining, synaptophysin is positive. In some cases, NeuN is positive. Usually GFAP is negative. Ki67 labeling indices usually are very low. Values greater than 2–3 % are associated with a worse prognosis. By electron microscopy the cellular processes are rich in microtubules, dense core and clear vesicles and synapses.

15.10.34 Primitive/Embryonal Tumors

15.10.34.1 Medulloblastoma

This is the commonest malignant brain tumor in children [70, 71]. It is defined as an embryonal tumor of the cerebellum. Medulloblastoma may be associated with Gorlin (basal cell nevus) syndrome and adenomatosis polyposis coli (Turcot syndrome). These can present at any age from birth until the fifth decade; the peak age of presentation is 7 years. Symptoms are due to raised intracranial pressure and cerebellar dysfunction. Three-fourths of cases arise in the midline of the cerebellum (vermis), with the remainder arising in the cerebellar hemispheres. Metastatic spread in the craniospinal axis may occur. Histological features include a dense cellular tumor with either a diffuse or nodular architecture. Typically, the small cells have dense hyperchromatic and rounded or wedge-shaped (carrot-shaped) nuclei. Mitotic activity is usually present, but it is not unusual for mitotic figures to be very difficult to identify; apoptoses and coagulative necrosis are frequent. Homer-Wright rosettes show a circular arrangement of tumor cells surrounding a small acellular region of neuropil, lacking a central lumen. Flexner-Wintersteiner rosettes occur occasionally.

Nodular (desmoplastic) Medulloblastoma. This tumor has a biphasic nodular pattern with intra-nodular areas consisting of lower cellularity and more differentiated tumor cells set in neuropil. Inter-nodular areas are densely cellular, consisting of reticulin-rich, poorly differentiated cells with little intervening neuropil. Tumors showing a greater extent of nodularity carry a better prognosis, particularly in infants. Anaplastic medulloblastoma shows cellular anaplasia.

Melanotic Medulloblastma. This tumor is very rare and is characterized by the presence of melanotic differentiation in an otherwise unremarkable medulloblastoma. Reticulin stains highlight nodularity and desmoplasia in nodular medulloblastoma. The immunohistochemical stain INI-1 is positive distinguishing it from atypical teratoid/rhabdoid tumor. Synaptophysin positivity is usually present but is occasionally weak and patchy. GFAP is mostly negative or only positive in trapped reactive cells. True glial differentiation may be seen, particularly in nodular medulloblastomas. The Ki67 (proliferation index) is usually high (greater than 20 %). In older age groups, staining for lymphocyte markers and cytokeratin may be helpful in the exclusion of lymphoma and metastatic small cell carcinoma respectively. Nuclear staining for β-catenin is a good prognostic factor. Staging of medulloblastoma is of great prognostic value and depends predominantly on the surgical and radiological findings.

On molecular investigation, a number of chromosomal abnormalities may occur. In particular, C-myc and N-myc amplification are associated with a poor prognosis.

15.10.34.2 Supratentorial PNET/CNS-PNET

CNS-PNET should be distinguished from the unrelated EWS/PNET. The mean age of presentation is 5 years. The most common site is the cerebral hemispheres; in rare cases, it occurs in the spinal cord. Prognosis is generally poor.

Variable features include Homer-Wright rosettes, streams and palisading cells; calcification is relatively common along with microvascular proliferation and fibrous septae. Immunohistochemical staining is typically positive for neuronal markers including synaptophysin. Glial differentiation is common. GFAP staining is frequently seen. Ki67 labeling indices are generally high, and INI-1 staining is positive. Evidence of muscular and melanocytic differentiation may be seen. On electron microscopy, the tumor is very poorly differentiated. Presence of dense core vesicles should be regarded as diagnostic of cerebral neuroblastoma.

15.10.35 Atypical Teratoid/Rhabdoid Tumor

This is a malignant tumor of the CNS associated with mutations in the INI-1/hSNF5 gene. It may be sporadic or associated with the rhabdoid tumor syndrome. Germline mutations occur in the INI-1 gene on chromosome 22q11.2. For the majority of cases, occurrence is in children less than 6 years old, with most are under age 3. It is slightly more common above the tentorium, but no site is exempt. The prognosis is poor and most die within 2 years.

Typical rhabdoid cells show eccentric nuclei, vesicular chromatin, prominent nucleoli, and cytoplasmic eosinophilic globules. Evidence of mesenchymal and epithelial differentiation may be seen, and they may show papillary structures or resemble poorly differentiated carcinoma. Other non-specific features of a malignant tumor are frequent with high mitotic rate, necrosis, and hemorrhage. Immunohistochemical staining reveals the diagnostic feature of loss of the nuclear expression of INI-1. Lack of expression is also described in choroid plexus carcinoma and supratentorial PNET. INI-1 negative tumors in the brain are associated with a poor prognosis. Other immunostaining is highly variable, including EMA, vimentin, SMA, GFAP, neurofilament, and cytokeratin. Paranuclear staining for vimentin or other intermediate filaments is useful for the diagnosis. On electron microscopy, whorled intermediate filaments indent the nucleus in typical rhabdoid cells.

15.10.36 Medulloepithelioma

This tumor is WHO grade IV. Most occur before the age of 5 years, with 50 % of cases shown in children who are less than 2 years old. The most common cerebral site is periventricular, but these may also occur in peripheral nerve spinal cord and orbit. A large tumor and raised intracranial pressure are typical. Survival is usually less than 1 year. Histological features include pseudostratified epithelium resembling primitive neural tube. The architecture is papillary, trabecular, and tubular. The luminal surface may contain small blebs but should not be ciliated. The inner membrane sits along a primitive basement membrane. Mitotic figures are generally toward the luminal aspect in hyperchromatic anaplastic cells. On immunohistochemical staining, nestin and vimentin are positive in the neuroepithelial areas. Focal staining may also be seen with neurofilament, CK, and EMA in the neuroepithelial areas. Typically, neuroepithelial areas are GFAP and S100 negative. A Ki67 index is variable. On electron microscopy, prominent lateral cell junctions are present in the basal lamina on the outer surface of the neuroepithelium.

15.10.37 Ependymoblastoma

This tumor is WHO grade IV. Ependymoblastomas usually occur in young children and neonates. In addition, it is usually supratentorial, but it may occur at other sites. The prognosis is poor, and death usually occurs within 1 year of diagnosis. Histological features include ependymoblastic rosettes, comprised of multilayered neuroectodermal cells with a small central lumen. The tumor contains primitive neuroectodermal cells with a malignant cytology. On immunohistochemical staining, GFAP is positive; it is also usually positive with S100, vimentin, and cytokeratin. Neurofilament stains may be positive. On electron microscopy, rosette cells are joined by junctional complexes; abortive cilia and a few basal bodies may be seen near the lumen.

15.10.38 Pineocytoma

This is a low-grade intrinsic tumor of the pineal gland. It is WHO grade I with an excellent prognosis. Histological features include an architecture with moderate cellularity in sheets or ill-defined lobules. Pinecytomatous rosettes are relatively large compared with Homer Wright rosettes. Pineocytoma has low mitotic activity, and the Ki67 index is low. Silver stains (e.g., Bielschowsky) may demonstrate club-like protrusions at the end of cellular processes. A range of neuronal markers are positive but most consistent is synaptophysin. Retinal antigens (rhodopsin, retinal S antigen) may be positive. Neurofilaments may highlight the clubbed ends of the cell processes. Occasionally, glial differentiation is present, evidenced by GFAP positivity.

15.10.39 Pineoblastoma

This is a primitive malignant tumor of the pineal gland resembling a CNS-PNET. It is WHO grade IV. When pineoblastoma occurs in familial retinoblastoma

Table 15.5 Histologic types of meningioma WHO grade I

Meningothelial Meningioma	Meningothelial meningioma has lobules and nests of cells that are separated by thin strands of collagen. Uniform arachnoid cells and rare psammoma bodies or whorls are seen
Fibrous (Fibroblastic) Meningioma	This is a spindle cell tumor with rich collagenous matrix
Psammomatous Meningioma	This type typically occurs in middle-aged women, frequently in the thoracic cord. Psammoma bodies are the predominant feature, and they may contain confluent calcification
Angiomatous Meningioma	Vessels predominate over tumor cells
Secretory Meningioma	These have characteristic pseudo-psammoma bodies with focal epithelial differentiation forming intracellular lumina contain eosinophilic inclusions, which are PAS and CEA positive. Serum CEA may even be raised. Mast cells may be prominent in this variant
Lymphoplasmacytic-Rich Meningioma	This type is characterized by chronic inflammation that obscures the tumor. There is an occasional association with hematological disorders, including iron refractory anemia and hypergammaglobulinemia
Metaplastic Meningioma	This is characterized by prominent focal or diffuse mesenchymal differentiation with cartilage, bone, lipid, or skeletal muscle formation

(trilateral retinoblastoma), it carries a worse prognosis. Diffuse rosettes including Homer Wright and Flexner-Wintersteiner are present. Ironically, they do not have pineocytomatous rosettes.

15.10.40 Meningioma

Meningiomas that are WHO grade I include most morphological variants. WHO grade II types have defined cytological features (atypical meningioma) or are of a specific subtype, including chordoid and clear cell meningioma. WHO grade III meningioma has cytological features of malignancy and include rhabdoid and papillary subtypes. There is an increased frequency of neurofibromatosis type 2. The rare malignant cases may have metastasis. General histological features include a whorled architecture and pseudo-syncytial sheets. Arachnoidal cells are oval with relatively uniform nuclei, small indistinct nucleoli, and nuclear pseudo-inclusions. Histologic types of meningioma WHO grade I are shown in Table 15.5; types of meningioma grade II are shown in Table 15.6.

Meningioma staging for brain invasion is defined by breach of the pia mater and presence of individual tumor cells invading into the brain parenchyma. It must be distinguished from prominent extensions of tumor that may extend into the brain. Brain invasion is associated with an increased risk of recurrence. It may be easier to assess by GFAP immunostaining.

Table 15.6 Types of meningioma grade II

Chordoid Meningioma	**Chordoid Meningioma** is a tumor that resembles a chordoma. These are associated rarely with Castleman disease
Clear Cell Meningioma	**Clear Cell Meningioma** is a rare tumor, which occurs relatively more frequently in children and young adults. The cerebellopontine angle and the cauda equina are the most common sites. The clear cells are due to glycogen accumulation. Collagen deposition is often very prominent
Atypical Meningioma	**Atypical Meningioma** is any meningioma with either 4–20 mitotic figures per 10 high-power fields, a patternless sheet-like growth, high nuclear-cytoplasmic ratio, prominent nucleoli, or foci of spontaneous/geographic necrosis
Papillary Meningioma	**Papillary Meningioma** is rare and relatively more frequent in children. It has a pseudo-papillary pattern and a poor prognosis
Rhabdoid Meningioma	**Rhabdoid Meningioma** contains rhabdoid cells, which have eccentric nuclei, prominent nucleoli, and eosinophilic cytoplasmic inclusions. It has a high mitotic count and may be papillary. This variant carries a poor prognosis. It is not associated with INI-1 loss, unlike atypical teratoid rhabdoid tumor
Anaplastic (Malignant) Meningioma	**Anaplastic (Malignant) Meningioma** is any meningioma with severe anaplasia and is akin to poorly differentiated carcinoma or sarcoma. The mitotic count is greater than or equal to 20 per 10 high power fields. Anaplastic meningioma has a poor prognosis

15.10.41 Retinoblastoma

Retinoblastoma is the most common primary intraocular neoplasm of children. Children usually present with leukocoria and/or strabismus. Of all retinoblastoma cases, approximately 60–70 % are unilateral and 30–40 % are bilateral. In unilateral cases, typically one single tumor is present in the affected eye. In bilateral cases, multifocal tumors in both eyes are usual. The median age at presentation is approximately 12 months in children who have bilateral retinoblastoma and 24 months in those with unilateral disease. The tumor has a strong tendency to invade the optic nerve and brain and to metastasize widely. The growth pattern in retinoblastoma is endophytic, exophytic, or diffusely infiltrating. Endophytic growth is growth predominantly toward the vitreous. Exophytic growth is growth toward the subretinal space and leads to retinal detachment. The diffuse infiltrating variety exhibits a spread of the tumor diffusely throughout the retina with infiltration of adjacent structures. Spontaneously arrested retinoblastoma may be seen in unaffected family members. Most commonly it is asymptomatic and is seen clinically as a translucent retinal mass with calcification.

Second non-ocular cancers are common in patients with germline mutations. The incidence of second cancers is approximately 1 % per year of life. The most common second cancers are osteogenic sarcomas of the skull and long bones, other sarcomas, cutaneous melanomas, Hodgkin lymphomas, and breast carcinomas.

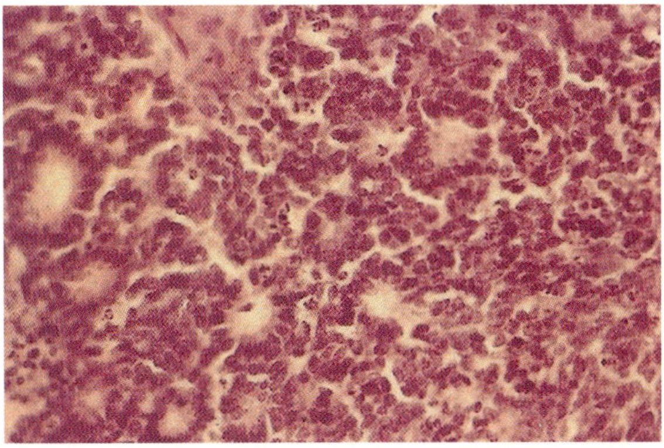

Fig. 15.8 Flexner-Wintersteiner rosettes of retinoblastoma with nearly empty central lumens (From Gilbert-Barness [56])

Trilateral retinoblastoma (pinealoblastoma) is a primitive neuroectodermal neoplasm occurring in the pineal region. Histologically, the tumor is composed of small, round, undifferentiated retinoblastoma cells with hyperchromatic nuclei and scant cytoplasm. Necrosis and calcification are often present. Several types of cellular patterns are seen. Flexner-Wintersteiner rosettes are specific for retinoblastoma but are not always seen (Fig. 15.8) Homer-Wright rosettes are indistinguishable from those found in neuroblastomas. Pseudorosettes are seen as viable tumor cells that cluster around blood vessels. Fleurettes are flower-like groupings of tumor cells that clearly show a differentiation into photoreceptor elements. Extensive necrosis is often present with calcification.

Retinoblastoma has been shown to result from loss or inactivation of both alleles present at the time of fertilization, but spontaneous mutations occur in which both the alleles become deleted or inactive in at least one immature retinal cell. Overall, only 6–7 % of newly diagnosed retinoblastoma patients have a family history of the disease; the vast majority of retinoblastoma cases are sporadic.

Retinoblastoma results from the effects of two independent mutations that cause a defective regulatory or suppressor gene at the chromosomal 13q14 locus. Tumors develop when both suppressor genes, one on each homologous chromosome, are inactivated. Hereditary retinoblastomas arise from a single mutagenic event (somatic mutation) in a cell that previously carried an inherited mutation (germinal mutation). Sporadic cases (non-heritable) require two somatic (postzygotic) mutations.

Retinoblastoma is inherited as an autosomal recessive disease at the cellular level, but clinically it behaves as if it has an autosomal dominant pattern of inheritance with almost complete penetrance.

15.11 Tumor-Associated Syndromes

Tumor-associated syndromes are listed in Tables 15.7 and 15.8.

Table 15.7 Some syndromes and congenital malformations associated with childhood tumors

Malformation or syndrome	Neoplasm
Beckwith-Wiedemann syndrome hemihypertrophy	Wilms' tumor
	Adrenocortical adenoma
	Adrenocortical carcinoma
	Hepatoblastoma
	Pancreatoblastoma
Aniridia	Wilms' tumor
Genitourinary system anomalies and Perlman syndrome	Nephroblastomatosis
	Wilms' tumor
Hirschsprung disease	Neuroblastoma
Poland syndrome	Leukemia
Drash syndrome	Wilms' tumor
Tuberous sclerosis	Cardiac rhabdomyoma
	Angiomyolipoma
	Astrocytoma
Multiple endocrine neoplasia (MEN2)	Thyroid medullary carcinoma
	Pheochromocytoma
	Submucosal neuromas
Nevoid basal cell carcinoma (Gorlin) syndrome	Basal cell carcinoma
	Medulloblastoma
	Ovarian fibroma
Wiskott-Aldrich syndrome	Lymphoma
Bloom syndrome	Leukemia

From: Isaacs [19]

Table 15.8 Some syndromes that Predispose to solid tumors

Syndromes	Chromosomal locus	Gene	Tumor
Neurofibromatosis type 1	17q11	*NF1*	Rhabdomyosarcoma
Beckwith-Wiedemann	11p15.5	Unknown	Wilms' tumor
			Hepatoblastoma
WAGR Denys-Drash	11p13	*WT1*	Wilms' tumor
Adenomatous polyposis coli	5q21	*APC*	Hepatoblastoma
Hereditary retinoblastoma	13q14	*RB1*	Retinoblastoma
			Osteosarcoma
Li-Fraumeni	17p13.1	*p53*	Osteosarcoma
	22q12.1		Rhabdomyosarcoma

From: Isaacs [72]

15.11.1 Beckwith-Wiedemann Syndrome

BWS and its related tumors are an excellent example of loss of imprinting. BWS is a clinically heterogeneous disorder of growth regulation manifesting as somatic overgrowth, congenital malformations, and tumor predisposition. The majority of cases are sporadic; however, a small number of pedigrees with autosomal dominant inheritance demonstrate linkage to 11p15.5 [73, 74]. Genomic imprinting in the phenotype was suggested by the preferential loss of maternal alleles in BWS and related tumors [75]. BWS is associated with abnormal transcription and regulation of genes associated with cell cycle and growth control in the imprinted domain on chromosome 11p15.5. The cluster of genes on chromosome 11p15.5 contains at least 12 imprinted genes. The chromosome 11p15.5 region has been divided into two distinct domains that are thought to be regulated by two imprinting centers separated by a non-imprinted region [76–81].

15.11.2 Central Nervous SystemTumor Syndromes

Although genetic factors account for only a minority of childhood CNS tumors, the incidences of particular types of CNS tumors are greatly increased in some tumor syndromes. All of these CNS tumor syndromes share autosomal dominant inheritance.

15.11.2.1 Neurofibromatosis Type 1

NF1 has an incidence of 1:4000. The responsible gene is located on chromosome 17q12 [82]. NF1 is frequently associated with optic pathway gliomas in children [83]. Histologically, the vast majority of these tumors are pilocytic astrocytomas, although diffuse astrocytoma and glioblastomas are also described.

15.11.2.2 Neurofibromatosis Type 2

Neurofibromatosis type 2 (NF2) is more commonly associated with adult CNS tumors than with pediatric CNS malignancies. The responsible gene is located on chromosome 22q12.2, encoding a product known as Merlin or schwannomin that functions as a tumor suppressor gene. Several types of mutations occur in the gene, leading to formation of a truncated product. A study by Evans et al. [84], showed that 18 % of patients with NF2 (61/334) presented in the pediatric (0–15 years) age group. Of these, 26 presented with vestibular schwannoma, 19 with meningioma, and 7 with spinal tumors.

15.11.2.3 Tuberous Sclerosis

Tuberous sclerosis is characterized by hamartomas and benign neoplastic lesions in the CNS and other organs. There is a locus heterogeneity in tuberous sclerosis with disease determining genes on chromosomes 9 and 16. The mutant genes occur in small regions of telomeric chromosome bands at 9q34.3, designated as TSC1 (encodes for protein hamartin) and at 16p13.3, designated as TSC2 (encodes for protein tuberin) [85, 86]. Hamartin complexes with tuberin to regulate the cell cycle. Tuberin participates in normal brain development and cardiomyocyte terminal differentiation [87]. The most common CNS neoplasm in tuberous sclerosis is the subependymal giant cell astrocytoma arising from the wall of the lateral ventricles. Other tumors associated with tuberous sclerosis include facial angiofibromas, cardiac rhabdomyoma, retinal nodular hamartomas, lymphangiomyomatosis, renal angiomyolipoma, and hamartomatous rectal polyps. The giant cell astrocytoma rarely becomes malignant (glioblastoma).

15.11.2.4 Von Hippel-Lindau Disease

This disease is caused by the mutation of the VHL gene. It is characterized by angiomatosis retinae and hemangioblastomas of the CNS and retina. Hemangioblastomas may also involve the face, adrenals, lungs, and liver. Other pathological lesions are renal cell carcinoma, pheochromocytoma, and visceral cysts [6].

15.11.2.5 Turcot Syndrome

This is a heterogenous group of disorders; both autosomal dominant and recessive inheritance have been described. This syndrome is characterized by the coexistence of colorectal neoplasms with either medulloblastoma (predominantly) or glioblastoma. Some cases are variants of FAP syndrome, whereas others are variants of the hereditary non-polyposis colorectal carcinoma syndrome [88]. At least two defined clinical groupings can be seen within Turcot syndrome. In the first, medulloblastoma is associated with FAP. In these cases, there is mutation in the APC gene on chromosome 5q21. The gene encodes a 300 kDa protein that is ubiquitously expressed and modifies the interaction between the beta-catenin protein and E-cadherin cell adhesion molecule. In the second clinical group, glioblastoma is seen in patients without FAP, some of whom have hereditary non-polyposis colorectal carcinoma and mutations in DNA mismatch repair genes.

15.11.2.6 Gorlin Syndrome (Nevoid Basal Cell Carcinoma Syndrome)

This syndrome is characterized by nevoid basal cell carcinomas and jaw keratocysts, palmar and plantar pits, skeletal abnormalities, ectopic calcifications, and ovarian fibromas. The characteristic associated CNS tumor is medulloblastoma and tends to be the desmoplastic variant [89, 90]. The affected gene is PTCH, which lies on chromosome 9q31.

15.11.2.7 Cowden Syndrome

This is a rare syndrome associated with hamartomatous and neoplastic lesions such as dysplastic gangliocytoma of the cerebellum (Lhermitte-Duclos disease), verrucous skin lesions, trichilemmomas, oral mucosa fibromas, hamartomatous colon polyps, thyroid neoplasms, and breast cancer. The affected gene is PTEN/MMAC1, located on chromosome 10q23. The gene product may be involved in cell growth and differentiation [91].

15.11.2.8 Li-Fraumeni Syndrome

Li-Fraumeni syndrome is characterized by the presence of bone or soft tissue sarcomas presenting before the age of 45 years, with presence of other cancers in first-degree relatives presenting before age 45 years. The pediatric brain tumors associated with Li-Fraumeni syndrome are medulloblastoma/PNET, choroid plexus tumor, and ependymoma. There are two genetic determinants of Li-Fraumeni syndrome. The first is a germline mutation of the p53 gene at chromosome 17P13.1. This gene plays a key role in cell cycle control and apoptosis. The second gene is CHEK2 (checkpoint kinase 2) on chromosome 22q. It has been shown that the gene product of CHEK2 directly phosphorylates p53, indicating its involvement in p53 regulation of DNA damage [92].

15.12 Conclusions

Neoplasms in the fetus and infant very frequently are of embryonal origin from cells that fail to mature and differentiate. Wilms tumors are derived from the metanephric blastema that has lost its propensity for differentiation. Neuroblastomas arise from the sympathetic nervous system in the neural crest and wander usually into the adrenal gland early in embryonic life. Other tumors occur predominantly in the first year of life and have certain features of embryonic growth and include embryonic sarcomas, yolk sac tumors of the testis, and heptaoblastomas. They are characterized by various chromosomal alternations. The growth, prognostic features, and clinical course have been addressed.

References

1. Bader JL, Miller RW (1979) US cancer incidence and mortality in the first year of life. Am J Dis Child 133:157–159
2. Bolande RP (1971) Benignity of neonatal tumors and concept of cancer repression in early life. Am J Dis Child 122:12–14
3. Bolande RP (1976) Neoplasia of early life and its relationships to teratogenesis. Perspect Pediatr Pathol 3:145–183

4. Crist W, Pullen J, Boyett J, Falletta J, van Eys J, Borowitz M, Jackson J, Dowell B, Frankel L, Quddus F et al (1986) Clinical and biologic features predict a poor prognosis in acute lymphoid leukemias in infants: a Pediatric Oncology Group Study. Blood 67:135–140
5. Young JL Jr, Ries LG, Silverberg E, Horm JW, Miller RW (1986) Cancer incidence, survival, and mortality for children younger than age 15 years. Cancer 58(2 Suppl):598–602
6. Gilbert-Barness E (ed) (2007) Potter's pathology of the fetus, infant and child, 2nd edn. Mosby-Elsevier, Philadelphia
7. Reaman G (1993) Special considerations for the infant with cancer, 2nd edn. Lippincott, Philadelphia
8. Reaman G, Zeltzer P, Bleyer WA, Amendola B, Level C, Sather H, Hammond D (1985) Acute lymphoblastic leukemia in infants less than one year of age: a cumulative experience of the Children's Cancer Study Group. J Clin Oncol 3:1513–1521
9. Willis RA (1962) The borderland of embryology and pathology. Butterworths, London
10. Fernbach DJ, Vietti TJ (1991) General aspects of childhood cancer, 3rd edn. Mosby, St. Louis
11. Isaacs HJ (1993) Tumors of the fetus and infant-an atlas. Springer, New York
12. Berry PJ (1993) Congenital tumors, 2nd edn. Springer, Berlin
13. Broadbent VA (1992) Malignant disease in the neonate, 2nd edn. Churchill Livingstone, Edinburgh
14. Gale GB, D'Angio GJ, Uri A, Chatten J, Koop CE (1982) Cancer in neonates: the experience at the children's hospital of Philadelphia. Pediatrics 70:409–413
15. Isaacs H Jr (1983) Neoplasms in infants: a report of 265 cases. Pathol Annu 18(Pt 2):165–214
16. Werb P, Scurry J, Ostor A, Fortune D, Attwood H (1992) Survey of congenital tumors in perinatal necropsies. Pathology 24:247–253
17. Mulvihill JJ (1993) Childhood cancer environment and hereditary, 2nd edn. JB Lippincott, Philadelphia
18. Isaacs H Jr (2007) Introduction to tumors. In: Gilbert-Barness E (ed) Potter's pathology of fetus, infant and child, 2nd edn. Elsevier, Philadelphia
19. Isaacs H Jr (1997) Tumors. In: Gilbert-Barness E (ed) Potter's pathology of fetus, infant and child. Mosby Year Book, Philadelphia
20. Lengauer C (2003) Cancer. An unstable liaison. Science 300:442–443
21. Kinzler KW, Vogelstein B (2001) Familial cancer syndromes the role of caretakers an gatekeepers, 8th edn. McGraw-Hill, New York
22. Feinberg AP (2004) The epigenetics of cancer etiology. Semin Cancer Biol 14:427–432
23. Falls JG, Pulford DJ, Wylie AA, Jirtle RL (1999) Genomic imprinting: implications for human disease. Am J Pathol 154:635–647
24. Hall JG (1990) Genomic imprinting: review and relevance to human diseases. Am J Hum Genet 46:857–873
25. Hark AT, Schoenherr CJ, Katz DJ, Ingram RS, Levorse JM, Tilghman SM (2000) CTCF mediates methylation-sensitive enhancer-blocking activity at the H19/Igf2 locus. Nature 405:486–489
26. Barlow DP (1994) Imprinting: a gamete's point of view. Trends Genet 1994(10):194–199
27. Villavicencio EH, Walterhouse DO, Iannaccone PM (2000) The sonic hedgehog-patched-gli pathway in human development and disease. Am J Hum Genet 67:1047–1054
28. Hooper JE, Scott MP (2005) Communicating with hedgehogs. Nat Rev Mol Cell Biol 6:306–317
29. Yuspa SH, Epstein EH Jr (2005) Cancer. An anchor for tumor cell invasion. Science 307:1727–1728
30. Meder D, Simons K (2005) Cell biology. Ras on the roundabout. Science 307:1731–1733
31. Fodde R, Smits R (2002) Cancer biology. A matter of dosage. Science 298:761–763
32. Wilkin F, Gagne N, Paquette J, Oligny LL, Deal C (2000) Pediatric adrenocortical tumors: molecular events leading to insulin-like growth factor II gene overexpression. J Clin Endocrinol Metab 85:2048–2056
33. Grier DG, Thompson A, Kwasniewska A, McGonigle GJ, Halliday HL, Lappin TR (2005) The pathophysiology of HOX genes and their role in cancer. J Pathol 205:154–171
34. Levine AJ (1997) p53, the cellular gatekeeper for growth and division. Cell 88:323–331

35. Guo W, Giancotti FG (2004) Integrin signaling during tumour progression. Nat Rev Mol Cell Biol 5:816–826
36. Knudson AG Jr (1986) Genetics of human cancer. Annu Rev Genet 20:231–251
37. Cooper WN, Luharia A, Evans GA, Raza H, Haire AC, Grundy R, Bowdin SC, Riccio A, Sebastio G, Bliek J et al (2005) Molecular subtypes and phenotypic expression of Beckwith-Wiedemann syndrome. Eur J Hum Genet 13:1025–1032
38. DeBaun MR, Niemitz EL, McNeil DE, Brandenburg SA, Lee MP, Feinberg AP (2002) Epigenetic alterations of H19 and LIT1 distinguish patients with Beckwith-Wiedemann syndrome with cancer and birth defects. Am J Hum Genet 70:604–611
39. McTaggart SJ, Algar E, Chow CW, Powell HR, Jones CL (2001) Clinical spectrum of Denys-Drash and Frasier syndrome. Pediatr Nephrol 16:335–339
40. Pelletier J, Bruening W, Kashtan CE, Mauer SM, Manivel JC, Striegel JE, Houghton DC, Junien C, Habib R, Fouser L et al (1991) Germline mutations in the Wilms' tumor suppressor gene are associated with abnormal urogenital development in Denys-Drash syndrome. Cell 67:437–447
41. Porteus MH, Narkool P, Neuberg D, Guthrie K, Breslow N, Green DM, Diller L (2000) Characteristics and outcome of children with Beckwith-Wiedemann syndrome and Wilms' tumor: a report from the National Wilms Tumor Study Group. J Clin Oncol 18:2026–2031
42. Call KM, Glaser T, Ito CY, Buckler AJ, Pelletier J, Haber DA, Rose EA, Kral A, Yeger H, Lewis WH et al (1990) Isolation and characterization of a zinc finger polypeptide gene at the human chromosome 11 Wilms' tumor locus. Cell 60:509–520
43. Haber DA, Englert C, Maheswaran S (1996) Functional properties of WT1. Med Pediatr Oncol 27:453–455
44. Gessler M, Poustka A, Cavenee W, Neve RL, Orkin SH, Bruns GA (1990) Homozygous deletion in Wilms tumours of a zinc-finger gene identified by chromosome jumping. Nature 343:774–778
45. Gashler AL, Bonthron DT, Madden SL, Rauscher FJ 3rd, Collins T, Sukhatme VP (1992) Human platelet-derived growth factor A chain is transcriptionally repressed by the Wilms tumor suppressor WT1. Proc Natl Acad Sci USA 89:10984–10988
46. Drummond IA, Madden SL, Rohwer-Nutter P, Bell GI, Sukhatme VP, Rauscher FJ 3rd (1992) Repression of the insulin-like growth factor II gene by the Wilms tumor suppressor WT1. Science 257:674–678
47. Morrison DJ, English MA, Licht JD (2005) WT1 induces apoptosis through transcriptional regulation of the proapoptotic Bcl-2 family member Bak. Cancer Res 65:8174–8182
48. Scott J, Cowell J, Robertson ME, Priestley LM, Wadey R, Hopkins B, Pritchard J, Bell GI, Rall LB, Graham CF et al (1985) Insulin-like growth factor-II gene expression in Wilms' tumour and embryonic tissues. Nature 317:260–262
49. Fraizer GE, Bowen-Pope DF, Vogel AM (1987) Production of platelet-derived growth factor by cultured Wilms' tumor cells and fetal kidney cells. J Cell Physiol 133:169–174
50. Eccles MR, Wallis LJ, Fidler AE, Spurr NK, Goodfellow PJ, Reeve AE (1992) Expression of the PAX2 gene in human fetal kidney and Wilms' tumor. Cell Growth Differ 3:279–289
51. Little MH, Prosser J, Condie A, Smith PJ, Van Heyningen V, Hastie ND (1992) Zinc finger point mutations within the WT1 gene in Wilms tumor patients. Proc Natl Acad Sci USA 89:4791–4795
52. Feinberg AP (1996) Multiple genetic abnormalities of 11p15 in Wilms' tumor. Med Pediatr Oncol 27:484–489
53. Li M, Squire JA, Weksberg R (1997) Molecular genetics of Beckwith-Wiedemann syndrome. Curr Opin Pediatr 9:623–629
54. Huff V, Amos CI, Douglass EC, Fisher R, Geiser CF, Krill CE, Li FP, Strong LC, McDonald JM (1997) Evidence for genetic heterogeneity in familial Wilms' tumor. Cancer Res 57:1859–1862
55. Rahman N, Abidi F, Ford D, Arbour L, Rapley E, Tonin P, Barton D, Batcup G, Berry J, Cotter F et al (1998) Confirmation of FWT1 as a Wilms' tumour susceptibility gene and phenotypic characteristics of Wilms' tumour attributable to FWT1. Hum Genet 103:547–556

56. Gilbert-Barness EF (ed) (1998) Potter's atlas of developmental and infant pathology. Mosby Year Book, Philadelphia
57. Sebire NJ, Malone M, Ashworth M, Jacques TS (2010) Diagnostic pediatric surgical pathology. Churchill-Livingstone/Elsevier, Philadelphia
58. Argani P, Fritsch M, Kadkol SS, Schuster A, Beckwith JB, Perlman EJ (2000) Detection of the ETV6-NTRK3 chimeric RNA of infantile fibrosarcoma/cellular congenital mesoblastic nephroma in paraffin-embedded tissue: application to challenging pediatric renal stromal tumors. Mod Pathol 13:29–36
59. Schwab M, Westermann F, Hero B, Berthold F (2003) Neuroblastoma: biology and molecular and chromosomal pathology. Lancet Oncol 4:472–480
60. Ara T, DeClerck YA (2006) Mechanisms of invasion and metastasis in human neuroblastoma. Cancer Metastasis Rev 25:645–657
61. Lastowska M, Cullinane C, Vriend S, Cotterill S, Brown N, O'Neill S, Mazzocco K, Roberts P, Nicholson J, Ellershaw C, Pearson AD, Jackson MS, United Kingdom Children Cancer Study Group and the United Kingdom Cancer Cytogenetics Group (2001) Comprehensive genetic and histopathologic study reveals three types of neuroblastoma tumors. J Clin Oncol 19:3080–3090
62. Shimada H (2003) The international neuroblastoma pathology classification. Pathologica 95:240–241
63. Gilbert-Barness E (2007) Potter's pathology of the fetus, infant and child, vol 1 and 2, 2nd edn. Elsevier, Philadelphia
64. Peuchmaur M, d'Amore ES, Joshi W, Hata J, Roald B, Dehner LP, Gerbing RB, Stram DO, Lukens JN, Matthay KK, Shimada H (2003) Revision of the international neuroblastoma pathology classification: confirmation of favorable and unfavorable prognostic subsets in ganglioneuroblastoma, nodular. Cancer 98:2274–2281
65. Lakhani VT, You YN, Wells SA (2007) The multiple endocrine neoplasia syndromes. Annu Rev Med 58:253–265
66. Tognon C, Knezevich SR, Huntsman D et al (2002) Expression of the ETV6-NTRK3 gene fusion as a primary event in human secretory breast carcinoma. Cancer Cell 2:367–376
67. Rajan PB, Cranor ML, Rosen PP (1998) Cytosarcoma phyllodes in adolescent girls and young women: a study of 45 patients. Am J Surg Pathol 22:64–69
68. Barrio AV, Clark BD, Goldberg JI et al (2007) Clinicopathologic features and long-term outcomes of 293 phyllodes tumors of the breast. Ann Surg Oncol 14:2961–2970
69. Pelizzo G, Conoscenti G, Kalache KD et al (2003) Antenatal manifestation of congenital pancreatoblastoma in a fetus with Beckwith-Wiedemann syndrome. Prenat Diagn 23:292–294
70. Eberhart CG, Kepner JL, Goldthwaite PT et al (2004) Histopathological and molecular prognostic markers in medulloblastoma: c-myc, N-myc, TrkC, and anaplasia. J Neuropathol Exp Neurol 63:441–449
71. Lamont JM, McManamy CS, Pearson AD, Clifford SC, Ellison DW (2004) Combined histopathological and molecular cytogenetic stratification of medulloblastoma patients. Clin Cancer Res 10:5482–5493
72. Isaacs H Jr (1997) Tumors. In: Gilbert-Barness EF (ed) Potter's pathology of the fetus and infant. Mosby Year Book, Philadelphia
73. Ping AJ, Reeve AE, Law DJ, Young MR, Boehnke M, Feinberg AP (1989) Genetic linkage of Beckwith-Wiedemann syndrome to 11p15. Am J Hum Genet 44:720–723
74. Wu NF, Kushnick T (1974) The Beckwith-Wiedemann syndrome. The exomphalos-macroglossia-gigantism syndrome. Clin Pediatr (Phila) 13:452–457
75. Henry I, Bonaiti-Pellie C, Chehensse V, Beldjord C, Schwartz C, Utermann G, Junien C (1991) Uniparental paternal disomy in a genetic cancer-predisposing syndrome. Nature 351:665–667
76. Dao D, Walsh CP, Yuan L, Gorelov D, Feng L, Hensle T, Nisen P, Yatnashiro DJ, Bestor TH, Tycko B (1999) Multipoint analysis of human chromosome 11p15/mouse digital chromosome 7: inclusion of H19/IGF2 in the minimal WT2 region, gene specificity of H19 silencing in Wilms' tumorigenesis and methylation hyper-dependence of H19 imprinting. Hum Mol Genet 8:1337–1352

77. Lee MP, DeBaun MR, Mitsuya K, Galonek HL, Brandenburg S, Oshimura M, Feinberg AP (1999) Loss of imprinting of a paternally expressed transcript, with antisense orientation to KVLQT1, occurs frequently in Beckwith-Wiedemann syndrome and is independent of insulin-like growth factor II imprinting. Proc Natl Acad Sci USA 96:5203–5208
78. Morison IM, Reeve AE (1998) A catalogue of imprinted genes and parent-of-origin effects in humans and animals. Hum Mol Genet 7:1599–1609
79. Onyango P, Miller W, Lehoczky J, Leung CT, Birren B, Wjeelan S, Dewar K, Feinberg AP (2000) Sequence and comparative analysis of the mouse 1-megabase region orthologous to the human 11p15 imprinted domain. Genome Res 10:1697–1710
80. Paulsen M, Davies KR, Bowden LM, Villar AJ, Franck I, Fuermann M, Dean WL, Moore TF, Rodrigues N, Davies KE et al (1998) Syntenic organization of the mouse distal chromosome 8 imprinting cluster and the Beckwith-Wiedemann syndrome region in chromosome 11p15.5. Hum Mol Genet 7:1149–1159
81. Xin Z, Soejima H, Higashimoto K, Yatsuki H, Zhu X, Satoh Y, Miasaki Z, Kaneko Y, Jimo Y, Fukuzawa R et al (2000) A novel imprinted gene, KCNQ1DN, within the WT2 critical region of human chromosome 11p15.5 and its reduced expression in Wilms' tumors. J Biochem (Toyko) 128:847–853
82. Seizinger BR, Rouleau GA, Ozelius LJ, Lane AH, Faryniarz AG, Chao MV, Huson S, Korf BR, Parry DM, Pericak-Vance MA et al (1987) Genetic linkage of von Recklinghausen neurofibromatosis to the nerve growth factor receptor gene. Cell 49:589–594
83. Listernick R, Charrow J, Gutmann DH (1999) Intracranial gliomas in neurofibromatosis type 1. Am J Med Genet 89:38–44
84. Evans DG, Birch JM, Ramsden RT (1999) Paediatric presentation of type 2 neurofibromatosis. Arch Dis Child 81:496–499
85. Brook-Carter PT, Peral B, Ward CJ, Thompson P, Hughes J, Maheshwar MM, Nellist M, Gamble V, Harris PC, Sampson JR (1994) Deletion of the TSC2 and PKD1 genes associated with severe infantile polycystic kidney disease-a contiguous gene syndrome. Nat Genet 8:328–332
86. Crino PB, Nathanson KL, Henskie EP (2006) The tuberous sclerosis complex. N Engl J Med 355:1345–1356
87. Vinaitheerthan M, Wei J, Mizuguchi M, Greco A, Barness EG (2004) Tuberous sclerosis: immunohistochemistry expression of tuberin and hamartin in a 31-week gestational fetus. Fetal Pediatr Pathol 23:241–249
88. Cavenee WK (1997) Turcot syndrome. International Agency for Research on Cancer, Lyon
89. Schofield D, West DC, Anthony DC, Marshal R, Sklar J (1995) Correlation of loss of heterozygosity at chromosome 9q with histological subtype in medulloblastomas. Am J Pathol 146:472–480
90. Cowan R, Hoban P, Kelsey A, Birch JM, Gattamaneni R, Evans DG (1997) The gene for the nevoid basal cell carcinoma syndrome acts as a tumour-suppressor gene in medulloblastoma. Br J Cancer 76:141–145
91. Wiestler OD, Kleihues P, Vital A, Padberg GW (1997) Cowden disease and dysplastic gangliocytoma of the cerebellum/Lhermitte-Duclos disease. International Agency for Research on Cancer, Lyon
92. Marsh D, Zori R (2002) Genetic insights into familial cancers-update and recent discoveries. Cancer Lett 181:125–164

Chapter 16
Molecular Pathology and Diagnostics of Cutaneous Malignancy

Sudeep Gaudi, Patricia M. McNab, Timothy W. McCardle, and Jane L. Messina

Contents

Abstract Advances and discoveries in molecular genetics over the past decade have literally changed the face of diagnosis and treatment decisions for patients with melanoma and non-melanoma skin cancer. These include genetic analysis of skin biopsies as a diagnostic aid, genotyping of tumors from patients with malignant melanoma for personalized treatment of metastatic disease, and discovery of

S. Gaudi • P.M. McNab • T.W. McCardle • J.L. Messina, M.D. (✉)
H. Lee Moffitt Cancer Center and Research Institute,
12902 Magnolia Drive, Tampa, FL 33612, USA
e-mail: jane.messina@moffitt.org

D. Coppola (ed.), *Molecular Pathology and Diagnostics of Cancer*,
Cancer Growth and Progression 16, DOI 10.1007/978-94-007-7192-5_16,

a new virus thought to play a role in the pathogenesis of Merkel cell carcinoma. Initiated by the discovery of a familial cancer gene in patients with familial melanoma and atypical nevi over three decades ago, molecular pathology techniques now play a central role in genetic testing for melanoma risk, in evaluation of melanocytic proliferations with uncertain biologic potential, and in stratifying patients with metastatic melanoma for treatment with targeted therapeutic agents, driving the search for better markers of prognosis and response to therapy. Targeted therapy is now available for treatment of unresectable or metastatic basal cell carcinoma. It is likely that continual improvements in techniques for analyzing blood and fresh and archival tumor tissue will uncover the pathogenesis of skin tumors related and unrelated to sun exposure, spawn the development of vaccinations or chemopreventive agents for these tumors, and enable physicians to customize treatment based on unique patient and tumor characteristics. This chapter will highlight relevant information concerning the molecular pathogenesis of melanoma, basal and squamous cell carcinoma, and Merkel cell carcinoma. Sections on molecular techniques available for diagnosis, prognosis, and treatment selection, emphasizing melanoma where this is most highly developed, are included

Keywords Nonmelanoma skin cancer • Molecular genetics of cutaneous malignancy • Melanoma prognosis • Prognostic biomarkers • Merkel cell carcinoma pathogenesis

Abbreviations

AE	Aloe-emodin
ASIP	Agouti signaling protein
BCC	Basal cell carcinoma
CGH	Comparative genomic hybridization
EGFR	Epidermal growth factor receptor
ERK	Extracellular signal-regulated kinase
FISH	Fluorescent in situ hybridization
GST	Glutathione S-transferase
GWASs	Genome-wide association studies
Hh	Hedgehog
MAPK	Mitogen-activated protein kinase
MC1R	Melanocortin 1 receptor
McPyV	Merkel cell polyomavirus
MEK	MAPK extracellular signal-regulated kinase
PCR	Polymerase chain reaction
SCC	Squamous cell carcinoma
SNP	Single nucleotide polymorphism
UV	Ultraviolet

16.1 Introduction

An estimated 76,250 new cases of cutaneous melanoma will have been diagnosed in the United States in 2012 [1], and this disease will claim the lives of approximately 9,000 American men and women this same year [1]. In contrast, greater than two million new cases of nonmelanoma skin cancer are anticipated to occur in the United States in 2012, while deaths from these malignancies are projected to be less than 1,000 [2]. Given the disproportionate mortality of melanoma compared to other skin cancers, detection of early-stage disease constitutes a major effort in all diagnostic endeavors. Many of the strides made in the molecular biologic analysis of melanoma have been aimed at increasing diagnostic accuracy. This is an important goal, especially in light of the number of skin biopsies performed to rule out melanoma—estimated to be more than one to two million in the United States in 2008 alone [3]. While histopathologic examination of suspicious pigmented lesions remains the "gold standard" for diagnosis, and the vast majority of malignancies can be readily distinguished from melanocytic nevi on the basis of histopathology, cases not so easily discernable can wreak havoc. The consequences of both false negative and false positive diagnoses are considerable: false positive diagnosis may subject the patient to undue mental anguish, financial burden, difficulties in attaining health insurance, and disfiguring surgical as well as toxic medical interventions. False negative diagnosis of melanoma, in addition to delaying appropriate treatment, is the single most common cause of medical malpractice lawsuits against a pathologist [4]. There have been numerous studies focusing on diagnostic discrepancy rates in melanocytic lesions [5–16]. In one illustrative example, experienced dermatopathologists considered experts in their field rendered opposing histopathologic diagnoses in as many as 25 % of cases reviewed [14].

Current molecular diagnostic tests, employed for the purpose of increased diagnostic accuracy and selection of targeted therapy, are informed by the earliest research into the molecular pathogenesis of melanoma. Therefore, this section will highlight current knowledge into the molecular basis for the disease, followed by discussion of established and emerging molecular techniques that may assist in the diagnosis and treatment of melanoma.

16.2 Familial Melanoma

Familial melanoma accounts for only 10 % of melanoma cases [17] but formed the basis for the earliest studies on genetic abnormalities in this disease, specifically mutations in p14/ARF, p16/INK4a, and CDK4. The best-characterized high-penetrance susceptibility gene predisposing to melanoma is CDKN2A, located on chromosome 9p21 [18–23]. This gene encodes two distinct tumor suppressor proteins (p14/ARF and p16/INK4a), implicated in the oncogenesis of melanoma.

The former hinders neoplasia through its indirect effect on p53 by binding to and inhibiting the function of human homolog of murine Mdm2 (HDM2), a protein that tags other proteins for ubiquitination. In mutated form, p14/ARF cannot bind to and suppress HDM2, allowing it to mark p53 for ubiquitination. With less p53 available to identify damaged DNA, genomic instability results, predisposing the afflicted individual to the development of melanoma. p16/INK4a functions in concert with retinoblastoma protein, a tumor suppressor protein, to regulate the G_1 phase of the cell cycle. In familial melanoma patients, compromised expression of p16 allows for uninhibited phosphorylation of retinoblastoma protein. This leads to transcription of genes encoding cyclin E, a protein that is required for the initiation of DNA replication in the S phase. CDK4 is another high penetrance but low-frequency melanoma susceptibility gene identified in linkage studies [19–22]. Located on chromosome 12q14, CDK4 encodes cyclin-dependent kinase 4 protein, a constituent of the CDK4/6 complex discussed above. Germline mutations that activate this gene occur at codon 24 (Arg24Cys and Arg24His) and render the CDK4/6 complex resistant to p16 inhibition. Thus, mutations in the p15/INK4a and CDKN2A genes produce a similar effect.

Additional genes involved in cases of familial melanoma have been identified through the use of genome-wide association studies (GWASs). While linkage studies have allowed the identification of the aforementioned high-penetrance, low-frequency genetic variants implicated in familial melanoma, GWASs have enabled high-powered searches for low-penetrance, high-frequency melanoma susceptibility genes. The melanoma genetics consortium, GenoMEL, performed the largest of these studies with the purpose of identifying common genetic variants contributing to melanoma risk across populations of European ancestry residing at varying altitudes [24]. This study found the strongest association in a single nucleotide polymorphism (SNP) that is a likely variant of the MC1R (melanocortin 1 receptor) gene, located on chromosome 16q24. This SNP was also discovered to be associated with hair color and skin pigmentation in a separate GWAS [25]. The link between pigmentation phenotype and melanoma susceptibility has long been established by epidemiological studies [26]. Thus, the relationship between allelic variants of the MC1R gene and both pigmentation phenotype and melanoma risk is not unexpected. The GenoMEL study also corroborated other previously suggested melanoma associations—locus 11q14-21 encompassing tyrosinase and locus 20q11.22, near ASIP (agouti signaling protein)—as well as two SNPs, for which prior associations with melanoma were not made. These latter two variants were located on chromosome 9p21, respectively, within the methylthioadenosine phosphorylase gene, which flanks CDK2NA, and ANRIL, an antisense noncoding mRNA that overlaps with the promoter of the p14ARF transcript of the CDK2NA gene and the transcribed sequence of CDK2NB.

A separate GWAS of nevus count using cohorts from the UK and Australia identified alleles at two strongly associated loci: 9p21 (MATP) and 22q13.1 (PLA2G6, a member of the phospholipase A2 superfamily of genes) [27]. The authors of this study were then able to associate the SNPs at these loci with melanoma susceptibility by analyzing two melanoma case-control samples. Interestingly, the signals within 9p21 of this GWAS overlapped with those of the GenoMEL study. Furthermore, the authors of the GenoMEL study were able to replicate the association between the SNPs at 22q13 and melanoma risk as well. Given these associations of the SNPs identified in the nevus study with melanoma, as well as the well-known positive correlation between number of melanocytic nevi and risk for melanoma, it is reasonable to assume that the risk of developing melanoma at these loci with these SNPs is, at least in part, mediated through nevus count [28, 29]. The discovery of these and additional susceptibility genes may yield further insight into the biological pathways involved in melanomagenesis.

At present, there are no formal guidelines for genetic testing of melanoma patients, their kindred, or their tumor samples for the p16/CDKN2A mutation. Potential benefits of such testing include the possibility of increased compliance in preventive programs with a positive test result. A negative test result in a patient with relatives who have died from melanoma or pancreatic cancer with the germline mutation could be reassuring. Those opposed to such testing cite the lack of identifiable germline mutations in known high-risk genes in affected members of known melanoma families. Conversely, non-gene carriers in CDKN2A-positive families may still develop dysplastic nevus syndrome and develop melanoma. Thus, negative test results could confer a false sense of reassurance and be a disincentive to continued participating in screening/prevention activities. Finally, it is difficult to assign an absolute risk for development of disease in individuals who do have a germline mutation identified [30]. It is reasonable to conclude that genetic testing for germline CDKN2a mutations should be performed only in patients that have a significant risk of having a positive test result (i.e., those with three or more affected members) and only in conjunction with a thorough explanation of the limitations of the test, in conjunction with qualified genetic counseling and education [31].

16.3 Sporadic Melanoma

Research into the molecular basis of sporadic melanoma has implicated many genes, particularly those encoding proteins involved in the mitogen-activated protein kinase (MAPK) pathway [19, 20, 22, 23, 32, 33]. With up to 90 % of melanomas harboring constitutive activation of this pathway, great interest lies in detailing the precise mechanisms involved, with the hope of intervening at key junctions in an effort to thwart melanomagenesis and/or progression [33]. The MAPK pathway regulates cellular proliferation through signal transduction along the cascade of RAS, RAF, MAPK extracellular signal-regulated kinase (MEK), and extracellular signal-regulated kinase (ERK). Activated ERK induces several proliferative and survival processes, one of which is activation of the cyclin D-CDK4/6 complex (discussed above) upon translocation to the nucleus. Mutational analyses have yielded key aberrations in crucial players in the MAPK pathway, including BRAF, NRAS, c-Kit, and epidermal growth factor receptor (EGFR).

16.4 Molecular Diagnostic Tests

16.4.1 BRAF

There are three mammalian RAF proto-oncogenes—ARAF, BRAF, and CRAF. However, of these, only activating mutations of BRAF have thus far been shown to be present in a significant percentage of human malignancies, with the highest rate occurring in melanoma [19, 20, 22, 23]. BRAF-mutated melanomas tend to occur at anatomic sites exposed to intermittent, rather than chronic, sun damage. With approximately 70 % of cases harboring such a mutation, BRAF is the most commonly mutated proto-oncogene in cutaneous melanoma. Furthermore, a significant proportion of both benign and dysplastic melanocytic nevi have been shown to harbor mutations of BRAF as well, suggesting a relatively early event in melanomagenesis [19, 22, 23, 34].

Greater than 90 % of BRAF mutations in melanoma result from a single base missense mutation (T→A) at codon 1799 that leads to the substitution of valine in favor of glutamic acid at position 600 of the BRAF protein [35]. This alteration introduces a conformational change in BRAF's kinase domain, which can lead to a 480-fold increase in kinase activity when compared to wild-type BRAF [36]. This mutated BRAF induces uncontrolled proliferation in melanoma. Ongoing research of this molecule includes its role in inducing senescence of benign melanocytic nevi, the mechanisms involved in bypassing this senescent response in the development of melanoma from such nevi, and the mechanisms for acquired resistance to targeted inhibition of this molecule in patients undergoing anti-BRAF therapy [37–48].

A major breakthrough in the treatment of metastatic melanoma has been the successful treatment of BRAF-mutant melanoma with selective BRAF inhibitors such as vemurafenib and dabrafenib [49]. Since this agent shows tenfold greater activity for V600E-mutant melanoma compared to wild-type melanoma, most current clinical trials require pre-treatment assessment for the presence of this mutation [50]. The mutation is ascertained by means of a polymerase chain reaction (PCR) assay (TaqMan, Applied Biosystems), which involves hybridizing a probe specific to the 1799T->A substitution with DNA isolated from formalin-fixed, paraffin-embedded tumor tissue and determining the presence or absence of amplification after repeated chain-reaction cycles [51]. This assay is now routinely available at most major commercial reference laboratories. There is also a commercially available monoclonal antibody (VE1) that can be used to assess for the BRAF V600E mutation immunohistochemically. This antibody was 100 % sensitive and specific for the mutation compared to the gold standard of molecular analysis in a recent series of 44 cases [52]. There have also been attempts at predicting BRAF mutation status by analyzing various clinical and histologic features of primary tumors. In a recent study of 302 primary melanomas, groupings of various combinations of 17 such factors revealed that phenotypic features such as increased upward scatter, intraepidermal nesting, epidermal thickening, sharp lateral demaracation of the tumor, and the presence of rounded, highly pigmented tumor cells were distinct features of melanomas with BRAF mutation. In this study, classification tree analysis showed that BRAF mutation status could be correctly predicted in up to 82 % of tumors using certain variables [53]. While there is certainly great interest in correlating easily analyzed clinicopathologic variables with mutation status, and active research aimed at this goal, at present, however, the gold standard for assessing tumors for BRAF status remains mutation analysis.

16.4.2 c-KIT

c-KIT, a proto-oncogene that encodes the type III receptor tyrosine kinase KIT, was first identified in 1987 as a result of sequence similarity to the Hardy-Zuckerman 4 feline sarcoma virus oncogene, v-KIT [54]. Upon binding its ligand, stem cell factor, KIT undergoes receptor dimerization, autophosphorylation, and activation of its intracellular tyrosine kinase domain [18, 55]. Once activated, KIT is capable of stimulating downstream signaling pathways, such as MAPK [18, 55, 56].

Activating mutations and/or gene amplification of KIT have been described in distinct subsets of melanoma [57–61]. In one study, aberrations were found in 39 % of mucosal melanomas, 36 % of acral melanomas, and 28 % of melanomas arising in chronically sun-damaged skin (as defined by the presence of solar elastosis on review of histopathology)—anatomic sites at which BRAF mutations occur far less frequently [60].

The most prevalent KIT mutations in melanoma occur in exons 11, 13, and 17 [62]. These mutations are thought to promote the constitutive activation of KIT either through precluding the protein from assuming its default autoinhibited conformation or by promoting its dimerization in the absence of stem cell factor [63, 64]. The precise manner in which constitutive KIT activation promotes melanomagenesis remains unclear. Nonetheless, recognizing activating mutations of KIT as well as copy number gains can be of great consequence, as this subtype of melanoma may respond the receptor tyrosine kinase imatinib [65–67]. Since the initial case report of a dramatic response to imatinib in c-KIT-mutated melanomas [65], interest has been raised in treating patients with acral and mucosal melanoma with this agent, leading to several ongoing phase II clinical trials (ClinicalTrials.gov) of imatinib and other c-KIT blockers such as sunitinib, dasatinib, and sorafenib. These studies require documentation of mutation or amplification of the c-kit gene. Currently, therefore, it seems reasonable that subgroups of patients with metastatic melanoma prone to c-kit mutations, such as primary mucosal or acral lentiginous tumors, be analyzed for KIT mutation status. If mutated, a therapeutic trial with a c-KIT blocking agent has been suggested. Testing, using PCR following by sequencing analysis of exons 11, 13, and 17 can be performed at several reference laboratories, including ARUP, as well as university laboratories such as those at University of Washington and University of Michigan.

16.4.3 N-RAS

The RAS proto-oncogene family is at the initiating point of the MAPK pathway, and theoretically activating mutations of these molecules should provide the affected cell with continuous growth signals in the absence of extracellular stimuli. Indeed, RAS molecules have documented roles in melanomagenesis [18–20, 22, 23, 33]. Of the three members of this family (H-RAS, K-RAS, and N-RAS), only the latter has been shown to sustain activating mutations in melanocytes, as well as nearly one third of all melanomas [19, 23, 33]. The most commonly documented N-RAS aberration in melanoma is a missense mutation at codon 61 (Q61R), which results in the substitution of arginine in place of glutamine and impairs GTP hydrolysis, locking the protein in a state of constitutive activation [68]. However, therapeutic attempts at blocking the farnesylation, which is required for proper function of the molecule, using farnesyltransfer inhibitors, have yielded disappointing results [56, 69].

There has been a resurgent interest in the role of the N-RAS pathway in sustaining melanoma growth in the wake of the phenomenon of acquired resistance to BRAF inhibitors. Specifically, investigations into this phenomenon in cell lines have revealed that hyperactivation of the MEK-ERK1/2 pathway occurs rapidly after treatment with the BRAF inhibitor PLX4032, and this has been noted most prominently in cell lines containing the activating N-RAS mutation, which demonstrated resistance to apoptosis [70, 71]. Therefore, future trials of targeted therapies may require genotyping for N-RAS to stratify treatment.

16.4.4 Epidermal Growth Factor Receptor (EGFR)

EGFR is yet another receptor tyrosine kinase that is involved in activation of the MAPK and PI3K/Akt signal transduction pathways. The latter pathway is also activated by RAS and results in decreased apoptosis [19]. The selective expression of this receptor in human melanoma cells harboring an extra copy of chromosome 7 was first studied in 1985 [72]. Numerous studies have since investigated the importance of this receptor in melanomagenesis and/or progression with contradictory results. More recently, however, researchers have shown an association between polysomy 7 and EGFR gene amplification by fluorescent in situ hybridization (FISH), with significantly higher amplification in tumors that metastasized within 2 years of surgical excision of the primary lesion [73]. Implying a poorer prognosis in this latter subset of patients, further studies into the potential benefit of anti-EGFR therapy for those with EGFR alterations have been recommended. However, at this time there appears to be no clinical utility to testing tumors for EGFR overexpression.

16.4.5 Comparative Genomic Hybridization

The technique of comparative genomic hybridization (CGH), wherein lesional DNA as well as normal control DNA are hybridized to either normal metaphase chromosomes or an array of thousands of defined DNA probes (array CGH) in order to detect copy number changes, has been used to examine differences between melanoma and benign melanocytic lesions. Specifically, gains of chromosomes 1q, 6p, 7p, 7q, 8q, 17q, and 20q and losses of chromosomes 6q, 9p, 9q, 10p, 10q, and 11q have been observed in greater than 95 % of melanomas [74]. Loss of chromosome 9, an early and common aberration in melanomagenesis, typically involves deletion of the distal region of the p arm that encompasses the 9p21 locus [75]. Of note, gain of 6p is a frequent aberration in both primary and malignant melanomas and may confer a poorer outcome [76, 77].

Melanocytic nevi rarely demonstrate chromosomal aberrations, with the exception of Spitz nevi, which may harbor gains on occasion [74, 78–80]. A gain of the entire short arm of chromosome 11 is the most commonly encountered aberration in Spitz nevus and is an abnormality not detected in primary cutaneous melanomas. Although most congenital nevi are readily distinguished from melanoma according to established histopathologic criteria, atypical nodular proliferations that arise in congenital nevi can be problematic [78]. These lesions simulate nodular melanomas microscopically, but tend to regress within a few months. CGH offers diagnostic aid in this area [78, 80]. While cases of atypical nodular proliferations show chromosomal aberrations by CGH, the pattern of involvement is distinct from that created by melanoma. Abnormalities in the former group involve only entire chromosomes. While gains or losses of entire chromosomes can frequently occur in melanoma as well, 95 % of such cases are paralleled by gains or losses of chromosomal fragments.

CGH has also underscored significant genetic differences between acral melanoma and superficial spreading melanoma [81], justifying the distinction between these subtypes by demonstrating disparity in pattern of chromosomal aberration between the two [80, 81]. While acral melanomas have been shown to invariably harbor gene amplifications (defined as greater than a threefold increase in copy number), superficial spreading melanomas, of comparable tumor thickness and patient age, contain an amplicon in less than 15 % of cases. The amplified regions frequently consist of areas containing known oncogenes. Study of the amplicons not harboring obvious candidate genes may provide further insight into the mechanisms of melanomagenesis.

Isolated melanocytes located beyond the microscopically-designated free margins of resection have been shown to harbor these genetic amplifications as well [80, 81]. Researchers believe that these field cells represent unrecognized radial growth of the acral melanoma and are likely responsible for local recurrences. If further studies support such a notion, then CGH may play an instrumental role in shaping future guidelines pertaining to the attainment of clear margins of resection.

16.4.6 Fluorescent In Situ Hybridization

A multiprobe fluorescent in situ hybridization (FISH) assay against several of the aforementioned chromosomal abnormalities detected in CGH studies has been developed and tested in several studies with promising results [3, 82]. The assay identifies copy number alterations in chromosomes 6p25 (RREB1), 6q23 (MYB), and 11q13 (cyclin D1) as well as centromere 6. Results of these preliminary studies have demonstrated high sensitivity (~87 %) as well as specificity (~95 %) in distinguishing benign melanocytic nevi from melanomas using this particular panel of probes.

Therefore, this technique plays a potential role in classifying problematic melanocytic lesions. The area of most intense investigation of the applicability of this technique is in the distinction between spitzoid melanoma and benign Spitz nevus. Two recent studies have demonstrated sensitivity and specificity of 43–60 % and 50–80 % for determination of malignancy in ambiguous Spitzid lesions, using metastatic behavior as the gold standard [83, 84]. In another recent, albeit small, study evaluating the efficacy of FISH in distinguishing nodular nevoid melanomas from mitotically active melanocytic nevi with probes targeting these same for four loci, chromosomal aberrations were detected in each of the nevoid melanomas and in none of the melanocytic nevi [85]. Other scenarios for which FISH has shown potential benefit include distinguishing epithelioid blue nevus from blue nevus-like cutaneous melanoma metastasis [86], distinguishing intranodal nevus from metastatic melanoma [87], classifying superficial melanocytic neoplasms with pagetoid melanocytosis [88], and the microstaging of melanoma arising in association with a nevus [89]. Several commercial laboratories now offer this test for use in formalin-fixed, paraffin-embedded tissue using probes developed by Abbott Laboratories (Caris Life Sciences, Neogenomics Laboratories).

16.4.7 Immunohistochemical Staining for Prognostic Biomarkers

There has been abundant research aimed at identifying biomarkers for prognosis as well as treatment response. The widespread availability of immunohistochemical staining makes this technique one of the most widely investigated, because it can characterize patterns of protein expression while maintaining preservation of tissue and cellular architecture. There have been literally thousands of manuscripts devoted to potential molecular markers of melanoma that could identify patients at greatest risk for recurrence, or most likely to benefit from adjuvant therapy. Two recent systematic reviews of published data on immunohistochemistry-based prognostic molecular markers for cutaneous melanoma have been performed [90, 91]. The first of two reviews sought to report on associations between immunohistochemical expression of protein biomarkers and survival outcomes in cases of cutaneous melanoma. Molecular markers were then scored according to the protein's major biological function, as categorized by a modified Hanahan-Weinberg functional capabilities scheme. This review identified effectors of DNA replication, cyclin-dependent kinase inhibitors, growth-promoting transcription factors, and regulators of tissue invasion and metastasis as having a statistically significant impact on patient outcome. Ki-67, proliferating cell nuclear antigen, metallothionein, Ku70,

Ku80, and microtubule-associated protein-2 were consistently associated with disease-free as well as overall survival. Interestingly, cyclins and cyclin-dependent kinases were not associated with melanoma prognosis. More recently, a significant association between Ki-67 expression and melanoma-specific mortality—in addition to dermal mitoses, which remain a significant and independent prognostic factor—has been shown in a large and representative population of patients diagnosed with thin ($\leq$ 1 mm in thickness) cutaneous melanomas [92]. With external validation in a similar population-based sample, it is possible that Ki-67 may be formally adopted into routine clinical practice, either as a prognostic factor for disease recurrence or a predictive factor of positive sentinel lymph node biopsy.

Expression of cyclin-dependent kinase inhibitors was significantly associated with mortality. For example, increased levels of p16 were associated with decreased all-cause and melanoma-specific mortalities, while increased levels of p27, which typically cause cells to arrest in the G_1 phase of the cell cycle, are paradoxically associated with increased mortality. The rationale behind this observation lies in the activation of p27 through cytoplasmic sequestration, rather than protein degradation. Cytoplasmic accumulation of p27 has been associated with metastatic potential [93]. Among proteins involved in growth signaling, statistically significant associations were most frequent among transcription factors, ATF-2 and AP-2α, and transcriptional coactivators, NCOA3/AIB-1. This observation suggests altered transcriptional regulation as a crucial step in regulation of melanoma-specific survival. Increased expression of three cellular adhesion molecules was shown to be associated with statistically significant worsening of disease-free survival: the melanocyte-specific melanoma cell adhesion molecule (MCAM/MUC18), neuron-specific L1 cell adhesion molecule (L1-CAM), and glandular tissue-associated carcinoembryonic antigen-related cell adhesion molecule 1 (CEACAM-1). These molecules are thought to promote tumor infiltration and distant spread through abnormal tumor-stroma interactions [94–97]. Also, elevated levels of osteopontin and tenascin-C—members of the matricellular protein family, which consists of secreted molecules that interface between cell surface receptors and the extracellular matrix [98]—were associated with statistically significant worsening of melanoma-specific mortality and disease-free survival, respectively. Among proteases, increased levels of tissue plasminogen activator and matrix metalloproteinase-2 were statistically significant for mortality outcomes.

16.5 Basal Cell Carcinoma

Basal cell carcinoma (BCC) is the most common invasive cancer in the Western world, and it accounts for 75 % of skin malignancies overall with increasing rates worldwide [99–101]. Ultraviolet (UV) radiation, more specifically of the UV B-wavelength, is the dominant etiologic agent thought to be responsible for most skin carcinomas [99, 102]. It does so by genetically altering genes involved in initiation, promotion, and progression of both melanoma and non-melanoma skin cancers. Since the discovery of the hedgehog gene and its influence on the development of carcinoma in certain populations, great strides have been made in uncovering other genetic abnormalities and the possible use of specific inhibitors in treatment of the disease [103, 104]. These emerging genetic alterations, originally studied in inheritable disorders, such as xeroderma pigmentosum and nevoid basal cell carcinoma syndrome (also known as Gorlin syndrome), have offered new insight into its molecular basis.

16.5.1 Inherited Forms of Basal Cell Carcinoma

There are several major mechanisms involved in inherited forms of BCC: defects in detoxifying proteins, DNA repair, and embryonic signaling pathways. Defects in these pathways cause well-recognized skin cancer syndromes, including xeroderma pigmentosum, Gorlin syndrome, and familial cylindromatosis, and play a role in sporadic BCC as well. One of the most important components that protect the skin against oxidative stress after UV irradiation is the glutathione S-transferase (GST) enzyme system [105]. In humans, GST is expressed in melanomas, but only weakly in BCC [106]. Several GST polymorphisms have been identified in patients with high UV sensitivity and increased risk for BCC [105]. Impaired DNA repair, especially in patients with xeroderma pigmentosum, predisposes to non-melanoma skin cancer, preferentially of the squamous cell carcinoma (SCC) type (discussed later in this chapter). Of the embryonic signaling pathways, the most important is the hedgehog (Hh) signaling pathway.

PTCH1 gene is a member of the Hh signaling pathway, which encodes for a membrane receptor for three extracellular ligands: sonic hedgehog, Indian hedgehog, and desert hedgehog [103, 107]. Located on chromosome 9q22, this gene inhibits the Hh signaling pathway in its unbound configuration, thus functioning as a tumor suppressor gene. Over 90 % of sporadic BCCs harbor mutations on at least one allele. Malignant cells may also contain mutations in the trans-membrane protein Smoothened (Smo), normally inhibited by the unbound Hh receptor, allowing for decreased effectiveness of the PTCH1 gene [103, 108, 109]. In normal situations, Hh binding allows for the relocation of Smo to the cilium and subsequent activation of signal transduction. The end result of this unregulated pathway is the upregulation of the Gli family of transcription factors known as Gli [103, 108–110]. Since PTCH1 is overexpressed in BCC (up to 11-fold in one study) but not in other nonmelanoma skin cancers; it may be utilized as a tumor marker via in situ hybridization or reverse transcription-PCR to asses for elevated levels of either PTCH1 or Gli1 mRNA [107, 111]. In addition, Hatta et al. [112] found that both BCCs and trichoeptheliomas may be distinguished from other basaloid neoplasms using reverse transcription-PCR quantifications of Gli1 levels. There were consistently higher levels detected in these two tumors, with almost non-existent levels in others.

It has been shown that interruption of the Hh pathway in concert with chemotherapy enhances tumor response in animal models of pancreatic cancer [110, 113, 114]. Several small molecular inhibitors of Hh signaling pathway are under investigation, and vismodegib was approved by the FDA in 2012 for patients with recurrent, locally advanced, or metastatic basal cell carcinoma. The targeted areas include Smo antagonists, Hh inhibitors, and Gli inhibitors, including cyclopamine, GDC-0449 (Phase I and II), IPI-926 (Phase I), LDE225 (Phase II), and BMS-833923 (Phase I) [110, 115, 116]. An in-depth discussion of Smo inhibitors on the horizon can be found in the recent review article by Peukert and Miller-Mosin [110].

Numerous Gli-mediated transcription inhibitors, as well as inhibitors targeting the Hh protein itself have been tested in animal models; however, these have not yet been brought to clinical trial. [110, 117, 118]. Because these mutations are so ubiquitous in sporadic BCC and always present in inherited BCC, there is no role for pre-treatment testing for their presence.

16.5.2 Sporadic Forms of Basal Cell Carcinoma

UV-induced mutations in both p53 and PTCH1 genes are thought to be the most common elements that induce the development of BCC [119]. The p53 gene is responsible for regulating the cell cycle and apoptosis induction in irreversible damaged cells, and mutations of the protein have been detected in 50–60 %% of BCCs [107, 119]. Although the usefulness of p53 is limited as a molecular diagnostic aid in BCC because it is overexpressed in numerous malignancies, levels are substantially increased in tumors with aggressive growth patterns [105]. This information may prove useful in determining prognosis or directing further medical management.

BCL-2 encodes for a protein that participates the regulation of cell death by blocking apoptosis [120]. In both BCC and SCC, overexpression has been noted, allowing for increased cell susceptibility to accumulation of harmful mutations. In contrast to the situation with SCC, where BCL-2 levels demonstrate a slow, graduated increase as lesions progress from an actinic keratosis to invasive carcinoma, in BCCs, BCL-2 expression is lost with increasing tumor progression or aggressiveness. Other studies have also attempted to characterize additional mutational events involved in basal carcinomas on a molecular level utilizing whole genome microarray, the details of which are beyond the scope of this chapter [111, 121]. The clinical implications of these new discoveries will be of great importance, impacting the diagnosis, treatment, and prevention of a variety of benign and malignant skin conditions.

16.6 Squamous Cell Carcinoma

Squamous cell carcinoma (SCC), the second most common skin malignancy, is postulated to demonstrate different pathogenetic mechanisms than BCC. While BCC generally develops de novo, SCC goes through a multistep process of development. Although p53 has been postulated to play a major role, the major signaling transduction pathway(s) is presently unknown. SCCs display a great number of chromosomal aberrations; therefore, chromosomal instability likely plays a key role in its progression. Also, the differing frequencies of these tumors in organ-transplant patients compared to non-immunosuppressed (SCC being more common in the former) raise the probability that defects in immune surveillance play a much more important role in SCC development than in BCC [122].

SCC demonstrates alterations in several major areas, including p53 and RAS, as well as DNA repair mechanisms in xeroderma pigmentosum. p53 tumor suppressor gene mutations are present in approximately 40–50 % of cases, while RAS genes carry an incidence of 10–30 %. In addition, infection with human papillomavirus is also felt to play a large role in the development of SCC [123–125].

One study found that point mutations in the p53 gene were seen early in tumorigenesis and complete allelic loss correlated with progression to higher grade lesions [126]. More specifically, it has been shown that gain-of-function mutations may shift development into a more aggressive, spindle cell variant [127]. However, another study by Jensen et al. showed no difference in p53 activity [128]. Obviously, more investigations are needed before the role of p53 in tumor prognosis and progression is fully elucidated.

Although more than 100 HPV subtypes have been identified in cervical SCC, only a subgroup of high-risk types, including HPV-16, 18, 31, 33, 35 and 58, are believed to be a causative agent in the development of cervical cancer. The product of the viral gene *E6* is able to effect proteasomal degradation of p53, inhibiting cell cycle arrest and/or apoptosis. HPV DNA is frequently detected in skin carcinomas and is found in both immunocompetent (47 %) as well as immunosuppressed patients (75 %). However, no high-risk subtypes have yet been identified in cutaneous SCC [129]. Recently, attention has turned to HPV38, which has been detected in ~50 % of skin carcinomas but only in 10 % of healthy skin. HPV38 was also demonstrated in 43 % of actinic keratoses, as well as 13 % and 16 % of SCCs and BCCs, respectively. At this point, however, the high frequency of HPV DNA in normal skin and hair follicles and the fact that more than one type of HPV may be found simultaneous in normal and tumor tissues make the role of HPV38 in skin carcinogenesis still elusive [129].

Recent insight into possible additional genetic markers with novel diagnostic or prognostic implications is included here for completeness. These include alterations in the c-Jun NH_2-terminal kinase (JNK) signaling cascade, MUC4, and collagen XVII protein. Emerging research by Ke et al. [130] has shown that the c-Jun NH_2-terminal kinase (JNK) signaling cascade is activated in at least 70 % of SCCs, and its interaction with RAS is necessary for glycolysis. In addition, they found that inhibition of JNK2 counteracts successful tumorigenesis of epithelial cells. MUC4, a high molecular weight glycoprotein, has been recognized as possible biomarker or prognostic indicator for several malignancies. A recent study has revealed its overexpression in cutaneous SCC, well to moderately differentiated, while it is only weakly expressed or negative in BCC and melanoma and normal cutaneous epithelium [131].

In late 2009, Chou et al. [132] published data concerning the effects of aloe-emodin (AE) on non-melanoma skin cancers. It was found that malignant cells were selectively targeted and destroyed through induced apoptosis via elevation of p53 levels and ultimate reduction in BCl-2 levels. In addition, the utilization of both AE and 5-fluorouracil resulted in significantly higher cell death in mutated cell lines in human epidermoid carcinoma (A431) and human head and neck SCC (SCC25) cells than only the use of AE or 5-fluorouracil alone. In the future, interference in the aforementioned genetic aberrations may have therapeutic implications.

16.7 Merkel Cell Carcinoma

The discovery that viral gene sequences were integrally incorporated into the genome of a significant percentage of Merkel cell carcinomas was revolutionary for our understanding of the pathogenesis of this tumor. Although this rare neuroendocrine malignancy was known to have a strong association with immunosuppression and a predilection for areas of chronic sun exposure, the role of a virus was only discovered in 2008. Feng and colleagues were the first to demonstrate the presence of a fusion transcript between a previously unrecognized viral T antigen and a human receptor tyrosine phosphatase in 8 of 10 Merkel cell tumors tested. They performed sequence analysis and identified a 5387-base pair genome of a polyomavirus they named Merkel cell polyomavirus (McPyV) [133]. Since then, numerous publications have documented the presence of this virus not only in a significant portion (approximately 70–80 %) of tumor tissues but in other tumors, as well as normal tissue. The mechanism of viral pathogenesis is believed to be the result of integration of the virus into band 3p14 at the human protein tyrosine phosphatase, receptor type, G gene, a tumor suppressor gene. The viral T antigen is expressed as large T and small T antigens, and integrated MCPyV large T protein is truncated due to the deletion of the carboxyl terminal, which then suppresses autonomous viral replication [134]. However, much remains unknown concerning the modes of transmission and replication of the virus, as well as the associations between seropositivity and viral presence in tumor tissues. In particular, further research into the interplay between viral integration and further mutations, probably related to UV radiation, is needed.

Soon after the discovery of the MCPyV, a series of studies were undertaken to determine if the presence of viral genes was associated with outcome. The evidence from these studies has been conflicting, with some data suggesting that patients with viral gene-positive Merkel cell carcinoma experience better survival, some not showing a difference, and some indicating worse survival. Bhatia et al. demonstrated that patients with ≥0.06 viral copies per cell experienced higher median survival than those with ≤0.0035 viral copies per cell (86 months versus 20 months, $P=0.015$) [135]. Sihto et al. also confirmed a positive association with viral load and outcome in a study of 114 Finnish Merkel cell carcinoma patients, reporting the 5-year survival to be 45 % for patients with virus-positive tumors versus 13 % for those with virus-negative tumors ($P<0.001$) [136]. After adjusting for gender and the presence of nodal metastases, the presence of viral DNA was significantly associated with improved survival (hazard ratio 0.42, 95 % confidence interval 0.25–0.71). In contrast, Garneski et al. evaluated the outcome of 30 Merkel cell carcinoma patients based on the presence or absence of viral sequences by real-time quantitative PCR. Using Kaplan–Meier analysis, no survival difference was noted between virus-positive and virus-negative tumors [137]. Becker et al. analyzed 75 samples from 53 MCC patients for the presence of MCPyV by real-time PCR. Their clinical follow-up data suggested that patients whose tumors contained the viral genome displayed a more aggressive behavior, but after stratifying for tumor stage there was no statistically significant difference between the groups [138]. Numerous studies continue to unravel the role this polyomavirus plays in the pathogenesis, prognosis, and outcome of Merkel cell carcinoma, but at present the assessment of viral presence is solely for research purposes.

16.8 Conclusion

The era of targeted therapy has ushered in a plethora of diagnostic tests aimed at optimal selection of cancer patients for treatment with novel agents. Beginning with the elucidation of the role of the p16 gene mutation in familial melanoma kindreds, continuing with the discovery of the BRAF V600E mutation, and more recently focusing on smaller subsets of patients such as those with nRAS and cKIT mutations, the explosion of molecular knowledge in the field of melanoma has led to new hope in patients with this aggressive tumor. While malignant melanoma has been the subject of the most active research, other forms of skin cancer are also the subject of ongoing, more recent studies. The discovery of the role of the Hh signaling pathway in BCC has opened the door to studies of targeted inhibitors of this molecule. Infectious agents have been shown to play a role in subsets of SCC and Merkel cell carcinoma, leading to new understanding of the underlying pathogenesis of these diseases. Molecular diagnostic testing for these four most prevalent forms of cutaneous malignancy will continue to play a major role in clinical decision making for prognostic and treatment purposes.

References

1. Siegel R, Naishadham D, Jemal A (2012) Cancer statistics, 2012. CA Cancer J Clin 62:10–12
2. National Cancer Institute Skin Cancer. http://www.cancer.gov/cancertopics/types/skin. Accessed 25 July 2013
3. Gerami P, Jewell SS, Morrison LE, Blondin B, Schulz J, Ruffalo T, Matushek P 4th, Legator M, Jacobson K, Dalton SR, Charzan S, Kolaitis NA, Guitart J, Lertsbarapa T, Boone S, LeBoit PE, Bastian BC (2009) Fluorescence in situ hybridization (FISH) as an ancillary diagnostic tool in the diagnosis of melanoma. Am J Surg Pathol 33:1146–1156
4. Troxel DB (2006) Medicolegal aspects of error in pathology. Arch Pathol Lab Med 130:617–619

5. Brochez L, Verhaeghe E, Grosshans E, Haneke E, Piérard G, Ruiter D, Naeyaert JM (2002) Inter-observer variation in the histopathological diagnosis of clinically suspicious pigmented skin lesions. J Pathol 196:459–466
6. Heenan PJ, Matz LR, Blackwell JB, Kelsall GR, Singh A, ten Seldam RE, Holman CD (1984) Inter-observer variation between pathologists in the classification of cutaneous malignant melanoma in Western Australia. Histopathology 8:717–729
7. Shoo BA, Sagebiel RW, Kashani-Sabet M (2010) Discordance in the histopathologic diagnosis of melanoma at a melanoma referral center. J Am Acad Dermatol 62:751–756
8. van Dijk MC, Aben KK, van Hees F, Klaasen A, Blokx WA, Kiemeney LA, Ruiter DJ (2008) Expert review remains important in the histopathological diagnosis of cutaneous melanocytic lesions. Histopathology 52:139–146
9. Veenhuizen KC, De Wit PE, Mooi WJ, Scheffer E, Verbeek AL, Ruiter DJ (1997) Quality assessment by expert opinion in melanoma pathology: experience of the pathology panel of the Dutch Melanoma Working Party. J Pathol 182:266–272
10. Barnhill RL, Argenyi ZB, From L, Glass LF, Maize JC, Mihm MC Jr, Rabkin MS, Ronan SG, White WL, Piepkorn M (1999) Atypical Spitz nevi/tumors: lack of consensus for diagnosis, discrimination from melanoma, and prediction of outcome. Hum Pathol 30:513–520
11. Corona R, Mele A, Amini M, De Rosa G, Coppola G, Piccardi P, Fucci M, Pasquini P, Faraggiana T (1996) Interobserver variability on the histopathologic diagnosis of cutaneous melanoma and other pigmented skin lesions. J Clin Oncol 14:1218–1223
12. Farmer ER, Gonin R, Hanna MP (1996) Discordance in the histopathologic diagnosis of melanoma and melanocytic nevi between expert pathologists. Hum Pathol 27:528–531
13. Kempf W, Haeffner AC, Mueller B, Panizzon RG, Burg G (1998) Experts and gold standards in dermatopathology: qualitative and quantitative analysis of the self-assessment slide seminar at the 17th colloquium of the International Society of Dermatopathology. Am J Dermatopathol 20:478–482
14. Lodha S, Saggar S, Celebi JT, Silvers DN (1994) Discordance in the histopathologic diagnosis of difficult melanocytic neoplasms in the clinical setting. J Cutan Pathol 35:349–352
15. Piepkorn MW, Barnhill RL, Cannon-Albright LA et al (1994) A multiobserver, population-based analysis of histologic dysplasia in melanocytic nevi. J Am Acad Dermatol 30(5 Pt 1):707–714
16. Wechsler J, Bastuji-Garin S, Spatz A, Bailly C, Cribier B, Andrac-Meyer L, Vergier B, Fraitag S, Verola O, Wolkenstein P, French Cutaneous Cancerology Group (2002) Reliability of the histopathologic diagnosis of malignant melanoma in childhood. Arch Dermatol 138:625–628
17. Yeh I, Bastian BC (2009) Genome-wide associations studies for melanoma and nevi. Pigment Cell Melanoma Res 22:527–528
18. Calder KB, Morgan MB (2010) Carcinogenic pathway of malignant melanoma. In: Coppola D (ed) Mechanisms of oncogenesis, vol 12. Springer, Dordrecht, pp 149–157
19. Ibrahim N, Haluska FG (2009) Molecular pathogenesis of cutaneous melanocytic neoplasms. Annu Rev Pathol 4:551–579
20. Meyle KD, Guldberg P (2009) Genetic risk factors for melanoma. Hum Genet 126:499–510
21. Nelson AA, Tsao H (2009) Melanoma and genetics. Clin Dermatol 27:46–52
22. Palmieri G, Capone M, Ascierto ML, Gentilcore G, Stroncek DF, Casula M, Sini MC, Palla M, Mozzillo N, Ascierto PA (2009) Main roads to melanoma. J Transl Med 7(86)
23. Sekulic A, Jr Haluska P, Miller AJ, Genebriera De Lamo J, Ejadi S, Pulido JS, Salomao DR, Thorland EC, Vile RG, Swanson DL, Pockaj BA, Laman SD, Pittelkow MR, Markovic SN, Melanoma Study Group of Mayo Clinic Cancer Center (2008) Malignant melanoma in the 21st century: the emerging molecular landscape. Mayo Clin Proc 83:825–846
24. Bishop DT, Demenais F, Iles MM et al (2009) Genome-wide association study identifies three loci associated with melanoma risk. Nat Genet 41(8):920–925
25. Han J, Kraft P, Nan H, Guo Q, Chen C, Qureshi A, Hankinson SE, Hu FB, Duffy DL, Zhao ZZ, Martin NG, Montgomery GW, Hayward NK, Thomas G, Hoover RN, Chanock S, Hunter DJ (2008) A genome-wide association study identifies novel alleles associated with hair color and skin pigmentation. PLoS Genet 4(5):e1000074

26. Gudbjartsson DF, Sulem P, Stacey SN et al (2008) ASIP and TYR pigmentation variants associate with cutaneous melanoma and basal cell carcinoma. Nat Genet 40:886–891
27. Falchi M, Bataille V, Hayward NK, Duffy DL, Bishop JA, Pastinen T, Cervino A, Zhao ZZ, Deloukas P, Soranzo N, Elder DE, Barrett JH, Martin NG, Bishop DT, Montgomery GW, Spector TD (2009) Genome-wide association study identifies variants at 9p21 and 22q13 associated with development of cutaneous nevi. Nat Genet 41(8):915–919
28. Bataille V, Bishop JA, Sasieni P, Swerdlow AJ, Pinney E, Griffiths K, Cuzick J (1996) Risk of cutaneous melanoma in relation to the numbers, types and sites of naevi: a case-control study. Br J Cancer 73:1605–1611
29. Chang YM, Newton-Bishop JA, Bishop DT, Armstrong BK, Bataille V, Bergman W, Berwick M, Bracci PM, Elwood JM, Ernstoff MS, Green AC, Gruis NA, Holly EA, Ingvar C, Kanetsky PA, Karagas MR, Le Marchand L, Mackie RM, Olsson H, Østerlind A, Rebbeck TR, Reich K, Sasieni P, Siskind V, Swerdlow AJ, Titus-Ernstoff L, Zens MS, Ziegler A, Barrett JH (2009) A pooled analysis of melanocytic nevus phenotype and the risk of cutaneous melanoma at different latitudes. Int J Cancer 124:420–428
30. Hansson J (2008) Familial melanoma. Surg Clin North Am 88:897–916, viii
31. Platz A, Ringborg U, Hansson J (2000) Hereditary cutaneous melanoma. Semin Cancer Biol 10:319–326
32. Smalley KS (2010) Understanding melanoma signaling networks as the basis for molecular targeted therapy. J Invest Dermatol 130:28–37
33. Kong Y, Kumar SM, Xu X (2010) Molecular pathogenesis of sporadic melanoma and melanoma-initiating cells. Arch Pathol Lab Med 134:1740–1749
34. Pollock PM, Harper UL, Hansen KS, Yudt LM, Stark M, Robbins CM, Moses TY, Hostetter G, Wagner U, Kakareka J, Salem G, Pohida T, Heenan P, Duray P, Kallioniemi O, Hayward NK, Trent JM, Meltzer PS (2003) High frequency of BRAF mutations in nevi. Nat Genet 33:19–20
35. Puzanov I, Flaherty KT (2010) Targeted molecular therapy in melanoma. Semin Cutan Med Surg 29:196–201
36. Wan PT, Garnett MJ, Roe SM, Niculescu-Duvaz D, Good VM, Jones CM, Marshall CJ, Springer CJ, Barford D, Marais R, Cancer Genome Project (2004) Mechanism of activation of the RAF-ERK signaling pathway by oncogenic mutations of B-RAF. Cell 116:855–867
37. Benbow U, Tower GB, Wyatt CA, Buttice G, Brinckerhoff CE (2002) High levels of MMP-1 expression in the absence of the 2G single nucleotide polymorphism is mediated by p38 and ERK1/2 mitogen-activated protein kinases in VMM5 melanoma cells. J Cell Biochem 86:307–319
38. Cartlidge RA, Thomas GR, Cagnol S, Jong KA, Molton SA, Finch AJ, McMahon M (2008) Oncogenic BRAF (V600E) inhibits BIM expression to promote melanoma cell survival. Pigment Cell Melanoma Res 21:534–544
39. Eisenmann KM, VanBrocklin MW, Staffend NA, Kitchen SM, Koo HM (2003) Mitogen-activated protein kinase pathway-dependent tumor-specific survival signaling in melanoma cells through inactivation of the proapoptotic protein bad. Cancer Res 63:8330–8337
40. Huntington JT, Shields JM, Der CJ, Wyatt CA, Benbow U, Slingluff CL Jr, Brinckerhoff CE (2004) Overexpression of collagenase 1 (MMP-1) is mediated by the ERK pathway in invasive melanoma cells: role of BRAF mutation and fibroblast growth factor signaling. J Biol Chem 279:33168–33176
41. Kono M, Dunn IS, Durda PJ, Butera D, Rose LB, Haggerty TJ, Benson EM, Kurnick JT (2006) Role of the mitogen-activated protein kinase signaling pathway in the regulation of human melanocytic antigen expression. Mol Cancer Res 4:779–792
42. Kumar SM, Yu H, Edwards R, Chen L, Kazianis S, Brafford P, Acs G, Herlyn M, Xu X (2007) Mutant V600E BRAF increases hypoxia inducible factor-1alpha expression in melanoma. Cancer Res 67:3177–3184
43. Sharma A, Tran MA, Liang S, Sharma AK, Amin S, Smith CD, Dong C, Robertson GP (2006) Targeting mitogen-activated protein kinase/extracellular signal-regulated kinase

kinase in the mutant (V600E) B-Raf signaling cascade effectively inhibits melanoma lung metastases. Cancer Res 66:8200–8209
44. Sharma A, Trivedi NR, Zimmerman MA, Tuveson DA, Smith CD, Robertson GP (2005) Mutant V599EB-Raf regulates growth and vascular development of malignant melanoma tumors. Cancer Res 65:2412–2421
45. Soengas MS, Lowe SW (2003) Apoptosis and melanoma chemoresistance. Oncogene 22:3138–3151
46. Sumimoto H, Imabayashi F, Iwata T, Kawakami Y (2006) The BRAF-MAPK signaling pathway is essential for cancer-immune evasion in human melanoma cells. J Exp Med 203:1651–1656
47. Woods D, Cherwinski H, Venetsanakos E, Bhat A, Gysin S, Humbert M, Bray PF, Saylor VL, McMahon M (2001) Induction of beta3-integrin gene expression by sustained activation of the Ras-regulated Raf-MEK-extracellular signal-regulated kinase signaling pathway. Mol Cell Biol 21:3192–3205
48. Zhang XD, Borrow JM, Zhang XY, Nguyen T, Hersey P (2003) Activation of ERK1/2 protects melanoma cells from TRAIL-induced apoptosis by inhibiting Smac/DIABLO release from mitochondria. Oncogene 22:2869–2881
49. Luke JJ, Hodi FS (2013) The oncologist 18:717–725
50. Tsai J, Lee JT, Wang W et al (2008) Discovery of a selective inhibitor of oncogenic B-Raf kinase with potent antimelanoma activity. Proc Natl Acad Sci U S A 105:3041–3046
51. Koch WH (2004) Technology platforms for pharmacogenomic diagnostic assays. Nat Rev Drug Discov 3:749–761
52. Busam KJ, Hedva C, Pulitzer M, von Deimling A, Jungbluth AA (2013) Am J Surg Pathol 37:413–420
53. Viros A, Fridlyand J, Bauer J, Lasithiotakis K, Garbe C, Pinkel D, Bastian BC (2008) Improving melanoma classification by integrating genetic and morphologic features. PLoS Med 5(6):e120
54. Yarden Y, Kuang WJ, Yang-Feng T, Coussens L, Munemitsu S, Dull TJ, Chen E, Schlessinger J (1987) Human proto-oncogene c-kit: a new cell surface receptor tyrosine kinase for an unidentified ligand. EMBO J 6:3341–3351
55. Woodman SE, Davies MA (2010) Targeting KIT in melanoma: a paradigm of molecular medicine and targeted therapeutics. Biochem Pharmacol 80:568–574
56. Flaherty KT, Hodi FS, Bastian BC (2010) Mutation-driven drug development in melanoma. Curr Opin Oncol 22:178–183
57. Antonescu CR, Busam KJ, Francone TD, Wong GC, Guo T, Agaram NP, Besmer P, Jungbluth A, Gimbel M, Chen CT, Veach D, Clarkson BD, Paty PB, Weiser MR (2007) L576P KIT mutation in anal melanomas correlates with KIT protein expression and is sensitive to specific kinase inhibition. Int J Cancer 121:257–264
58. Ashida A, Takata M, Murata H, Kido K, Saida T (2009) Pathological activation of KIT in metastatic tumors of acral and mucosal melanomas. Int J Cancer 124:862–868
59. Beadling C, Jacobson-Dunlop E, Hodi FS, Le C, Warrick A, Patterson J, Town A, Harlow A, Cruz F 3rd, Azar S, Rubin BP, Muller S, West R, Heinrich MC, Corless CL (2008) KIT gene mutations and copy number in melanoma subtypes. Clin Cancer Res 14:6821–6828
60. Curtin JA, Busam K, Pinkel D, Bastian BC (2006) Somatic activation of KIT in distinct subtypes of melanoma. J Clin Oncol 24:4340–4346
61. Rivera RS, Nagatsuka H, Gunduz M, Cengiz B, Gunduz E, Siar CH, Tsujigiwa H, Tamamura R, Han KN, Nagai N (2008) C-kit protein expression correlated with activating mutations in KIT gene in oral mucosal melanoma. Virchows Arch 452:27–32
62. Smalley KS, Sondak VK, Weber JS (2009) c-KIT signaling as the driving oncogenic event in sub-groups of melanomas. Histol Histopathol 24:643–650
63. Lennartsson J, Blume-Jensen P, Hermanson M, Ponten E, Carlberg M, Ronnstrand L (1999) Phosphorylation of Shc by Src family kinases is necessary for stem cell factor

receptor/c-kit mediated activation of the Ras/MAP kinase pathway and c-fos induction. Oncogene 18:5546–5553

64. Mol CD, Dougan DR, Schneider TR, Skene RJ, Kraus ML, Scheibe DN, Snell GP, Zou H, Sang BC, Wilson KP (2004) Structural basis for the autoinhibition and STI-571 inhibition of c-Kit tyrosine kinase. J Biol Chem 279:31655–31663
65. Hodi FS, Friedlander P, Corless CL, Heinrich MC, Mac Rae S, Kruse A, Jagannathan J, Van den Abbeele AD, Velazquez EF, Demetri GD, Fisher DE (2008) Major response to imatinib mesylate in KIT-mutated melanoma. J Clin Oncol 26:2046–2051
66. Lutzky J, Bauer J, Bastian BC (2008) Dose-dependent, complete response to imatinib of a metastatic mucosal melanoma with a K642E KIT mutation. Pigment Cell Melanoma Res 21:492–493
67. Eton O, Billings L, Kim K et al (2004) Phase II trial of imatinib mesylate (STI-571) in metastatic melanoma (MM) [abstract]. J Clin Oncol 22(14S):7528
68. Platz A, Egyhazi S, Ringborg U, Hansson J (2008) Human cutaneous melanoma; a review of NRAS and BRAF mutation frequencies in relation to histogenetic subclass and body site. Mol Oncol 1:395–405
69. Margolin KA, Moon J, Flaherty LE et al (2010) Randomized phase II trial of sorafenib (SO) with temsirolimus (TEM) or tipifarnib (TIPI) in metastatic melanoma: Southwest Oncology Group Trial S0438 [abstract]. J Clin Oncol 28(15s):7528
70. Kaplan FM, Shao Y, Mayberry MM, Aplin AE (2011) Hyperactivation of MEK-ERK1/2 signaling and resistance to apoptosis induced by the oncogenic B-RAF inhibitor, PLX4720, in mutant N-RAS melanoma cells. Oncogene 30:366–371
71. Nazarian R, Shi H, Wang Q, Kong X, Koya RC, Lee H, Chen Z, Lee MK, Attar N, Sazegar H, Chodon T, Nelson SF, McArthur G, Sosman JA, Ribas A, Lo RS (2010) Melanomas acquire resistance to B-RAF(V600E) inhibition by RTK or N-RAS upregulation. Nature 468:973–977
72. Koprowski H, Herlyn M, Balaban G, Parmiter A, Ross A, Nowell P (1985) Expression of the receptor for epidermal growth factor correlates with increased dosage of chromosome 7 in malignant melanoma. Somat Cell Mol Genet 11:297–302
73. Rakosy Z, Vizkeleti L, Ecsedi S et al (2007) EGFR gene copy number alterations in primary cutaneous malignant melanomas are associated with poor prognosis. Int J Cancer 121(8):1729–1737
74. Bastian BC, Olshen AB, LeBoit PE, Pinkel D (2003) Classifying melanocytic tumors based on DNA copy number changes. Am J Pathol 163(5):1765–1770
75. Bastian BC, LeBoit PE, Hamm H, Brocker EB, Pinkel D (1998) Chromosomal gains and losses in primary cutaneous melanomas detected by comparative genomic hybridization. Cancer Res 58:2170–2175
76. Balazs M, Adam Z, Treszl A, Begany A, Hunyadi J, Adany R (2001) Chromosomal imbalances in primary and metastatic melanomas revealed by comparative genomic hybridization. Cytometry 46:222–232
77. Namiki T, Yanagawa S, Izumo T, Ishikawa M, Tachibana M, Kawakami Y, Yokozeki H, Nishioka K, Kaneko Y (2005) Genomic alterations in primary cutaneous melanomas detected by metaphase comparative genomic hybridization with laser capture or manual microdissection: 6p gains may predict poor outcome. Cancer Genet Cytogenet 157(1):1–11
78. Bastian BC, Xiong J, Frieden IJ, Williams ML, Chou P, Busam K, Pinkel D, LeBoit PE (2002) Genetic changes in neoplasms arising in congenital melanocytic nevi: differences between nodular proliferations and melanomas. Am J Pathol 161:1163–1169
79. Bastian BC, Wesselmann U, Pinkel D, Leboit PE (1999) Molecular cytogenetic analysis of Spitz nevi shows clear differences to melanoma. J Invest Dermatol 113:1065–1069
80. Bastian BC (2003) Understanding the progression of melanocytic neoplasia using genomic analysis: from fields to cancer. Oncogene 22:3081–3086
81. Bastian BC, Kashani-Sabet M, Hamm H, Godfrey T, Moore DH 2nd, Bröcker EB, LeBoit PE, Pinkel D (2000) Gene amplifications characterize acral melanoma and permit the detection of occult tumor cells in the surrounding skin. Cancer Res 60:1968–1973

82. Morey AL, Murali R, McCarthy SW, Mann GJ, Scolyer RA (2009) Diagnosis of cutaneous melanocytic tumours by four-colour fluorescence in situ hybridisation. Pathology 41:383–387
83. Gaiser T, Kutzner H, Palmedo G, Siegelin MD, Wiesner T, Bruckner T, Hartschuh W, Enk AH, Becker MR (2010) Classifying ambiguous melanocytic lesions with FISH and correlation with clinical long-term follow up. Mod Pathol 23:413–419
84. Vergier B, Prochazkova-Carlotti M, de la Fouchardiere A, Cerroni L, Massi D, De Giorgi V, Bailly C, Wesselmann U, Karlseladze A, Avril MF, Jouary T, Merlio JP (2011) Fluorescence in situ hybridization, a diagnostic aid in ambiguous melanocytic tumors: European study of 113 cases. Mod Pathol 24:613–623
85. Gerami P, Wass A, Mafee M, Fang Y, Pulitzer MP, Busam KJ (2009) Fluorescence in situ hybridization for distinguishing nevoid melanomas from mitotically active nevi. Am J Surg Pathol 33:1783–1788
86. Pouryazdanparast P, Newman M, Mafee M, Haghighat Z, Guitart J, Gerami P (2009) Distinguishing epithelioid blue nevus from blue nevus-like cutaneous melanoma metastasis using fluorescence in situ hybridization. Am J Surg Pathol 33:1396–1400
87. Dalton SR, Gerami P, Kolaitis NA, Charzan S, Werling R, LeBoit PE, Bastian BC (2010) Use of fluorescence in situ hybridization (FISH) to distinguish intranodal nevus from metastatic melanoma. Am J Surg Pathol 34:231–237
88. Gerami P, Barnhill RL, Beilfuss BA, LeBoit P, Schneider P, Guitart J (2010) Superficial melanocytic neoplasms with pagetoid melanocytosis: a study of interobserver concordance and correlation with FISH. Am J Surg Pathol 34:816–821
89. Newman MD, Lertsburapa T, Mirzabeigi M, Mafee M, Guitart J, Gerami P (2009) Fluorescence in situ hybridization as a tool for microstaging in malignant melanoma. Mod Pathol 22:989–995
90. Gould Rothberg BE, Bracken MB, Rimm DL (2009) Tissue biomarkers for prognosis in cutaneous melanoma: a systematic review and meta-analysis. J Natl Cancer Inst 101:452–474
91. Gould Rothberg BE, Rimm DL (2010) Biomarkers: the useful and the not so useful – an assessment of molecular prognostic markers for cutaneous melanoma. J Invest Dermatol 130:1971–1987
92. Gimotty PA, Guerry D (2010) Prognostication in thin cutaneous melanomas. Arch Pathol Lab Med 134:1758–1763
93. Denicourt C, Saenz CC, Datnow B, Cui XS, Dowdy SF (2007) Relocalized p27Kip1 tumor suppressor functions as a cytoplasmic metastatic oncogene in melanoma. Cancer Res 67:9238–9243
94. Briese J, Schulte HM, Bamberger CM, Loning T, Bamberger AM (2006) Expression pattern of osteopontin in endometrial carcinoma: correlation with expression of the adhesion molecule CEACAM1. Int J Gynecol Pathol 25:161–169
95. Gavert N, Sheffer M, Raveh S, Spaderna S, Shtutman M, Brabletz T, Barany F, Paty P, Notterman D, Domany E, Ben-Ze'ev A (2007) Expression of L1-CAM and ADAM10 in human colon cancer cells induces metastasis. Cancer Res 67:7703–7712
96. Thies A, Moll I, Berger J, Wagener C, Brümmer J, Schulze HJ, Brunner G, Schumacher U (2002) CEACAM1 expression in cutaneous malignant melanoma predicts the development of metastatic disease. J Clin Oncol 20:2530–2536
97. Watson-Hurst K, Becker D (2006) The role of N-cadherin, MCAM and beta3 integrin in melanoma progression, proliferation, migration and invasion. Cancer Biol Ther 5:1375–1382
98. Bornstein P, Sage EH (2002) Matricellular proteins: extracellular modulators of cell function. Curr Opin Cell Biol 14:608–616
99. Dessinioti C, Antoniou C, Katsambas A, Stratigos AJ (2010) Basal cell carcinoma: what's new under the sun. Photochem Photobiol 86:481–491
100. Gallagher RP, Hill GB, Bajdik CD, Fincham S, Coldman AJ, McLean DI, Threlfall WJ (1995) Sunlight exposure, pigmentary factors, and risk of nonmelanocytic skin cancer. I. Basal cell carcinoma. Arch Dermatol 131:157–163
101. Miller SJ (1991) Biology of basal cell carcinoma (Part I). J Am Acad Dermatol 24:1–13

102. Oberyszyn TM (2008) Non-melanoma skin cancer: importance of gender, immunosuppressive status and vitamin D. Cancer Lett 261:127–136
103. Epstein EH (2008) Basal cell carcinomas: attack of the hedgehog. Nat Rev Cancer 8:743–754
104. Bodak N, Queille S, Avril MF, Bouadjar B, Drougard C, Sarasin A, Daya-Grosjean L (1999) High levels of patched gene mutations in basal-cell carcinomas from patients with xeroderma pigmentosum. Proc Natl Acad Sci U S A 96:5117–5122
105. Tilli CM, Van Steensel MA, Krekels GA, Neumann HA, Ramaekers FC (2005) Molecular aetiology and pathogenesis of basal cell carcinoma. Br J Dermatol 152:1108–1124
106. Hanada K, Ishikawa H, Tamai K, Hashimoto I, Sato K (1991) Expression of glutathione S-transferase-pi in malignant skin tumors. J Dermatol Sci 2:18–23
107. Saldanha G, Fletcher A, Slater DN (2003) Basal cell carcinoma: a dermatopathological and molecular biological update. Br J Dermatol 148:195–202
108. Reifenberger J, Wolter M, Knobbe CB, Köhler B, Schönicke A, Scharwächter C, Kumar K, Blaschke B, Ruzicka T, Reifenberger G (2005) Somatic mutations in the PTCH, SMOH, SUFUH and TP53 genes in sporadic basal cell carcinomas. Br J Dermatol 152:43–51
109. Lindstrom E, Shimokawa T, Toftgard R, Zaphiropoulos PG (2006) PTCH mutations: distribution and analyses. Hum Mutat 27:215–219
110. Peukert S, Miller-Moslin K (2010) Small-molecule inhibitors of the hedgehog signaling pathway as cancer therapeutics. ChemMedChem 5:500–512
111. O'Driscoll L, McMorrow J, Doolan P, McKiernan E, Mehta JP, Ryan E, Gammell P, Joyce H, O'Donovan N, Walsh N, Clynes M (2006) Investigation of the molecular profile of basal cell carcinoma using whole genome microarrays. Mol Cancer 5:74
112. Hatta N, Hirano T, Kimura T, Hashimoto K, Mehregan DR, Ansai S, Takehara K, Takata M (2005) Molecular diagnosis of basal cell carcinoma and other basaloid cell neoplasms of the skin by the quantification of Gli1 transcript levels. J Cutan Pathol 32:131–136
113. Jimeno A, Feldmann G, Suarez-Gauthier A, Rasheed Z, Solomon A, Zou GM, Rubio-Viqueira B, García-García E, López-Ríos F, Matsui W, Maitra A, Hidalgo M (2009) A direct pancreatic cancer xenograft model as a platform for cancer stem cell therapeutic development. Mol Cancer Ther 8:310–314
114. Mueller MT, Hermann PC, Witthauer J, Rubio-Viqueira B, Leicht SF, Huber S, Ellwart JW, Mustafa M, Bartenstein P, D'Haese JG, Schoenberg MH, Berger F, Jauch KW, Hidalgo M, Heeschen C (2009) Combined targeted treatment to eliminate tumorigenic cancer stem cells in human pancreatic cancer. Gastroenterology 137:1102–1113
115. Von Hoff DD, LoRusso PM, Rudin CM, Reddy JC, Yauch RL, Tibes R, Weiss GJ, Borad MJ, Hann CL, Brahmer JR, Mackey HM, Lum BL, Darbonne WC, Marsters JC Jr, de Sauvage FJ, Low JA (2009) Inhibition of the hedgehog pathway in advanced basal-cell carcinoma. N Engl J Med 361:1164–1172
116. Dose finding and safety of oral LDE225 in patients with advanced solid tumors 2010. http://clinicaltrials.gov/ct2/show/NCT00880308. Accessed 25 July 2013
117. Hosoya T, Arai MA, Koyano T, Kowithayakorn T, Ishibashi M (2008) Naturally occurring small-molecule inhibitors of hedgehog/GLI-mediated transcription. Chembiochem 9:1082–1092
118. Mahindroo N, Connelly MC, Punchihewa C, Kimura H, Smeltzer MP, Wu S, Fujii N (2009) Structure-activity relationships and cancer-cell selective toxicity of novel inhibitors of glioma-associated oncogene homologue 1 (Gli1) mediated transcription. J Med Chem 52:4277–4287
119. Lacour JP (2002) Carcinogenesis of basal cell carcinomas: genetics and molecular mechanisms. Br J Dermatol 146(Suppl 61):17–19
120. Hussein MR (2005) Ultraviolet radiation and skin cancer: molecular mechanisms. J Cutan Pathol 32:191–205
121. Howell BG, Solish N, Lu C, Watanabe H, Mamelak AJ, Freed I, Wang B, Sauder DN (2005) Microarray profiles of human basal cell carcinoma: insights into tumor growth and behavior. J Dermatol Sci 39(1):39–51

122. Boukamp P (2005) Non-melanoma skin cancer: what drives tumor development and progression? Carcinogenesis 26:1657–1667
123. Lazar AJF, Murphy GF (2010) The skin. In: Kumar VM, Abul K, Abbas M, Nelson Fausto M, Jon C, Aster M (eds) Robbins and Cotran pathologic basis of disease, 8th edn. Elsevier, Philadelphia, pp 1178–1181
124. Harwood CA, Proby CM (2002) Human papillomaviruses and non-melanoma skin cancer. Curr Opin Infect Dis 15:101–114
125. Rubin AI, Chen EH, Ratner D (2005) Basal-cell carcinoma. N Engl J Med 353:2262–2269
126. Benjamin CL, Melnikova VO, Ananthaswamy HN (2008) P53 protein and pathogenesis of melanoma and nonmelanoma skin cancer. Adv Exp Med Biol 624:265–282
127. Owens DM (2007) p53, chemokines, and squamous cell carcinoma. J Clin Invest 117:1752–1755
128. Jensen V, Prasad AR, Smith A, Raju M, Wendel CS, Schmelz M, Leyva W, Warneke J, Krouse RS (2010) Prognostic criteria for squamous cell cancer of the skin. J Surg Res 159:509–516
129. Meyer T, Arndt R, Christophers E, Nindl I, Stockfleth E (2001) Importance of human papillomaviruses for the development of skin cancer. Cancer Detect Prev 25:533–547
130. Ke H, Harris R, Coloff JL, Jin JY, Leshin B, Miliani de Marval P, Tao S, Rathmell JC, Hall RP, Zhang JY (2010) The c-Jun NH2-terminal kinase 2 plays a dominant role in human epidermal neoplasia. Cancer Res 70:3080–3088
131. Chakraborty S, Swanson BJ, Bonthu N, Batra SK (2010) Aberrant upregulation of MUC4 mucin expression in cutaneous condyloma acuminatum and squamous cell carcinoma suggests a potential role in the diagnosis and therapy of skin diseases. J Clin Pathol 63:579–584
132. Chou TH, Liang CH (2009) The molecular effects of aloe-emodin (AE)/liposome-AE on human nonmelanoma skin cancer cells and skin permeation. Chem Res Toxicol 22:2017–2028
133. Feng H, Shuda M, Chang Y, Moore PS (2008) Clonal integration of a polyomavirus in human Merkel cell carcinoma. Science 319:1096–1100
134. Shuda M, Feng H, Kwun HJ, Chang Y, Moore PS (2008) T antigen mutations are a human tumor-specific signature for Merkel cell polyomavirus. Proc Natl Acad Sci U S A 105:16272–16277
135. Bhatia K, Goedert JJ, Modali R, Preiss L, Ayers LW (2010) Merkel cell carcinoma subgroups by Merkel cell polyomavirus DNA relative abundance and oncogene expression. Int J Cancer 126(9):2240–2246
136. Sihto H, Kukko H, Koljonen V, Sankila R, Bohling T, Joensuu H (2009) Clinical factors associated with Merkel cell polyomavirus infection in Merkel cell carcinoma. J Natl Cancer Inst 101:938–945
137. Garneski KM, Warcola AH, Feng Q, Kiviat NB, Leonard JH, Nghiem P (2009) Merkel cell polyomavirus is more frequently present in North American than Australian Merkel cell carcinoma tumors. J Invest Dermatol 129:246–248
138. Becker JC, Houben R, Ugurel S, Trefzer U, Pfohler C, Schrama D (2009) MC polyomavirus is frequently present in Merkel cell carcinoma of European patients. J Invest Dermatol 129:248–250

Chapter 17
Molecular Diagnostics of Lymphoid Neoplasms

Deniz Peker, Jianguo Tao, and Ling Zhang

Contents

Abstract According to 2008 World Health Organization (WHO) Classification of Tumors of Hematopoietic and Lymphoid Tissue, lymphoid neoplasms are divided into two, mature and immature (precursors), forms including mature B and T/NK cell leukemia/lymphomas and B and T-lymphoblastic leukemia/lymphomas (B-ALL/LBL, T-ALL/LBL). Nowadays a variety of molecular methods are introduced for the modern classification of lymphoid neoplasm system. Although morphological characteristics remain the cornerstone of the evaluation of lymphoid neoplasm, ancillary studies e.g. immunophenotyping and PCR study for T- and B-cell gene rearrangements are routinely implicated in daily service. Different from

D. Peker • J. Tao • L. Zhang, M.D. (✉)
Department of Pathology and Cell Biology, University of South Florida College of Medicine, 12901 Bruce B. Downs Blvd, Tampa, FL 33612, USA

Department of Hematopathology and Laboratory Medicine, Moffitt Cancer Center & Research Institute, 12902 Magnolia Drive, Tampa, FL 33612, USA
e-mail: ling.zhang@moffitt.org

D. Coppola (ed.), *Molecular Pathology and Diagnostics of Cancer*, Cancer Growth and Progression 16, DOI 10.1007/978-94-007-7192-5_17,

myeloid neoplasms, the application of molecular/genetic diagnosis and subclassification of lymphoid neoplasm are mainly limited in B-ALL. There are few known protooncogenes or cytogenetic abnormalities in the certain T/NK or B lymphoid malignancies. The chapter focuses on common molecular diagnostic approaches and molecules that implicated in therapeutic strategies, predicting prognosis and monitoring minimal residual disease.

Keywords Lymphoid malignancy • Cytogenetics • Molecular • Gene rearrangement • Diagnostic and prognostic implications • Novel molecular techniques

Abbreviations

ABC	Activated B cell-like type
ALK	Anaplastic large cell kinase
ALL	Acute lymphoblastic leukemias
ALTCL	Anaplastic large T cell lymphoma
ATM	Ataxia telangiectasia mutated gene
B-ALL	B-lymphoblastic leukemia/lymphoma
BL	Burkitt lymphoma
B-PLL	B-cell prolymphocytic leukemia
CDK6	Cyclin dependent kinase 6 gene
CLL/SLL	Chronic lymphocytic leukemia/small lymphocytic lymphoma
CNS	Central nervous system
CRA	Common region of amplification
DAPK1	Death-associated protein kinase 1
DLBCL	Diffuse large B-cell lymphoma
FFPE	Formalin-fixed and paraffin-embedded
FISH	Fluorescence in situ hybridization
FNA	Fine needle aspirate
GCB	Germinal center B-cell like
iAMP21	Intrachromosomal amplification of chromosome 21
LPL	Lymphoplasmacytic lymphoma
M-bcr	Major breakpoint cluster region
m-bcr	"minor" breakpoint cluster region
MF	Mycosis fungoides
MLPA	Multiplex ligation-dependent probe amplification
MRD	Minimal residual disease
NK	Natural killer
Non-GCB	Non-germinal center B-cell like
NPM	Nucleophosmin gene
PCR	Polymerase Chain Reaction
PTCL, NOS	Peripheral T cell lymphoma, not otherwise specified
RT-PCR	Reverse Polymerase Chain Reaction

SHM	Somatic hypermutation
SMZL	Splenic marginal zone lymphoma
SNP	Single Nucleotide Polymorphism Array
T-ALL	T-lymphoblastic leukemia/lymphoma
TCR	T cell gene rearrangement
TKI	Tyrosine kinase inhibitor
UDP	Uniparental disomy
WHO	World Health Organization

17.1 Introduction

Lymphoid neoplasms are clonal proliferation of mature or immature B cells, T cells and natural killer (NK) cells. According to 2008 World Health Organization (WHO) classification of hematopoietic and lymphoid neoplasms precursor T and B lymphoid neoplasms, mature B-cell neoplasms, mature T-cell and NK-cell neoplasms, Hodgkin lymphomas and immunodeficiency-associated lymphoproliferative disorders are defined in this group [1]. The classical diagnostic methods including histomorphology and immunophenotypic analysis have been widely used in diagnosis of lymphoid malignancies. In recent years, the advances in molecular techniques lead a better understanding of the role of genetic defects in the pathogenesis of neoplastic processes as a result of which molecular testing has become an important part of routine diagnostics including many leukemias and lymphomas. This chapter will address the key molecular tests used in diagnosis of lymphoid neoplasms as well as promising future diagnostic approaches.

17.2 Diagnostic Algorithms

A complete morphologic examination of involved tissues or body sites is the crucial first step of histopathologic evaluation of lymphoid neoplasms. A collection of substantial sample from fine needle aspirate (FNA), fine needle core biopsy or small resection biopsy is necessary in help of a diagnosis of lymphoid neoplasms. However, excisional biopsy of lymph node or extranodal tissue is recommended to more accurately assess the disease evolution or progression, to further subclassify lymphoid neoplasms as well as to identify composite neoplasms. A good quality of histology and staining technique prevents from misinterpretation, while a careful cytomorphologic examination of any single provided slide would avoid "tunnel-vision" or misdiagnosis.

Immunophenotyping refers to the technique of identifying the surface or cytoplasmic molecules or antigen that present in lymphoid cells. The three methods are commonly used for immunophenotyping including immunofluorescence, flow cytometry and immunohistochemistry. Using immunophenotyping strategy is able to identify the majority of lymphoma/leukemias, so as to subclassify them. Nevertheless, it might generally not useful in distinguishing some low grade lymphomas from high grade ones, predicting clinical course or prognostic outcome. In addition to morphologic and immunophenotypic evaluation, molecular analysis of lymphoid neoplasms has become more important in classification of certain T/NK or B-cell lymphomas/leukemias with implication of therapeutic strategies, predicting disease prognosis and monitoring minimal residual disease (MRD). The most common use of molecular techniques in lymphoid malignancies can be divided into three categories: (1) detection of karyotypic abnormalities including gain or loss of chromosome(s), chromosomal translocations, deletions, and insertions some of which have shown to be recurrent in certain neoplasms; (2) detection of individual mutations associated with the malignancy; and (3) defining clonality in lymphomas and leukemias based on gene rearrangements on T and B cells. 2008 WHO classification and the most recent studies indicate that the molecular and genetic diagnostic tools seem more applicable as a diagnostic tool in precursor B-cell lymphoid neoplasms, particularly with regard to defined recurrent cytogenetic abnormalities [1–6].

B-lymphoblastic leukemia/lymphoma (B-ALL) commonly involves peripheral blood and bone marrow while T- lymphoblastic leukemia/lymphoma (T-ALL) is usually tissue-based, most common in the mediastinum. For the majority of cases, morphologic and phenotypic evaluation is often sufficient for diagnosis of ALL and making the distinction between B-ALL and T-ALL. However, further cytogenetic and/or molecular testing is required for further subclassification of B-ALL. Furthermore, some certain cytogenetic abnormalities are of importance in terms of prognosis and rational therapy. Mature lymphoid neoplasms often involve the lymphoid tissue as well as other body sites including visceral organs, skin and brain. Although for many lymphomas, morphologic and phenotypic assessment is usually sufficient to render a diagnosis and molecular testing might not be demanded, clonality studies has been widely used especially to differentiate a neoplasm from a reactive process. It is clear that molecular techniques facilitate the diagnosis of difficult cases [7–11]. Molecular studies also allow further categorization of some lymphomas regarding the prognosis and tracking subsequent minimal residual disease (MRD) [12].

Nowadays molecular and genetic diagnosis has been, without a doubt, integrated into daily pathologic practice and play an important role in diagnostic algorithm to differentiate lymphoma/leukemia from the other reactive processes (Fig. 17.1).

17.2.1 Molecular Methods Commonly Used in Lymphoid Malignancies

17.2.1.1 Standard Chromosomal Analysis

Conventional karyotyping is one of standard chromosomal analyses that have been widely used in diagnosis of myeloid leukemias as well as lymphoid neoplasms. Discovery of the recurrent cytogenetic abnormality in Burkitt lymphoma with t(8; 14) and chronic myelogenous leukemia with t(9;22) in early 1960s. [13, 14], is

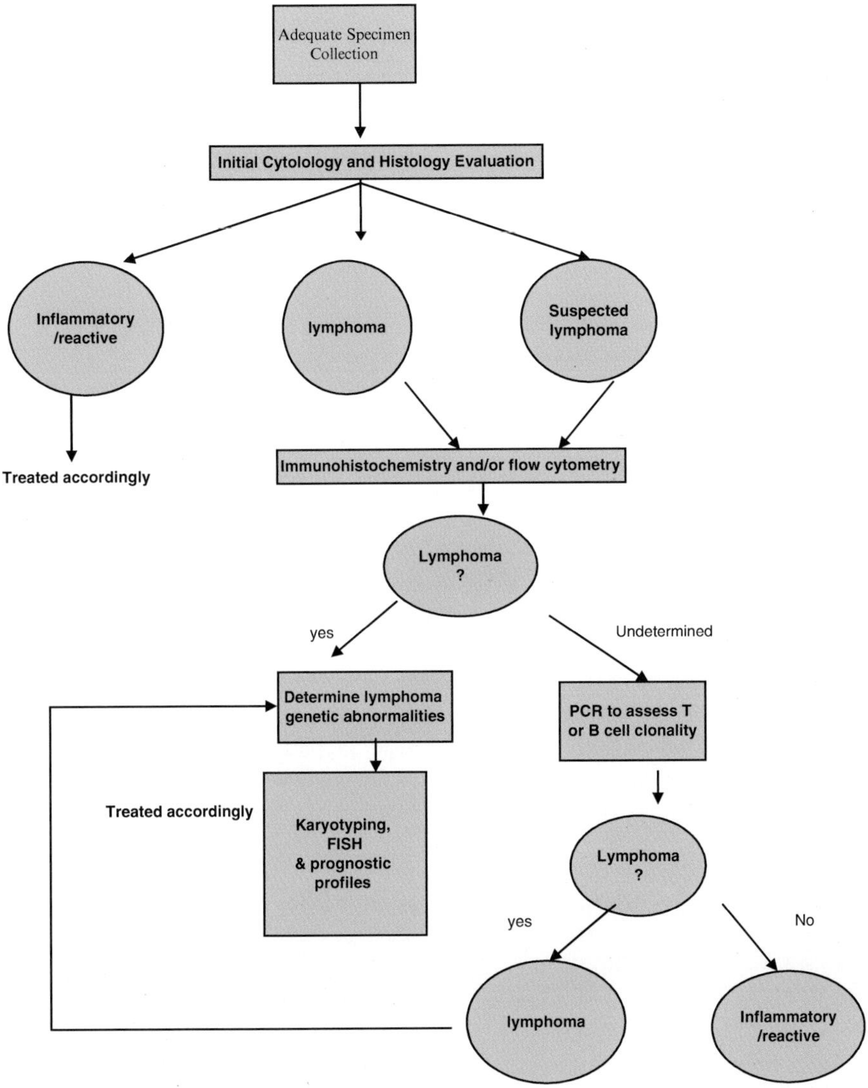

Fig. 17.1 The diagnostic algorithm for lymphoid malignancies commonly accepted in daily practice

followed by many chromosomal abnormalities described in lymphomas and leukemias. Up to date, certain precursor B lymphoid neoplasms, vast majority of the Burkitt lymphoma, mantle cell lymphoma, follicular lymphoma and a subset of marginal zone lymphomas are associated with recurrent translocations (Table 17.1) [1–3, 15, 16]. Diffuse large B cell lymphomas (DLBCL), can associate with single or multiple breakpoints and translocations, namely BCL6 at 3q and BCl-2 at 18q, "double or triple" hit lymphomas commonly involving *MYC* and *BCL2* and less

Table 17.1 The WHO classification of precursor lymphoid neoplasms

I. Precursor lymphoid neoplasms
B lymphoblastic leukemia/lymphoma, not otherwise specified (NOS)
B lymphoblastic leukemia/lymphoma, with recurrent genetic abnormalities
B lymphoblastic leukemia/lymphoma with t(9;22)(q34;q11.2); *BCR-ABL*
B lymphoblastic leukemia/lymphoma with t(v;11q23); *MLL* rearranged
B lymphoblastic leukemia/lymphoma with t(12;21)(p13;q22); *TEL-AML-1 (ETV6-RUNX1)*
B lymphoblastic leukemia/lymphoma with hyperdiploidy
B lymphoblastic leukemia/lymphoma with hypodiploidy (Hypodiploid ALL)
B lymphoblastic leukemia/lymphoma with t(5;14)(q31;q32); *IL3-IGH*
B lymphoblastic leukemia/lymphoma with t(1;19)(q23;p13.3); *E2A-PBX1(TCF3-PBX1)*
T lymphoblastic leukemia/lymphoma

frequently *BCL6* genes [17–20]. Nevertheless, only a minority of T cell lymphomas exhibit recurrent chromosomal translocations. Anaplastic large T cell lymphoma is a good example, often associated with t(2;5) involving *NPM1-ALK* gene fusion [21], though the other ALK partner genes also encountered.

Most cytogenetic abnormalities seen in lymphomas and leukemias are often detectable by conventional karyotyping by G-banding. Although it is considered to be the "gold standard" technique, some limitations prevent a wide use of this test, including the need to obtain a large volume of fresh tissue and rapid processing. Another problem encountered in cytogenetic testing is that the analysis requires high level of technical skills in culturing tissue, preparing the metaphase cells and analyzing complex karyograms which makes the method labor-intensive, expensive and time consuming [15].

17.2.1.2 Fluorescence In Situ Hybridization (FISH)

Fluorescence in situ hybridization (FISH) is widely used as an ancillary method in diagnosis of lymphomas and leukemias. It is applicable to cytospin preparations from fresh harvested tissue as well as formalin-fixed and paraffin-embedded (FFPE) tissue without requiring tissue culturing. Thus, FISH is a less complex and rapid molecular technique with shorter turnaround time. The main limitation of FISH is the probe specific testing only for specific abnormalities with no genome-wide analysis.

17.2.1.3 Polymerase Chain Reaction (PCR), Reverse Transcription-PCR (RT-PCR)

PCR tests are widely used in lymphomas and lymphoblastic leukemias for clonality analysis of the immunoglobulin genes and T cell receptors (TCR). The testing can be performed on either fresh tissues or FFPE materials. DNA or RNA materials are extracted from submitted specimen according to the study design. Quantitative

RT-PCR is also very useful in detecting of the chromosomal translocations that lead to the production of fusion mRNA transcripts. A good example of this fusion transcript and protein generation is cyclin D1-IgH resulting in mantle cell lymphoma [22]. An advantage of PCR in lymphoma and leukemias is that it enables to amplify the fusion transcript; therefore it is superior in detection of minimal residual disease (MRD). PCR analysis for clonality is particularly advantageous in certain circumstances; (1) if the tissue is limited (e.g. small needle biopsies or fine needle aspirations) for immunohistochemical analysis and/or flow cytometry cannot be performed (e.g. FFPE tissue); (2) some B cell lymphoma cells may lack surface light chain antigens so that clonality may be equivalent by flow cytometry. (3) Phenotypic clonality evaluation has not been established for T cell neoplasms, therefore, gene rearrangement studies are helpful determining T cell clonality; (4) differentiation of reactive hematogone response vs. residual/recurrent precursor lymphoid neoplasms with increased immature lymphoblasts [23–26]. On the other hand, there are some limitations when using PCR for diagnostic purposes. False positive gene rearrangement results can be observed especially when testing a small biopsy with small number of lymphocytes as well as various reactive and inflammatory conditions [27, 28]. Furthermore, some T cell lymphomas may have false immunoglobulin *(IG)* gene re-arrangement [28]. False negative results can also be seen mostly due to technical or biologic factors [29].

17.2.1.4 Single Nucleotide Polymorphism (SNP) Array

SNP array is the most recently introduced molecular method that can analyze the whole genome with higher resolution than the other techniques. An important advantage of SNP array is the ability to detect not only copy number changes but also the regions with loss of heterozygosity without DNA loss or gain. This indicates that the both alleles are homozygous and derived from one parent, "uniparental disomy" (UDP), which is important in certain lymphomas [30–32]. Regions of UDP may harbor one or more genes with inactivating mutations (classical tumor suppressor genes) and since both alleles will have the mutation, the Knudson two-hit rule is fulfilled [15]. The main problem with SNP array is the difficulty in distinguishing acquired abnormalities from polymorphism which may be resolved by comparing to the germline DNA from the same patient [33]. SNP is so far not the replacement of cytogenetics and FISH laboratory, however, it is usually ordered for those patients with normal karyotyping or FISH results when seeking a possible disease related genetic findings.

17.3 Precursor Lymphoid Neoplasms

Precursor lymphoid neoplasms, also termed acute lymphoblastic leukemias (ALL), are one of the most common hematopoietic malignancies affecting pediatric population and a major cause of co-morbidity in adult. The current WHO classification of ALL contains three main subgroups: (1) B-lymphoblastic leukemia/lymphoma (B-ALL), not otherwise specified, (2) B-ALL with recurrent cytogenetic abnormalities, and (3) T-lymphoblastic leukemia/lymphoma (T-ALL) [1] (Table 17.1). ALL is a greatly heterogeneous group of disorders with variety of associated genetic defects that have been defined recently or still unknown. The classical algorithm used in diagnosis of ALL includes a careful morphological examination of peripheral smear and/or bone marrow samples as well as involved tissue with appropriate phenotypic studies supported by relevant testing for karyotype analysis and molecular genetics. Cytogenetic abnormalities are seen in 60–80 % of ALL including recurrent genetic abnormalities.

17.3.1 B Lymphoblastic Leukemia/Lymphoma with Recurrent Genetic Abnormalities

This is a group of disease characterized by recurrent genetic abnormalities including chromosomal abnormalities and balanced translocations. The distinction of this B-ALL from other types is especially important as they have specific clinical and phenotypic features leading to important prognostic implications.

17.3.1.1 B Lymphoblastic Leukemia/Lymphoma with t(9;22)(q34;q11.2);BCR-ABL1

The Philadelphia (Ph) chromosome is the most common associated genetic anomaly in adult B-ALL, accounting for about 20–30 %. Only about 2–4 % of childhood leukemias harbor Ph chromosome. The lympho blasts have the translocation between the *BCR* gene on chromosome 22 and the *ABL* oncogene on chromosome 9 that creates the Ph chromosome. While the *ABL* breakpoint occurs in the same region (between exons a1 and a2) on chromosome 9, the *BCR* breakpoints on chromosome 22 can occur in two different regions. The m-bcr creates a fusion protein of 190 kDa (p190) and M-bcr results in a fusion protein of 210 kDa (p210) [34, 35]. The "minor" breakpoint cluster region (m-bcr) between exons 1 and 2 is present in vast majority of childhood Ph+ALL while a "major" breakpoint cluster region (M-bcr) spanning exons 12 to 16 is more common in adult Ph+ALL. The m-bcr creates a fusion protein of 190 kDa (p190) and M-bcr results in a fusion protein of 210 kDa (p210) [34, 35]. Phenotypically, Ph+B-ALL is typically CD10+, CD19+ and TdT+. The expression of myeloid antigens CD13 and CD33 is frequent. CD25 is highly associated with adult Ph+ALL [36].

Cytogenetics is still commonly used in detection of Ph chromosome. In cases of failed or normal cytogenetic results, FISH can be used as an alternative method. Quantitative RT-PCR is a rapid, accurate and sensitive method for the detection of *BCR/ABL* fusion transcripts. The advantage of test is to quantitatively track the copy number change of transcript before and after therapy. One major disadvantage is that this approach is highly specific and cooperating abnormalities cannot be simultaneously identified [37]. The presence of t(9;22) is a poorer prognostic factor in both children and adults. Combination of tyrosine kinase inhibitor (TKI) with established antileukemic agents is promising in management of these patients.

17.3.1.2 B Lymphoblastic Leukemia/Lymphoma with t(v;11q23); MLL Rearranged

This is a group of acute leukemias harboring translocation between *MLL* gene at band 11q23 and any of the fusion partners. MLL translocations generate a new chimeric gene, in which the NH2-terminal portion of MLL is fused to the COOH-terminal sequence from multiple different partners [38]. The common result of many of these rearrangements is the expression of a DNA-binding protein that recruits additional histone methyltransferases such as DOT1L and leads to ectopic histone H3 lysine 79-dimethylation [39, 40].

These lymphomas exhibit unique clinical and biologic feature. *MLL* translocation occurs up to 70 % of infant B-ALL and less frequently in older patients. Typically patients present with very high white blood cell counts and often central nervous system (CNS) involvement at diagnosis. A characteristic feature of ALL with *MLL* translocations, mostly t(4;11) ALL, is the absence of CD10 in pro-B blasts often expressing myeloid antigen CD15. The expression of chondroitin sulfate proteo-glycan neural-glial antigen 2 (NG2) is also typical in these leukemias. Many fusion genes have been described in ALL with *MLL* translocation. t(4;11)(q21;q23)/*MLL-AFF1* (previously known as *MLL-AF4*) comprise the largest group in ALL with *MLL*. Other common partner genes include *ENL* (19p13) and *AF9* (9p22). *FLT3* overexpression is also found in the presence of *MLL* translocations [41]. *MLL-AFF1* fusion is easily detectable by RT-PCR or cytogenetics. However, a more complex molecular analysis may be advantageous in detecting other common fusion partners. A dual color break-apart probe may provide detection of all chromosomal abnormalities involved in ALL with *MLL* translocations by FISH. Leukemias with *MLL* gene rearrangements usually have poor prognosis. The specific type B-ALL is also associated with adverse outcome, particularly when it occurred in infant <6 months.

17.3.1.3 B Lymphoblastic Leukemia/Lymphoma with t(12;21)(p13;q22); TEL-AML1 (ETV6-RUNX1)

This is the most common leukemia in childhood, accounting 25 % of all B-ALLs with a very favorable prognosis. It is not identified in infants and barely found in adults. It has similar clinical and phenotypic features to other types of ALL. CD13 myeloid antigen expression is common with no indication of mixed phenotype acute leukemia. t(12;21) results in the production of *TEL-AML1(ETV6-RUNX1)*, a fusion protein with important role in leukomogenesis [42]. The product protein acts in a dominant negative fashion to interfere with normal function of the transcription factor *RUNX1*. It has been shown that the translocation occurs early in life, prenatally, as "preleukemic clone" but leukemia develops many years later [43]. There is evidence that secondary changes are needed for overt leukemia including frequent additional changes include losses of the *EBF1, ETV6* and *PAX5* genes and gains of chromosome 21 and chromosome arm Xq [44]. The fusion protein can be detected by RT-PCR. As t(12;21)(p13;q22) is invisible at cytogenetic level, FISH is usually used to detect the translocation applying an extra signal or dual color fusion probe. Furthermore, detecting deletion of second *ETV6* allele and additional fusion signals is also important in this type of B-ALL, possibly leading a longer survival [45]. FISH provides information on the status of second *ETV6* homologue.

17.3.1.4 B Lymphoblastic Leukemia/Lymphoma with Hyperdiploidy

Hyperdiploid B-ALL is characterized by blasts containing 51–65 chromosomes, in the absence of translocations or other structural alterations. This subtype accounts for 25 % of B-ALL. It is common in children and has a good prognosis with a survival rate up to 80 % at 5 years. Hyperdiploid B-ALL has no unique features to distinguish it from other subtypes. Hyperdiploid is characterized by gain of chromosomes, typically + X, +4, +6, +10, +14,+17, +18, and +21. The best method for the detection of chromosomal gain in hyperdiploid B-ALL is the standard karyotyping. Cytogenetics may fail in a portion of cases [46, 47]. FISH with centromeric probes specific for the trisomies of chromosomes 4, 10, 17, and 18 may be helpful to identify hidden hyperdiploidy [48, 49]. Identified trisomy 4, 10, and 17 link to a good prognosis. Flow cytometry to measure DNA index analysis can also be used.

17.3.1.5 B Lymphoblastic Leukemia/Lymphoma with Hypodiploidy (Hypodiploid ALL)

Hypodiploid B-ALL is characterized by blasts containing < 44–45 chromosomes including near-haploid ones (23–29 chromosomes). It is seen in both children and adults, although near-haploid ones are more common in children. This subgroup is associated with a worse prognosis. The overall clinical, morphologic and phenotypic features are not distinguishable from other B-ALL. By definition, there is loss of from single or more chromosomes to near haploid with or without structural abnormalities in the remaining chromosomes. The structural anomalies including translocations are more common in the cases with chromosome number between 30 and 40. Detection of hypodiploidy in this group could be problematic. One characteristic feature is the gain of some specific chromosomes onto the haploid chromosomes and the presence of a population of cells with an exact doubling of this chromosome number [50]. This may result in a near diploid or even hyperdiploid karyotype. In such cases, standard karyotyping may dismiss the hypodiploid line. Flow cytometry can be used to detect hypodiploidy in these cases with the advantage of more rapid processing. Flow cytometry is also not affected by mitotic index of the cell population. However, flow cytometry does not identify the specific chromosomes with numeric changes, nor does show the additional structural anomalies which may have potential clinical and biologic importance [51]. Therefore, it is useful to use both techniques in tandem. FISH may also detect certain chromosomes with hypodiploidy; however, FISH detection may be difficult when near-haploid or doubled populations present.

In summary, hypodiploidy and near-haploidy in B-ALL carries a prognostic significance and molecular testing should be carefully applied in detecting chromosomal loss when this subgroup is clinically suspected.

17.3.1.6 B Lymphoblastic Leukemia/Lymphoma with t(5;14)(q31;q32);IL3-IGH

This subgroup is very rare and accounts for < 1 % of all ALL. It has been reported in all age groups. The eosinophilia is reactive and not part of the neoplastic process. The features and prognosis are otherwise similar to other B-ALL. The blast count has not shown to be a prognostic factor in this type of ALL. Patients typically have variable circulating eosinophilia due to overexpression of the *IL3* gene following the functional rearrangement between *IL3* gene and *IGH@* gene. The translocation may be detected using standard karyotyping, RT-PCR and/or less commonly FISH.

17.3.1.7 B Lymphoblastic Leukemia/Lymphoma with t(1;19)(q23;p13.3);E2A-PBX1 (TCF3-PBX1)

ALL with t(1;19) is fairly common in children, accounting for 6 % of all ALL. Clinical features are similar to those of other ALL patients. Although they used to be classified in the poor prognosis group, with therapeutic advances, they are regarded as standard risk [52, 53]. Although they do not differ morphologically from other types, blasts in this group are pre-B type and typically express CD19, CD10 and cytoplasmic μ (cμ) with less or no CD34. Strong CD9 expression is also characteristic. *TCF3* gene encodes two transcriptional proteins E12 and E47 which play a critical role in B-cell maturation while *PBX1* is a homeobox gene not expressed in B or T-cells [54]. Translocation between *TCF3* (previously *E2A*) gene, on chromosome 19, and *PBX1* gene, on chromosome 1, results in production of a fusion protein that has an oncogenic role. Recently, a variant subtype harboring translocation between *TCF3* and *HLF* genes related to a worse prognosis. Cytogenetics and FISH as well as RT-PCR are useful to detect the associated translocations in majority of the cases. The diagnosis of this subtype warrants the careful evaluation by both phenotypic features and translocation status, as an identical t(1;19) can be seen in a portion of B-ALL not necessarily associated with *TCF3-PBX1* translocation.

17.3.1.8 Other Cytogenetic Abnormalities Detected in B-ALL

Up to 50 % of all B-ALL show abnormalities involving genes associated with B cell development including *PAX5, TCF3,EBF1, LEF1, IKZF1* and *IKZF3* and cell cycle controlling genes such as *CDKN2A, CDKN1B* and *RB1* [55–59]. A cryptic translocation involving sex chromosomes, t(X;14)(p22;q32) or t(Y;14)(p11;q32), involving *IGH@* and *CRLF2* genes, and deletion within *PAR1,* resulting in *P2RY8-CRLF2* fusion has been reported [60–62]; possibly activating JAK-STAT signaling pathway and associated with a worse prognosis [63–65]. Intrachromosomal amplification of chromosome 21 (iAMP21) is a distinct chromosomal abnormality in B-ALL and associated with adverse prognosis and poor response to therapy [66]. Despite the variability between patients in the morphology of the abnormal chromosome 21, they consistently show multiple, extra copies of the *RUNX1 (AML1)* gene, tandemly repeated along the length of the abnormal chromosome [67]. Genomic and expression analysis has further characterized this abnormality, demonstrating a common region of amplification (CRA) between 33.192 and 39.796 Mb on chromosome 21 (which includes *RUNX1*) [68]. FISH can also be used to detect this abnormality.

17.3.1.9 B Lymphoblastic Leukemia/Lymphoma, NOS

Diagnosis of B-lymphoblastic leukemia/lymphoma (B-ALL), NOS is based on clinical, morphological and phenotypic findings when the aforementioned cytogenetic abnormalities are not indentified. Gene re-arrangement by PCR is a commonly used as a supportive diagnostic tool and also is also helpful in determining the minimal residual disease in some settings. Studies have showed that nearly all cases have clonal DJ rearrangements of the *IGH@* gene along with T cell gene rearrangement (TCR) in a majority of the cases (up to 70 %) [30, 69]. The B cell clonality in B-ALL can be detected by PCR amplification of the IG and/or TCR VDJ region. The secondary change of TCR gene in B-ALL is considered reactive with uncertainty in pathophysiology, being worthy of further investigation. SNP might be an alternative way to detect any underlying genetic aberration if it is applicable in clinical laboratory.

17.3.2 T Lymphoblastic Leukemia/Lymphoma

T lymphoblastic leukemia/lymphoma is a neoplasm of precursor T cells which are typically medium to large sized blasts with dispersed chromatin, inconspicuous nucleoli and scant cytoplasm. It involves bone marrow and blood (T-ALL) or lymphoid organs or extranodal sites (T-LBL). Both forms are more common in children than adults. The blasts usually express TdT with often T cell antigens CD2, cytoplasmic CD3, CD4, CD5, CD7, and CD8 and CD1a. Aberrant expression of myeloid markers (CD13 and CD33) can be seen in up to 30 % of the cases [70]. Coexpression of CD117 occurs less frequently but often associated with *FLT3* mutation [71]. Multiple genetic aberrations encounter in T-ALL, but none of them is T-ALL specific. Translocations involving *TCR* loci are the most common cytogenetic anomalies observed in T-ALL/LBL. t(7;10)(q34;q24) and t(10;14)(q24;q11) are most common in adults involving *HOX11(TLX1)* gene whereas t(5;14)(q35;q32) involving *HOX11L2 (TLX3)* gene is commonly found in children [6]. As reported, dysregulation of HOX-type transcription factors is found in 30–40 % of cases of T-ALL [72]. Characteristically, *HOX*-type T-ALLs often accompany with activating *NOTCH*1 mutations and *CDKN2A* loss of function, *NUP214-ABL* amplifications, *C-MYB* tandem duplications, *PHF6* mutations, *PTPN2* deletions, and *WT1* mutations [6, 72–78], which are not present in non-HOX-type T-ALL. However, the role of these genetic changes in leukemogenesis is not well understood. The unique genetic features are not only helpful in view of diagnosis but also guide future clinical therapy. An in vitro study has demonstrated that a blockade of both TLX1/HOX and NOTCH could inhibit cell cycle progression in TLX1 T-ALL cell line 9,490 cells (Lesley A. 2011). Mutations that may occur in T-ALL/LBL are important. Mutation of *NOTCH* oncogene is the most common mutation and is seen about 60 % of cases. NOTCH proteins are transmembrane receptors and are important regulators of T cell differentiation and activation. Recent studies showed that *MYC* is upregulated by activated *NOTCH1* in T-ALL which stimulates the growth of T-ALL cells [46, 79]. *N-RAS* and *FLT3* are other mutation seen in T-ALL [80, 81]. Another common rearrangement is the formation of fusion genes, mostly in children. *SIL/TAL1* fusion gene results from a cryptic deletion of chromosome 1 and is seen in up to 30 % of childhood T-ALL. Important translocations resulting in fusion gene formation includes t(10;11) involving *CALM/AF10* genes in 10 % of all cases and less frequently t(11;19) involving *MLL* gene. Other *MLL* gene translocations {t(6;11), t(10;11), t(X;11) and t(4;11)} seen in some T-ALL cases [6]. Philadelphia chromosome has also been reported in rare cases [82]. Deletions may be detected in as many as 30 % cases. 9p21 involving *p16* gene and del(6q) are the important ones. Almost all cases show clonality in T cell receptors with up to 20 % accompanying *IGH@* gene rearrangement [83].

17.4 Mature Lymphoid Neoplasms

Lymphoid neoplasms are clonal tumors with malignant transformation of normal lymphoid cells at various stages of differentiation and comprise the sixth most common group of malignancies worldwide in men and women. Although certain infectious agents, autoimmune disorders and immunosuppression-related conditions have been linked to some lymphomas, the etiology in the majority of lymphomas remains unclear. Morphology and immunophenotype are generally sufficient to make the diagnosis of most lymphomas. Genetic features have begun to play an important role in classification and diagnosis of mature lymphomas. The recent advances in molecular genetics have enlightened lymphoma biology and provide useful testing that can be integrated with the conventional diagnostic methods widely used in hematopathology. Although isolated use of molecular tests is not of any help in lymphoma diagnosis, the use of these tests has clear utility to facilitate the diagnosis, in particularly morphologically and phenotypically challenging cases. Also some molecular markers have prognostic implications in certain lymphomas. Mature B and T/NK cell lymphomas with recurrent cytogenetic abnormalities are discussed below.

17.4.1 Mature B Cell Neoplasms

Mature B cell lymphomas comprise over 90 % of lymphoid neoplasms worldwide. They are common in Western world and account for 4 % of new cancers each year [1]. The most common types are diffuse large B cell lymphoma and follicular lymphoma. The majority of the B cell lymphomas recapitulate the stages of normal B cell proliferation, except for some types, e.g. hairy cell leukemia, that do not correspond to any maturation stage (Table 17.2). Diagnosis of B cell lymphomas, like other mature lymphoid neoplasms, is usually based on histomorphologic and phenotypic features in conjunction with genetic and molecular profiles.

17.4.1.1 Chronic Lymphocytic Leukemia/Small Lymphocytic Lymphoma

Chronic lymphocytic leukemia/small lymphocytic lymphoma (CLL/SLL) is a neoplasm of monomorphic small B cells with a fairly unique phenotype. CLL is the most common leukemia in the Western world affecting mainly the elderly population. The neoplastic cells often coexpress CD5 and CD23 along with characteristically dim CD20, CD79b and dim surface immunoglobulin expression. CLL is the term used when long standing lymphocytosis ($\geq 5 \times 10^9$/L monoclonal lymphocytes for at least 3 months) is present in peripheral blood (PB) with or without bone marrow (BM) involvement [1]. The term SLL refers to the less frequent form with same phenotype to CLL but non-leukemic with the tissue morphology. The diagnosis of SLL requires lymphadenopathy, no cytopenias due to BM involvement by CLL/SLL and $<5 \times 10^9$/L peripheral blood B cells [1].

CLL is a heterogenous disease with variable clinical outcome in the light of variety of genetic abnormalities. Importantly, CLL has the highest familial genetic predisposition in all hematologic malignancies. A polymorphism in the death-associated protein kinase 1 (DAPK1) gene was associated with familial CLL in a single family, but this allele has not been found again in a larger number of cases [84]. The involved genes in genetically predisposed CLL are still yet to be defined. Approximately 80 % of cases have cytogenetic abnormalities. Although some of these abnormalities can be detected in about 40 % of cases by standard karyotyping, FISH is essential in evaluation [85]. The FISH CLL panel including probe CCND1 study is used to exclude mantle cell lymphoma and predict the prognosis of

Table 17.2 The WHO classification of mature B cell neoplasms

II. Mature B cell neoplasms
Chronic lymphocytic leukemia/small lymphocytic lymphoma
B-cell prolymphocytic leukemia
Splenic marginal zone lymphoma
Hairy cell leukemia
Splenic B-cell lymphoma/leukemia, unclassifiable
Splenic diffuse red pulp small B-cell lymphoma
Hairy cell leukemia-variant
Lymphoplasmacytic lymphoma
Heavy chain disease
Gamma heavy chain disease
Mμ heavy chain disease
Alpha heavy chain disease
Plasma cell neoplasms
Monoclonal gammopathy of undetermined significance (MGUS)
Plasma cell myeloma
Solitary plasmacytoma of bone
Extraosseous plasmacytoma
Monoclonal immunoglobulin deposition diseases
Extranodal marginal zone lymphoma of mucosa-associated lymphoid tissue (MALT lymphoma)
Nodal marginal zone lymphoma
Follicular lymphoma
Primary cutaneous follicle center lymphoma
Mantle cell lymphoma
Diffuse large B-cell lymphoma (DLBCL), NOS
T cell/histiocyte-rich large B-cell lymphoma
Primary DLBCL of the CNS
Primary cutaneous DLBCL, leg type
EBV positive DLBCL of the elderly
DLBCL associated with chronic inflammation
Lymphomatoid granulomatosis
Primary mediastinal (thymic) large B-cell lymphoma
Intravascular large B-cell lymphoma
ALK positive large B-cell lymphoma
Plasmablastic lymphoma
Large B-cell lymphoma arising in HHV8-associated multicentric Castleman disease
Primary effusion lymphoma
Burkitt lymphoma
B-cell lymphoma, unclassifiable, with features intermediate between DLBCL and Burkitt lymphoma
B-cell lymphoma, unclassifiable, with features intermediate between DLBCL and Hodgkin lymphoma

CLL. The most common recurrent abnormality seen in CLL is deletion of 13q14, approximately 55 % of cases, which is also associated with the best prognosis [86]. Twenty percentage of cases have deletion of 11q22-23which corresponds to loss of *ataxia* telangiectasia *mutated (ATM) gene*. This abnormality is associated with bulky lymphadenopathy and poor clinical outcome [87]. Deletion of 17p13 is seen in ~7 % of cases majority of which is related to loss or mutation of *TP53* tumor suppressor gene. Deletion 17p13 is often leads a poor prognosis with chemotherapy, particularly Fludarabine resistance in these patients [88–90]. *TP53* mutation with or without del(17p13) is associated with a worse prognosis [91, 92] CLL with trisomy 12 often has an atypical morphology and bright aberrant expression of CD11c on the neoplastic B-cells. FISH is sufficient in detecting the chromosomal anomalies but not gene mutations A novel molecular technique, Multiplex Ligation-dependent Probe Amplification (MLPA), can be used to complement FISH [16].

Status of immunoglobulin variable domain genes, Ig VH gene, in remains the "gold standard" prognostic feature in CLL patients. Presence of *IGH* variable domain gene somatic hypermutation (SHM) is seen 50–60 % of cases; whereas unmutated cases comprise 40–50 % with a worse prognosis [93]. Despite the prognostic importance, the test cannot be performed widely due to its complexity. In this case, the mutation status can be analyzed through a surrogate marker, such as ZAP-70 expression using flow cytometry or infrequently immunohistochemistry. The expression of ZAP-70 corresponds to the absence of *IGH* SHM in the vast majority of the cases [94, 95]. Recent studies also demonstrated *NOTCH1* activating mutations associated with worse prognosis in CLL [96].

17.4.1.2 B Cell Prolymphocytic Leukemia

B cell prolymphocytic leukemia (B-PLL) is the neoplasm of prolymphocytes involving peripheral blood, bone marrow and often spleen. Diagnosis requires prolymphocytes exceeding 55 % of the lymphocytes in the blood. It can be transformed from CLL. The typical morphology of prolymphocytes includes medium size with round nuclei and a prominent central nucleolus. Neoplastic cells strongly express surface immunoglobin, along with B cell antigens (CD19 and CD20). B-cells show often loss of CD23. B-cells with CD5 and CD23 co-expression are seen about 20 % of cases. Variable FMC-7 expression is noted. ZAP-70 and CD38 are expressed in half of the cases with no correspondence to *IGH* mutation status [97].

Immunoglobulin genes are clonally rearranged in half of the cases. Deletion of 17p and related *TP53* mutation has been demonstrated in 50 % of cases associated with poor prognosis and therapy resistant disease [98, 99]. Some case may also have 13q14 by FISH [97].

Initially, t(11;14)(q13;q32) had been demonstrated in "B-PLL"; however these cases are now considered leukemic forms of mantle cell lymphoma [100].

17.4.1.3 Splenic Marginal Zone Lymphoma

According to the WHO classification, splenic marginal zone lymphoma (SMZL) is neoplasm of small B lymphocytes which expansion of splenic white pulp, efface the follicle mantle zone and emerge with marginal zone of larger cells; both small and large cells invade the red pulp [1]. Splenic hilar lymph nodes and bone marrow are usually involved as well as peripheral blood by circulating lymphoma cells with villous projections, usually with polar orientation. Lymphoma cells express surface IgM and often IgD along with B cell markers. Annexin A1 and cyclin D1 are negative with rare CD103 expression. Immunoglobulin heavy and light chains are often re-arranged with somatic hypermutation (SHM). Allelic loss of chromosome 7q31-32 has been reported in up to half of the cases [101]. Overexpression of cyclin dependent kinase 6 (*CDK6)* genes through chromosome 7q21 has been reported in few cases with possible role in lymphomagenesis [102]. *BCL2* and t(14;18) are absent. The presence of 7q deletion and unmutated IgVH in SMZL are possibly associated with adverse clinical outcome [103, 104].

17.4.1.4 Lymphoplasmacytic Lymphoma

Lymphoplasmacytic lymphoma (LPL) is characterized by clonal small B cells, plasmacytoid and plasma cells involving bone marrow and less frequently nodes and spleen. The neoplastic cells are typically IgM-secreting and clinically associated with hyperviscosity, autoimmune disorder, and cryoglobulinerimia. Phenotypically, LPL express both B-cell and plasma cell (subset) markers. *Immunoglobulin* genes are usually clonally arranged with hypermutation. No specific recurrent cytogenetic abnormality has been described in LPL. Deletion of chromosome 6q may be seen but not consistently and minority of patients showed trisomy 3 or 18 [105, 106]. Recently, Treson et al. reported that MYD88 L265P somatic mutation is detected in LPL/Waldenström's macroglobulinemia, which can be useful in distinguishing LPL from the other B-cell lymphoma with similar morphologic and immunophenotypic features [107]

17.4.1.5 Plasma Cell Myeloma

Plasma cell myeloma is the neoplasm of mature and clonal plasma cells involving bone marrow with widespread symptoms and findings from asymptomatic to prominent end-organ damage. Clinical, histomorphologic and phenotypic findings are often sufficient for a definitive diagnosis. Genetic evaluation is particularly important as for the prognosis and therapy effectiveness. Immunoglobin heavy and light chains are clonally arranged in myeloma patients. Plasma cell myeloma arises from post-germinal center B cells resulting in *IGH* SHM.

Standard karyotyping may reveal cytogenetic abnormalities in about one third of myelomas [108, 109]. The main difficulty in karyotype analysis of myeloma is the low-yield metaphases generated from myeloma cells due to low proliferation rate. Therefore; FISH is more commonly used in detecting myeloma related cytogenetics and reveals more than 90 % of the abnormalities [110–112]. When able to analyze sufficient sample, the karyotype in these patients is usually complex, mostly hyperdiploidy. Hyperdiploidy has been defined in 40–65 % of myelomas [109, 113]. These gains in the chromosomes are random and often involve chromosomes with odd numbers including 3, 5, 7, 9, 11, 15, 19 and 21 [114]. Other less common type of karyotype abnormality includes structural re-arrangements in the absence of hyperdiploidy. Most of these cases include specific rearrangements involving the *IGH* gene located at 14q32 and comprise 55–70 % of all cases [115–118]. These rearrangements are typical reciprocal translocations with various chromosomal partners leading to upregulation of the target genes. The most frequent 14q32 partners are 11q13 (involving *CCND1 (CyclinD1)*; 20 % of patients) [119, 120], 4p16 (involving both *FGFR3* and *MMSET*; 15 % of patients) [121, 122], as well as 16q23 and 20q11 (targeting *MAF* genes; 2–5 % of patients each) [123–125]. Both *IGH@* translocations and hyperdiploidy appear to be early events in the oncogenesis in plasma cell neoplasms, unified by upregulation of various *cyclin D* genes (D1, D2, and/or D3) [126, 127].

Other chromosomal changes seen in myeloma include monosomy 13 which may be seen in about half of the cases considered an early event in the pathogenesis [110, 117, 128]. Additional two secondary events are also recurrent: gains of the long arm of chromosome 1 (1q21), in one third of patients, and del 17p, observed in approximately 10 % of patients which are related to disease progression from MGUS to myeloma as well as disease relapse [129, 130].

Activating mutations of *KRAS*- or *N-RAS* may be present in up to 40 % of cases and are likely associated with disease progression [117, 131]. Translocations involving *MYC* gene and activation of NF-kappa B pathway have also been shown in myeloma patients [132, 133]. Chapman et al. recently showed 4 % *BRAF* mutation in myeloma patients, a novel discovery in myeloma suggesting therapeutic implication [134]. Recent studies also emphasized the significance of Phosphatidylinositide 3-kinase (PI3K)/protein kinase B (PKB) pathway, also known as the Akt pathway, in myeloma [135]. The PKB/Akt kinase family includes 3 isoforms (PKBα/Akt1, PKBβ/Akt2, and PKBγ/Akt3) that are encoded by separate genes and that are involved in the regulation of apoptosis, proliferation, motility, and energy metabolism. In many tumors including myeloma, activation of Akt is usually indicative of poor prognosis [136].

17.4.1.6 Extranodal Marginal Zone Lymphoma of Mucosa-Associated Lymphoid Tissue (MALT Lymphoma)

This is an often indolent extranodal lymphoma composed of heterogenous small B cells associated with various precursor lesions described, e.g. Helicobacter pylori gastritis and autoimmune diseases. Neoplastic lymphoid cells infiltrate the epithelium causing destruction of normal architecture and are characterized as "lymphoepithelial lesion". There is several recurrent cytogenetic changes described in MALT lymphoma. The t(11;18)(q21;q21) resulting in fusion of *API2* and *MALT1* genes is detected in approximately one third of cases by standard karyotyping. RT-PCR or FISH studies are helpful in detecting this defect and can be performed on either fresh cells or PEFF tissue [46]. Importantly, the cases with t(11;18) are resistant to therapy targeting *H. pylori* [137]. Other described translocations associated with MALT lymphoma include t(1;14)(p22;q32), t(14;18)(q32;q21), (3;14)(p14.1;q32) and t(1;14) (p22;q32), showing fusion of the N-terminus of the API2 gene to the C-terminus of the MALT1 gene or trancriptional gene deregulation in BCL10, MALT1 or FOXP1 [138, 139, and 140]. t(1;14) (p22;q32), involving *BCL10* gene is usually seen in MALT lymphoma of lung and stomach [139, 140]. Immunohistochemical evaluation of BCL10 protein nuclear staining can be correlated with the presence of translocation [141]. t(14;18)(q32;q21), resulting fusion of IGH/MALT1, is associated with transcriptional dysregulation of *MALT1* and accumulation of cytoplasmic BCL10 [138]. This translocation is most common in parotid, liver and ocular MALT lymphoma [139, 140]. The translocation by karyotyping seems indistinguishable from that seen in follicular lymphoma and an attention should be paid when diagnosing MALT lymphoma. MALT lymphoma arising in thyroid, ocular adnexa and skin can be associated with t(3;14) (p14.1;q32) involving *FOXP1* and *IGH@* [140, 142]. Trisomy 3, 18, and less commonly other chromosomes may be seen less frequently in MALT lymphomas. *BCL6* translocation can also rarely be seen resulting in fusion to the *IGH@* gene [143].

17.4.1.7 Follicular Lymphoma

Follicular lymphoma (FL) is a clonal neoplasm of germinal center B cells including both small centrocytes and large centroblasts with a variable morphology and grading at the diagnosis. Approximately 90 % of the cases harbor the characteristic translocation, t(14;18), involving *BCL2* and *IGH@* genes. That can be detected by cytogenetic analysis or FISH as a more sensitive tool. *BCL2* overexpression results in decreased apoptosis in the lymphoma cells. Importantly, a subportion of cases, mostly high grade FL, may lack *BCL2* rearrangement [144]. A special attention needs to be paid in the situation in order to avoid a misinterpretation of "reactive germinal center cells". Morphologic features by devoiding of "tangible body macrophage", loss of normal polarity and significantly increased centroblasts are diagnostic clues when lack of the specific gene/protein expression. Furthermore, some FL, usually seen in elderly population, may lack *BCL2* but harbor *BCL6* re-arrangement. These cases have a different phenotype than typical FL; CD10-, BCL2- and BCL6+ as well as MUM1+ [145, 146]. The *BCL2* re-arrangement status may vary depending on the localization of primary FL. For instance, primary cutaneous FL is frequently BCL2 negative and often lack IgH-BCL2 fusion product/t(14;18) when analyzed by FISH [147]. Pediatric FL also lacks BCL2 and the translocation.

Other common cytogenetic abnormalities seen in 90 % of FL include 1p-, 6q-, 17p-, +7, +8, +12 and+X [148, 149]. Deletions of 6q25-q27 and 9p21 are associated with poor prognosis [150].

Transformation to a more aggressive lymphoma from FL has been described. Translocations resulting in inactivation of *TP53* and *p16* and activation of *MYC* are associated with transformation to a higher grade disease [151–154]. Per literature, the majority of FL transforms into diffuse large B-cell lymphoma (DLBCL). Transformation to Burkitt-type lymphomas or precursor B-cell lymphoblastic lymphoma is also reported in a small subset of FL [155, 156].

17.4.1.8 Mantle Cell lymphoma

Mantle cell lymphoma (MCL) is a neoplasm of small to medium sized B cells with typical CD5 co-expression and *(CCND1)* translocation. Translocation between *CCND1* on chromosome 11 and *IGH@* on chromosome 14 leading to overexpression of *CCND1* is characteristic and seen in almost all cases. *CCND1* gene encodes a cell cycle protein, dysregulation of which by *IGH@* gene enhancer region results in possibly overcoming the cell cycle suppressors leading to MCL development [157, 158]. FISH analysis of *CCND1* is the preferred and commonly used method in diagnosis of MCL. Rare cases of MCL do not overexpress cyclin D, in which a higher expression of cyclin D2 and cyclin D3 is present and these cases have identical clinical and morphologic features and same genomic profile [159]. A subset of these cases harbor t(2;12)(p12;p13) or t(12;14)(p13;q32) fusing cyclin D2 to kappa light chain (*IGK@) or* IGH@, respectively. RT-PCR is superior in assessing cyclin D2 translocations. Several other recurrent genetic abnormalities have been demonstrated in MCL, including losses of 9p21.3, 11q22-q23, and 22q11.22, and gains of 10p11.23 and 13q31.3 [160, 161]. Specific mutations and deletions in *TP53 (*17p13), *p16 (CDKN2A), ATM,* and *CHEK2* have also been frequently noted in MCL [162, 163]. The cases with *TP53* are rather in blastoid morphology compared to conventional MCL and associated with poor prognosis. Deletion of 13q14 and trisomy 12 also can be seen in MCL [164]. MCL is often encountered as an aggressive lymphoma by nature. Recent studies demonstrated an indolent variant sharing a common genomic profile with conventional MCL. *SOX11* gene, which has a role in cell differentiation, is found to be associated with indolent variant MCL [165, 166]. Immunohistochemical testing is available to evaluate *SOX11* protein.

17.4.1.9 Diffuse Large B Cell Lymphoma

Diffuse large B cell lymphoma, not otherwise specified (DLBCL, NOS) is a very heterogenous neoplasm of large B cells with variable localization, morphology and clinical behavior. DLBCL, NOS accounts for 25–30 % of adult non-Hodgkin lymphomas and common in elderly population. It can arise as the primary or as transformation or progression from a lower grade lymphoma and clinically presents a rapidly enlarging mass. A subset of cases may be associated with EBV infection in the absence of immunodeficiency. DLBCL may arise in the nodal or extranodal sites, with gastrointestinal tract being the most common extranodal site. Common morphological variants include centroblastic, immunoblastic, and anaplastic as well as rare variants, e.g. with spindle morphology [1]. By immunohistochemical features,

DLBCL, NOS is divided into three groups; (1) CD5-positive DLBCL; (2) germinal center B-cell-like (GCB) and (3) non-germinal center B-cell-like (non-GCB). Molecular subgroups include germinal center B-cell-like (GCB) type and activated B cell-like (ABC) type [1].

Certainly, karyotyping and/or FISH study is useful in molecular subgrouping of DLBCL, differentiating between DLBCL and Burkitt lymphoma or hybrized variants. For example, detection of t(14;18) or BCL-2 gene rearrangement in DLBCL suggests follicular center origin (GCB type) while ABC type DLBCL often acquires gains of 3q, 18q21-q22 and losses of 6q21-q22 [167–169].

However, beyond aforementioned functions, cytogenetics study also helps to identify a subset of them with more aggressive clinical features. Abnormalities of *BCL6* gene on chromosome 3q27 is the most common cytogenetic change in DLBCL and is seen in approximately 40–45 % of cases [170]. *BCL6* is a transcription factor required for germinal center formation in B cells. Translocation of *BCL6* occurs in approximately 30 % while 10 % of cases have BCL6 targeted by somatic hypermutation [171–173]. *BCL6* related translocations involve multiple partner genes and prognosis is usually worse in non-*IG/BCL6* gene fusion [174, 175]. Translocations of *BCL2* and *BCL10* genes are the other common changes, seen in 30 % and 15 % of DLBCL, respectively [171, 176]. Translocation involving *MYC* gene also occurs up to 15 % of cases [171, 177, 178]. It has been shown that *MYC* translocation can be seen in *de novo* DLBCL, transformed DLBCL from an underlying low grade lymphoma or in the recently characterized B cell lymphoma unclassifiable, with features intermediate between diffuse large B cell lymphoma and Burkitt lymphoma (formerly atypical Burkitt lymphoma or Burkitt-like lymphoma) associated with poor prognosis [171, 179–181]. FISH testing is a valuable tool in detecting *MYC* amplification/translocation in large B cell lymphomas. Recent studies have been focusing on the implication of measuring Myc protein by immunohistochemical methods. Although some authors suggest that Myc protein may predict the *MYC* gene translocation status [182], it is still unclear if Myc protein is enough to evaluate the gene status requiring further studies. *MYC* translocation has also been found in HIV associated diffuse large B cell lymphomas with plasmablastic features [183]. Recently, "double hit" and "triple hit" lymphomas have been introduced to define DLBCL with often complex cytogenetics involving combinations of *MYC* gene rearrangement with *BCL2 and/or BCL6* gene detected by FISH [17–20]. These are considered high grade or aggressive lymphomas often associated with high proliferation fraction. They require intensive chemotherapy.

17.4.1.10 Other Large B Cell Lymphomas

Primary mediastinal (thymic) large B cell lymphoma (PMBL) is a subgroup of DLBCL that is usually seen in younger age females and associated with a favorable prognosis. Since the lymphoma is putative thymic B-cell origin, it differs from the other *de novo* DLBCL by its own pathohistologic and genetic features.

The genes involved in PMBL include *MAL, FIG 1, PDL1, PDL2, JAK2,* and *BCL11A* [184–187] but rarely BCL2, BCL-6, and c-MYC gene rearrangements are detected. Interestingly, PMBL overlaps with classical Hodgkin lymphoma (CHL) by morphology and sometimes it is difficult to distinguish between these two lymphomas. Recent studies investigated the gene profile of PMBL and CHL and found out PMBL showed the molecular gene-expression signature reminiscent of nodular sclerosis subtype of CHL; both lymphomas were shown to harbor 2p *(REL)* and 9p *(JAK-2)* amplification [188]. ALK-positive DLBCL is another rare subgroup of DLBCL. In contrast to its T cell counterpart ALK-positive anaplastic large T cell lymphoma which characteristically harbors t(2;5) with fusion between *ALK* and often *NMP1*, ALK-positive DLBCL shows fusion between *ALK* gene and *CLTC* (Clathrin) gene associated with t(2;17)(p23:q23) [189]. There are less than 1 % of ALK-positive anaplastic large T cell lymphoma having the same translocation [1]. As known, some cell markers (CD4, CD43 and MUM1) can also be aberrantly expressed in ALK-positive DLBCL, which could result in diagnostic challenging. Since karyotyping might not be requested on the submitted tissue sample, FISH positive for ALK gene rearrangement by using ALK break-apart probe could mislead to a diagnosis of anaplastic large T-cell lymphoma.

17.4.1.11 Burkitt Lymphoma

Burkitt lymphoma (BL) is a very high grade B cell lymphoma characteristically associated with t(8;14)(q24;q32) involving *MYC* gene. *MYC* translocation located at 8q24 region often involves immunoglobulin heavy chain at 14q32 region. Less frequently translocations between *MYC* and immunoglobulin light chains can be observed; at 22q11 region for kappa, t(8;22) or 2p12 region for lambda, t(2;8). FISH is the most valuable test to detect *MYC* gene translocations, however a small portion of cases, up to 10 %, may be negative by FISH [190, 191]. As a result of this finding, the recent studies have focused on alternative mechanisms resulting *MYC* deregulation. E2F1 is a transcription factor loss of which impairs *MYC*-mediated proliferation and lymphomagenesis [192]. Another mechanism that has been recently investigated is miRNA-related dysregulation of *MYC* without translocation [193]. Leucci et al. showed that down-regulation of hsa-miR-34b is associated with *MYC* negativity in BL [193]. Clinically, it is critical to distinguish between Burkitt's lymphoma and diffuse large-B-cell lymphoma in MYC negative cases by FISH since these two lymphomas require different treatments. In this setting, miRNA expression profiling appears to be promising diagnostic tool in highly suspected but *MYC* translocation negative BL cases.

A subset of Burkitt lymphoma demonstrates more than one gene aberration, also called complex abnormalities besides *MYC* [1]. Other genetic abnormalities involving Burkitt lymphoma include *p16*^{INK4a}, *TP53, p53, BAX, p130/RB2* and *BCL6* and chromosome 1q abnormalities [46], Despite the additional genetic changes do not alter the original diagnosis as Burkitt lymphoma when the other diagnostic criteria meet, the clinical significance of these additional cytogenetic abnormalities is still

Table 17.3 The WHO classification of mature T/NK cell neoplasms

Mature T- and NK-cell neoplasms
T-cell prolymphocytic leukemia
T-cell large granular lymphocytic leukemia
Chronic lymphoproliferative disorder of NK cells
Aggressive NK cell leukemia
Epstein-Barr virus (EBV) positive T-cell lymphoproliferative diseases of childhood
Systemic EBV + T-cell lymphoproliferative disease of childhood
Hydroa vacciniforme-like lymphoma
Adult T-cell leukemia/lymphoma
Extranodal NK-T-cell lymphoma, nasal type
Enteropathy associated T-cell lymphoma
Hepatosplenic T-cell lymphoma
Subcutaneous panniculitis-like T-cell lymphoma
Mycosis fungoides
Sezary syndrome
Primary cutaneous CD30 positive T-cell lymphoproliferative disorders
Primary cutaneous peripheral T cell lymphomas, rare subtypes
Primary cutaneous gamma-delta T-cell lymphoma
Primary cutaneous CD8 positive aggressive epidermotropic cytotoxic T-cell lymphoma
Primary cutaneous CD4 positive small/medium T-cell lymphoma
Peripheral T-cell lymphoma, NOS
Angioimmunoblastic T-cell lymphoma
Anaplastic large T-cell lymphoma, ALK positive
Anaplastic large T-cell lymphoma, ALK negative

of further exploration. Under certain circumstances, a careful distinction between "double-hit" lymphoma and Burkitt lymphoma with complex cytogenetics is clinically warranted since these two different entities can greatly overlap by morphology, phenotype and genetically.

17.4.2 Mature T/NK Cell Neoplasms

T/Natural killer (NK) cell lymphomas are relatively uncommon with a significant variation in incidence in different geographical regions and racial populations [1]. The diagnosis of mature T/NK cell neoplasms, as in mature B cell neoplasms, is often based on histomorphologic and phenotypic features. In contrast to B cell counterpart, only anaplastic large T cell lymphoma has been associated with recurrent cytogenetic abnormalities with diagnostic implication up to date [12]. However, a variety of mostly random genetic abnormalities have been described in various mature T cell neoplasms. This section mainly focuses on the frequent genetic abnormalities in some T/NK cell lymphomas (Table 17.3).

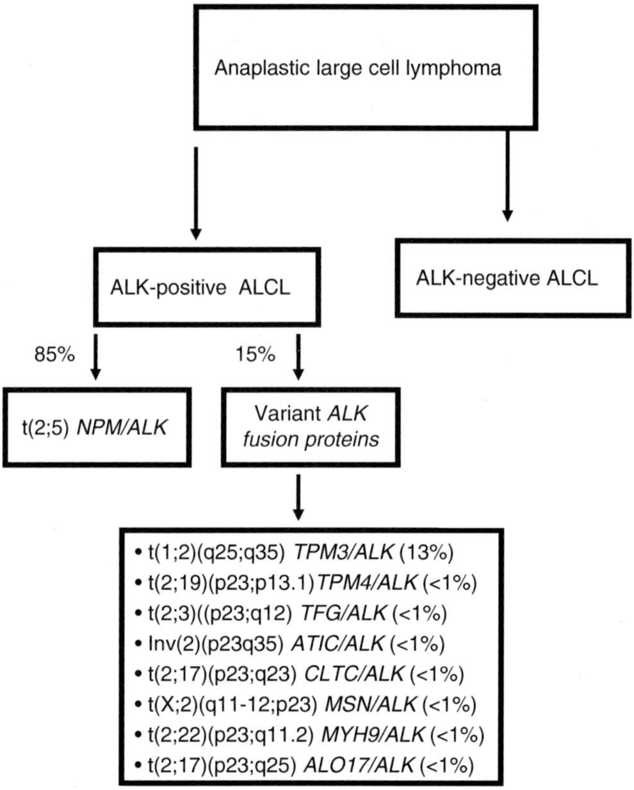

Fig. 17.2 The commonly detected partner genes to *ALK* gene in anaplastic large T-cell lymphoma

17.4.2.1 Anaplastic Large T Cell Lymphoma (ALTCL)

Anaplastic large T cell lymphoma (ALTCL) is characterized by CD30 expressing mostly large atypical T-cells, often displaying pleomorphic morphology and "C-shaped" or "horseshoe-shaped nuclei". Based on the genetic background, ALTCL can be divided into two subcategories by presence or absence of *ALK* (anaplastic large cell kinase) gene abnormality [21].

Anaplastic large T cell lymphoma (ALTCL), ALK positive, is a T cell lymphoma with defined recurrent cytogenetic abnormality. The most frequent translocation seen is t(2;5)(p23;q35) between *ALK* gene and often nucleophosmin (*NPM*) genes, found nearly 84 % of ALTCL [1]. This translocation can be detected by FISH using ALK break apart probe or karyotyping. There are also many other less frequent partners to *ALK* genes located on various chromosomes including *TPM3, TPM4, TFG, ATIC, CLTC, MOESIN, MYH9* and *ALO17* [1, 194–200] (Fig. 17.2). *ALK* gene rearrangement, with different translocations beyond t(2;5)(p23;q35), can also be found in the other hematopoietic or non-hematopoietic neoplasms e.g. ALK+DLBCL involving t(2;17), non-small cell lymphoma, involving ALK fused to EML4 in an inv(2)(p21p23), and inflammatory myofibroblastic tumors involving t(1;2)(q25;p23).

A molecular diagnosis of ALK-negative ALTCL is challenging due to lack of recurrent primary cytogenetic aberration [1]. Careful examination of morphohistology and immunphenotyping are essentially needed to diagnose ALK-negative ALTCL. Notable efforts should be made in characterizing ALK-negative ALCL with gene profile.

17.4.2.2 T-Prolymphocytic Leukemia

T cell prolymphocytic leukemia (T-PLL) is an aggressive T cell neoplasm often associated with inversion of chromosome 14. The incidence of inv(14q) in T-PLL is high, approximately 80 % of cases, while 10 % of cases show a reciprocal translocation of chromosome 14 (t(14;14)(q11;q32) [179]. t(X;14) can rarely be seen [201]. As the results of inversion or translocation of 14q11, TCL1A and TCL1B oncogenes at the break region are activated [202]. Because of TCL1 is not present in mature T-cells and has a -high frequency found in T-PLL (70–80 % of patients) [202], identification of TCL1 activation by genetic or molecular tools helps a diagnosis of a T-PLL. In addition, a study showed that increased TCL1 is not only useful in diagnosis of T-PLL but also indicates a high proliferation in a subset of T-PLL in conjunction with intact T-cell receptor signaling [203]. Abnormalities of chromosome 8 and deletions of 11q23 are other rare genetic inactivation of *CDKN2A* as well as *PTEN* is described with possible association with disease progression [46, 204–206]. In addition, deletions or point mutations of *ATM* gene alleles have been demonstrated in some T-PLL cases suggesting that the dysfunction of this tumor suppressor gene play a role in the pathogenesis of this tumor [207].

17.4.2.3 The Other T Cell Lymphomas

There are sporadic cytogenetic changes noted in the other T-cell lymphomas, which have no known implications in diagnosis or prognosis of these T-cell lymphomas. As discussed in above, clonal T-cell gene rearrangement remains the sole molecular approach, though with low specificity.

Peripheral T cell lymphoma, not otherwise specified (PTCL, NOS) is usually associated with a complex karyotypes with recurrent chromosomal gains in chromosomes 7q, 8q, 17q, and 22q as well as recurrent losses in chromosomes 4q, 5q, 6q, 9p, 10q, 12q and 13q [1].

Mycosis fungoides (MF) is another T cell lymphoma of cutaneous origin. MF is often associated with complex karyotype, such as structural and numerical changes of chromosomes. Activation of *STAT3 and* inactivation of *CDKN2A* as well as *PTEN* are described with possible association with disease progression [46, 204–206].

References

1. Swerdlow SH, I.A.f.R.o. Cancer, WHO (2008) *WHO classification of tumours of haematopoietic and lymphoid tissues*2008. International Agency for Research on Cancer
2. Harrison CJ, Foroni L (2002) Cytogenetics and molecular genetics of acute lymphoblastic leukemia. Rev Clin Exp Hematol 6(2):91–113, discussion 200–2
3. Harrison CJ (2009) Cytogenetics of paediatric and adolescent acute lymphoblastic leukaemia. Br J Haematol 144(2):147–156
4. Mullighan CG, Downing JR (2009) Global genomic characterization of acute lymphoblastic leukemia. Semin Hematol 46(1):3–15
5. Pui CH, Relling MV, Downing JR (2004) Acute lymphoblastic leukemia. N Eng J Med 350(15):1535–1548
6. Graux C et al (2006) Cytogenetics and molecular genetics of T-cell acute lymphoblastic leukemia: from thymocyte to lymphoblast. Leukemia 20(9):1496–1510
7. Rezuke WN, Abernathy EC, Tsongalis GJ (1997) Molecular diagnosis of B- and T-cell lymphomas: fundamental principles and clinical applications. Clin Chem 43(10):1814–1823
8. Cossman J et al (1991) Gene rearrangements in the diagnosis of lymphoma/leukemia. Guidelines for use based on a multiinstitutional study. Am J Clin Pathol 95(3):347–354
9. van Krieken JH et al (2007) Improved reliability of lymphoma diagnostics via PCR-based clonality testing: report of the BIOMED-2 concerted action BHM4-CT98-3936. Leukemia 21(2):201–206
10. Langerak AW et al (2007) Polymerase chain reaction-based clonality testing in tissue samples with reactive lymphoproliferations: usefulness and pitfalls. A report of the BIOMED-2 concerted action BMH4-CT98-3936. Leukemia 21(2):222–229
11. van Dongen JJ et al (2003) Design and standardization of PCR primers and protocols for detection of clonal immunoglobulin and T-cell receptor gene recombinations in suspect lymphoproliferations: report of the BIOMED-2 concerted action BMH4-CT98-3936. Leukemia 17(12):2257–2317
12. Bagg A (2004) Molecular diagnosis in lymphoma. Curr Oncol Rep 6(5):369–379
13. Jacobs PA, Tough IM, Wright DH (1963) Cytogenetic studies in Burkitt's lymphoma. Lancet 2(7318):1144–1146
14. Nowell PC, Hungerford DA (1960) Chromosome studies on normal and leukemic human leukocytes. J Natl Cancer Inst 25:85–109
15. Kluin P, Schuuring E (2011) Molecular cytogenetics of lymphoma: where do we stand in 2010? Histopathology 58(1):128–144
16. Roullet M, Bagg A (2010) The basis and rational use of molecular genetic testing in mature B-cell lymphomas. Adv Anat Pathol 17(5):333–358
17. Aukema SM et al (2011) Double-hit B-cell lymphomas. Blood 117(8):2319–2331
18. Li S et al (2012) B-cell lymphomas with MYC/8q24 rearrangements and IGH@BCL2/t(14;18)(q32;q21): an aggressive disease with heterogeneous histology, germinal center B-cell immunophenotype and poor outcome. Mod Pathol 25(1):145–156
19. Lindsley RC, Lacasce AS (2012) Biology of double-hit B-cell lymphomas. Curr Opin Hematol 19(4):299–304
20. Pedersen MO et al (2012) Double-hit BCL2/MYC translocations in a consecutive cohort of patients with large B-cell lymphoma – a single centre's experience. Eur J Haematol 89(1):63–71
21. Falini B, Martelli MP (2009) Anaplastic large cell lymphoma: changes in the world health organization classification and perspectives for targeted therapy. Haematologica 94(7):897–900
22. Bijwaard KE et al (2001) Quantitative real-time reverse transcription-PCR assay for cyclin D1 expression: utility in the diagnosis of mantle cell lymphoma. Clin Chem 47(2):195–201
23. Vianello F et al (1998) Detection of B-cell monoclonality in fine needle aspiration by PCR analysis. Leuk Lymphoma 29(1–2):179–185

24. Isaacson PG et al (1989) Immunoproliferative small-intestinal disease. An immunohistochemical study. Am J Surg Pathol 13(12):1023–1033
25. Griesser H (1995) Gene rearrangements and chromosomal translocations in T cell lymphoma–diagnostic applications and their limits. Virchows Arch 426(4):323–338
26. Kallakury BV et al (1999) Posttherapy surveillance of B-cell precursor acute lymphoblastic leukemia. Value of polymerase chain reaction and limitations of flow cytometry. Am J Clin Pathol 111(6):759–766
27. Elenitoba-Johnson KS et al (2000) PCR analysis of the immunoglobulin heavy chain gene in polyclonal processes can yield pseudoclonal bands as an artifact of low B cell number. J Mol Diagn 2(2):92–96
28. Diss TC et al (1995) The polymerase chain reaction in the demonstration of monoclonality in T cell lymphomas. J Clin Pathol 48(11):1045–1050
29. Bagg A et al (2002) Immunoglobulin heavy chain gene analysis in lymphomas: a multicenter study demonstrating the heterogeneity of performance of polymerase chain reaction assays. J Mol Diagn 4(2):81–89
30. Bea S et al (2009) Uniparental disomies, homozygous deletions, amplifications, and target genes in mantle cell lymphoma revealed by integrative high-resolution whole-genome profiling. Blood 113(13):3059–3069
31. O'Shea D et al (2009) Regions of acquired uniparental disomy at diagnosis of follicular lymphoma are associated with both overall survival and risk of transformation. Blood 113(10):2298–2301
32. Schwindt H et al (2009) Chromosomal imbalances and partial uniparental disomies in primary central nervous system lymphoma. Leukemia 23(10):1875–1884
33. Heinrichs S, Li C, Look AT (2010) SNP array analysis in hematologic malignancies: avoiding false discoveries. Blood 115(21):4157–4161
34. Cazzaniga G et al (2002) Prospective molecular monitoring of BCR/ABL transcript in children with Ph+acute lymphoblastic leukaemia unravels differences in treatment response. Br J Haematol 119(2):445–453
35. Scrideli CA et al (2003) Gene expression profile unravels significant differences between childhood and adult Ph+acute lymphoblastic leukemia. Leukemia 17(11):2234–2237
36. Owaidah TM et al (2008) Expression of CD66c and CD25 in acute lymphoblastic leukemia as a predictor of the presence of BCR/ABL rearrangement. Hematol Oncol Stem Cell Ther 1(1):34–37
37. Harrison CJ et al (2010) Detection of prognostically relevant genetic abnormalities in childhood B-cell precursor acute lymphoblastic leukaemia: recommendations from the biology and diagnosis committee of the international Berlin-Frankfurt-Munster study group. Br J Haematol 151(2):132–142
38. Harper DP, Aplan PD (2008) Chromosomal rearrangements leading to MLL gene fusions: clinical and biological aspects. Cancer Res 68(24):10024–10027
39. Krivtsov AV, Armstrong SA (2007) MLL translocations, histone modifications and leukaemia stem-cell development. Nat Rev Cancer 7(11):823–833
40. Krivtsov AV et al (2008) H3K79 methylation profiles define murine and human MLL-AF4 leukemias. Cancer Cell 14(5):355–368
41. Armstrong SA et al (2003) Inhibition of FLT3 in MLL. Validation of a therapeutic target identified by gene expression based classification. Cancer Cell 3(2):173–183
42. Romana SP et al (1995) High frequency of t(12;21) in childhood B-lineage acute lymphoblastic leukemia. Blood 86(11):4263–4269
43. Wiemels JL et al (1999) Prenatal origin of acute lymphoblastic leukaemia in children. Lancet 354(9189):1499–1503
44. Davidsson J et al (2009) The DNA methylome of pediatric acute lymphoblastic leukemia. Hum Mol Genet 18(21):4054–4065
45. Konn ZJ et al (2010) Cytogenetics of long-term survivors of ETV6-RUNX1 fusion positive acute lymphoblastic leukemia. Genes Chromosomes Cancer 49(3):253–259

46. Chan WC et al (2009) T-Cell large granular lymphocytic leukemia. WHO classification of tumours of haematopoietic and lymphoid tissues. International Agency for Research on Cancer
47. Harrison CJ et al (2005) Interphase molecular cytogenetic screening for chromosomal abnormalities of prognostic significance in childhood acute lymphoblastic leukaemia: a UK cancer cytogenetics group study. Br J Haematol 129(4):520–530
48. Moorman AV et al (2003) Outcome heterogeneity in childhood high-hyperdiploid acute lymphoblastic leukemia. Blood 102(8):2756–2762
49. Schultz KR et al (2007) Risk- and response-based classification of childhood B-precursor acute lymphoblastic leukemia: a combined analysis of prognostic markers from the pediatric oncology group (POG) and children's cancer group (CCG). Blood 109(3):926–935
50. Harrison CJ et al (2004) Three distinct subgroups of hypodiploidy in acute lymphoblastic leukaemia. Br J Haematol 125(5):552–559
51. Pui CH et al (1990) Clinical presentation, karyotypic characterization, and treatment outcome of childhood acute lymphoblastic leukemia with a near-haploid or hypodiploid less than 45 line. Blood 75(5):1170–1177
52. Burmeister T et al (2010) Clinical features and prognostic implications of TCF3-PBX1 and ETV6-RUNX1 in adult acute lymphoblastic leukemia. Haematologica 95(2):241–246
53. Kager L et al (2007) Incidence and outcome of TCF3-PBX1-positive acute lymphoblastic leukemia in Austrian children. Haematologica 92(11):1561–1564
54. Bain G, Maandag ECR, te Riele HPJ, Feeney AJ, Sheehy A, Schlissel M, Shinton SA, Hardy RR, Murre C (1997) Both E12 and E47 allow commitment to the B cell lineage. Immunity 6:145–154
55. Kuiper RP et al (2007) High-resolution genomic profiling of childhood ALL reveals novel recurrent genetic lesions affecting pathways involved in lymphocyte differentiation and cell cycle progression. Leukemia 21(6):1258–1266
56. Strefford JC et al (2007) Genome complexity in acute lymphoblastic leukemia is revealed by array-based comparative genomic hybridization. Oncogene 26(29):4306–4318
57. Put N et al (2011) FOXP1 and PAX5 are rare but recurrent translocations partners in acute lymphoblastic leukemia. Cancer Genet 204(8):462–464
58. Perez-Vera P, Reyes-Leon A, Fuentes-Panana EM (2011) Signaling proteins and transcription factors in normal and malignant early B cell development. Bone Marrow Res 2011:502751
59. Tasian SK, Loh ML (2011) Understanding the biology of CRLF2-overexpressing acute lymphoblastic leukemia. Crit Rev Oncog 16(1–2):13–24
60. Hertzberg L et al (2010) Down syndrome acute lymphoblastic leukemia, a highly heterogeneous disease in which aberrant expression of CRLF2 is associated with mutated JAK2: a report from the international BFM study group. Blood 115(5):1006–1017
61. Mullighan CG et al (2009) Rearrangement of CRLF2 in B-progenitor- and down syndrome-associated acute lymphoblastic leukemia. Nat Genet 41(11):1243–1246
62. Russell LJ et al (2009) A novel translocation, t(14;19)(q32;p13), involving IGH@ and the cytokine receptor for erythropoietin. Leukemia 23(3):614–617
63. Chapiro E et al (2010) Activating mutation in the TSLPR gene in B-cell precursor lymphoblastic leukemia. Leukemia 24(3):642–645
64. Yoda A et al (2010) Functional screening identifies CRLF2 in precursor B-cell acute lymphoblastic leukemia. Proc Natl Acad Sci USA 107(1):252–257
65. Cario G et al (2010) Presence of the P2RY8-CRLF2 rearrangement is associated with a poor prognosis in non-high-risk precursor B-cell acute lymphoblastic leukemia in children treated according to the ALL-BFM 2000 protocol. Blood 115(26):5393–5397
66. Moorman AV et al (2007) Prognosis of children with acute lymphoblastic leukemia (ALL) and intrachromosomal amplification of chromosome 21 (iAMP21). Blood 109(6):2327–2330
67. Harewood L et al (2003) Amplification of AML1 on a duplicated chromosome 21 in acute lymphoblastic leukemia: a study of 20 cases. Leukemia 17(3):547–553
68. Strefford JC et al (2006) Complex genomic alterations and gene expression in acute lymphoblastic leukemia with intrachromosomal amplification of chromosome 21. Proc Natl Acad Sci USA 103(21):8167–8172

69. van der Velden VH et al (2004) TCRB gene rearrangements in childhood and adult precursor-B-ALL: frequency, applicability as MRD-PCR target, and stability between diagnosis and relapse. Leukemia 18(12):1971–1980
70. Khalidi HS et al (1999) Acute lymphoblastic leukemia. Survey of immunophenotype, French-American-British classification, frequency of myeloid antigen expression, and karyotypic abnormalities in 210 pediatric and adult cases. Am J Clin Pathol 111(4):467–476
71. Hoehn D et al (2012) CD117 expression is a sensitive but nonspecific predictor of FLT3 mutation in T acute lymphoblastic leukemia and T/myeloid acute leukemia. Am J Clin Pathol 137(2):213–219
72. Ferrando AA et al (2002) Gene expression signatures define novel oncogenic pathways in T cell acute lymphoblastic leukemia. Cancer Cell 1(1):75–87
73. Kleppe M et al (2010) Deletion of the protein tyrosine phosphatase gene PTPN2 in T-cell acute lymphoblastic leukemia. Nat Genet 42(6):530–535
74. Lahortiga I et al (2007) Duplication of the MYB oncogene in T cell acute lymphoblastic leukemia. Nat Genet 39(5):593–595
75. Rakowski LA, Lehotzky EA, Chiang MY (2011) Transient responses to NOTCH and TLX1/HOX11 inhibition in T-cell acute lymphoblastic leukemia/lymphoma. PLoS One 6(2):e16761
76. Tosello V et al (2009) WT1 mutations in T-ALL. Blood 114(5):1038–1045
77. Van Vlierberghe P et al (2010) PHF6 mutations in T-cell acute lymphoblastic leukemia. Nat Genet 42(4):338–342
78. Weng AP et al (2004) Activating mutations of NOTCH1 in human T cell acute lymphoblastic leukemia. Science 306(5694):269–271
79. Weng AP et al (2006) c-Myc is an important direct target of Notch1 in T-cell acute lymphoblastic leukemia/lymphoma. Genes Dev 20(15):2096–2109
80. Paietta E et al (2004) Activating FLT3 mutations in CD117/KIT(+) T-cell acute lymphoblastic leukemias. Blood 104(2):558–560
81. Yokota S et al (1998) Mutational analysis of the N-ras gene in acute lymphoblastic leukemia: a study of 125 Japanese pediatric cases. Int J Hematol 67(4):379–387
82. Prebet T et al (2009) Presence of a minor Philadelphia-positive clone in young adults with de novo T-cell ALL. Leuk Lymphoma 50(3):485–487
83. Pilozzi E et al (1999) Gene rearrangements in T-cell lymphoblastic lymphoma. J Pathol 188(3):267–270
84. Raval A et al (2007) Downregulation of death-associated protein kinase 1 (DAPK1) in chronic lymphocytic leukemia. Cell 129(5):879–890
85. Dohner H et al (1999) Chromosome aberrations in B-cell chronic lymphocytic leukemia: reassessment based on molecular cytogenetic analysis. J Mol Med 77(2):266–281
86. Dohner H et al (2000) Genomic aberrations and survival in chronic lymphocytic leukemia. N Engl J Med 343(26):1910–1916
87. Dickinson JD et al (2006) 11q22.3 deletion in B-chronic lymphocytic leukemia is specifically associated with bulky lymphadenopathy and ZAP-70 expression but not reduced expression of adhesion/cell surface receptor molecules. Leuk Lymphoma 47(2):231–244
88. Byrd JC et al (2006) Select high-risk genetic features predict earlier progression following chemoimmunotherapy with fludarabine and rituximab in chronic lymphocytic leukemia: justification for risk-adapted therapy. J Clin Oncol 24(3):437–443
89. Grever MR et al (2007) Comprehensive assessment of genetic and molecular features predicting outcome in patients with chronic lymphocytic leukemia: results from the US intergroup phase III trial E2997. J Clin Oncol 25(7):799–804
90. Sellmann L et al (2012) P53 protein expression in chronic lymphocytic leukemia. Leuk lymphoma 53(7):1282–1288
91. Rossi D et al (2009) The prognostic value of TP53 mutations in chronic lymphocytic leukemia is independent of Del17p13: implications for overall survival and chemorefractoriness. Clin Cancer Res 15(3):995–1004
92. Zenz T et al (2010) TP53 mutation and survival in chronic lymphocytic leukemia. J Clin Oncol 28(29):4473–4479

93. Hamblin TJ et al (1999) Unmutated Ig V(H) genes are associated with a more aggressive form of chronic lymphocytic leukemia. Blood 94(6):1848–1854
94. Orchard JA et al (2004) ZAP-70 expression and prognosis in chronic lymphocytic leukaemia. Lancet 363(9403):105–111
95. Cruse JM et al (2007) Zap-70 and CD38 as predictors of IgVH mutation in CLL. Exp Mol Pathol 83(3):459–461
96. Rosati E et al (2009) Constitutively activated Notch signaling is involved in survival and apoptosis resistance of B-CLL cells. Blood 113(4):856–865
97. Del Giudice I et al (2006) IgVH genes mutation and usage, ZAP-70 and CD38 expression provide new insights on B-cell prolymphocytic leukemia (B-PLL). Leukemia 20(7):1231–1237
98. Lens D et al (1997) p53 abnormalities in B-cell prolymphocytic leukemia. Blood 89(6): 2015–2023
99. Krishnan B, Matutes E, Dearden C (2006) Prolymphocytic leukemias. Semin Oncol 33(2): 257–263
100. Wong KF, So CC, Chan JK (2002) Nucleolated variant of mantle cell lymphoma with leukemic manifestations mimicking prolymphocytic leukemia. Am J Clin Pathol 117(2):246–251
101. Mateo M et al (1999) 7q31-32 allelic loss is a frequent finding in splenic marginal zone lymphoma. Am J Pathol 154(5):1583–1589
102. Corcoran MM et al (1999) Dysregulation of cyclin dependent kinase 6 expression in splenic marginal zone lymphoma through chromosome 7q translocations. Oncogene 18(46):6271–6277
103. Algara P et al (2002) Analysis of the IgV(H) somatic mutations in splenic marginal zone lymphoma defines a group of unmutated cases with frequent 7q deletion and adverse clinical course. Blood 99(4):1299–1304
104. Traverse-Glehen A et al (2005) Analysis of VH genes in marginal zone lymphoma reveals marked heterogeneity between splenic and nodal tumors and suggests the existence of clonal selection. Haematologica 90(4):470–478
105. Buckley PG et al (2009) Genome-wide microarray-based comparative genomic hybridization analysis of lymphoplasmacytic lymphomas reveals heterogeneous aberrations. Leuk Lymphoma 50(9):1528–1534
106. Braggio E et al (2009) High-resolution genomic analysis in Waldenstrom's macroglobulinemia identifies disease-specific and common abnormalities with marginal zone lymphomas. Clin Lymphoma Myeloma 9(1):39–42
107. Treon SP, Xu L, Yang G, Zhou Y, Liu X, Cao Y, Sheehy P, Manning RJ, Patterson CJ, Tripsas C, Arcaini L, Pinkus GS, Rodig SJ, Sohani AR, Harris NL, Laramie JM, Skifter DA, Lincoln SE, Hunter ZR (2012) MYD88 L265P somatic *mutation* in Waldenström's macroglobulinemia. N Engl J Med 367(9):826–833
108. Dewald GW et al (1985) The clinical significance of cytogenetic studies in 100 patients with multiple myeloma, plasma cell leukemia, or amyloidosis. Blood 66(2):380–390
109. Sawyer JR et al (1995) Cytogenetic findings in 200 patients with multiple myeloma. Cancer Genet Cytogenet 82(1):41–49
110. Avet-Loiseau H et al (2007) Genetic abnormalities and survival in multiple myeloma: the experience of the Intergroupe Francophone du Myelome. Blood 109(8):3489–3495
111. Chng WJ et al (2005) A validated FISH trisomy index demonstrates the hyperdiploid and nonhyperdiploid dichotomy in MGUS. Blood 106(6):2156–2161
112. Konigsberg R et al (2000) Predictive role of interphase cytogenetics for survival of patients with multiple myeloma. J Clin Oncol 18(4):804–812
113. Calasanz MJ et al (1997) Cytogenetic analysis of 280 patients with multiple myeloma and related disorders: primary breakpoints and clinical correlations. Genes Chromosomes Cancer 18(2):84–93
114. Chng WJ et al (2007) Molecular dissection of hyperdiploid multiple myeloma by gene expression profiling. Cancer Res 67(7):2982–2989

115. Ackermann J et al (1998) Absence of p53 deletions in bone marrow plasma cells of patients with monoclonal gammopathy of undetermined significance. Br J Haematol 103(4):1161–1163
116. Avet-Loiseau H et al (2002) Oncogenesis of multiple myeloma: 14q32 and 13q chromosomal abnormalities are not randomly distributed, but correlate with natural history, immunological features, and clinical presentation. Blood 99(6):2185–2191
117. Fonseca R et al (2004) Genetics and cytogenetics of multiple myeloma: a workshop report. Cancer Res 64(4):1546–1558
118. Nishida K et al (1997) The Ig heavy chain gene is frequently involved in chromosomal translocations in multiple myeloma and plasma cell leukemia as detected by in situ hybridization. Blood 90(2):526–534
119. Chesi M et al (1996) Dysregulation of cyclin D1 by translocation into an IgH gamma switch region in two multiple myeloma cell lines. Blood 88(2):674–681
120. Fonseca R et al (2002) Myeloma and the t(11;14)(q13;q32); evidence for a biologically defined unique subset of patients. Blood 99(10):3735–3741
121. Chesi M et al (1997) Frequent translocation t(4;14)(p16.3;q32.3) in multiple myeloma is associated with increased expression and activating mutations of fibroblast growth factor receptor 3. Nat Genet 16(3):260–264
122. Santra M et al (2003) A subset of multiple myeloma harboring the t(4;14)(p16;q32) translocation lacks FGFR3 expression but maintains an IGH/MMSET fusion transcript. Blood 101(6):2374–2376
123. Chesi M et al (1998) Frequent dysregulation of the c-maf proto-oncogene at 16q23 by translocation to an Ig locus in multiple myeloma. Blood 91(12):4457–4463
124. Hurt EM et al (2004) Overexpression of c-maf is a frequent oncogenic event in multiple myeloma that promotes proliferation and pathological interactions with bone marrow stroma. Cancer Cell 5(2):191–199
125. Hanamura I et al (2001) Ectopic expression of MAFB gene in human myeloma cells carrying (14;20)(q32;q11) chromosomal translocations. Jpn J Cancer Res 92(6):638–644
126. Bergsagel PL et al (2005) Cyclin D dysregulation: an early and unifying pathogenic event in multiple myeloma. Blood 106(1):296–303
127. Kuehl WM, Bergsagel PL (2005) Early genetic events provide the basis for a clinical classification of multiple myeloma. Hematology Am Soc Hematol Educ Program 2005:346–352
128. Agnelli L et al (2007) Integrative genomic analysis reveals distinct transcriptional and genetic features associated with chromosome 13 deletion in multiple myeloma. Haematologica 92(1):56–65
129. Drach J et al (1998) Presence of a p53 gene deletion in patients with multiple myeloma predicts for short survival after conventional-dose chemotherapy. Blood 92(3):802–809
130. Hanamura I et al (2006) Frequent gain of chromosome band 1q21 in plasma-cell dyscrasias detected by fluorescence in situ hybridization: incidence increases from MGUS to relapsed myeloma and is related to prognosis and disease progression following tandem stem-cell transplantation. Blood 108(5):1724–1732
131. Rasmussen T et al (2005) Possible roles for activating RAS mutations in the MGUS to MM transition and in the intramedullary to extramedullary transition in some plasma cell tumors. Blood 105(1):317–323
132. Annunziata CM et al (2007) Frequent engagement of the classical and alternative NF-kappaB pathways by diverse genetic abnormalities in multiple myeloma. Cancer Cell 12(2):115–130
133. Chng WJ et al (2011) Clinical and biological implications of MYC activation: a common difference between MGUS and newly diagnosed multiple myeloma. Leukemia 25(6): 1026–1035
134. Chapman MA et al (2011) Initial genome sequencing and analysis of multiple myeloma. Nature 471(7339):467–472
135. Zollinger A et al (2008) Combined functional and molecular analysis of tumor cell signaling defines 2 distinct myeloma subgroups: Akt-dependent and Akt-independent multiple myeloma. Blood 112(8):3403–3411

136. Bellacosa A et al (2005) Activation of AKT kinases in cancer: implications for therapeutic targeting. Adv Cancer Res 94:29–86
137. Liu H et al (2001) Resistance of t(11;18) positive gastric mucosa-associated lymphoid tissue lymphoma to Helicobacter pylori eradication therapy. Lancet 357(9249):39–40
138. Ye H et al (2005) MALT lymphoma with t(14;18)(q32;q21)/IGH-MALT1 is characterized by strong cytoplasmic MALT1 and BCL10 expression. J Pathol 205(3):293–301
139. Streubel B et al (2004) Variable frequencies of MALT lymphoma-associated genetic aberrations in MALT lymphomas of different sites. Leukemia 18(10):1722–1726
140. Remstein ED et al (2006) The incidence and anatomic site specificity of chromosomal translocations in primary extranodal marginal zone B-cell lymphoma of mucosa-associated lymphoid tissue (MALT lymphoma) in North America. Am J Surg Pathol 30(12):1546–1553
141. Sagaert X et al (2006) MALT1 and BCL10 aberrations in MALT lymphomas and their effect on the expression of BCL10 in the tumour cells. Mod Pathol 19(2):225–232
142. Streubel B et al (2005) T(3;14)(p14.1;q32) involving IGH and FOXP1 is a novel recurrent chromosomal aberration in MALT lymphoma. Leukemia 19(4):652–658
143. Ye H et al (2008) Chromosomal translocations involving BCL6 in MALT lymphoma. Haematologica 93(1):145–146
144. Ott G et al (2002) Cytomorphologic, immunohistochemical, and cytogenetic profiles of follicular lymphoma: 2 types of follicular lymphoma grade 3. Blood 99(10):3806–3812
145. Karube K et al (2007) CD10-MUM1+ follicular lymphoma lacks BCL2 gene translocation and shows characteristic biologic and clinical features. Blood 109(7):3076–3079
146. Karube K et al (2008) BCL6 gene amplification/3q27 gain is associated with unique clinicopathological characteristics among follicular lymphoma without BCL2 gene translocation. Mod Pathol 21(8):973–978
147. Kim BK et al (2005) Clinicopathologic, immunophenotypic, and molecular cytogenetic fluorescence in situ hybridization analysis of primary and secondary cutaneous follicular lymphomas. Am J Surg Pathol 29(1):69–82
148. Cook JR, Shekhter-Levin S, Swerdlow SH (2004) Utility of routine classical cytogenetic studies in the evaluation of suspected lymphomas: results of 279 consecutive lymph node/extranodal tissue biopsies. Am J Clin Pathol 121(6):826–835
149. Hoglund M et al (2004) Identification of cytogenetic subgroups and karyotypic pathways of clonal evolution in follicular lymphomas. Genes Chromosomes Cancer 39(3):195–204
150. Schwaenen C et al (2009) Microarray-based genomic profiling reveals novel genomic aberrations in follicular lymphoma which associate with patient survival and gene expression status. Genes Chromosomes Cancer 48(1):39–54
151. Davies AJ et al (2007) Transformation of follicular lymphoma to diffuse large B-cell lymphoma proceeds by distinct oncogenic mechanisms. Br J Haematol 136(2):286–293
152. Elenitoba-Johnson KS et al (1998) Homozygous deletions at chromosome 9p21 involving p16 and p15 are associated with histologic progression in follicle center lymphoma. Blood 91(12):4677–4685
153. Mannouji K et al (2009) Transformation from follicular lymphoma to high-grade B-cell lymphoma/leukemia with additional t(2;8)(p12;q24), with inverse expressions of c-MYC and BCL-2, and light-chain switch. Pathol Int 59(4):261–264
154. Sander CA et al (1993) p53 mutation is associated with progression in follicular lymphomas. Blood 82(7):1994–2004
155. Young KH et al (2008) Transformation of follicular lymphoma to precursor B-cell lymphoblastic lymphoma with c-myc gene rearrangement as a critical event. Am J Clin Pathol 129(1):157–166
156. Li L et al (2006) Serial cytogenetic alterations resulting in transformation of a low-grade follicular lymphoma to Burkitt lymphoma. Cancer Genet Cytogenet 170(2):140–146
157. Quintanilla-Martinez L et al (2003) Sequestration of p27Kip1 protein by cyclin D1 in typical and blastic variants of mantle cell lymphoma (MCL): implications for pathogenesis. Blood 101(8):3181–3187

158. Williams ME, Swerdlow SH, Meeker TC (1993) Chromosome t(11;14)(q13;q32) breakpoints in centrocytic lymphoma are highly localized at the bcl-1 major translocation cluster. Leukemia 7(9):1437–1440
159. Fu K et al (2005) Cyclin D1-negative mantle cell lymphoma: a clinicopathologic study based on gene expression profiling. Blood 106(13):4315–4321
160. Salaverria I et al (2007) Specific secondary genetic alterations in mantle cell lymphoma provide prognostic information independent of the gene expression-based proliferation signature. J Clin Oncol 25(10):1216–1222
161. Hartmann EM et al (2010) Pathway discovery in mantle cell lymphoma by integrated analysis of high-resolution gene expression and copy number profiling. Blood 116(6):953–961
162. Perez-Galan P, Dreyling M, Wiestner A (2011) Mantle cell lymphoma: biology, pathogenesis, and the molecular basis of treatment in the genomic era. Blood 117(1):26–38
163. Camacho E et al (2002) ATM gene inactivation in mantle cell lymphoma mainly occurs by truncating mutations and missense mutations involving the phosphatidylinositol-3 kinase domain and is associated with increasing numbers of chromosomal imbalances. Blood 99(1):238–244
164. Bigoni R et al (2001) Secondary chromosome changes in mantle cell lymphoma: cytogenetic and fluorescence in situ hybridization studies. Leuk Lymphoma 40(5–6):581–590
165. Wang X et al (2010) Gene expression profiling and chromatin immunoprecipitation identify DBN1, SETMAR and HIG2 as direct targets of SOX11 in mantle cell lymphoma. PLoS One 5(11):e14085
166. Gustavsson E et al (2010) SOX11 expression correlates to promoter methylation and regulates tumor growth in hematopoietic malignancies. Mol Cancer 9:187
167. Huang JZ et al (2002) The t(14;18) defines a unique subset of diffuse large B-cell lymphoma with a germinal center B-cell gene expression profile. Blood 99(7):2285–2290
168. Tagawa H et al (2005) Comparison of genome profiles for identification of distinct subgroups of diffuse large B-cell lymphoma. Blood 106(5):1770–1777
169. Bea S et al (2005) Diffuse large B-cell lymphoma subgroups have distinct genetic profiles that influence tumor biology and improve gene-expression-based survival prediction. Blood 106(9):3183–3190
170. Lo Coco F et al (1994) Rearrangements of the BCL6 gene in diffuse large cell non-Hodgkin's lymphoma. Blood 83(7):1757–1759
171. Kramer MH et al (1998) Clinical relevance of BCL2, BCL6, and MYC rearrangements in diffuse large B-cell lymphoma. Blood 92(9):3152–3162
172. Tibiletti MG et al (2009) BCL2, BCL6, MYC, MALT 1, and BCL10 rearrangements in nodal diffuse large B-cell lymphomas: a multicenter evaluation of a new set of fluorescent in situ hybridization probes and correlation with clinical outcome. Hum Pathol 40(5):645–652
173. Tzankov A et al (2009) Prognostic importance of BCL6 rearrangements in diffuse large B-cell lymphoma with respect to Bcl6 protein levels and primary lymphoma site. Hum Pathol 40(7):1055–1056, author reply 1056
174. Akasaka H et al (2000) Molecular anatomy of BCL6 translocations revealed by long-distance polymerase chain reaction-based assays. Cancer Res 60(9):2335–2341
175. Akasaka T et al (2000) Nonimmunoglobulin (non-Ig)/BCL6 gene fusion in diffuse large B-cell lymphoma results in worse prognosis than Ig/BCL6. Blood 96(8):2907–2909
176. Kawasaki C et al (2001) Rearrangements of bcl-1, bcl-2, bcl-6, and c-myc in diffuse large B-cell lymphomas. Leuk Lymphoma 42(5):1099–1106
177. Barrans S et al (2010) Rearrangement of MYC is associated with poor prognosis in patients with diffuse large B-cell lymphoma treated in the era of rituximab. J Clin Oncol 28(20):3360–3365
178. Obermann EC et al (2009) Aberrations of the MYC gene in unselected cases of diffuse large B-cell lymphoma are rare and unpredictable by morphological or immunohistochemical assessment. J Clin Pathol 62(8):754–756
179. Scandurra M et al (2010) Genomic profiling of Richter's syndrome: recurrent lesions and differences with de novo diffuse large B-cell lymphomas. Hematol Oncol 28(2):62–67

180. McClure RF et al (2005) Adult B-cell lymphomas with burkitt-like morphology are phenotypically and genotypically heterogeneous with aggressive clinical behavior. Am J Surg Pathol 29(12):1652–1660
181. Lin P et al (2012) Prognostic value of MYC rearrangement in cases of B-cell lymphoma, unclassifiable, with features intermediate between diffuse large B-cell lymphoma and Burkitt lymphoma. Cancer 118(6):1566–1573
182. Green TM et al (2012) High levels of nuclear MYC protein predict the presence of MYC rearrangement in diffuse large B-cell lymphoma. Am J Surg Pathol 36(4):612–619
183. Bogusz AM et al (2009) Plasmablastic lymphomas with MYC/IgH rearrangement: report of three cases and review of the literature. Am J Clin Pathol 132(4):597–605
184. Guiter C et al (2004) Constitutive STAT6 activation in primary mediastinal large B-cell lymphoma. Blood 104(2):543–549
185. Joos S et al (1996) Primary mediastinal (thymic) B-cell lymphoma is characterized by gains of chromosomal material including 9p and amplification of the REL gene. Blood 87(4):1571–1578
186. Weniger MA et al (2007) Gains of REL in primary mediastinal B-cell lymphoma coincide with nuclear accumulation of REL protein. Genes Chromosomes Cancer 46(4):406–415
187. Weniger MA et al (2006) Gains of the proto-oncogene BCL11A and nuclear accumulation of BCL11A(XL) protein are frequent in primary mediastinal B-cell lymphoma. Leukemia 20(10):1880–1882
188. Savage KJ (2006) Primary mediastinal large B-cell lymphoma. Oncologist 11(5):488–495
189. De Paepe P et al (2003) ALK activation by the CLTC-ALK fusion is a recurrent event in large B-cell lymphoma. Blood 102(7):2638–2641
190. Haralambieva E et al (2005) Clinical, immunophenotypic, and genetic analysis of adult lymphomas with morphologic features of Burkitt lymphoma. Am J Surg Pathol 29(8):1086–1094
191. Hummel M et al (2006) A biologic definition of Burkitt's lymphoma from transcriptional and genomic profiling. N Engl J Med 354(23):2419–2430
192. Baudino TA et al (2003) Myc-mediated proliferation and lymphomagenesis, but not apoptosis, are compromised by E2f1 loss. Mol Cell 11(4):905–914
193. Leucci E et al (2008) MYC translocation-negative classical Burkitt lymphoma cases: an alternative pathogenetic mechanism involving miRNA deregulation. J Pathol 216(4):440–450
194. Cools J et al (2002) Identification of novel fusion partners of ALK, the anaplastic lymphoma kinase, in anaplastic large-cell lymphoma and inflammatory myofibroblastic tumor. Genes Chromosomes Cancer 34(4):354–362
195. Falini B et al (1999) Lymphomas expressing ALK fusion protein(s) other than NPM-ALK. Blood 94(10):3509–3515
196. Hernandez L et al (1999) TRK-fused gene (TFG) is a new partner of ALK in anaplastic large cell lymphoma producing two structurally different TFG-ALK translocations. Blood 94(9):3265–3268
197. Lamant L et al (1999) A new fusion gene TPM3-ALK in anaplastic large cell lymphoma created by a (1;2)(q25;p23) translocation. Blood 93(9):3088–3095
198. Lamant L et al (2003) Non-muscle myosin heavy chain (MYH9): a new partner fused to ALK in anaplastic large cell lymphoma. Genes Chromosomes Cancer 37(4):427–432
199. Pulford K et al (2004) The emerging normal and disease-related roles of anaplastic lymphoma kinase. Cell Mol Life Sci 61(23):2939–2953
200. Tort F et al (2001) Molecular characterization of a new ALK translocation involving moesin (MSN-ALK) in anaplastic large cell lymphoma. Lab Invest 81(3):419–426
201. Stern MH et al (1993) MTCP-1: a novel gene on the human chromosome Xq28 translocated to the T cell receptor alpha/delta locus in mature T cell proliferations. Oncogene 8(9):2475–2483
202. Soulier J et al (2001) A complex pattern of recurrent chromosomal losses and gains in T-cell prolymphocytic leukemia. Genes Chromosomes Cancer 31(3):248–254

203. Herling M et al (2008) High TCL1 expression and intact T-cell receptor signaling define a hyperproliferative subset of T-cell prolymphocytic leukemia. Blood 111(1):328–337
204. Navas IC et al (2000) p16(INK4a) gene alterations are frequent in lesions of mycosis fungoides. Am J Pathol 156(5):1565–1572
205. Scarisbrick JJ et al (2000) Loss of heterozygosity on 10q and microsatellite instability in advanced stages of primary cutaneous T-cell lymphoma and possible association with homozygous deletion of PTEN. Blood 95(9):2937–2942
206. Sommer VH et al (2004) In vivo activation of STAT3 in cutaneous T-cell lymphoma. Evidence for an antiapoptotic function of STAT3. Leukemia 18(7):1288–1295
207. Stilgenbauer S et al (1997) Biallelic mutations in the ATM gene in T-prolymphocytic leukemia. Nat Med 3(10):1155–1159

Chapter 18
Molecular Diagnostics of Myeloid Neoplasms

Xiaohui Zhang and Ling Zhang

Contents

X. Zhang, M.D., Ph.D.
Department of Hematopathology and Laboratory Medicine, H. Lee Moffitt Cancer Center & Research Institute, 12902 Magnolia Drive, Tampa, FL 33612, USA

L. Zhang, M.D. (✉)
Department of Pathology and Cell Biology, College of Medicine,
University of South Florida, 12902 Magnolia Drive, Tampa, FL 33612, USA

Department of Hematopathology and Laboratory Medicine, H. Lee Moffitt Cancer Center & Research Institute, 12902 Magnolia Drive, Tampa, FL 33612, USA
e-mail: ling.zhang@moffitt.org

D. Coppola (ed.), *Molecular Pathology and Diagnostics of Cancer*,
Cancer Growth and Progression 16, DOI 10.1007/978-94-007-7192-5_18,

Abstract According to 2008 World Health Organization (WHO) Classification of Tumors of Hematopoietic and Lymphoid Tissue, myeloid neoplasms include (1) myeloproliferative neoplasms (MPN), (2) myeloid and lymphoid neoplasms with eosinophilia and abnormalities of PDGFRA, PFGFRB, or FGFR1, (3) myelodysplastic/myeloproliferative neoplasms (MDS/MPN), (4) myelodysplastic syndromes (MDS), and (5) acute myeloid leukemia (AML) and related precursor neoplasms. The diagnosis and subclassification of myeloid neoplasms is critical and approaches are multifaceted. In an era of advanced molecular biology, the diagnosis of myeloid neoplasms requires an integration of morphology, clinical presentation, laboratory results and immunophenotying with cytogenetics and molecular studies. Emerging novel molecular genetic technologies e.g. DNA microarray, single nucleotide polymorphism (SNP) array, whole genomic sequencing will aid further subclassification and characterization of disease entities of myeloid neoplasm. The common or fundamental molecular markers and associated cytogenetic aberrations, together with the diagnostic approaches are emphasized and reviewed in this chapter.

Keywords Myeloid neoplasm • Myeloproliferative neoplasm • Myelodysplastic syndrome • Acute myeloid leukemia • Molecular diagnosis

Abbreviations

aCML	Atypical chronic myeloid leukemia
ALL	Acute lymphoblastic leukemia
AML	Acute myeloid leukemia
APL	Acute promyelocytic leukemia
B-ALL	B lymphoblastic leukemia
CARs	Commonly affected regions
CBBF	Core binding factor translocations
CBF	Core-binding factor
CDR	Common deletion region
CEL	Chronic eosinophilic leukemia
CML	Chronic myelogenous leukemia
CMML	Chronic myelomonocytic leukemia
CyR	Cytogenetic response
DIC	Disseminated intravascular coagulation
EMH	Extramedullary hematopoiesis
ET	Essential thrombocythemia
FAB	French-American-British
FGFR1	Febroblast growth factor receptor 1

FISH	Fluorescence in-situ hybridization
GEP	Gene expression profiling
GIST	Gastrointestinal stromal tumors
HR	Hematological response
JMML	Juvenile myelomonocytic leukemia
MDS	Myelodysplastic syndromes
MPN	Myeloproliferative neoplasms
MR	Molecular response
MPN-U	Myeloproliferative neoplasms, unclassifiable
MR	Molecular response
MS	Mastocytosis
NOS	Not otherwise specified
PDGFR	Platelet derived growth factor receptor
PMF	Primary myelofibrosis
PML	Promyelocytic leukemia
PV	Polycythemia vera
RAEB	Refractory anemia with excess blasts
RARA	Retinoic acid receptor gene, alpha
RARS	Refractory anemia with ring sideroblasts
RCMD	Refractory cytopenia with multilineage dysplasia
RCUD	Refractory cytopenia with unilineage dysplasia
RFLP	Restricted fragment length polymorphism
SM-AHNMD	Systemic mastocytosis with associated clonal hematopoetic non-mast cell lineage disease
SPOC	Spen paralog and ortholog C-terminal
T-ALL	T-lymphoblastic leukemia
WHO	World Health Organization

18.1 Introduction

According to 2008 World Health Organization (WHO) classification of hematopoietic and lymphoid neoplasms [1], myeloid neoplasms include myeloproliferative neoplasms (MPN), myeloid and lymphoid neoplasms with eosinophilia and abnormalities of PDGFRA, PFGFRB, or FGFR1, myelodysplastic/myeloproliferative neoplasms (MDS/MPN), myelodysplastic syndromes (MDS), and acute myeloid leukemia (AML) and related precursor neoplasms (Table 18.1). In recent years, there have been significant advances in hematopathology, making the diagnosis rely not only on morphology, but also heavily on immunophenotying, cytogenetics, and molecular studies. This is significantly different from the previous classification known as the French-American-British (FAB) classification, which

Table 18.1 The 2008 WHO classification of myeloid neoplasms

Myeloproliferative neoplasms
Chronic myelogenous leukemia, *BCR-ABL1*-positive
Chronic neutrophilic leukemia
Polycythemia vera
Primary myelofibrosis
Essential thrombocythemia
Chronic eosinophilic leukemia, NOS
Mastocytosis
Myeloproliferative neoplasm, unclassifiable
Myeloid and lymphoid neoplasms with eosinophilia and abnormalities of *PDGFRA*, *PDGFRB* or *FGFR1*
Myelodysplastic/myeloproliferative neoplasms
Chronic myelomonocytic leukemia
Atypical chronic myeloid leukemia, *BCR-ABL1* negative
Juvenile myelomonocytic leukemia
Myelodysplastic/myeloproliferative neoplasm, unclassifiable
Myelodysplastic syndromes
Refractory cytopenia with unilineage dysplasia
Refractory anemia with ring sideroblasts
Refractory cytopenia with multilineage dysplasia
Refractory anemia with excess blasts
Myelodysplastic syndrome associated with isolated del(5q)
Myelodysplastic syndrome, unclassifiable
Childhood myelodysplastic syndrome
Acute myeloid leukemia (AML) and related precursor neoplasms
AML with recurrent genetic abnormalities
AML with t(8;21)(q22;q22); *RUNX1-RUNX1T1*
AML with inv(16)(p13.1q22) or t(16;16)(p13.1;q22); *CBFβ-MYH11*
Acute promyelocytic leukemia with t(15;17)(q22;q21); *PML-RARA*
AML with t(9;11)(p22;q23); *MLLT3-MLL*
AML with t(6;9)(p23;q34); *DEK-NUP214*
AML with inv(3)(q21q26.2) or t(3;3)(q21;q26.2); *RPN1-EVI1*
AML (megakaryoblastic) with t(1;22)(p13;q13); *RBM15-MKL1*
AML with mutated *NPM1*
AML with mutated *CEBPA*
AML with myelodysplasia-related changes
Therapy-related myeloid neoplasms
Acute myeloid leukemia, not otherwise specified
AML with minimal differentiation
AML without maturation
AML with maturation
Acute myelomonocytic leukemia
Acute monoblastic and monocytic leukemia
Acute erythroid leukemia
Acute megakaryoblastic leukemia
Acute basophilic leukemia
Acute panmyelosis with myelofibrosis
Myeloid sarcoma
Myeloid proliferations related to down syndrome
Blastic plasmacytoid dendritic cell neoplasm

was based on morphology and cytochemical stains. Besides, the approaches to prognostication and therapeutic guidance have been transformed and have been increasingly useful molecular markers for clinical practice. Since the molecules involved in myeloid neoplasms are extensive, we will address only those molecular markers that have been widely used or will be potentially used in practical hematopathology.

18.2 Diagnostic Algorithms

The morphologic examinations on peripheral blood smears, bone marrow smears and bone marrow biopsies are always the first step on diagnostic algorithms, which are followed by immunophenotyping, cytogenetics, molecular cytogenetics and molecular genetics studies. The initial morphologic evaluation of the available specimen including peripheral blood and/or bone marrow aspirate is critical for the subsequent ordering of ancillary studies.

Generally, the presence of 20 % or more blasts in bone marrow or peripheral blood warrants the diagnosis of acute leukemia. However, when certain cytogenetic changes e.g. t(8;12)(q22;q22), inversion 16/t(16;16)(p13.1;q22), t(15:17)/(q22;q12) are confirmed, the diagnosis of leukemia can be made even when the blast count is less than 20 %. Careful assessment of morphology of blast with monocytic differentiation is needed since monoblasts and promonocytes are both counted as blasts, while atypical monocytes are not. Blasts with bilobed, or cup-shape or concaved nuclei with or without fine azurophic granules and blasts with Auer rods in cytoplasm are also important to recognize, which could suggest acute promyelocytic leukemia (APL). In this situation, a laboratory work up for disseminated intravascular coagulopathy (DIC) is warranted and molecular genetic study of t(15;17)(q22;q12)/*PML-RARA* should be performed to confirm the diagnosis. Blasts with perinuclear hofs and chunky orange, or salmon-pink cytoplasmic granules are also important to recognize, not to be misinterpreted as myelocytes, which are unique features of acute leukemia with t(8;21)(q22;q22)/*RUNX1-RUNX1T1*. An overt increase of abnormal eosinophils with large, basophilic granules, along with increased myeloblasts, are features of acute leukemia with inv(16)(p13.1q22) or t(16;16)(p13.1;q22)/*CBFB-MYH11*. Immunophenotyping by flow cytometry is required to define the lineage differentiation of the blast cell population. Cytogenetic studies by conventional karyotyping or FISH analysis should be performed to detect the recurrent cytogenetic abnormalities. According to studies, approximately 55 % of acute myeloid leukemia cases have various kinds of cytogenetic changes [2]. Some of the cytogenetic aberrations also predict disease prognosis. Mutation analysis of certain genes, such as NPM1, CEBPA, FLT3 internal tandem duplications (FLT3-ITDs) and FLT3 kinase domain mutation (FLT3-TKD), have been included in the 2008 WHO classification, and these mutations are not only related to the nature of AML but also tend to be considered as important prognostic markers. Moreover, clinical findings should be integrated into the diagnosis consideration, as in patients with myeloid proliferations related to Down syndrome and therapy-related myeloid neoplasms. Schematic algorithms of clinical and genetic diagnostic approaches for acute myeloid leukemia is

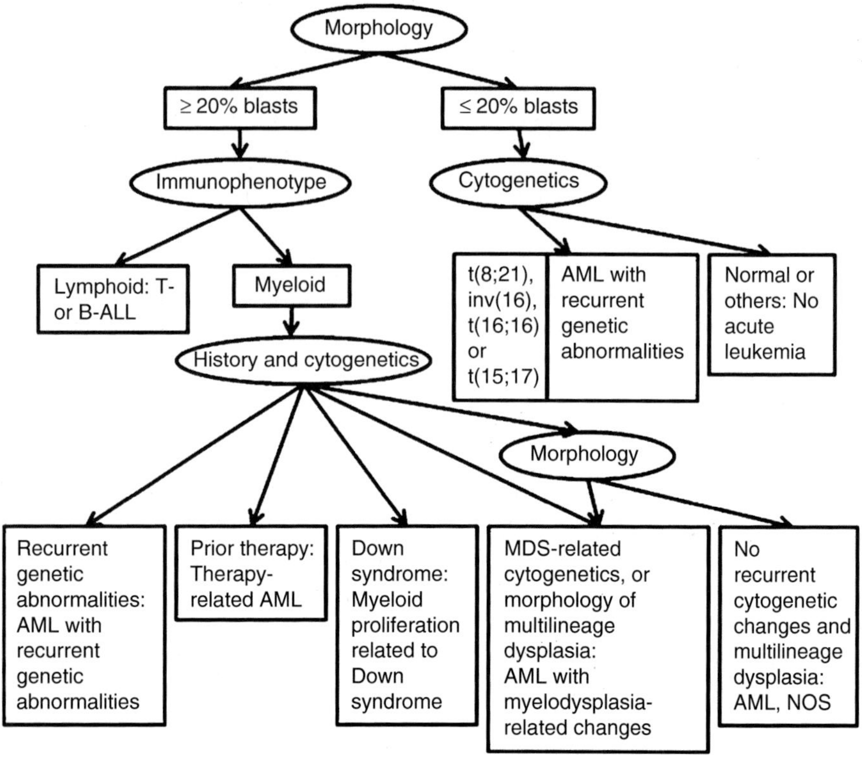

Fig. 18.1 Algorithmic approach to the classification of acute leukemia (Modified from http://www.uscap.org/site~/98th/pdf/companion21h02.pdf)

summarized below (Fig. 18.1) (modified from http://www.uscap.org/site~/98th/pdf/companion21h02.pdf; accessed Jan 10, 2011) [3].

For myeloproliferative neoplasm (MPN), myelodysplastic syndromes/myeloproliferative neoplasm (MDS/MPN), and myelodysplastic syndrome (MDS), the diagnostic algorithms integrate clinical and laboratory data, histologic findings, and molecular markers. The 2008 WHO classification criteria combine all three factors [1]. Clinical and laboratory data are important. For example, in patients with hemoglobin level greater than 18.5 g/dL in men or 16.5 g/dL in women, polycythemia vera (PV) would be suspected if the patients do not have any other etiology that could cause a secondary erythrocytosis or elevated hemoglobin, and testing JAK2 mutation (V671F, or exon 12) is needed to confirm the diagnosis. A patient with essential thrombocythemia would have a platelet count of more than 450×10^9/L, persistent, often accompanying thrombotic episodes. Bone marrow morphology is an important diagnostic tool, which is non-replaceable to distinguish among the categories of MPN, MDS/MPN, and MDS, but plays only a minor role in distinguishing between reactive and clonal myeloproliferation [1]. True MPN could be distinguished from MDS and MDS/MPN by the absence of dyserythropoiesis, dysgranulopoiesis and monocytosis, and the morphology of hyperplastic megakaryocytes provides important diagnostic clues [4]. MDS will be considered when morphologic dysplasia is present in one or more major myeloid cell lineages with associated cytopenia. The availability of molecular markers, namely, BCR-ABL1, JAK2 V617F, JAK2 exon 12, MPL 515L/K, c-Kit D816V are widely applied in the diagnosis of myeloproliferative neoplasm. Among them, detection of t(9;22)(q34;q11.2)/*BCR-ABL1* translocation is necessary to diagnose chronic myelogenous leukemia (CML), which makes the diagnostic criteria dramatically different from other categories of myeloid disorder. Different from the prior versions of WHO classification, novel 2008 WHO classification has conjunction with the cytogenetic aberration and certain molecular markers into major diagnostic criteria of many categories of myeloid disorders [5]. We will discuss the important diagnostic features and correlated clinicopathologic findings, and prognostic outcomes of myeloid neoplasm as below in this chapter.

18.3 Myeloproliferative Neoplasms (MPN)

The MPN are clonal hematopoietic stem cell disorders characterized by proliferation of one or more of the myeloid lineage [1]. The bone marrow is hypercellular with effective hematopoietic maturation and the peripheral blood has increased numbers of granulocytes, red blood cells, and/or platelets. This category includes eight entities: Chronic myelogenous leukemia (CML), BCR-ABL1-positive, chronic neutrophilic leukemia, polycythemia vera (PV), primary myelofibrosis (PMF), essential thrombocythemia (ET), chronic eosinophilic leukemia (CEL), NOS, mastocytosis (MS), and myeloproliferative neoplasm, unclassifiable (MPN, U).

18.3.1 BCR-ABL and Chronic Myelogenous Leukemia (CML)

CML is a clonal proliferation of myeloid cells at all stages of differentiation with the chromosome translocation t(9;22)(q34;q11.2) leading to the formation of the *BCR-ABL* fusion gene. Patients usually present with marked leukocytosis and basophilia in the peripheral blood and bone marrow with splenomegaly. An initial chronic phase usually lasts for 3–5 years and the disease progresses to accelerated phase and blast phase, which have increased blast counts. The blast phase has more than 20 % of blasts and it can be of myeloid or lymphoid lineage or mixed lineages.

As early as the 1960s, Philadelphia (Ph) chromosome, a minute chromosome 22 resulting from a translocation of chromosome 22q11.2 to chromosome 9q34 [t(9;22)(q34;q11.2)], was identified and has been associated with CML since 1973 [6, 7]. Reportedly 90–95 % of CML cases have this translocation at diagnosis [1],

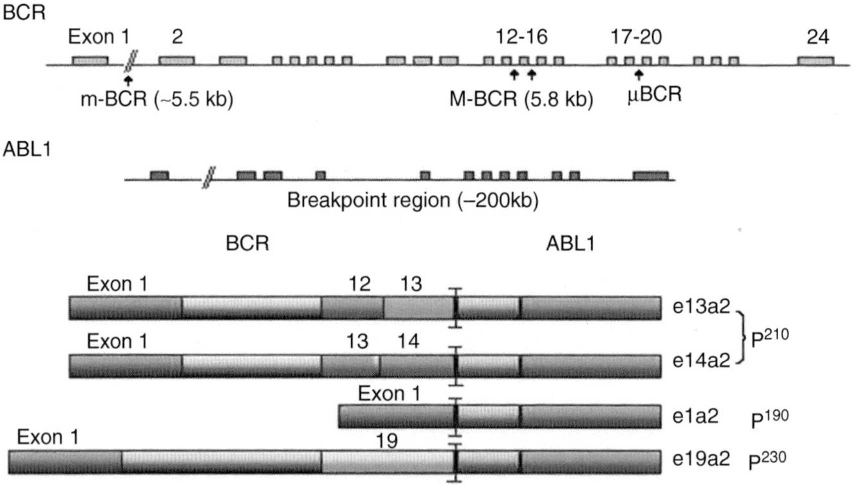

Fig. 18.2 Schematic BCR-ABL1 fusion proteins. *Arrows* indicate breakpoint sites for M-BCR (p210), m-BCR (p190), and **μ**-BCR (p230). The breakpoints in BCR are variable and can occur in the major (M-BCR), minor (m-BCR), or micro (**μ**-BCR) breakpoint cluster region. The breakpoint in ABL1 occurs upstream of 2a. The resulting fusion transcripts are e13a2, e14a2, e1a2, e19a2 encoding p210, p190, and p230, respectively

and the remaining cases have either variant translocations involving chromosome other than chromosomes 22 and 9, or cryptic translocations which cannot be identified by conventional cytogenetic analysis. All of these cases have molecular level detectable BCR-ABL1 transcript, a fusion product of *BCR* gene on chromosome 22 with *ABL1* gene on chromosome 9 [8]. The *BCR-ABL1* fusion gene is present in CML by definition, and has been designated in 2008 WHO classification as CML, *BCR-ABL1* positive. However, *BCR-ABL1* gene rearrangement is not specific for CML, as it is also found in acute lymphoblastic leukemia (ALL), AML, and rarely, MDS [9–12].

As known, the wild-type *BCR* gene encodes a serine/threonine kinase and might be involved in signal transduction pathways [13]. The wild-type *ABL1* gene product is a tyrosine kinase involved in cell cycle regulation [14]. The *BCR-ABL1* fusion gene produces a chimeric oncoprotein, BCR-ABL1, which is an aberrantly activated tyrosine kinase and activates several different growth factor mediated signaling pathways including RAS, STAT, NFκB, PI3K/AKT, and MAPK pathways [15].

The breakpoint in the *BCR* gene may occur at three different sites: major (M-BCR), minor (m-BCR), and micro (μ-BCR). M-BCR spans exons 12–16, and encodes an abnormal protein, p210. M-BCR is the most common site in CML, occurring in 95 % of CML patients. m-BCR, spanning exons 1–2, encodes a shorter protein, p190. μ-BCR occurs rarely; it spans exons 17–20 and encodes a larger fusion protein, p230 (Fig. 18.2). μ-BCR (p230) is associated with prominent neutrophilic maturation and/or conspicuous thrombocytosis [1]. m-BCR (p190) is most frequently associated with Ph chromosome positive ALL. However, p190 can be seen in rare cases of CML with monocytosis which resembles chronic myelomonocytic leukemia and a small amount of p190 can be seen in the majority of p210 CML as a result of alternative splicing [1]. A more recent study reported p190 BCR-ABL CML, although rare, is associated with a poor outcome and irresponsive to tyrosine kinase inhibitor therapy [17].

To diagnose CML, it needs a correlation of clinical features, laboratory findings, bone marrow morphology, and cytogenetic and molecular studies. Detection of Ph chromosome or *BCR-ABL1* fusion gene is required. Conventional cytogenetics has been the gold standard, but fluorescence in-situ hybridization (FISH) and reverse transcriptase PCR (RT-PCR) methods are more sensitive for diagnosing the disease and monitoring for minimal residual disease. FISH can detect a cryptic translocation as well as deletions of derivative chromosome [18]. RT-PCR is most sensitive and real-time PCR methods can be used for quantification [19, 20].

18.3.2 CML Transformation, Therapy Monitoring and Imatinib Resistance

The accelerated and blast phases of CML frequently demonstrate secondary cytogenetic changes, including extra Ph chromosome, +8, +19, or i(17q) [1]. Translocations characteristic of *de novo* AML are occasionally detected in blast phase of CML, such as t(8;21)(q22;22), t(3;21)(q26;q22), t(7;11)(p15;p15), inv16(p13q22), and t(15;17)(q22;q12-21), which are, though with the same chromosome breakpoints, not associated with a better prognosis as they are noted in *de novo* AML. Associated gene changes include *TP53, RB1, MYC, p16INK4a, RAS, AML1 and EVI-1,* but their significance in diagnostics is unknown [1].

Targeted on the BCR-ABL1 tyrosine kinase activity, imatinib mesylate is very effective to control CML, particularly when used early in the chronic phase. Imatinib mesylate induces hematologic remission in nearly all CML patients [21]. The evaluation of response to treatment is based on the hematologic, cytogenetic, and molecular criteria. A hematological response (HR) is indicated by normal peripheral blood cell counts and bone marrow morphology. Complete, major, minor, and minimal cytogenetic response (CyR) can be achieved by detection of 0 %,<35 %, 36–65 % and 66–95 % Ph chromosome positive (Ph+) bone marrow cells [21]. Molecular response (MR) is defined by reduction in the *BCR-ABL1* transcript, which can be measured by quantitative RT-PCR. The real-time technology provides sensitive and reproducible results. A ratio of the *BCR-ABL1* to control genes, usually ABL1, is reported, and the treatment plan is changed accordingly [22].

Resistance to imatinib mesylate occurs when subclones of CML cells acquire point mutations on ABL1 kinase domain that prevent the binding of imatinib mesylate to the kinase. Up to 90 % of the resistant patients have detectable mutations, and more than 35 mutations have been described [23]. Detection of emerging mutations can be analyzed by PCR followed by direct sequencing of the *BCR-ABL1* kinase domain. However, it should be pointed out that kinase mutation independent imatinib-resistance also exists in CML, e.g. LYN kinase overexpression, and increased

BCR-ABL1 expression [24, 25]. A study demonstrates a role of constitutive activation of the PI3K/AKT1 pathway in *BCR-ABL1*-independent imatinib resistance [26]. Additionally, some patients are resistant to imatinib primarily, which is defined by inability to achieve complete hematologic response by 3 months or molecular complete response by 6 months of imatinib treatment, and the molecular mechanism remains unclear.

18.3.3 JAK2 and MPN

In 2005, several groups independently identified *JAK2* V617F as the major molecular mutation event in *BCR-ABL1* negative MPNs. This somatic mutation is found in more than 95 % of PV patients, and 40–50 % of ET and PMF patients [27–30]. With this regard, PV, ET and PMF may be considered as a spectrum of diseases sharing a common molecular etiology. There is also a rare *JAK2* exon 12 mutation which has similar functional effects as *JAK2* V617F [1, 31].

JAK2 (Janus Kinase 2) is a tyrosine kinase that mediates activation of receptors for erythropoietin, thrombopoietin, granulocyte-macrophage colony-stimulating factor, and granulocyte colony-stimulating factor. It is also involved in signaling by receptors with tyrosine kinase activity, such as *KIT* [32]. *JAK2* mutations can activate the downstream signaling pathways (STAT, ERK1/2, MAPK, PI3K/AKT) and cause uninhibited growth, independent of cytokines [33, 34].

Virtually all patients with PV have either *JAK2* V617F or *JAK2* exon 12 mutation, thus, it is a sensitive diagnostic marker for PV. Homozygous mutation of *JAK2* V617F has been more frequently detected in PV and associated with the clinical picture of classic PV and with a higher tendency to secondary myelofibrosis but without increased leukemia [35]. For ET or PMF, only about half of patients have the *JAK2* mutation and a small portion of patients (5 %) have *MPL* mutation (*MPL* W515K/L) [36], so the diagnostic use of *JAK2* mutation is limited. *JAK2* V167F is not specific to any of the MPNs and its absence does not exclude MPN; at the same time, its presence does support the diagnosis of an MPN if other clinical and laboratory data are supportive. Importantly, its presence excludes reactive myeloproliferative causes [4]. In addition, concurrent *MPL* and *JAK2* V617F mutations have also been reported, which indicate that these two mutations may have functional complementation in myeloproliferative disease [36]. Of note as well, *JAK2* mutation could occasionally be seen in MDS [37], MDS/MPN [38] and rarely coexist with CML [39].

For the diagnosis of PV, ET and PMF, an initial *JAK2* V617F test is routinely performed. If the result comes back negative, a *JAK2* exon12 mutation test can be done if PV is still suspected, while an *MPL* W515K/L mutation should be performed if ET or PMF is suspected. Either DNA or RNA from the peripheral blood or bone marrow aspirate is applicable for the mutation analysis. Qualitative as well as quantitative methods, including restricted fragment length polymorphism (RFLP), direct Sanger sequencing, and real time PCR, can be selected. Real time PCR is a preferred method with better sensitivity.

18.3.4 Polycythemia Vera (PV)

PV is characterized by increased red blood cell production independent of the mechanisms that normally regulate erythropoiesis. The proliferation involves not only the erythroid lineage but also the granulocytes and megakaryocytes. The diagnosis of PV is based on clinical and laboratory parameters. According to 2008 WHO classification, PV is suspected in patients with hemoglobin levels greater than 18.5 g/dL in men or 16.5 g/dL in women, or hemoglobin greater than 17 g/dL in men or 15 g/dL in women if associated with a documented and sustained increase of at least 2 g/dL from a previous base line [1]. Serum erythropoietin level is usually lower than that in the other pseudo PVs and also below the normal range in healthy patients (3.3 IU/L) [40]. Bone marrow biopsy shows marked hypercellularity with pan-hyperplasia. Lack of stainable iron particles is a common phenomenon noted in marrow aspirate from PV patient. *JAK2* V617F or other functionally similar mutations such as *JAK2* exon 12 mutation is a required molecular test. Identification of an abnormal karyotype would be helpful but not necessary for a diagnosis since only about 20 % of patients with PV have cytogenetic abnormalities. Presence of Ph chromosome and/or *BCR-ABL* fusion excludes PV. The most common recurring cytogenetic abnormalities include +8, +9, del (20q), del (13q) and del (9p); sometimes +8 and +9 are found together [41].

18.3.5 Essential Thrombocythemia (ET)

ET is characterized by sustained thrombocytosis > 450×10^9/L in the peripheral blood and increased numbers of large, mature megakaryocytes in the bone marrow. Bone marrow cellularity usually retains in normal range. There is no significant erythrocytosis or leukocytosis with left shifted mutation. Clinically the patients usually have episodes of thrombosis and/or hemorrhage. The diagnosis is after exclusion of other causes of reactive or neoplastic thrombocytosis, including other MPN, inflammatory, iron deficiency anemia, infectious or non-hematopoietic neoplastic disorders. The presence of a *BCR-ABL1* fusion gene excludes the diagnosis of ET. As mentioned above, approximately 40–50 % of ET patients have the *JAK2* V617F or a functionally similar mutation. It has been recently found that carrying homozygous *JAK2* V617F mutation in patients with ET increased a risk of recurrent thrombosis [42]. *MPL* mutation, namely *MPL* W515K/L, has been found in 1 % of cases of *JAK2* V617K negative ET [1]. *MPL* is a thrombopoietin receptor, and it is spontaneously activated by the mutation in amino acid position 515 (*MPL* W515K/L). The mutation leads to thrombocytosis and myelofibrosis [36]. Worthy of mention is that W515L/K has not been detected in patients with PV according to a large series of studies including 1,182 patients with myeloproliferative and other myeloid disorders [6]. Thus, presence of W515L/K narrows the diagnosis down to ET or PMF. Presence of *JAK2* or *MPL* mutation helps to make the diagnosis, nevertheless, neither *JAK2* nor *MPL* mutations is specific for ET.

There is no consistent karyotypic abnormalities noted in ET, but +8, abnormalities of 9q, and del (20q) have been reported [43].

18.3.6 Primary Myelofibrosis (PMF)

PMF is characterized by a proliferation of predominantly megakaryocytes and granulocytes in the bone marrow associated with excess reticulin and collagen deposition and extramedullary hematopoiesis (EMH). In cellular phase, PMF is often associated with myeloid preponderance, with less intensive myelofibrosis besides atypical megakaryocytic proliferation. Historically, PMH should have no other myeloproliferative neoplasm diagnosed before and no *BCR-ABL1* fusion gene documented. As aforementioned, approximately 50 % of patients with PMF have the *JAK2* V617F mutation [27–30]. Up to 5 % of PMF cases have *MPL* W515K/L mutation [27–30, 36], although none of the mutations are specific to the disease entity. Similar to ET, the presence of *JAK2* V617F or MPL mutation is helpful to rule out reactive marrow fibrosis, e.g. chronic inflammatory condition, autoimmune disorder, and drug-related situations. Exclusion of other primary and secondary malignancies with secondary myelofibrosis, namely lymphoma, metastatic carcinoma, is also needed.

Approximately 30 % of patients have cytogenetic changes, including partial trisomy 1q, 13q deletion, 20q deletion, trisomy 8, and chromosomes 1, 7, and 9 abnormalities [44–46]. The presence of either del(13)(q12–22) or der(6)t(1;6)(q21–23;p21.3) is strongly suggestive but not diagnostic of PMF [44, 47].

Since some cytogenetic abnormalities, e.g. 20q deletion and trisomy 8, can also be associated with MDS, differential diagnosis should include fibrotic MDS. A careful morphologic assessment and correlation with clinical presentation would be helpful. In general, splenomegaly is less commonly associated with MDS. Presence of characteristic syncytial clustering of megakaryocytes, extrasinasoidal hematopoiesis and osterosclerosis favors PMF over fibrotic MDS.

18.3.7 Mastocytosis

Mastocytosis is a new addition to the MPN category in 2008 WHO classification. It is a clonal proliferation of mast cells that accumulate in one or more organ systems, and it is characterized by the presence of multifocal compact clusters or cohesive aggregates/infiltrates of abnormal mast cells [1]. Cutaneous and systemic mastocytosis are the two most common clinicopathologic settings. Systemic mastocytosis with associated clonal hematopoetic non-mast cell lineage disease (SM-AHNMD) has been observed and considered a variant of systemic mastocytosis [1]. Mastocytosis is separated from mast cell hyperplasia by distinct morphological and/or molecular characteristics.

KIT mutations at codon 816 in exon 17, most commonly D816V, have been reported in 95 % or more of adult patients with systemic mastocytosis or one third of cutaneous mastocytosis in pediatric patients [48]. The *KIT* mutation results in a constitutively activated kinase, signaling from which appears to be essential for the survival and proliferation of mast cell precursors in the marrow. The D816V mutation also confers resistance to imatinib therapy [49]. Other mutations on *KIT* including D816Y, D816H and D816F are rarely seen. The latter (D816F) is reported and relatively more common in the pediatric group [50]. Pyrosequencing or mutation-specific quantitative PCR on DNA extracted from microdissected bone marrow or skin biopsy specimens, or from sorted mast cells from bone marrow aspirates are recommended methods [51, 52].

In the setting of SM-AHNMD, seeking additional disease specific cytogenetic or molecular abnormalities is warranted. For example, *JAK2* mutation can be detected in MPN. In addition, since D816V is also observed in cases of AML, particularly in tumors with core binding factor (CBF) translocations [53, 54], correlation with clinical information and morphologic findings is suggested before a final diagnosis is rendered.

18.3.8 Chronic Neutrophilic Leukemia (CNL)

CNL is very rare, characterized by persistent neutrophilia (>80 % of white blood cells, white blood cells at least $>25\times10^9$/L) in peripheral blood, bone marrow hypercellularity and hepatosplenomegaly. Diagnosis is made by exclusion of other causes of neutrophilic leukocytosis. There is no Philadelphia chromosome or *BCR-ABL1* fusion gene. No *PDGFRA, PDGFRB, FGFR1* gene rearrangements are detected. *JAK2* mutation has been found in 20 % of patients [55]. In the presence of *JAK2* mutation, further investigation is requested to completely exclude any *JAK2* positive MPN as well as MDS/MPN.

18.4 Myeloid and Lymphoid Neoplasms with Eosinophilia and Abnormalities of *PDGFEA, PDGFB,* or *FGFR1*

Myeloproliferative and lymphoid neoplasms associated with rearrangement of *PDGFRA, PDGFRB* and *FGFR1* includes three rare diseases. They have some shared clinical and pathological features and all of them have chromosomal rearrangement of one of three tyrosine kinases: platelet-derived growth factor receptor *(PDGFR) alpha (A), PDGFR beta (B)*, or fibroblast growth factor receptor 1 (*FGFR1*) [1]. The fusion genes encode aberrant tyrosine kinases. Eosinophilia is characteristic but not invariable. All three diseases could represent as AML, MDS/

MPN or MPN, depending upon their partnership. The most common partner genes involved are *FIP1L1, ETV6/TEL*, and *ZNF198* for PDGFRA, PDGFRB, and *FGFR1*, respectively [56]. Cytogenetic and molecular genetic analysis should be performed. *FIP1L1-PDGFRA* fusion gene usually results from a cryptic del(4)(q12). Clinically, the specific gene fusion is representative of a picture of chronic eosinophilic leukemia (CEL) with eosinophilia with dysplasia. *ETV6-PDGFRB* results from t(5;12)(q31 ~ 33;p12), which has hematological features resembling CMML, CEL, aCML with eosinophilia and MPN with eosinophilia [57–59]. Translocations involving an 8p11 breakpoint lead to a fusion gene with *FGFR1* [1]. There are multiple partner genes associated with *FGFR1*. Among them, one of the partners located at 6q27 creates a fusion gene, *FGFR1OP1/FGFR1*, is observed in some patients with PV [60]

To diagnose *PDGFR* or *FGFR* related disorder, FISH or PCR should be performed. FISH analysis with any *PDGFA, PDGFRB* or *FGFR1* probe is widely accepted to identify the gene rearrangement. PCR is an alternative approach. Recently, generic quantitative RT-PCR has also been developed to detect diverse *PDGFRA* or *PDGFRB* [61].

18.5 Myelodysplastic/Myeloproliferative Neoplasms (MDS/MPN)

MDS/MPN neoplasms have both MDS and MPN features, comprising chronic myelomonocytic leukemia (CMML), atypical chronic myeloid leukemia, *BCR-ABL1* negative (aCML), juvenile myelomonocytic leukemia (JMML), and MDS/MPN, unclassifiable.

The manifestation of CMML is persistent peripheral monocytosis greater than 1×10^9/L and fewer than 20 % blasts (including promonocytes). Philadelphia Chromosome/BCR-ABL1 gene or rearrangement of *PDGFRA* or *PDGFRB* should be absent. Dysplasia involves one or more myeloid lineages. Dysplasia is not a necessary condition for diagnosis of CMML if the other criteria are met. The other diagnostic criteria include a persistent monocytosis lasting over 3 months without any other explainable reactive process, or a clonal cytogenetic or molecular genetic aberration is acquired. The most common numerical and structural chromosome abnormalities associated with CMML are trisomy 8, deletion of 7 or 7q and 12p. In view of molecular changes, as many as 40 % of patients with CMML have *RAS* gene point mutations [62, 63].

However, the diagnosis of CMML is based on clinical, laboratory and morphological observations. Nonspecific cytogenetic changes are found in 20–40 % of patients [1]. It is important to know that cases with abnormalities of 11q23 suggest the diagnosis of AML instead of CMML. Cases with p190 *BCR-ABL1* is classified as CML, regardless of persistent high monocyte count over 10 % of WBCs or 1×10^9/L [64].

Atypical chronic myelogneous leukemia (aCML) is characterized by leukocytosis with dysplastic neutrophils and their precursors. *BCR-ABL1* fusion gene is absent. *PDGFA* or *PDGFB* genes are also excluded. Similar to *BCR-ABL1* positive CML, patients with aCML commonly present with elevated WBC count with granulocytic predominance and splenomegaly. It is distinguished from CML by dysgranulopoiesis with nuclear aberrations and cytoplasmic hypogranulation [64, 65] and from CMML by less than 10 % monocytes [64]. About 30 % of cases have acquired mutations of *NRAS* or *KRAS* [66]. Cytogenetic abnormalities have been reported in up to 80 % of patients with aCML, most commonly +8 and del(20q).

JMML affects children of 0–14 years of age. There is no *BCR-ABL1* fusion gene. PTPN11 mutations occur in 35 % of patients [67, 68], and oncogenic mutation of the *RAS, NRAS, KRAS*, and *NF1* are each seen in approximately 20 % of patients. Most of the patients with JMML (65 %) have normal karyotype. Monosomy 7 is found in about 25 % of patients. Other cytogenetic abnormalities are also noted in 10 % of patients [1].

18.6 Myelodysplastic Syndrome (MDS)

MDS is a group of clonal hematopoietic stem cell diseases characterized by cytopenia, dysplasia in one or more of the major myeloid cell lines, ineffective hematopoiesis, and increased risk to transform to AML. According to 2008 WHO classification, the diseases include refractory cytopenias with unilineage dysplasia (RCUD), refractory anemia with ring sideroblasts (RARS), refractory cytopenia with multilineage dysplasia (RCMD), refractory anemia with excess blasts (RAEB), myelodysplastic syndrome – unclassified (MDS-U), and MDS associated with isolated del(5q). This classification integrates prognostically different subgroups, and certain chromosome aberrations, which have prognostic significance and may predict response to therapeutic drugs. For example, MDS associated with isolated del(5q), which usually has a favorable prognosis and may benefit from lenalidomide therapy [69, 70].

Cytogenetic abnormalities have been found in approximately 50 % of patients with MDS. Table 18.2 shows the common recurring chromosomal changes. The presence of these chromosomal abnormalities and refractory cytopenia of undetermined origin could suggest a diagnosis of presumptive MDS if no convincing morphologic evidence of dysplasia. Exceptions are sole +8, −Y or del(20q), which are not sufficient for a diagnosis of MDS if morphological criteria are not met. These recurring changes can also be used in monitoring of the disease during follow up. It is known that certain cytogenetic changes are associated with some characterized clinical or morphologic features. For example, del(5q) occurs primarily in elderly women with refractory macrocytic anemia, and the associated MDS is characterized by megakaryocytes with non-lobated or hypolobated nuclei, and has a favorable clinical course. Loss of 17p is associated with pseudo Pelger-Huët anomaly, small vacuolated neutrophils, TP53 mutation and unfavorable clinical course [1, 71]. Inversion of 3q21q26 or t(3;3;)(q21;q26.2) is often associated with atypical megakaryocytic hyperplasia [72]. Complex karyotype which is defined by at least three independent chromosomal

Table 18.2 Common recurring cytogenetic abnormalities and their frequency [1]

Cytogenetic abnormalities	Frequency in MDS	Frequency in t-MDS
Unbalanced		
+8	10 %	
−7 or del(7q)	10 %	50 %
−5 or del(5q)	10 %	40 %
del(20q)	5–8 %	
−Y	5 %	
i(17q) or t(17p)	3–5 %	
−13 or del(13q)	3 %	
del(11q)	3 %	
del(12p) or t(12p)	3 %	
del(9q)	1–2 %	
idic(X)(q13)	1–2 %	
Balanced		
t(11;16)(q23;p13.3)		3 %
t(3;21)(q26.2;q22.1)		2 %
t(1;3)(p36.3;q21.2)	1 %	
t(2;11)(p21;q23)	1 %	
inv(3)(q21q26.2)	1 %	
t(6;9)(p23;q34)	1 %	

t-MDS therapy-related MDS

abnormalities, typically includes chromosomes 5 and/or 7 [−5/del(5q), −7/del(7q)], and is associated with an unfavorable clinical course [1, 73].

Molecular defects associated with the cytogenetic changes are largely unknown. Often times, the breakpoints are not clustered in a small area, but are distributed in a relatively large commonly affected regions (CARs) [74]. Only a few molecular markers have been identified.

Genes located at 5q- have been investigated. In common deletion region (CDR), there is many tumor suppressor genes identified. For example, *RPS14* has been identified as a del(5q) related gene [75], and *SPARC* may also be involved in the pathogenesis of 5q- syndrome and response to lenalidomide [76].

MDS1/EVI1 gene in 3q26 is found to be involved in translocations like inv(3)(q21q26), t(3;3)(q21;q26), and t(3;21)(q26;q22). It can form a fusion gene with *AML1* gene in 21q22, or overexpression may be the consequence of the translocations [77–79].

Unrelated to the cytogenetics, many gene mutations have been reported in MDS, including *TET, KIT, G-CSFR, PDGFRB, FLT3, FMS, N-RAS, K-RAS, JAK2, RUNX1, CEBPA, PU.1, GATA-1, p53* and *MLL* [74]. It is noteworthy that *JAK2* V617F can be found in MDS, most often associated with marrow fibrosis and thrombocytosis [80, 81], however, it is less frequent than in MPN or MDS/MPN [82]. A small subset of patients with isolated del(5q) may show a concomitant *JAK2* V617F mutation [83]. *JAK2* has been found frequently in refractory anemia with ring sideroblasts associated with marked thrombocytosis (RARS-T), which belongs to MDS/MPN, and should be distinguished from pure RARS. Despite the progress to date, the molecular markers are mostly under research and they have not been widely accepted in diagnosis and therapy of MDS.

18.7 Acute Myeloid Leukemia (AML)

AML represents a group of hematopoietic stem cell disorders characterized by clonal proliferation of immature hematopoietic cells, or blasts that accumulate in bone marrow, and interfere with normal hematopoietic function. It can develop *de novo*, or secondary to myelodysplastic syndrome, myeloproliferative neoplasm, chemotherapy or radiation. In 2008 WHO classification, AML and related precursor neoplasms consists of seven subcategories: (1) AML with recurrent genetic abnormalities; (2) AML with myelodysplasia-related changes; (3) therapy-related myeloid neoplasms; (4) acute myeloid leukemia, not otherwise specified (NOS), which is essentially a modified FAB classification predominantly based on traditional morphologic and cytochemical criteria; (5) myeloid sarcoma; (6) myeloid proliferations related to Down syndrome and (7) blastic plasmacytoid dendritic cell neoplasm [1].

Besides AML with recurrent genetic abnormalities, cytogenetics and molecular studies are also an integral part of 2008 WHO classification for those AML under the remaining six subcategories and are recommended for risk stratification in disease progression. In addition, cytogenetics and gene mutation status have been used to stratify the patients into favorable, intermediate, and poor prognostic groups, and are also used to predict the patient's response to therapies [84].

18.7.1 AML with Recurrent Genetic Abnormalities

This category includes seven neoplasms associated with specific genetic abnormalities. These genetic abnormalities have prognostic significance and are correlated with morphology and immunophenotypes in most types. The most common abnormalities are balanced chromosomal translocations including t(8;21)(q22;q22), inv(16)(p13.1q22)/t(16;16)(p13.1;q22), t(15;17)(q22;q12) and t(9;11)(p22;q23) [1]. As mentioned earlier, the presence of t(8;21), inv(16), or t(15;17) is diagnostic of acute leukemia even when the blasts are less than 20 %. The fusion genes resulted from the translocations can be detected by FISH, and RT-PCR. RT-PCR is a more sensitive method.

18.7.1.1 t(8;21)(q22;q22); *RUNX1-RUNX1T1*

The t(8;21) (q22;q22) is observed in 8 % of AML cases. The translocation results in a fusion gene involving the *RUNX1* (also known as core-binding factor α, and *AML1*) gene and *RUNX1T1* (also known as *ETO*) gene. The *RUNX1-RUNX1T1* fusion gene product represses normal transcriptional activity of *RUNX1* which contributes to the leukemic transformation. Cases with t(8;21) have distinct morphological and immunophenotypic features, with long, thin Auer rods and salmon-colored cytoplasmic granules (AML-M2 in FAB classification), and expression of B cell lineage markers (CD19) [1]. AML with t(8;21) is one of the core-binding factor (CBF) leukemias, along with inv(16) and t(3;21) in AML and t(12;21) in pediatric acute lymphoblastic leukemia (ALL). These CBF leukemias have a favorable prognosis [85].

18.7.1.2 inv(16)(p13.1q22) or t(16;16)(p13.1;q22); *CBFβ-MYH11*

The inv(16)(p13.1q22) or t(16;16)(p13.1;q22) is observed in 10 % of adult and approximately 6 % of childhood AML cases. Both of the inv(16)(p13.1q22) and t(16;16)(p13.1;q22) result in a fusion protein composed of β subunit of the core-binding factor (*CBFβ*) and smooth muscle myosin heavy chain (*MYH11*). *CBFβ-MYH11* acts as a transcriptional repressor [86]. The characteristic morphology is acute myelomonocytic leukemia with abnormal eosinophils (AML-M4Eo in FAB classification). The inv(16)(p13.1q22)/t(16;16)(p13.1;q22) is a subtle rearrangement by conventional cytogenetic analysis, therefore FISH and RT-PCR may be necessary to detect the changes. This type of AML has favorable prognosis.

18.7.1.3 t(15;17)(q22;q21); *PML-RARA*

This translocation is present exclusively in acute promyelocytic leukemia (APL) (AML-M3 in FAB classification). APL patients commonly present with coagulopathy, due to disseminated intravascular coagulation (DIC), thus a prompt diagnosis is essential. Therefore, morphologic recognition or molecular detection of genetic abnormalities is important. Detection of the genetic changes alone is diagnostic, regardless of the blast count

There are two types of APL identified, hypergranular and hypogranular variants. Hypergranular APL represents 60–70 % of cases. The abnormal promyelocytes have numerous large cytoplasmic red to purple granules and Auer rods. Hypogranular or microgranular APL (AML-M3v in FAB classification) promyelocytes have fine granules and often bilobed ("apple-core" or "butterfly" shaped) nuclei.

The translocation results in fusion of the promyelocytic (*PML*) gene with the retinoic acid receptor, alpha (*RARA*) gene. The break point in *RARA* occurs consistently within intron 2. The breakpoints in the *PML* gene occur in three different sites, introns 6, 3 and exon 6. Accordingly, three forms of *PML-RARA* may be formed: long form (bcr-1), short form (bcr-3) and variable form (bcr-2) [87] (Fig. 18.3).

Wild-type *PML* functions as a tumor suppressor gene, and *RARA* has been shown to promote differentiation and to suppress growth. The fused *PML-RARA* acts as a dominant negative regulator preventing transcription of genes, thus interfering with myeloid maturation [88].

Cytogenetic analysis, FISH, or RT-PCR is necessary for detection of the *PML-RARA* fusion. In FISH, APL leukemic cells have a "microspeckled" pattern in

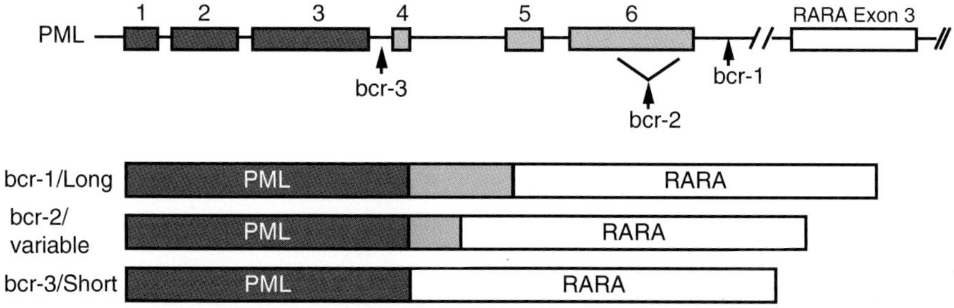

Fig. 18.3 Schematic representation of *PML* breakpoints and *PML-RARA* fusion transcripts. The 3 PML breakpoint cluster regions (bcr−1, −2, and −3) are indicated by *arrows*, and the resultant long, variable, and short *PML-RARA* isoforms are diagrammed

contrast to the normal speckled or macrospeckled pattern of staining for PML protein. RT-PCR is also a sensitive method for minimal residual disease monitoring.

18.7.1.4 t(9;11)(p22;q23); *MLLT3-MLL*

Translocations involving the MLL gene on chromosome 11q23 are associated with more than 70 different partner genes [89]. They are observed in approximately 6 % of AML cases [84]. The MLL protein is a histone methyltransferase that assembles in protein complexes that regulate gene transcription [1]. The t(9;11)(p22;q23) is associated with AML with monocytic features. It typically occurs in children with an intermediate prognosis. Using Southern blot or FISH, MLL probe can detect most translocations involving 11q23. PCR is not used routinely because of the large number of partner genes, but can be used for minimal residual disease, and multiplex RT-PCR is developed using multiple primers [90].

18.7.1.5 t(6;9)(p23;q34); *DEK-NUP214*

The t(6;9)(p23;q34) is observed in approximately 1 % of AML cases. The translocation results in a fusion of *DEK* with *NUP214*, and the fusion protein acts as an aberrant transcription factor and also affects transport factors. AML with t(6;9)(p23;q34); *DEK-NUP214* may have blasts with Auer rods and may exhibit monocytic features. It is often associated with basophilia and multilineage dyspoiesis [91].

18.7.1.6 inv(3)(q21q26.2) or t(3;3)(q21;q26.2); *RPN1-EVI1*

The inv(3)(q21q26.2) or t(3;3)(q21;q26.2) occurs in 1–2 % of AML cases. The translocation involves the oncogene *EVI1*, or its longer form *MDS1-EVI1*, and *RPN1*. *RPN1* acts as an enhancer of *EVI1* expression, resulting in increased cell proliferation, and impaired cell differentiation [1]. High expression of *EVI* also suggests a poor prognosis. The morphologies are variable, including AML-M1, M4, and M7 subtypes in FAB classification. Cytogenetics may not be able to detect the cryptic changes, which can be identified by FISH [92].

18.7.1.7 t(1;22)(p13;q13); *RBM15-MKL1*

The t(1;22) occurs rarely in infantile AML, taking approximately 1 % of childhood AML. The translocation results in a fusion of RNA binding motif protein-15 (*RBM15*), which encodes RNA recognition motifs and a spen paralog and ortholog C-terminal (SPOC) domain, and megakaryocyte leukaemia-1 (*MKL1*), which encodes a DNA-binding motif involved in chromatin organization [1]. The fusion protein may modulate chromatin organization, HOX-induced differentiation and extracellular signaling pathways [1]. The blasts show typical features of megakaryoblasts with a small amount of agranular cytoplasm with budding or blebs [84].

18.7.2 Other AML Subtypes

Among the other AML subtypes are AML with myelodysplasia-related changes, therapy-related myeloid neoplasms, and AML, not otherwise specified (NOS). AML with myelodysplasia-related changes has morphological features of myelodysplasia or a prior history of myelodysplastic syndrome (MDS) or myelodysplastic/myeloproliferative neoplasm (MDS/MPN), or MDS-related cytogenetic abnormalities. There are no specific genetic abnormalities. Cytogenetic changes are similar to MDS. Therapy-related myeloid neoplasms include therapy-related acute myeloid leukemia (t-AML), myelodysplastic syndrome (t-MDS) and myelodysplastic/myeloproliferative neoplasms (t-MDS/MPN) occurring as late complications of cytotoxic chemotherapy and/or radiation therapy. Following a long latent period after alkylating agent and/or radiation therapy, unbalanced chromosomal aberrations develop, mostly involving whole or partial loss of chromosomes 5 and/or 7, and are often associated with additional chromosomal abnormalities. These changes compose of 70 % of the patients. In contrast, following a short period after therapy, balanced chromosomal translocations may develop, including rearrangements of 11q23 and other abnormalities such as t(15;17) and inv(16). These happen in the remaining 20–30 % of the patients [1].

AML, NOS, includes AML categories based on morphologic and cytochemical criteria modified from FAB classification. The cases should not have recurrent genetic abnormalities, a history of prior therapy, or Down syndrome [1].

18.7.3 Molecular Markers in AML

Specific gene mutations in AML include frequent mutations of *FLT3* (fms-like tyrosine kinase 3), *NPM1* (nucleophosmin), *CEBPA* (CCAAT/enhancer-binding protein alpha), *KIT, MLL* (mixed lineage leukemia), *WT1* (Wilm's tumor 1), *N-RAS* and *K-RAS*. By WHO classification, mutations can be divided into two classes: class I and class II mutations. Class I mutations constitute *FLT-3, KIT* and *RAS*, while class II mutations include mutation of *CEBPA* and probably *NPM1* [1]. Class I mutations occur late in AML or relapsed AML, integrating to more than one subtype of AML and play roles in predicting prognosis. Class II mutations, also including *PML-RARA*, *RUNX-1-RUNX1T1*, *CBFB-MYH11*, appear to be in earlier AML and affect hematopoietic differentiation and subsequent apoptosis [1]. Among aforementioned, mutations of *FLT3, NPM1* and *CEBPA* have been known to have a great impact on prognosis.

18.7.3.1 FLT3

FLT3 is located on chromosome 13q12, and it encodes a receptor tyrosine kinase. It is primarily expressed on normal myeloid and lymphoid progenitors as well as on the blast cells in AML [93]. An activation of FLT3 regulates a number of different cellular processes, including transcription, proliferation and apoptosis, and it plays critical roles in normal hematopoiesis and stem cell proliferation [94].

There are two distinct FLT3 mutations in juxtamembrane and kinase domains. Internal tandem duplications (FLT3-ITD) has been identified in a high proportion of patients with AML (75–80 %) [95]. The second most common (20–35 %) mutation involves codons 835 or 836 of the tyrosine kinase domain at exon 20 (FLT3-TKD, D835 or D836) [96].

FLT3-ITD mutations are duplication of a fragment within the juxtamembrane domain coding region, exons 14 and 15. The length of duplicated DNA can be between 3 and more than 400 base pairs [97]. The mutations lead to the receptor activation, and further stimulate cell proliferation [98, 99]. FLT3-ITD is the most common mutation in hematologic malignancies, occurring in AML (20–40 %), as well as in CML (5–10 %) and MDS (5–10 %) [1, 100]. In AML, it is most commonly in AML with t(6;9)(p23;q34), acute promyelocytic leukemia and AML with a normal karyotype [101, 102].

Importantly, FLT3-ITD is a significant prognostic factor, which is associated with an adverse clinical outcome. FLT3-TKD mutation remains controversial [1]. Detection of FLT3-ITD is critical to predict the prognosis of most cytogenetically normal AML.

18.7.3.2 *NPM1*

NPM1 is located on chromosome 5q35, and is a nucleocytoplasmic shuttling protein. It has multiple functions, including regulating *p53* and *ALK* tumor suppressors [103]. It can be involved in several translocations, such as *NPM-ALK*, *NPM-RARA*, and *NPM-MLF1* [104]. The mutations most commonly occur in exon 12, and rarely in exon 9 and exon 11. In exon 12, the mutations are usually duplications of TCTG tetranucleotide at position 956–959. There are more than 40 *NPM1* mutation variants detected [105]. *NPM1* mutations occur in about one third of adult AML and in approximately 50–60 % of adult AML with normal karyotype [106, 107].

The presence of *NPM1* mutation, as an independent factor without combining *FLT3-ITD*, suggests a good prognosis and improved response to chemotherapy, while *NPM1* mutation combined with *FLT3-ITD* suggests an intermediate prognosis [108]. A provisional entity of AML with mutated *NPM1* is proposed in 2008 WHO classification [1]. In this AML type, blasts show monocytic differentiation and lack of CD34 expression, and are largely (85 %) with normal karyotype. It has a good response to induction therapy [105, 109]. Genetic features of AML with mutated *NPM1* include: It is specific for AML, mostly *de novo* AML; Usually all leukemic cells carry the mutation; It is mutually exclusive with other AML with recurrent genetic abnormalities; It is consistently retained at relapse; It usually precedes other associated mutations (e.g., *FLT3-ITD*); It has unique gene expression profiling (GEP) signature and distinct microRNA profile.

18.7.3.3 *CEBPA*

CEBPA (CCAAT/enhancer-binding protein-α) is located on chromosome 19q13.1, and it is a basic leucine zipper (bZIP) transcription factor. The normal protein functions in control of proliferation and differentiation of myeloid progenitors [110]. There are two types of *CEBPA* mutation: N-terminal nonsense mutations resulting in a truncated isoform with dominant negative activity, and C-terminal mutations in the bZIP domain interfering with DNA binding and homodimerization of the transcription factor [110]. *CEBPA* mutations are observed in 6–15 % of all AML [1]. Like *NPM1* mutations, *CEBPA* mutations are also frequently observed in AML with a normal karyotype.

CEBPA mutations are associated with a favorable prognosis in AML with normal karyotype. The clinical significance of combined *FLT3-ITD* and *CEBPA* mutations is still uncertain. A provisional entity of AML with mutated *CEBPA* is proposed in 2008 WHO classification. The AML subtype is equivalent to AML with maturation or AML without maturation and characterized with high blast count in peripheral blood.

18.7.3.4 Other Markers

C-KIT is a tyrosine kinase receptor of the platelet-derived growth factor family, located at 4q11-12. Gain-of-function mutations of *C-KIT* occur in multiple diseases, including gastrointestinal stromal tumors (GIST), germ cell tumors, mastocytosis and AML. The most frequent *KIT* mutations reported are point mutations at codon 816 of exon 17 and insertions/deletions in exon 8. Exon 17 mutations of *KIT* are associated with poor prognosis in AML with t(8;21)(q22;q22) and inv(16)(p13.1q22)/t(16;16)(p13.1;q22) [111]. The relevance of exon 8 mutations is still not clear.

Wilm's Tumor 1 (*WT1*) gene mutations have been observed in approximately 10 % of AML with normal karyotype, and the patients are usually younger than 60 years old [112]. *WT1* mutations are associated with poor prognosis in AML patients with a normal karyotype.

Mixed Lineage Leukemia (*MLL*) gene, located on chromosome 11q23, is involved in multiple chromosomal translocations with 71 partner genes [113]. *MLL* related hematologic malignancies are found in patients with AML related to topoisomerase II inhibitor therapy [114], as well as in ALL, MDS/tMDS, *de novo* AML, and acute leukemias of ambiguous lineage [115]. *MLL*-rearranged leukemias represent about 10 % of all leukemia cases [113]. The mechanism of *MLL*-related AML is largely elusive [113]. Speaking of mutation, a partial tandem duplication of *MLL* has been reported in 5–10 % of AML with normal karyotype and in patients with isolated trisomy 11 [1]. Presence of *MLL* gene has an adverse prognostic significance in AML with normal karyotype.

RAS mutations occur in 12–27 % of AML patients [116]. *NRAS* is mutated and constitutively activated in 10–20 % of AMLs, *KRAS* in 5–15 % of patients, and *HRAS* is rarely mutated [117]. *RAS* mutations do not have consistent prognostic significance.

Furthermore, the expression levels of *BAALC* gene (Brain And Acute Leukemia, Cytoplasmic), *ERG* (ETS-related gene), MN1 (Meningioma 1), and *CXCR4* genes, as well as gene expression profiles and microRNA expression patterns may also provide useful markers for AML [97].

18.8 Future Perspectives

The last decade saw the rapid progress in myeloid neoplasm diagnosis, response prediction, monitoring of minimal residual disease, and prognosis. Molecular studies are playing more and more important roles in the diagnosis and management of the patients with myeloid neoplasms. It is very likely that in the coming years, more genetic abnormalities, molecular markers or prognostic factors will be identified and the stratification of the diseases will change accordingly.

In a view of technological aspect, gene expression profiling (GEP) and microRNA profiling are the emerging diagnostic tools which may lead to more precise classification, with their enormous capacity to simultaneously quantify the expression of tens of thousands of genes [118, 119]. Moreover, these approaches may also contribute to prognostic stratification, targeted therapy and the detection of new molecular markers.

References

1. Swerdlow S, Campo E, Harris N, Jaffe E, Pileri S, Stein H, Thiele J, Vardiman J (2008) WHO classification of tumours of haematopoietic and lymphoid tissues, 4th edn. International Agency for Research on Cancer press, Lyon
2. Mrozek K, Heerema NA, Bloomfield CD (2004) Cytogenetics in acute leukemia. Blood Rev 18(2):115–136

3. Betz BL, Hess JL (2010) Acute myeloid leukemia diagnosis in the 21st century. Arch Pathol Lab Med 134(10):1427–1433
4. Wadleigh M, Tefferi A (2010) Classification and diagnosis of myeloproliferative neoplasms according to the 2008 World Health Organization criteria. Int J Hematol 91(2):174–179
5. Tefferi A, Vardiman JW (2008) Classification and diagnosis of myeloproliferative neoplasms: the 2008 World Health Organization criteria and point-of-care diagnostic algorithms. Leukemia 22(1):14–22
6. Randolph TR (2005) Chronic myelocytic leukemia–Part I: history, clinical presentation, and molecular biology. Clin Lab Sci 18(1):38–48
7. Rowley JD (1973) Letter: a new consistent chromosomal abnormality in chronic myelogenous leukaemia identified by quinacrine fluorescence and Giemsa staining. Nature 243(5405):290–293
8. Bartram CR, de Klein A, Hagemeijer A, van Agthoven T, Geurts van Kessel A, Bootsma D, Grosveld G, Ferguson-Smith MA, Davies T, Stone M et al (1983) Translocation of c-abl oncogene correlates with the presence of a Philadelphia chromosome in chronic myelocytic leukaemia. Nature 306(5940):277–280
9. Zhang L, Bennett JM, Zhang X, Moscinski L, Ibarz-Pinilla J, List AF, Komrokji R (2010) Uncommon of the uncommon: low-grade myelodysplastic syndrome evolving into chronic myelogenous leukemia. J Clin Oncol 29:434–436
10. Fine BM, Stanulla M, Schrappe M, Ho M, Viehmann S, Harbott J, Boxer LM (2004) Gene expression patterns associated with recurrent chromosomal translocations in acute lymphoblastic leukemia. Blood 103(3):1043–1049
11. Bacher U, Haferlach T, Alpermann T, Zenger M, Hochhaus A, Beelen DW, Uppenkamp M, Rummel M, Kern W, Schnittger S, Haferlach C (2011) Subclones with the t(9;22)/BCR-ABL1 rearrangement occur in AML and seem to cooperate with distinct genetic alterations. Br J Haematol 152(6):713–720
12. Villegas A, Anguita E, Gonzalez FA, Ferro MT, San Roman C (1998) Occurrence of BCR-ABL rearrangement in a Philadelphia chromosome-negative patient with 5q and 13q deletions and myeloproliferative syndrome. Cancer Genet Cytogenet 100(1):1–4
13. Kurzrock R, Kantarjian HM, Druker BJ, Talpaz M (2003) Philadelphia chromosome-positive leukemias: from basic mechanisms to molecular therapeutics. Ann Intern Med 138(10):819–830
14. McWhirter JR, Wang JY (1993) An actin-binding function contributes to transformation by the Bcr-Abl oncoprotein of Philadelphia chromosome-positive human leukemias. EMBO J 12(4):1533–1546
15. Deininger MW, Goldman JM, Melo JV (2000) The molecular biology of chronic myeloid leukemia. Blood 96(10):3343–3356
16. Pane F, Frigeri F, Sindona M, Luciano L, Ferrara F, Cimino R, Meloni G, Saglio G, Salvatore F, Rotoli B (1996) Neutrophilic-chronic myeloid leukemia: a distinct disease with a specific molecular marker (BCR/ABL with C3/A2 junction). Blood 88(7):2410–2414
17. Verma D, Kantarjian HM, Jones D, Luthra R, Borthakur G, Verstovsek S, Rios MB, Cortes J (2009) Chronic myeloid leukemia (CML) with P190 BCR-ABL: analysis of characteristics, outcomes, and prognostic significance. Blood 114(11):2232–2235
18. Wan TS, Ma SK, Au WY, Chan LC (2003) Derivative chromosome 9 deletions in chronic myeloid leukaemia: interpretation of atypical D-FISH pattern. J Clin Pathol 56(6):471–474
19. Thorn I, Botling J, Hermansson M, Lonnerholm G, Sundstrom C, Rosenquist R, Barbany G (2009) Monitoring minimal residual disease with flow cytometry, antigen-receptor gene rearrangements and fusion transcript quantification in Philadelphia-positive childhood acute lymphoblastic leukemia. Leuk Res 33(8):1047–1054
20. Emig M, Saussele S, Wittor H, Weisser A, Reiter A, Willer A, Berger U, Hehlmann R, Cross NC, Hochhaus A (1999) Accurate and rapid analysis of residual disease in patients with CML using specific fluorescent hybridization probes for real time quantitative RT-PCR. Leukemia 13(11):1825–1832

21. Kantarjian H, Sawyers C, Hochhaus A, Guilhot F, Schiffer C, Gambacorti-Passerini C, Niederwieser D, Resta D, Capdeville R, Zoellner U, Talpaz M, Druker B, Goldman J, O'Brien SG, Russell N, Fischer T, Ottmann O, Cony-Makhoul P, Facon T, Stone R, Miller C, Tallman M, Brown R, Schuster M, Loughran T, Gratwohl A, Mandelli F, Saglio G, Lazzarino M, Russo D, Baccarani M, Morra E (2002) Hematologic and cytogenetic responses to imatinib mesylate in chronic myelogenous leukemia. N Engl J Med 346(9):645–652
22. Aguayo A, Couban S (2009) State-of-the-art in the management of chronic myelogenous leukemia in the era of the tyrosine kinase inhibitors: evolutionary trends in diagnosis, monitoring and treatment. Leuk Lymphoma 50(Suppl 2):1–8
23. Hughes T, Deininger M, Hochhaus A, Branford S, Radich J, Kaeda J, Baccarani M, Cortes J, Cross NC, Druker BJ, Gabert J, Grimwade D, Hehlmann R, Kamel-Reid S, Lipton JH, Longtine J, Martinelli G, Saglio G, Soverini S, Stock W, Goldman JM (2006) Monitoring CML patients responding to treatment with tyrosine kinase inhibitors: review and recommendations for harmonizing current methodology for detecting BCR-ABL transcripts and kinase domain mutations and for expressing results. Blood 108(1):28–37
24. Donato NJ, Wu JY, Stapley J, Gallick G, Lin H, Arlinghaus R, Talpaz M (2003) BCR-ABL independence and LYN kinase overexpression in chronic myelogenous leukemia cells selected for resistance to STI571. Blood 101(2):690–698
25. Donato NJ, Wu JY, Stapley J, Lin H, Arlinghaus R, Aggarwal BB, Shishodia S, Albitar M, Hayes K, Kantarjian H, Talpaz M (2004) Imatinib mesylate resistance through BCR-ABL independence in chronic myelogenous leukemia. Cancer Res 64(2):672–677
26. Quentmeier H, Eberth S, Romani J, Zaborski M, Drexler HG (2011) BCR-ABL1-independent PI3Kinase activation causing imatinib-resistance. J Hematol Oncol 4(1):6
27. James C, Ugo V, Le Couedic JP, Staerk J, Delhommeau F, Lacout C, Garcon L, Raslova H, Berger R, Bennaceur-Griscelli A, Villeval JL, Constantinescu SN, Casadevall N, Vainchenker W (2005) A unique clonal JAK2 mutation leading to constitutive signalling causes polycythaemia vera. Nature 434(7037):1144–1148
28. Baxter EJ, Scott LM, Campbell PJ, East C, Fourouclas N, Swanton S, Vassiliou GS, Bench AJ, Boyd EM, Curtin N, Scott MA, Erber WN, Green AR (2005) Acquired mutation of the tyrosine kinase JAK2 in human myeloproliferative disorders. Lancet 365(9464):1054–1061
29. Levine RL, Wadleigh M, Cools J, Ebert BL, Wernig G, Huntly BJ, Boggon TJ, Wlodarska I, Clark JJ, Moore S, Adelsperger J, Koo S, Lee JC, Gabriel S, Mercher T, D'Andrea A, Frohling S, Dohner K, Marynen P, Vandenberghe P, Mesa RA, Tefferi A, Griffin JD, Eck MJ, Sellers WR, Meyerson M, Golub TR, Lee SJ, Gilliland DG (2005) Activating mutation in the tyrosine kinase JAK2 in polycythemia vera, essential thrombocythemia, and myeloid metaplasia with myelofibrosis. Cancer Cell 7(4):387–397
30. Kralovics R, Teo SS, Buser AS, Brutsche M, Tiedt R, Tichelli A, Passamonti F, Pietra D, Cazzola M, Skoda RC (2005) Altered gene expression in myeloproliferative disorders correlates with activation of signaling by the V617F mutation of Jak2. Blood 106:3374–3376
31. Scott LM, Tong W, Levine RL, Scott MA, Beer PA, Stratton MR, Futreal PA, Erber WN, McMullin MF, Harrison CN, Warren AJ, Gilliland DG, Lodish HF, Green AR (2007) JAK2 exon 12 mutations in polycythemia vera and idiopathic erythrocytosis. N Engl J Med 356(5):459–468
32. Delhommeau F, Jeziorowska D, Marzac C, Casadevall N (2010) Molecular aspects of myeloproliferative neoplasms. Int J Hematol 91(2):165–173
33. Kota J, Caceres N, Constantinescu SN (2008) Aberrant signal transduction pathways in myeloproliferative neoplasms. Leukemia 22(10):1828–1840
34. Kralovics R, Passamonti F, Buser AS, Teo SS, Tiedt R, Passweg JR, Tichelli A, Cazzola M, Skoda RC (2005) A gain-of-function mutation of JAK2 in myeloproliferative disorders. N Engl J Med 352(17):1779–1790
35. Bellucci S, Michiels JJ (2006) The role of JAK2 V617F mutation, spontaneous erythropoiesis and megakaryocytopoiesis, hypersensitive platelets, activated leukocytes, and endothelial

cells in the etiology of thrombotic manifestations in polycythemia vera and essential thrombocythemia. Semin Thromb Hemost 32(4 Pt 2):381–398
36. Pardanani AD, Levine RL, Lasho T, Pikman Y, Mesa RA, Wadleigh M, Steensma DP, Elliott MA, Wolanskyj AP, Hogan WJ, McClure RF, Litzow MR, Gilliland DG, Tefferi A (2006) MPL515 mutations in myeloproliferative and other myeloid disorders: a study of 1182 patients. Blood 108(10):3472–3476
37. Jekarl DW, Han SB, Kim M, Lim J, Oh EJ, Kim Y, Kim HJ, Min WS, Han K (2010) JAK2 V617F mutation in myelodysplastic syndrome, myelodysplastic syndrome/myeloproliferative neoplasm, unclassifiable, refractory anemia with ring sideroblasts with thrombocytosis, and acute myeloid leukemia. Korean J Hematol 45(1):46–50
38. Schmitt-Graeff AH, Teo SS, Olschewski M, Schaub F, Haxelmans S, Kirn A, Reinecke P, Germing U, Skoda RC (2008) JAK2V617F mutation status identifies subtypes of refractory anemia with ringed sideroblasts associated with marked thrombocytosis. Haematologica 93(1):34–40
39. Ho K, Valdez F, Garcia R, Tirado CA (2010) JAK2 translocations in hematological malignancies: review of the literature. J Assoc Genet Technol 36(3):107–109
40. Mossuz P, Girodon F, Donnard M, Latger-Cannard V, Dobo I, Boiret N, Lecron JC, Binquet C, Barro C, Hermouet S, Praloran V (2004) Diagnostic value of serum erythropoietin level in patients with absolute erythrocytosis. Haematologica 89(10):1194–1198
41. Andrieux JL, Demory JL (2005) Karyotype and molecular cytogenetic studies in polycythemia vera. Curr Hematol Rep 4(3):224–229
42. De Stefano V, Za T, Rossi E, Vannucchi AM, Ruggeri M, Elli E, Mico C, Tieghi A, Cacciola RR, Santoro C, Vianelli N, Guglielmelli P, Pieri L, Scognamiglio F, Cacciola E, Rodeghiero F, Pogliani EM, Finazzi G, Gugliotta L, Leone G, Barbui T (2010) Increased risk of recurrent thrombosis in patients with essential thrombocythemia carrying the homozygous JAK2 V617F mutation. Ann Hematol 89(2):141–146
43. Hirose Y, Masaki Y, Sugai S (2002) Leukemic transformation with trisomy 8 in essential thrombocythemia: a report of four cases. Eur J Haematol 68(2):112–116
44. Reilly JT, Snowden JA, Spearing RL, Fitzgerald PM, Jones N, Watmore A, Potter A (1997) Cytogenetic abnormalities and their prognostic significance in idiopathic myelofibrosis: a study of 106 cases. Br J Haematol 98(1):96–102
45. Reilly JT (2005) Cytogenetic and molecular genetic abnormalities in agnogenic myeloid metaplasia. Semin Oncol 32(4):359–364
46. Strasser-Weippl K, Steurer M, Kees M, Augustin F, Tzankov A, Dirnhofer S, Fiegl M, Simonitsch-Klupp I, Gisslinger H, Zojer N, Ludwig H (2006) Prognostic relevance of cytogenetics determined by fluorescent in situ hybridization in patients having myelofibrosis with myeloid metaplasia. Cancer 107(12):2801–2806
47. Dingli D, Grand FH, Mahaffey V, Spurbeck J, Ross FM, Watmore AE, Reilly JT, Cross NC, Dewald GW, Tefferi A (2005) Der(6)t(1;6)(q21-23;p21.3): a specific cytogenetic abnormality in myelofibrosis with myeloid metaplasia. Br J Haematol 130(2):229–232
48. Lim KH, Pardanani A, Tefferi A (2008) KIT and mastocytosis. Acta Haematol 119(4):194–198
49. Hungness SI, Akin C (2007) Mastocytosis: advances in diagnosis and treatment. Curr Allergy Asthma Rep 7(4):248–254
50. Yanagihori H, Oyama N, Nakamura K, Kaneko F (2005) c-kit Mutations in patients with childhood-onset mastocytosis and genotype-phenotype correlation. J Mol Diagn 7(2): 252–257
51. Zhao W, Bueso-Ramos CE, Verstovsek S, Barkoh BA, Khitamy AA, Jones D (2007) Quantitative profiling of codon 816 KIT mutations can aid in the classification of systemic mast cell disease. Leukemia 21(7):1574–1576
52. Corless CL, Harrell P, Lacouture M, Bainbridge T, Le C, Gatter K, White C Jr, Granter S, Heinrich MC (2006) Allele-specific polymerase chain reaction for the imatinib-resistant KIT D816V and D816F mutations in mastocytosis and acute myelogenous leukemia. J Mol Diagn 8(5):604–612
53. Beghini A, Ripamonti CB, Cairoli R, Cazzaniga G, Colapietro P, Elice F, Nadali G, Grillo G, Haas OA, Biondi A, Morra E, Larizza L (2004) KIT activating mutations: incidence in adult

and pediatric acute myeloid leukemia, and identification of an internal tandem duplication. Haematologica 89(8):920–925
54. Goemans BF, Zwaan CM, Miller M, Zimmermann M, Harlow A, Meshinchi S, Loonen AH, Hahlen K, Reinhardt D, Creutzig U, Kaspers GJ, Heinrich MC (2005) Mutations in KIT and RAS are frequent events in pediatric core-binding factor acute myeloid leukemia. Leukemia 19(9):1536–1542
55. Hellmann A (2008) Myeloproliferative syndromes: diagnosis and therapeutic options. Pol Arch Med Wewn 118(12):756–760
56. Cross NC, Reiter A (2008) Fibroblast growth factor receptor and platelet-derived growth factor receptor abnormalities in eosinophilic myeloproliferative disorders. Acta Haematol 119(4):199–206
57. Golub TR, Barker GF, Lovett M, Gilliland DG (1994) Fusion of PDGF receptor beta to a novel ets-like gene, tel, in chronic myelomonocytic leukemia with t(5;12) chromosomal translocation. Cell 77(2):307–316
58. Bain BJ, Fletcher SH (2007) Chronic eosinophilic leukemias and the myeloproliferative variant of the hypereosinophilic syndrome. Immunol Allergy Clin North Am 27(3):377–388
59. Steer EJ, Cross NC (2002) Myeloproliferative disorders with translocations of chromosome 5q31-35: role of the platelet-derived growth factor receptor beta. Acta Haematol 107(2):113–122
60. Vizmanos JL, Hernandez R, Vidal MJ, Larrayoz MJ, Odero MD, Marin J, Ardanaz MT, Calasanz MJ, Cross NC (2004) Clinical variability of patients with the t(6;8)(q27;p12) and FGFR1OP-FGFR1 fusion: two further cases. Hematol J 5(6):534–537
61. Erben P, Gosenca D, Muller MC, Reinhard J, Score J, Del Valle F, Walz C, Mix J, Metzgeroth G, Ernst T, Haferlach C, Cross NC, Hochhaus A, Reiter A (2010) Screening for diverse PDGFRA or PDGFRB fusion genes is facilitated by generic quantitative reverse transcriptase polymerase chain reaction analysis. Haematologica 95(5):738–744
62. Hirsch-Ginsberg C, LeMaistre AC, Kantarjian H, Talpaz M, Cork A, Freireich EJ, Trujillo JM, Lee MS, Stass SA (1990) RAS mutations are rare events in Philadelphia chromosome-negative/bcr gene rearrangement-negative chronic myelogenous leukemia, but are prevalent in chronic myelomonocytic leukemia. Blood 76(6):1214–1219
63. Tefferi A, Gilliland DG (2007) Oncogenes in myeloproliferative disorders. Cell Cycle 6(5):550–566
64. Orazi A, Germing U (2008) The myelodysplastic/myeloproliferative neoplasms: myeloproliferative diseases with dysplastic features. Leukemia 22(7):1308–1319
65. Vannucchi AM, Guglielmelli P, Tefferi A (2009) Advances in understanding and management of myeloproliferative neoplasms. CA Cancer J Clin 59(3):171–191
66. Vardiman JW (2004) Myelodysplastic/myeloproliferative diseases. Cancer Treat Res 121:13–43
67. Loh ML, Vattikuti S, Schubbert S, Reynolds MG, Carlson E, Lieuw KH, Cheng JW, Lee CM, Stokoe D, Bonifas JM, Curtiss NP, Gotlib J, Meshinchi S, Le Beau MM, Emanuel PD, Shannon KM (2004) Mutations in PTPN11 implicate the SHP-2 phosphatase in leukemogenesis. Blood 103(6):2325–2331
68. Tartaglia M, Niemeyer CM, Fragale A, Song X, Buechner J, Jung A, Hahlen K, Hasle H, Licht JD, Gelb BD (2003) Somatic mutations in PTPN11 in juvenile myelomonocytic leukemia, myelodysplastic syndromes and acute myeloid leukemia. Nat Genet 34(2):148–150
69. List A, Dewald G, Bennett J, Giagounidis A, Raza A, Feldman E, Powell B, Greenberg P, Thomas D, Stone R, Reeder C, Wride K, Patin J, Schmidt M, Zeldis J, Knight R (2006) Lenalidomide in the myelodysplastic syndrome with chromosome 5q deletion. N Engl J Med 355(14):1456–1465
70. Giagounidis AA, Germing U, Aul C (2006) Biological and prognostic significance of chromosome 5q deletions in myeloid malignancies. Clin Cancer Res 12(1):5–10
71. Lai JL, Preudhomme C, Zandecki M, Flactif M, Vanrumbeke M, Lepelley P, Wattel E, Fenaux P (1995) Myelodysplastic syndromes and acute myeloid leukemia with 17p deletion.

An entity characterized by specific dysgranulopoiesis and a high incidence of P53 mutations. Leukemia 9(3):370–381
72. Jotterand Bellomo M, Parlier V, Muhlematter D, Grob JP, Beris P (1992) Three new cases of chromosome 3 rearrangement in bands q21 and q26 with abnormal thrombopoiesis bring further evidence to the existence of a 3q21q26 syndrome. Cancer Genet Cytogenet 59(2):138–160
73. Haase D, Germing U, Schanz J, Pfeilstocker M, Nosslinger T, Hildebrandt B, Kundgen A, Lubbert M, Kunzmann R, Giagounidis AA, Aul C, Trumper L, Krieger O, Stauder R, Muller TH, Wimazal F, Valent P, Fonatsch C, Steidl C (2007) New insights into the prognostic impact of the karyotype in MDS and correlation with subtypes: evidence from a core dataset of 2124 patients. Blood 110(13):4385–4395
74. Valent P, Wieser R (2009) Update on genetic and molecular markers associated with myelodysplastic syndromes. Leuk Lymphoma 50(3):341–348
75. Ebert BL, Pretz J, Bosco J, Chang CY, Tamayo P, Galili N, Raza A, Root DE, Attar ESR, Golub TR (2008) Identification of RPS14 as a 5q- syndrome gene by RNA interference screen. Nature 451(7176):335–339
76. Pellagatti A, Jadersten M, Forsblom AM, Cattan H, Christensson B, Emanuelsson EK, Merup M, Nilsson L, Samuelsson J, Sander B, Wainscoat JS, Boultwood J, Hellstrom-Lindberg E (2007) Lenalidomide inhibits the malignant clone and up-regulates the SPARC gene mapping to the commonly deleted region in 5q- syndrome patients. Proc Natl Acad Sci USA 104(27):11406–11411
77. Morishita K, Parganas E, William CL, Whittaker MH, Drabkin H, Oval J, Taetle R, Valentine MB, Ihle JN (1992) Activation of EVI1 gene expression in human acute myelogenous leukemias by translocations spanning 300-400 kilobases on chromosome band 3q26. Proc Natl Acad Sci USA 89(9):3937–3941
78. Suzukawa K, Parganas E, Gajjar A, Abe T, Takahashi S, Tani K, Asano S, Asou H, Kamada N, Yokota J et al (1994) Identification of a breakpoint cluster region 3' of the ribophorin I gene at 3q21 associated with the transcriptional activation of the EVI1 gene in acute myelogenous leukemias with inv(3)(q21q26). Blood 84(8):2681–2688
79. Vinatzer U, Mannhalter C, Mitterbauer M, Gruener H, Greinix H, Schmidt HH, Fonatsch C, Wieser R (2003) Quantitative comparison of the expression of EVI1 and its presumptive antagonist, MDS1/EVI1, in patients with myeloid leukemia. Genes Chromosomes Cancer 36(1):80–89
80. Steensma DP, Dewald GW, Lasho TL, Powell HL, McClure RF, Levine RL, Gilliland DG, Tefferi A (2005) The JAK2 V617F activating tyrosine kinase mutation is an infrequent event in both "atypical" myeloproliferative disorders and myelodysplastic syndromes. Blood 106(4):1207–1209
81. Gattermann N, Billiet J, Kronenwett R, Zipperer E, Germing U, Nollet F, Criel A, Selleslag D (2007) High frequency of the JAK2 V617F mutation in patients with thrombocytosis (platelet count>600×109/L) and ringed sideroblasts more than 15% considered as MDS/MPD, unclassifiable. Blood 109(3):1334–1335
82. Della Porta MG, Malcovati L, Boveri E, Travaglino E, Pietra D, Pascutto C, Passamonti F, Invernizzi R, Castello A, Magrini U, Lazzarino M, Cazzola M (2009) Clinical relevance of bone marrow fibrosis and CD34-positive cell clusters in primary myelodysplastic syndromes. J Clin Oncol 27(5):754–762
83. Ingram W, Lea NC, Cervera J, Germing U, Fenaux P, Cassinat B, Kiladjian JJ, Varkonyi J, Antunovic P, Westwood NB, Arno MJ, Mohamedali A, Gaken J, Kontou T, Czepulkowski BH, Twine NA, Tamaska J, Csomer J, Benedek S, Gattermann N, Zipperer E, Giagounidis A, Garcia-Casado Z, Sanz G, Mufti GJ (2006) The JAK2 V617F mutation identifies a subgroup of MDS patients with isolated deletion 5q and a proliferative bone marrow. Leukemia 20(7):1319–1321
84. Heerema-McKenney A, Arber DA (2009) Acute myeloid leukemia. Hematol Oncol Clin North Am 23(4):633–654

85. Paschka P (2008) Core binding factor acute myeloid leukemia. Semin Oncol 35(4):410–417
86. Kundu M, Liu PP (2001) Function of the inv(16) fusion gene CBFB-MYH11. Curr Opin Hematol 8(4):201–205
87. Lo Coco F, Diverio D, Falini B, Biondi A, Nervi C, Pelicci PG (1999) Genetic diagnosis and molecular monitoring in the management of acute promyelocytic leukemia. Blood 94(1):12–22
88. Degos L (2003) The history of acute promyelocytic leukaemia. Br J Haematol 122(4):539–553
89. Meyer C, Hofmann J, Burmeister T, Gröger D, Park TS, Emerenciano M, Pombo de Oliveira M, Renneville A, Villarese P, Macintyre E, Cavé H, Clappier E, Mass-Malo K, Zuna J, Trka J (2013) The MLL recombinome of acute leukemias in 2013. Leukemia doi: 10.1038/leu.2013.135 [Epub ahead of print]
90. Repp R, Borkhardt A, Haupt E, Kreuder J, Brettreich S, Hammermann J, Nishida K, Harbott J, Lampert F (1995) Detection of four different 11q23 chromosomal abnormalities by multiplex-PCR and fluorescence-based automatic DNA-fragment analysis. Leukemia 9(1):210–215
91. Alsabeh R, Brynes RK, Slovak ML, Arber DA (1997) Acute myeloid leukemia with t(6;9)(p23;q34): association with myelodysplasia, basophilia, and initial CD34 negative immunophenotype. Am J Clin Pathol 107(4):430–437
92. Lugthart S, van Drunen E, van Norden Y, van Hoven A, Erpelinck CA, Valk PJ, Beverloo HB, Lowenberg B, Delwel R (2008) High EVI1 levels predict adverse outcome in acute myeloid leukemia: prevalence of EVI1 overexpression and chromosome 3q26 abnormalities underestimated. Blood 111(8):4329–4337
93. Rosnet O, Buhring HJ, Marchetto S, Rappold I, Lavagna C, Sainty D, Arnoulet C, Chabannon C, Kanz L, Hannum C, Birnbaum D (1996) Human FLT3/FLK2 receptor tyrosine kinase is expressed at the surface of normal and malignant hematopoietic cells. Leukemia 10(2):238–248
94. Ray RJ, Paige CJ, Furlonger C, Lyman SD, Rottapel R (1996) Flt3 ligand supports the differentiation of early B cell progenitors in the presence of interleukin-11 and interleukin-7. Eur J Immunol 26(7):1504–1510
95. Nakao M, Yokota S, Iwai T, Kaneko H, Horiike S, Kashima K, Sonoda Y, Fujimoto T, Misawa S (1996) Internal tandem duplication of the flt3 gene found in acute myeloid leukemia. Leukemia 10(12):1911–1918
96. Kiyoi H, Naoe T (2002) FLT3 in human hematologic malignancies. Leuk Lymphoma 43(8):1541–1547
97. Motyckova G, Stone RM (2010) The role of molecular tests in acute myelogenous leukemia treatment decisions. Curr Hematol Malig Rep 5(2):109–117
98. Kiyoi H, Ohno R, Ueda R, Saito H, Naoe T (2002) Mechanism of constitutive activation of FLT3 with internal tandem duplication in the juxtamembrane domain. Oncogene 21(16):2555–2563
99. Mizuki M, Fenski R, Halfter H, Matsumura I, Schmidt R, Muller C, Gruning W, Kratz-Albers K, Serve S, Steur C, Buchner T, Kienast J, Kanakura Y, Berdel WE, Serve H (2000) Flt3 mutations from patients with acute myeloid leukemia induce transformation of 32D cells mediated by the Ras and STAT5 pathways. Blood 96(12):3907–3914
100. Meshinchi S, Appelbaum FR (2009) Structural and functional alterations of FLT3 in acute myeloid leukemia. Clin Cancer Res 15(13):4263–4269
101. Kottaridis PD, Gale RE, Linch DC (2003) Flt3 mutations and leukaemia. Br J Haematol 122(4):523–538
102. Wagner K, Damm F, Thol F, Gohring G, Gorlich K, Heuser M, Schafer I, Schlegelberger B, Heil G, Ganser A, Krauter J (2011) FLT3-internal tandem duplication and age are the major prognostic factors in relapsed acute myeloid leukemia with normal karyotype. Haematologica 96(5):681–686
103. Rau R, Brown P (2009) Nucleophosmin (NPM1) mutations in adult and childhood acute myeloid leukaemia: towards definition of a new leukaemia entity. Hematol Oncol 27(4):171–181

104. Falini B, Nicoletti I, Martelli MF, Mecucci C (2007) Acute myeloid leukemia carrying cytoplasmic/mutated nucleophosmin (NPMc+AML): biologic and clinical features. Blood 109(3):874–885
105. Falini B, Martelli MP, Bolli N, Sportoletti P, Liso A, Tiacci E, Haferlach T (2011) Acute myeloid leukemia with mutated nucleophosmin (NPM1): is it a distinct entity? Blood 117(4):1109–1120
106. Schlenk RF, Dohner K, Krauter J, Frohling S, Corbacioglu A, Bullinger L, Habdank M, Spath D, Morgan M, Benner A, Schlegelberger B, Heil G, Ganser A, Dohner H (2008) Mutations and treatment outcome in cytogenetically normal acute myeloid leukemia. N Engl J Med 358(18):1909–1918
107. Falini B, Sportoletti P, Martelli MP (2009) Acute myeloid leukemia with mutated NPM1: diagnosis, prognosis and therapeutic perspectives. Curr Opin Oncol 21(6):573–581
108. Gale RE, Green C, Allen C, Mead AJ, Burnett AK, Hills RK, Linch DC (2008) The impact of FLT3 internal tandem duplication mutant level, number, size, and interaction with NPM1 mutations in a large cohort of young adult patients with acute myeloid leukemia. Blood 111(5):2776–2784
109. Falini B, Lenze D, Hasserjian R, Coupland S, Jaehne D, Soupir C, Liso A, Martelli MP, Bolli N, Bacci F, Pettirossi V, Santucci A, Martelli MF, Pileri S, Stein H (2007) Cytoplasmic mutated nucleophosmin (NPM) defines the molecular status of a significant fraction of myeloid sarcomas. Leukemia 21(7):1566–1570
110. Marcucci G, Maharry K, Radmacher MD, Mrozek K, Vukosavljevic T, Paschka P, Whitman SP, Langer C, Baldus CD, Liu CG, Ruppert AS, Powell BL, Carroll AJ, Caligiuri MA, Kolitz JE, Larson RA, Bloomfield CD (2008) Prognostic significance of, and gene and microRNA expression signatures associated with, CEBPA mutations in cytogenetically normal acute myeloid leukemia with high-risk molecular features: a Cancer and Leukemia Group B Study. J Clin Oncol 26(31):5078–5087
111. Cairoli R, Beghini A, Grillo G, Nadali G, Elice F, Ripamonti CB, Colapietro P, Nichelatti M, Pezzetti L, Lunghi M, Cuneo A, Viola A, Ferrara F, Lazzarino M, Rodeghiero F, Pizzolo G, Larizza L, Morra E (2006) Prognostic impact of c-KIT mutations in core binding factor leukemias: an Italian retrospective study. Blood 107(9):3463–3468
112. Paschka P, Marcucci G, Ruppert AS, Whitman SP, Mrozek K, Maharry K, Langer C, Baldus CD, Zhao W, Powell BL, Baer MR, Carroll AJ, Caligiuri MA, Kolitz JE, Larson RA, Bloomfield CD (2008) Wilms' tumor 1 gene mutations independently predict poor outcome in adults with cytogenetically normal acute myeloid leukemia: a cancer and leukemia group B study. J Clin Oncol 26(28):4595–4602
113. Meyer C, Kowarz E, Hofmann J, Renneville A, Zuna J, Trka J, Ben Abdelali R, Macintyre E, De Braekeleer E, De Braekeleer M, Delabesse E, de Oliveira MP, Cave H, Clappier E, van Dongen JJ, Balgobind BV, van den Heuvel-Eibrink MM, Beverloo HB, Panzer-Grumayer R, Teigler-Schlegel A, Harbott J, Kjeldsen E, Schnittger S, Koehl U, Gruhn B, Heidenreich O, Chan LC, Yip SF, Krzywinski M, Eckert C, Moricke A, Schrappe M, Alonso CN, Schafer BW, Krauter J, Lee DA, Zur Stadt U, Te Kronnie G, Sutton R, Izraeli S, Trakhtenbrot L, Lo Nigro L, Tsaur G, Fechina L, Szczepanski T, Strehl S, Ilencikova D, Molkentin M, Burmeister T, Dingermann T, Klingebiel T, Marschalek R (2009) New insights to the MLL recombinome of acute leukemias. Leukemia 23(8):1490–1499
114. Whitman SP, Liu S, Vukosavljevic T, Rush LJ, Yu L, Liu C, Klisovic MI, Maharry K, Guimond M, Strout MP, Becknell B, Dorrance A, Klisovic RB, Plass C, Bloomfield CD, Marcucci G, Caligiuri MA (2005) The MLL partial tandem duplication: evidence for recessive gain-of-function in acute myeloid leukemia identifies a novel patient subgroup for molecular-targeted therapy. Blood 106(1):345–352
115. Naghashpour M, Lancet J, Moscinski L, Zhang L (2011) Mixed phenotype acute leukemia with t(11;19)(q23;p13.3)/MLL-MLLT1(ENL), B/T-lymphoid type: a first case report. Am J Hematol 85(6):451–454
116. Neubauer A, Maharry K, Mrozek K, Thiede C, Marcucci G, Paschka P, Mayer RJ, Larson RA, Liu ET, Bloomfield CD (2008) Patients with acute myeloid leukemia and RAS mutations

benefit most from postremission high-dose cytarabine: a Cancer and Leukemia Group B study. J Clin Oncol 26(28):4603–4609

117. Valk PJ, Verhaak RG, Beijen MA, Erpelinck CA, van Waalwijk B, van Doorn-Khosrovani S, Boer JM, Beverloo HB, Moorhouse MJ, van der Spek PJ, Lowenberg B, Delwel R (2004) Prognostically useful gene-expression profiles in acute myeloid leukemia. N Engl J Med 350(16):1617–1628
118. Bacher U, Kohlmann A, Haferlach T (2009) Current status of gene expression profiling in the diagnosis and management of acute leukaemia. Br J Haematol 145(5):555–568
119. Marcucci G, Radmacher MD, Maharry K, Mrozek K, Ruppert AS, Paschka P, Vukosavljevic T, Whitman SP, Baldus CD, Langer C, Liu CG, Carroll AJ, Powell BL, Garzon R, Croce CM, Kolitz JE, Caligiuri MA, Larson RA, Bloomfield CD (2008) MicroRNA expression in cytogenetically normal acute myeloid leukemia. N Engl J Med 358(18):1919–1928

Author Index

D. Coppola (ed.), *Molecular Pathology and Diagnostics of Cancer*, Cancer Growth and Progression 16, DOI 10.1007/978-94-007-7192-5_1,

X

Y

Z

Subject Index

D. Coppola (ed.), *Molecular Pathology and Diagnostics of Cancer*, Cancer Growth and Progression 16, DOI 10.1007/978-94-007-7192-5_1,

Printed by Printforce, the Netherlands